Theodore H. Schwartz • Doo-Sik Kong
Kris S. Moe
Editors

Endoscopic Transorbital Surgery of the Orbit, Skull Base and Brain

Springer

Editors
Theodore H. Schwartz
Department of Neurosurgery
Weill Cornell Medicine
NewYork–Presbyterian Hospital
New York, NY, USA

Doo-Sik Kong
Department of Neurosurgery
Samsung Medical Center
Seoul, Korea (Republic of)

Kris S. Moe
Division of Facial Plastic Surgery
Departments of Otolaryngology and
Neurological Surgery
University of Washington
School of Medicine
Seattle, WA, USA

ISBN 978-3-031-59503-5 ISBN 978-3-031-59504-2 (eBook)
https://doi.org/10.1007/978-3-031-59504-2

This Springer imprint is published by the registered company Springer Nature Switzerland AG
The registered company address is: Gewerbestrasse 11, 6330 Cham, Switzerland

I dedicate this book to my mentor and friend, Vijay K. Anand, MD, who taught me how to hold an endoscope and introduced me to the brave new world of minimal access neurosurgery.

—Theodore H. Schwartz, MD

I dedicate this book to my wife, Hee Jeong, and my three children, Seo Hyun, Seo-Jin, Min-Jun.

—Doo-Sik Kong, MD

I dedicate this book to my wife, Stephanie, and our children, Grady, Rainier, and Madeleine. And to my mentors, Roger E. Moe, MD, FACS, and Ernest A. Weymuller, Jr., MD, who encouraged me to continue my work in this field when few others saw its future.

—Kris S. Moe, MD

Foreword

"Modern" orbital surgery dates to the 1888 publication by Swiss ophthalmologist Kronlein, who described his lateral orbitotomy, and yet neurosurgeons of the twentieth century developed a fondness for the transcranial approach to orbital disease; Walter Dandy published a series of such cases in 1941. Unable to keep their hands to themselves, the otorhinolaryngologists, who, in all fairness, had been EENTs, pushed their way into the orbit, as documented by Walsh and Ogura's transantral approach.

In 1976, my mentors, neurosurgeon Joe Maroon and surgical neuro-ophthalmologist Jack Kennerdell, published their experience with transorbital craniotomy by an extended lateral orbital approach, aided by employment of the surgical microscope. Indeed, they were a model multidisciplinary team.

The popularization of functional endoscopic sinus surgery (FESS) in the 1980s, initially without the employment of intraoperative navigation, unfortunately, led to some therapeutic misadventures, with unintended intrusions into the intracranial or intraorbital spaces with untoward consequences. Thankfully, the 1980s were also the early years of multidisciplinary skull base surgery, and, as often has been the case in the history of medicine and surgery, the FESS misadventures led to flashes of genius in the minds of some, who reasoned that if you can easily get there unintentionally, perhaps transnasal endoscopic intraorbital and intracranial surgery may be done in a safe, guided manner, with efficacious outcomes. In 1994, Drs. Metson, Dallow, and Shore published their experience in endoscopic orbital decompression, and in 1997, Drs. Jho and Carrau published their landmark paper on endoscopic endonasal transsphenoidal surgery.

It has been said, "the eyes are the window of the soul," and yet they are also windows into the brain, wherein observations, images, and scans of retina and optic nerve are in regular use in the evaluation and management of brain disorders. Similarly, windows made in the orbital bones allow direct observation and instrumentation into the intracranial space. Thus, this exceptional book is compiled, edited and contributed to by many of the pioneers of transorbital endoscopic skull base and intracranial surgery. *Endoscopic Transorbital Surgery of the Orbit, Skull Base and Brain* will rapidly bring you up to today's state of the art, and then some, with authors and works which establish safety and efficacy, and, at the same time, push ahead into unchartered waters, undoubtedly yielding more novel, safe and efficacious therapeutic interventions ahead, thanks to the combined multidisciplinary efforts of our medical and surgical colleagues and our partners in biomedical technology, ever-improving the tools they place before us. I trust you will be as excited to read and reread this book as will I!

Howard R. Krauss
Director, Eye, Ear & Skull Base Center
Pacific Neuroscience Institute
Santa Monica, CA, USA

Foreword

Paradigm shifts in surgery are often driven by advances in technology. A technology that has transformed all the surgical disciplines is the development of the Hopkins rod lens endoscope. Within otolaryngology, rigid endoscopy enabled minimally invasive approaches with new surgical corridors through the nasal cavity. Battles were waged over the merits of open versus endoscopic surgery for sinus disease. When the dust had settled, there was a clear winner. Endoscopic surgery, despite some limitations and growing pains, emerged as the new standard for sinonasal pathology. The adoption of endoscopic techniques played a major role in the growth of rhinology as a subspecialty within otolaryngology.

It wasn't long before the nasal endoscope was applied to skull base pathology and a new war was waged within neurosurgery. The outcome was predictable for those of us who had witnessed the battles within rhinology. Similarly, the endoscope transformed skull base surgery, providing new corridors for hard-to-reach places within the ventral skull base with less morbidity for patients. Endoscopic endonasal skull base surgery continues to evolve with further refinements in technique and testing of limits.

It is only natural that the endoscope would be applied to the orbit, a black box for most non-ophthalmologic surgeons. Like the skull base, the orbit is at the crossroads of multiple specialties and brings together ophthalmologists, otolaryngologists, neurosurgeons, plastic/reconstructive surgeons, and maxillofacial surgeons. Early pioneers such as Kris Moe defined a new paradigm of TONES (transorbital neuroendoscopic surgery). TONES expands the limits of orbital surgery, using the orbit as a corridor to intracranial pathology of the anterior cranial fossa, middle cranial fossa, and lateral cavernous sinus. It fosters multidisciplinary collaboration and is a rapidly evolving discipline. The indications and limits of TONES are still being defined.

The editors of this book bring together many of the pioneers and leaders of transorbital endoscopic skull base surgery to provide a comprehensive and authoritative review of the state of the art of this new frontier. This is an opportune time for such a work since early exuberance has now been tempered by the realities of experience. The wealth of experience of the editors and authors provides the necessary foundation for discussions of indications, surgical technique, decision-making, and limitations. *Endoscopic Transorbital*

Surgery of the Orbit, Skull Base and Brain is an essential addition to the library of all endoscopic skull base surgeons.

Carl H. Snyderman
Professor of Otolaryngology and Neurosurgery
University of Pittsburgh Medical Center
Pittsburgh, PA, USA

Preface

The advent of endoscopic transorbital surgery (ETOS) marks a significant developmental milestone and paradigm shift in the approach to treatment of pathology of the periorbital skull base and adjacent brain. This textbook is designed to serve as a comprehensive guide for neurosurgeons, otolaryngologists, ophthalmologists, and skull base surgeons who are beginning to venture into the intricate world of ETOS, offering a detailed overview of the surgical techniques, anatomical considerations, and clinical applications associated with this innovative approach.

The journey of ETOS from its conceptualization to clinical application reflects a remarkable synergy of multidisciplinary expertise, technological advancements, and a deep understanding of skull base anatomy. The minimal invasiveness, enhanced visual access to the skull base, and the potential for reduced patient morbidity associated with ETOS present a compelling case for its adoption into clinical practice. However, the complexity of orbital anatomy and the proximity to critical neurovascular structures necessitate a thorough educational foundation and hands-on training for surgeons adopting this technique.

This textbook is structured to bridge the knowledge gap, providing a step-by-step guide to ETOS procedures, from patient selection and preoperative planning to postoperative care and complication management. Each chapter is meticulously crafted by leading experts in the field, combining theoretical knowledge with practical insights gained from extensive clinical experience.

Key features of this textbook include:

Foundational Concepts: An introduction to the principles of endoscopic skull base surgery, including a historical overview, the evolution of ETOS, and its integration into current surgical practice.

Anatomical Atlas: A detailed examination of the orbital and skull base anatomy through high-quality illustrations and endoscopic images, providing a solid foundation for understanding the surgical corridor and the relationship with critical structures.

Surgical Technique: Comprehensive coverage of the ETOS procedure, including instrumentation, surgical steps, and intraoperative navigation, supported by illustrative case studies and operative videos.

Clinical Applications: An exploration of the indications, benefits, and limitations of ETOS for various skull base lesions, supported by evidence-based outcomes and case series.

Complication Management: Insightful discussions on the recognition, prevention, and management of potential complications associated with ETOS, emphasizing patient safety and surgical efficacy.

Future Directions: A look ahead at the potential innovations in technology, surgical techniques, and multidisciplinary collaboration that may further enhance the role of ETOS in skull base surgery.

Intended for surgeons at all levels, ranging from novice to expert, this textbook aims to cultivate a deep understanding of the many applications of ETOS, foster the development of surgical skills that can improve patient outcomes, and expand the horizons of skull base surgery. As the field continues to grow, this book will serve as a pivotal resource for ongoing education, research, and clinical excellence in endoscopic transorbital surgery.

We hope that this textbook will inspire and equip surgeons to navigate the complexities of ETOS with confidence and precision, contributing to the advancement of skull base surgery and improving the lives of patients worldwide.

New York, NY, USA — Theodore H. Schwartz
Seoul, Republic of Korea — Doo-Sik Kong
Seattle, WA, USA — Kris S. Moe

Contents

Contributors

Waleed M. Abuzeid Division of Rhinology and Endoscopic Skull Base Surgery, Department of Otolaryngology: Head and Neck Surgery, University of Washington, Seattle, WA, USA

Hanna N. Algattas Department of Neurological Surgery, University at Buffalo Neurosurgery, Buffalo, NY, USA

Joao Paulo Almeida Department of Neurological Surgery, Mayo Clinic, Jacksonville, FL, USA

Isam Alobid Rhinology Unit and Smell Clinic, ENT Department, Hospital Clínic de Barcelona, Barcelona, Spain

Diana C. Alvarez Caicedo Department of Neurological Surgery, Mayo Clinic, Jacksonville, FL, USA

Alberto Daniele Arosio Division of Otorhynolaryngology, Department of Biotechnology and Life Sciences, "Ospedale di Circolo e Fondazione Macchi", University of Insubria, Varese, Italy

Evan D. Bander Department of Neurosurgery, Weill Cornell Medical College, NewYork Presbyterian Hospital, New York, NY, USA

Christopher Bergeron Division of Otolaryngology/Division of Neurosurgery, Scripps Clinic and Scripps Green Hospital, La Jolla, CA, USA

Randall A. Bly Department of Otolaryngology-Head and Neck Surgery, University of Washington, Seattle Children's Hospital, Seattle, WA, USA

Ernest Bobeff Department of Neurosurgery, Weill Cornell Medicine, New York Presbyterian Hospital, New York, NY, USA

Department of Neurosurgery, Barlicki University Hospital, Lodz, Poland

Department of Sleep Medicine and Metabolic Disorders, Medical University of Lodz, Lodz, Poland

Joseph A. Carnevale Department of Neurological Surgery, Weill Cornell Medicine/New York Presbyterian Hospital, New York, NY, USA

Ricardo L. Carrau Department of Otolaryngology-Head & Neck Surgery, Ohio State University, Columbus, OH, USA

Department of Neurosurgery, Ohio State University, Columbus, OH, USA

Paolo Castelnuovo ENT Department, University of Insubria, Varese, Italy

Division of Otorhynolaryngology, Department of Biotechnology and Life Sciences, "Ospedale di Circolo e Fondazione Macchi", University of Insubria, Varese, Italy

Head and Neck & Forensic Dissection Research Center (HNS&FDRc), Department of Biotechnology and Life Sciences, University of Insubria, Varese, Italy

Research Center for Pituitary Adenomas and Sellar Pathology, University of Insubria, Varese, Italy

John K. Chae Department of Neurological Surgery, Weill Cornell Medicine/New York Presbyterian Hospital, New York, NY, USA

Jeremy N. Ciporen Department of Neurosurgery, Scripps Clinic Medical Group-Scripps Green Hospital, La Jolla, CA, USA

Allison Coombs Department of Ophthalmology, Weill Cornell Medical College, New York, NY, USA

Francesco Corrivetti Laboratory of Neuroanatomy, EBRIS Foundation, European Biomedical Research Institute of Salerno, Salerno, Italy

Department of Neurosurgery, San Luca Hospital, Vallo della Lucania, Salerno, Italy

Lodovica Cristofani Mencacci ENT Unit, Azienda Ospedaliero-Universitaria Pisana, Pisa, Italy

Iacopo Dallan ENT Unit, Azienda Ospedaliero-Universitaria Pisana, Pisa, Italy

Matteo de Notaris Laboratory of Neuroanatomy, EBRIS Foundation, European Biomedical Research Institute of Salerno, Salerno, Italy

Unit of Neurosurgery, San Giovanni di Dio and Ruggi D'Aragona Hospital, University of Salerno, Salerno, Italy

Andrea De Rosa Division of Neurosurgery, Department of Neurosciences, Reproductive and Odontostomatological Sciences, Università degli Studi di Napoli "Federico II", Naples, Italy

Alberto Di Somma Department of Neurological Surgery, Hospital Clínic de Barcelona, Barcelona, Spain

Joaquim Enseñat Department of Neurological Surgery, Hospital Clínic de Barcelona, University of Barcelona, Barcelona, Spain

Giacomo Fiacchini ENT Unit, Azienda Ospedaliero-Universitaria Pisana, Pisa, Italy

Paul A. Gardner Department of Neurological Surgery, School of Medicine, University of Pittsburgh, Pittsburgh, PA, USA

Kyle J. Godfrey Department of Ophthalmology and Neurosurgery, Weill Cornell Medicine, New York, NY, USA

Division of Oculoplastic Surgery, Department of Ophthalmology, Weill Cornell Medicine/New York Presbyterian Hospital, New York, NY, USA

Giulia Guizzardi Department of Neurological Surgery, Hospital Clínic de Barcelona, Barcelona, Spain

Chang-Ki Hong Department of Neurosurgery, Asan Medical Center, Ulsan University College of Medicine, Seoul, South Korea

Ian M. Humphreys Department of Otolaryngology—Head and Neck Surgery, University of Washington School of Medicine, Seattle, WA, USA

Sayyada Hyder Department of Ophthalmology, Weill Cornell Medical College, New York, NY, USA

Basit A. Jawad Department of Otolaryngology-Head & Neck Surgery, Ohio State University, Columbus, OH, USA

Chiman Jeon Department of Neurosurgery, Korea Universtiy Ansan Hospital, Korea University College of Medicine, Ansan, Republic of Korea

Patricia G. Johnson Division of Otolaryngology—Head and Neck Surgery, Allegheny Health Network, Pittsburgh, PA, USA

Eui Hyun Kim Department of Neurosurgery, Yonsei University College of Medicine, Seoul, South Korea

Brain Tumor Center, Endoscopic Skull Base Center, Severance Hospital, Seoul, South Korea

Doo-Sik Kong Department of Neurosurgery, Sungkyunkwan University School of Medicine, Samsung Medical Center, Seoul, South Korea

Lili Laleva Department of Neurosurgery, Acibadem City Clinic University Hospital Tokuda, Sofia, Bulgaria

Won-Jae Lee Department of Neurosurgery, Sungkyunkwan University School of Medicine, Samsung Medical Center, Seoul, South Korea

Jaejoon Lim Department of Neurosurgery, Bundang CHA Medical Center, CHA University College of Medicine, Seongnam, Republic of Korea

Maximilian Linxweiler Department of Otorhinolaryngology, Head and Neck Surgery, Saarland University Medical Center, Homburg, Saar, Germany

Davide Locatelli Division of Neurosurgery, Department of Biotechnology and Life Sciences, "Ospedale di Circolo e Fondazione Macchi", University of Insubria, Varese, Italy

Head and Neck & Forensic Dissection Research Center (HNS&FDRc), Department of Biotechnology and Life Sciences, University of Insubria, Varese, Italy

Research Center for Pituitary Adenomas and Sellar Pathology, University of Insubria, Varese, Italy

Davide Longo Department of Neurosurgery, Weill Cornell Medicine, NewYork–Presbyterian Hospital, New York, NY, USA

Darlene Lubbe Division of Otolaryngology, Department of Surgery, University of Cape Town, Cape Town, South Africa

Division of Otorhinolaryngology, Groote Schuur Hospital, University of Cape Town, Cape Town, South Africa

Brandon Lucke-Wold Department of Neurosurgery, University of Florida, Gainesville, FL, USA

Justin Maldonado Department of Neurosurgery, School of Medicine, Emory University, Atlanta, GA, USA

Dimitrios Mathios Department of Neurosurgery, Weill Cornell Medicine, NewYork–Presbyterian Hospital, New York, NY, USA

Kris S. Moe Division of Facial Plastic Surgery, Departments of Otolaryngology and Neurological Surgery, University of Washington School of Medicine, Seattle, WA, USA

Kittichai Mongkolkul Department of Otolaryngology-Head & Neck Surgery, Ohio State University, Columbus, OH, USA

Ju Hyung Moon Department of Neurosurgery, Endoscopic Skull Base Center, Severance Hospital, Yonsei University College of Medicine, Seoul, Republic of Korea

Alejandra Mosteiro Department of Neurological Surgery, Hospital Clínic de Barcelona, Barcelona, Spain

Hamzah Mustak Division of Ophthalmology, Groote Schuur Hospital, University of Cape Town, Cape Town, South Africa

Hun Ho Park Department of Neurosurgery, Gangnam Severance Hospital, Yonsei University, Seoul, South Korea

J. Nathaniel Perkins Department of Otolaryngology-Head and Neck Surgery, University of Washington, Seattle Children's Hospital, Seattle, WA, USA

Miriana Picariello ENT Unit, Azienda Ospedaliero-Universitaria Pisana, Pisa, Italy

Edoardo Porto Department of Neurosurgery, School of Medicine, Emory University, Atlanta, GA, USA

Gustavo Pradilla Department of Neurosurgery, School of Medicine, Emory University, Atlanta, GA, USA

Alberto Prats-Galino Laboratory of Surgical Neuroanatomy, Universitat de Barcelona, Barcelona, Spain

Daniel M. Prevedello Department of Otolaryngology-Head & Neck Surgery, Ohio State University, Columbus, OH, USA

Department of Neurosurgery, Ohio State University, Columbus, OH, USA

J. Manuel Revuelta Barbero Department of Neurosurgery, School of Medicine, Emory University, Atlanta, GA, USA

Luis Reyes Department of Neurological Surgery, Hospital Clínic de Barcelona, Barcelona, Spain

Alejandra Rodas Department of Otolaryngology, School of Medicine, Emory University, Atlanta, GA, USA

Tae Hoon Roh Department of Neurosurgery, Ajou University Hospital, Ajou University School of Medicine, Suwon, Gyeonggi-Do, Republic of Korea

Kate U. Rosen Department of Neurosurgery, Weill Cornell Medical College, NewYork Presbyterian Hospital, New York, NY, USA

Jacob Ruzevick Department of Neurological Surgery, University of Washington, Seattle Children's Hospital, Seattle, WA, USA

Theodore H. Schwartz Department of Neurosurgery, Weill Cornell Medicine, NewYork–Presbyterian Hospital, New York, NY, USA

Dhruv Sharma Department of Otolaryngology: Head and Neck Surgery, University of Louisville, Louisville, KY, USA

Dong-Won Shin Department of Neurosurgery, Brain Tumor Center, Gil Medical Center, College of Medicine, Gachon University, Incheon, South Korea

Giorgio Sileo Division of Otorhynolaryngology, Department of Biotechnology and Life Sciences, "Ospedale di Circolo e Fondazione Macchi", University of Insubria, Varese, Italy

Carl H. Snyderman Department of Otolaryngology, School of Medicine, University of Pittsburgh, Pittsburgh, PA, USA

C. Arturo Solares Department of Otolaryngology, School of Medicine, Emory University, Atlanta, GA, USA

Toma Spiriev Department of Neurosurgery, Acibadem City Clinic University Hospital Tokuda, Sofia, Bulgaria

S. Tonya Stefko Departments of Ophthalmology, Otolaryngology, and Neurological Surgery, University of Pittsburgh Medical Center, Pittsburgh, PA, USA

Department of Ophthalmology, School of Medicine, University of Pittsburgh, Pittsburgh, PA, USA

Kyoung Su Sung Department of Neurosurgery, Dong-A University Hospital, Dong-A University College of Medicine, Busan, Republic of Korea

Laura Tiedemann Department of Ophthalmology, University of Pittsburgh Medical Center, Pittsburgh, PA, USA

Murat Ulutas Department of Neurosurgery, Sanko University School of Medicine, Konukoglu Hospital, Gaziantep, Turkey

Pierlorenzo Veiceschi Division of Neurosurgery, Department of Biotechnology and Life Sciences, "Ospedale di Circolo e Fondazione Macchi", University of Insubria, Varese, Italy

Eric W. Wang Department of Otolaryngology, School of Medicine, University of Pittsburgh, Pittsburgh, PA, USA

Umut Yilmaz Department of Neuroradiology, Saarland University Medical Center, Homburg, Saar, Germany

In-Sik Yun Department of Oculoplastic Surgery, Gangnam Severance Hospital, Yonsei University, Seoul, South Korea

Georgios A. Zenonos Department of Neurological Surgery, School of Medicine, University of Pittsburgh, Pittsburgh, PA, USA

1 Transorbital Neuroendoscopic Surgery

Kris S. Moe, Doo-Sik Kong, and Theodore H. Schwartz

Introduction

Transorbital neuroendoscopic surgery, or TONES, refers to a group of surgical approaches that access the skull base and brain through the bone of the orbit (Figs. 1.1 and 1.2). The field of transorbital skull base and brain surgery has gained rapid adoption and popularity since its inception nearly 15 years ago. The growth of these minimally disruptive, scarless procedures has benefitted from the overall trend in skull base surgery away from large, open-field procedures toward operations that minimize the brain retraction and collateral damage of open craniotomies. The result of this trend is diminished hospital stays, lower healthcare costs, and a more rapid return of the patient to preoperative lifestyle.

It was the earlier development and rapid adoption of transnasal endoscopic skull base surgery that paved the way for the advent of transorbital

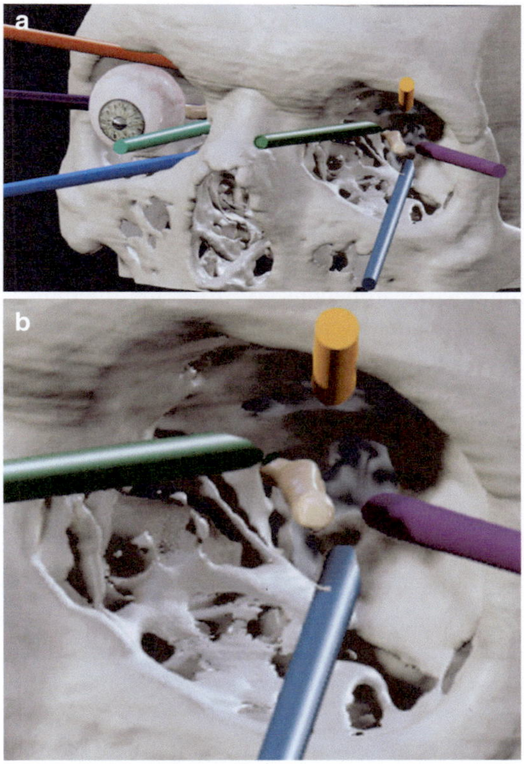

Fig. 1.1 Transorbital neuroendoscopic approaches. *Fused three-dimensional CT/MRI reconstructions.* (**a**) *the four primary endoscopic transorbital approaches. Right orbit, the globe and optic nerve demonstrate relation of potential pathways to key structures. Left orbit, the globe has been removed, demonstrating identical pathways.* (**b**) *enlarged image of the left orbit and optic nerve demonstrating potential pathways around the optic nerve and superior orbital fissure. Superior approach, orange; lateral approach, purple; inferior approach, blue; medial approach, green*

K. S. Moe (✉)
Division of Facial Plastic Surgery, Departments of Otolaryngology and Neurological Surgery, University of Washington School of Medicine, Seattle, WA, USA

D.-S. Kong
Department of Neurosurgery, Samsung Medical Center, Seoul, Korea (Republic of)

T. H. Schwartz
Department of Neurosurgery, Weill Cornell Medicine, NewYork–Presbyterian Hospital, New York, NY, USA

T. H. Schwartz et al. (eds.), *Endoscopic Transorbital Surgery of the Orbit, Skull Base and Brain*,
https://doi.org/10.1007/978-3-031-59504-2_1

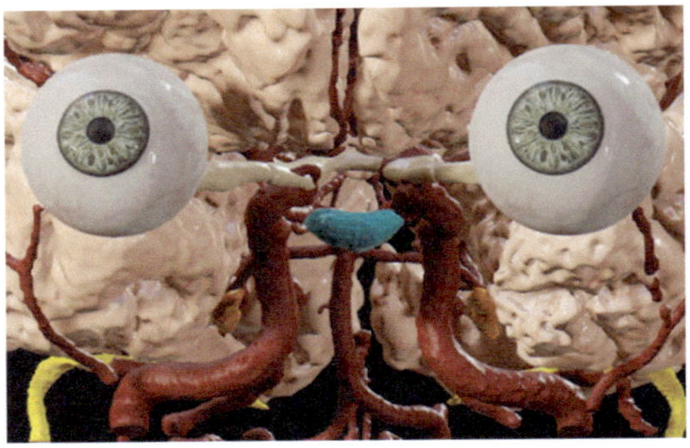

Fig. 1.2 Deep structures related to transorbital approaches. *Three-dimensional MRI reconstruction demonstrating the anatomy of critical neurovascular structures around the transorbital approaches. Brain and optic nerves and chiasm, tan; pituitary gland, blue; facial nerves, yellow. Note the position of the globes anterior to the temporal and frontal lobes and their location relative to the course of the internal carotid arteries*

approaches. The surgical techniques are largely the same, as are many of the skills, technology, and context. Yet, the orbit remained for some time compartmentalized from the multidisciplinary collaboration that is the hallmark of skull base surgery. Ophthalmologists, long experts in the regional anatomy and surgical techniques of orbital surgery, were understandably consumed by pathology within the orbit rather than adjacent structures. Otolaryngologists, focusing on the adjacent sinuses and skull base, considered the orbit a region to avoid with the concern of causing surgical complications. Neurosurgeons, while occasionally working with ophthalmologists on brain and skull base pathology entering the orbit, have not considered that region within their primary domain or training.

The development of transorbital skull base and brain procedures thus required transgressing traditional boundaries between specialties and anatomy in ways that had eluded most surgeons' education. Yet the logic for doing this was strong. While transnasal endoscopic approaches are excellent for the interorbital skull base, sella, clivus, and pterygopalatine fossa, they are not appropriate for the entire skull base. The central and lateral frontal sinus, though partially visible through transnasal endoscopy, cannot be instrumented effectively from that route. Pathologies within the superior orbit and supraorbital anterior cranial fossa are likewise challenging to treat from a transnasal approach, as are regions lateral and posterior to the orbit, in the middle fossa, and in the lateral infratemporal fossa. As reports of accessing these regions transorbitally using mono- or multiportal techniques [1, 2] (combined with transnasal or other portals) became available, the transorbital approach was eventually introduced at national meetings and courses to now become incorporated in resident education. Traditional boundaries have been diminished, with ophthalmologists and otolaryngologists further partnering (as they had before separation of the training of those specialties in 1947) and collaborating with neurosurgeons to provide cross-disciplinary care to achieve the best possible outcomes for their patients. For an interesting and comprehensive history of the development of transorbital endoscopic surgery, see Houlihan [3].

Today, the applications of transorbital skull base and brain surgery are diverse and growing. These include the treatment of pathology in the paranasal sinuses, orbit, skull base (anterior, middle, and posterior cranial fossa, temporal bone [petrous apex]), and brain (frontal and temporal lobes, Sylvian fissure, insula) in adults and children (Table 1.1). There are several excellent reviews of the literature describing international multidisciplinary experience with these procedures [4–6].

One of the most common concerns of those learning transorbital approaches is, understandably, the risk to vision of placing a retractor, instruments, and an endoscopic within the orbit. The safety of the transorbital pathway, as dem-

Table 1.1 Pathology addressed through transorbital neuroendoscopic approaches

• Aneurysm clipping
• Angiofibroma (juvenile nasopharyngeal)
• Carcinoma (sebaceous gland, squamous cell, adenoid cystic)
• Cavernous sinus thrombosis
• Chondrosarcoma
• Craniopharyngioma
• CSF leak
• Dermoid
• Epidural abscess, brain abscess
• Epilepsy (mesial temporal lobe)
• Epistaxis
• Fibrous dysplasia
• Foreign body removal
• Fracture frontal bone, frontal sinus
• Gliosis, glioblastoma
• Hemangioma, cavernous
• Hematoma epidural, subdural
• Infection (orbital abscess, frontal abscess, frontal sinusitis, epidural abscess, brain abscess)
• Lymphatic malformation
• Meningocele, meningoencephalocele, meningioma
• Metastatic osteosarcoma, olfactory neuroblastoma, clear cell renal carcinoma
• Mucocele, mucopyocele (frontal lobe, orbitofrontal)
• Orbit decompression
• Orbital apex syndrome
• Olfactory neuroblastoma
• Optic nerve decompression
• Osteoma, osteosarcoma, osteoblastoma
• Paget disease
• Peripheral nerve sheath tumor (benign, malignant)
• Pituitary adenoma
• Plasmacytoma
• Pseudotumor
• Schwannoma (benign, malignant)
• Seizure (mesial temporal lobe)
• Tension pneumocephalus
• Teratoma

onstrated by the numerous cases reported in the literature, is not unexpected giving the following observations. The orbital volume is 30 cc on average, reaching its maximal diameter 1 cm behind the orbital rim. Minor variations based on gender and race are reported. In addition, larger globes are associated with increased orbital volume [7], as is geography, with those living at higher latitudes having larger orbital volumes than those living near the equator [8]. On average, the globe occupies between one fifth and one third of the orbital volume [9] (Fig. 1.3). The average volume of the orbital component of the lateral surgical corridor was 2.75 cc on computer analysis [10]. Thus, the average approach comprises less than 10% of the total orbital volume.

In addition, the typical retraction of orbital contents measures <9 mm from the orbital wall [10], and reports have shown that less than 1 cm of retraction is safe during endoscopic orbital approaches [11, 12]. Furthermore, the optic nerve measures 40 mm in length, 25 mm of which is intraorbital, 4–10 mm is intracanalicular, and 10 mm is intracranial on average. Thus, the intraorbital component of the nerve is the longest and offers considerable redundancy to allow displacement of the globe.

If compression of the globe is a concern due to tumor occupying a portion of the volume, medial orbital decompression can be done at the outset before tumor resection to gain additional space for instrumentation. Although not required in all cases, Goncalvez and Lubbe routinely perform a medial decompression before resection of sphenoid wing meningiomas with excellent results [13].

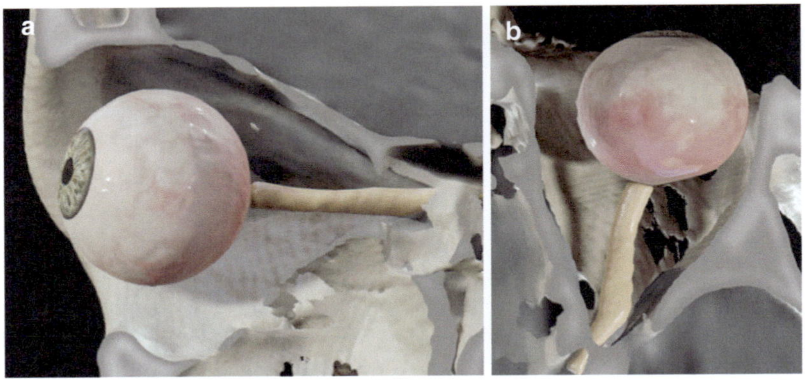

Fig. 1.3 Globe size relative to orbital volume. Fused CT/MRI three-dimensional reconstructions. (**a**) medial to lateral view of the right orbit, orbital contents removed other than globe and optic nerve. (**b**) superior to inferior view of same structures. Note the significant volume within the orbital bone within which the globe can be displaced

Terminology

Given the rapid growth of papers on the subject and nuances of the techniques that are presented here and elsewhere, it is relevant to review important terminology used on this subject. While it would be ideal if there were standardization of terminology for reporting on techniques, outcome studies, and meta-analyses, individual groups have adopted their own terms.

The term **transorbital neuroendoscopic surgery** (TONES) was originally introduced in 2010 to describe the four transorbital approaches to the anterior (ACF) and middle (MCF) cranial fossae, adjacent skull base structures, and brain [1]. There is a primary approach for each V-shaped quadrant of the orbit: superior, medial, inferior, and lateral. The term "transorbital" indicates that the pathways pass through the bone of the orbit to access extra-orbital structures. The term "neuroendoscopic" is used to differentiate these from transorbital procedures that do not involve a neurologic target; the latter procedures are referred to as **transorbital endoscopic surgery**. These are further differentiated from endoscopic surgery that addresses pathology confined to the orbit, which we refer to as **endoscopic orbital surgery**. However, use of the term "neuroendoscopic" implies that an endoscope is *required* for these approaches, which it is not. One can employ a microscope, or an exoscope, depending on one's preferences. Nevertheless, most of these procedures are done with an endoscope since the pathway is narrow and visualization may not be ideal without it. Other terms used in the literature include "transorbital approach" (TOA), "transorbital endoscopic approach (TOEA), "endoscopic transorbital approach" (ETOA), and others.

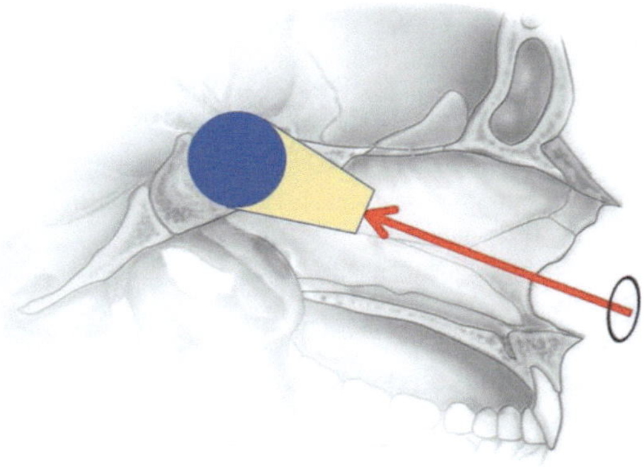

Fig. 1.4 Components of an endoscopic approach. *Black circle: portal (representing nostril). Red arrow: pathway. Tan: optical cavity. Blue circle: target pathology*

The terminology relating to the components of transorbital endoscopic procedures is also somewhat varied (Fig. 1.4). An endoscopic approach requires an entry into the body, which we refer to as the **portal**. This may require a skin incision or may pass through a natural orifice such as a nostril. The portal leads into the surgical **pathway**. A pathway may make use of an open lumen such as a nasal cavity, referred to as a "corridor" if it does not require dissection to create. At the distal end of the pathway where the **pathology** or **target** is located, an **optical cavity**

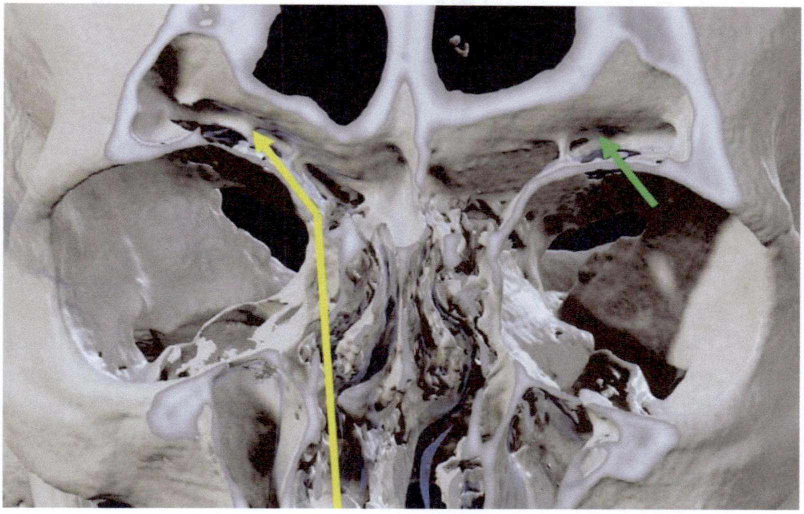

Fig. 1.5 Biplanar vs. coplanar approach to the lateral recess of frontal sinus

is required. The optical cavity is a space naturally open or created by a retractor, of sufficient volume to allow adequate visualization and instrumentation of the pathology [14].

Another important concept to consider is whether the portal, pathway, and target share a common plane. When these all lie in one plane, the procedure is termed **coplanar**. Coplanar approaches allow more efficacious access with improved visualization and instrumentation of the target, theoretically less collateral damage, and reduced requirement for angled endoscopy compared to **biplanar approaches** (Fig. 1.5).

Note that the transnasal (yellow) approach on the patient's right side is biplanar due to obstruction by the orbit while the superior transorbital approach (green) on the patient's left is coplanar and unobstructed.

The surgical approach is typically named by the pathway. A lateral transorbital approach, for example, may be accessed by several portals and may be used to reach multiple targets, but it is named after the approach rather than the portal or pathology. Similarly, an endoscopic approach through the nose to a target within the orbit is referred to as a transnasal, or endonasal, approach rather than transorbital. There may be multiple possible portals to access a pathway; similarly, multiple approaches may be available to access a target. When two or more approaches are used to access pathology, this is referred to as **multiportal surgery** [2, 15, 16] which will be discussed below. When describing multiportal surgery, additional pathways on the ipsilateral side of the midline coronal plane are referred to as **paraportal approaches**, while additional pathways from the contralateral side are referred to as **contraportal approaches** [1, 17–20].

When published in 2010, the four transorbital approaches were termed superior eyelid crease (to the superior quadrant); precaruncular approach (to the medial quadrant); preseptal lower eyelid (to the inferior quadrant); and lateral retrocanthal (to the inferior quadrant). In subsequent publications [20], the authors changed their terminology to reflect the relevant orbital quadrant for simplicity and clarity, given the panoply of techniques and portals to reach each quadrant. This chapter's authors concur and thus refer to the **superior, medial, inferior, and lateral transorbital approaches** (Fig. 1.1).

We consider these approaches to be minimally disruptive rather than minimally invasive. Invasiveness is dictated by the location of the pathology, not by the approach. There are two types of surgical damage: that caused by creation and use of the pathway to the target and that incurred during manipulation of the pathology. Morbidities caused by manipulation of the pathology are due in large part to its characteristics such as consistency and adherence to adjacent structures. Manipulation trauma is difficult to minimize, other than by using adequate exposure and appropriate instrument selection. However, pathway-associated injury caused by creating and transiting the approach is collateral damage, and every effort should be made to minimize this damage. This effort is the rationale and goal of transorbital neuroendoscopic surgery.

While some experts state that an approach should allow "four-handed" surgery (two surgeons working synchronously), the number of hands working is not as significant as the number of functions being performed. One must employ as many functions as are required to get the job done safely and effectively. The number of tasks typically performed synchronously during a narrow corridor endoscopic procedure are four: visualization, illumination, tissue resection, and aspiration, which can currently be performed with as few as two instruments (an endoscope and microdebrider) by one surgeon. Whether the endoscope is held and fluidly moved about by a second surgeon or held and intermittently relocated via a scope holder (manual, robotic, or pneumatic) is the choice of the surgical team.

Choice of Endoscopic Approach: Surgical Planning

The correct choice of surgical approach is one of the most important determinants of surgical outcome. In the case of skull base pathology, the options include open, endoscopic, and hybrid (combined open craniotomy and endoscopic approaches). These decisions are highly complex [20–24] and should be made in conjunction with a multidisciplinary tumor board. Factors to consider include the overall health of the patient and any comorbidities. When transorbital approaches are considered, it is important to take the ophthalmologic history into account including the patient's visual acuity, complaints such as dry eye, and any prior orbital or periorbital surgery. For recurrent tumors, a history of prior radiation therapy is important to consider as this can affect tumor handling and influence postoperative healing. Important pathway considerations include:

- Creation and reconstruction of the pathway must be technically feasible.
- The pathway should not cross critical neurovascular structures in a manner that can cause compression or other trauma.
- The pathway should be short, direct, and as straight as possible to minimize collateral damage.
- The pathway must allow target visualization unobstructed by instruments or tissue.
- The angle of approach must allow surgical task completion including comfortable passage and use of instruments and the endoscope (up to 6-function surgery if required).
- The collateral damage (morbidity) caused by pathway creation should be the least possible.
- The surgical team must have adequate experience to safely use the chosen pathway.
- Patient preference should figure strongly in the choice.

It may be challenging to evaluate whether a surgical approach will fulfill these criteria. To determine this, careful analysis of preoperative imaging (CT and MRI at a minimum) is required. Surgical planning software is available that allows labelling of the surgical target and the portal, which allows analysis so that the precise vector and its associated anatomic structures can be studied through means such as virtual endoscopy.

When considering endoscopic approaches, it is important to evaluate the pathway globally rather than in a single-plane (coronal) analysis. This is important both for understanding the global target landscape that can be accessed with transorbital approaches and for investigating which quadrant might be ideal for accessing a given target. As demonstrated in Fig. 1.6, each of the four quadrant approaches can be utilized with varying pathway angulation, depending on the adjacent structures that the surgeon wishes to transgress or avoid. For example, in accessing a frontal lobe target, multiple vectors are available depending on whether the frontal sinus will be used as an optical cavity (Fig. 1.6c). Similarly, global anatomic analysis will show all structures that may lie within or adjacent to the potential pathway for risk stratification. While critical neurovascular structures may be crossed during a procedure, it is critical to do so in a manner that will ensure a safety zone between that structure and transiting instrumentation. Either CT or MRI with contrast is typically sufficient for this analysis.

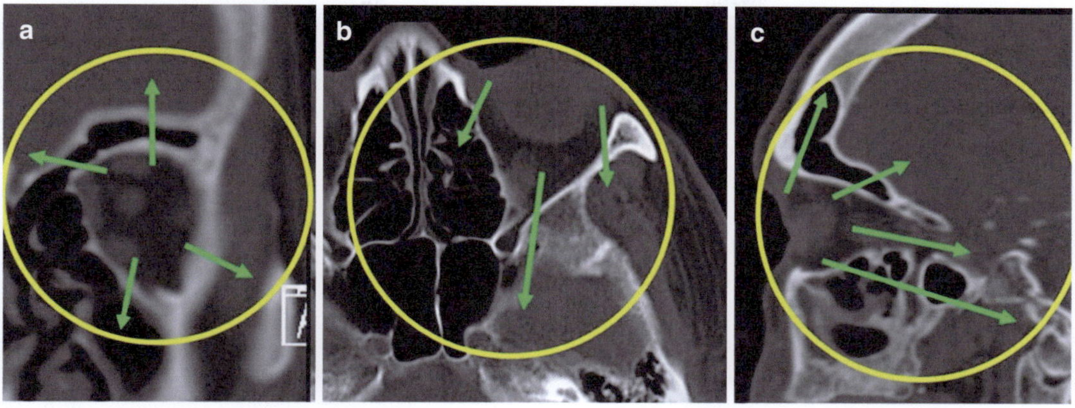

Fig. 1.6 Global analysis of transorbital endoscopic approaches, CT scan. (**a**) coronal; (**b**), axial; and (**c**), sagittal planes. Note that each orbital quadrant offers multiple approach pathways and vectors, depending on the intended surgical target. Detailed anatomical analysis must be undertaken in each plane to understand that structures that will be passed or transgressed and whether critical neurovascular structures will be placed at undue risk by a given strategy. Green arrows: potential approach vectors. Yellow circles, global target region that may be accessed transorbitally

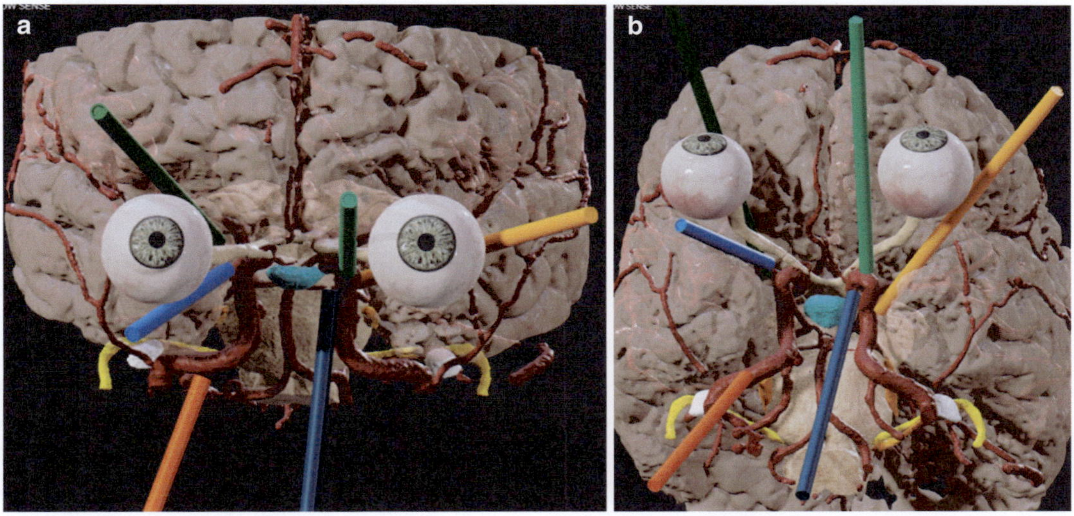

Fig. 1.7 Role of optic nerve and internal carotid artery in pathway selection. Three-dimensional MRI reconstruction. Endoscopic pathways denoted by colored rods. Inferior right (orange, paramaxillary); inferior left (dark blue, transnasal); superior right (dark green, superior transorbital); inferior right (light blue, inferior transorbital); medial left (light green, medial transorbital); lateral right (light orange, lateral transorbital). (**a**) anterior view. (**b**) inferior view. Note that each approach optimizes access to a specific portion of the internal carotid artery while avoiding compressing the optic nerve

Detailed analysis of critical neurovascular structures within the region of the approach and target is mandatory for endoscopic procedures [23, 24]. For transorbital approaches, the location of the pathology relative to the optic nerve and internal carotid artery may play a vital role in choosing the pathway (Fig. 1.7).

It is important to create a surgical plan based on the location of the target pathology as the primary factor. The shape of the target is also important. For nonspherical targets, choosing a coplanar pathway perpendicular to the long axis of the mass will maximize the possibility of complete resection and minimize collateral damage. While it may be tempting to extend a favored portal or pathway beyond its comfortable reaches to access a given destination, it is in the patient's best interest to adhere to the criteria listed above.

Confirmation of the surgical plan before beginning the operation can also be useful (Fig. 1.8). In some instances, it may be challenging to decide between two adjacent approaches. By using a navigation system and probe when the patient is under general anesthesia, potential pathway vectors may be trialed to identify the ideal angulation and working space. In addition, pathway lengths can be measured, and the ideal portal position can be marked on the skin.

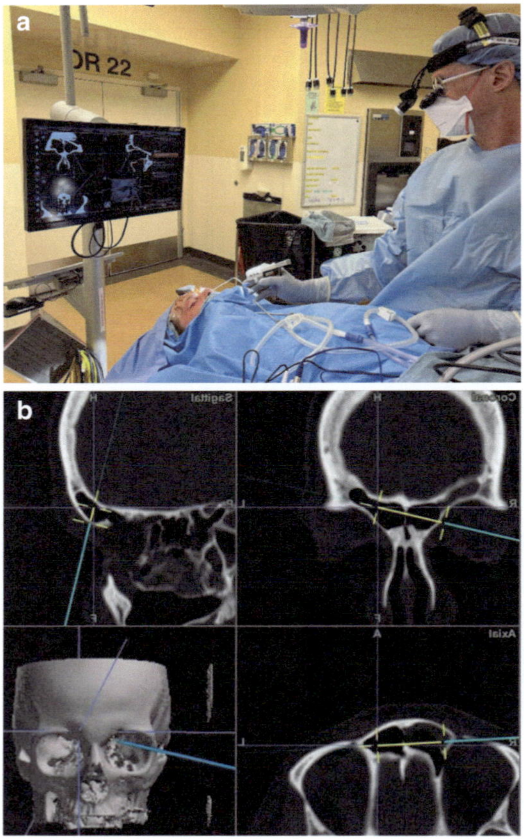

Fig. 1.8 Final pathway navigation analysis: Contraportal medial transorbital/transfrontal approach to ACF. (**a**) surgical setup demonstrating use of navigation probe to analyze and choose final approach vector and location of skin incision. (**b**) probe position demonstrated on navigation screen. Blue line represents probe; yellow line is a vector extension beyond the probe measuring distance and ability to reach the surgical target. Various approaches and vectors can be investigated in the final decision analysis and confirmation

Surgical Anatomy

The anatomy of the orbit and associated structures will be discussed in depth in a separate chapter. However, several concepts will be described in brief to allow technical discussion.

The critical surgical anatomy of transorbital approaches can be separated into superficial and deep components. The superficial structures (Fig. 1.9) include anterior soft tissue (eyelids, medial and lateral canthi, and tarsi), while the critical deeper anatomy relates to orbital bone (fissures and foramina). As the transorbital pathways are predominantly subperiosteal in their dissection planes, intraconal orbital structures are not typically visualized and are not discussed in this chapter.

The eyelids consist of the skin and orbicularis oculi muscle draped over the superior and inferior tarsi. The superior tarsus is supported vertically by the levator palpebrae muscle and aponeurosis. The inferior tarsus is supported by an analogous structure, the lower lid retractor, though this is functionally less important and can generally be transected without deleterious effects. Laterally, the tarsi are supported by the lateral canthal tendon (lateral retinaculum), which inserts several millimeters posterior to the lateral orbital rim, inferior to the frontozygomatic suture. Medially, the tarsi are supported by the medial canthal tendon. This structure splits around the lacrimal canaliculi and sac to form posterior and anterior limbs, which insert on the posterior and anterior lacrimal crests, respectively. The important posterior limb holds the lid posteriorly and superiorly, maintaining contact with the globe and holding the lacrimal puncta in position to drain tear fluid.

The critical deep orbital anatomy relates to the orbital apex. The superior orbital fissure contains

a

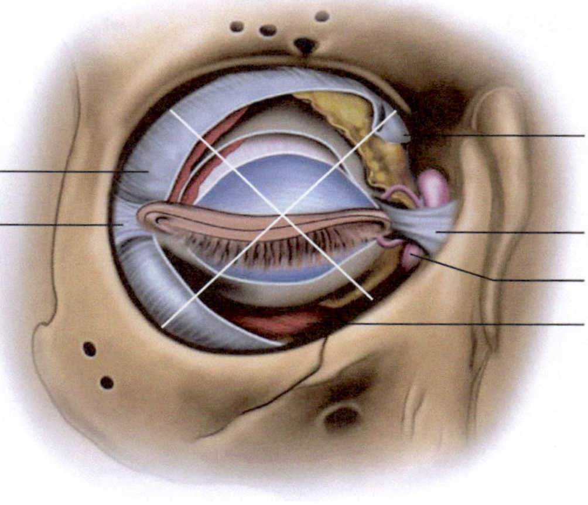

b

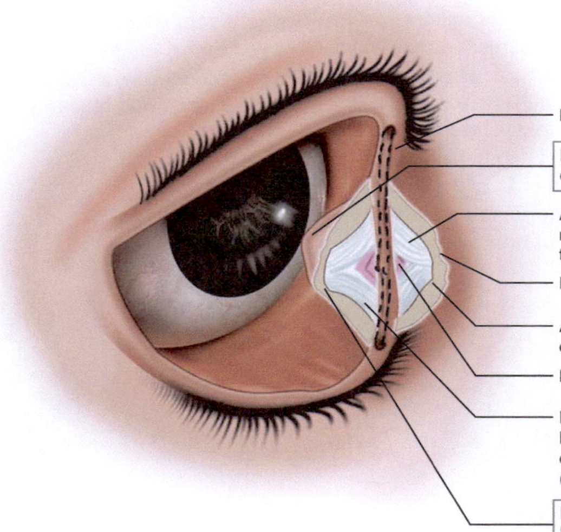

Fig. 1.9 Superficial orbital anatomy. (**a**) key anatomic structures of the superficial orbit. The septum is removed in the central and medial orbit to demonstrate the underlying structures. The medial and lateral canthal tendons provide the primary horizontal support, while the vertical support of the upper lid is provided by the levator muscle and aponeurosis. The lower lid retractors (not shown) are somewhat analogous to the levator muscle but function primarily in anteroposterior lid stabilization and can typically be transected without sequelae. Note the trochlea of the superior oblique at the medial superior orbit. The orbit is divided into quadrants as shown, with separate approaches for each region. (**b**) anatomy of the medial canthus. Note that the canaliculi travel through the medial upper and lower lids and thence to the lacrimal sac. The medial canthal tendon splits into anterior and posterior limbs which cover the sac in a dense membrane. The medial approach is entirely posterior to the lacrimal apparatus and medial canthus

cranial nerves III, IV, V1, and VI, as well as the ophthalmic vein and sympathetic innervation from the cavernous plexus. It is bound laterally by the greater wing of the sphenoid bone and medially by the lesser wing of the sphenoid. Superomedially to the superior fissure is the base of the anterior clinoid process, which extends posteriorly and medially as it courses over the optic nerve. Medial to the base of the anterior clinoid is the optic canal, and inferiorly, the optic strut extends laterally to comprise the inferior aspect of the optic canal (Figs. 1.10 and 1.11).

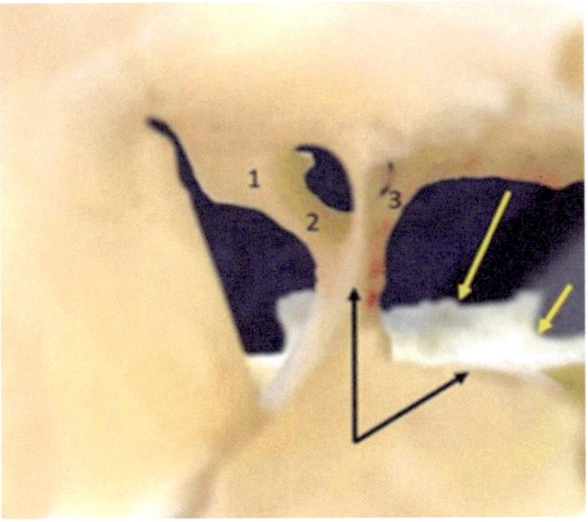

Fig. 1.10 Anatomy of right orbital apex. Photograph of dry skull, right orbital apex. Black arrows indicate posterior and inferior borders of the lamina papyracea, which has been removed up to the orbital roof. The face of the sella has been removed. Through the superior fissure and sella, the dorsum sella is visible (large yellow arrow) as is the position of the left posterior clinoid (small yellow arrow). 1, root of the anterior clinoid; 2, optic strut; 3, medial wall of optic canal. Note the superior fissure joining the inferior fissure at the inferior orbital apex

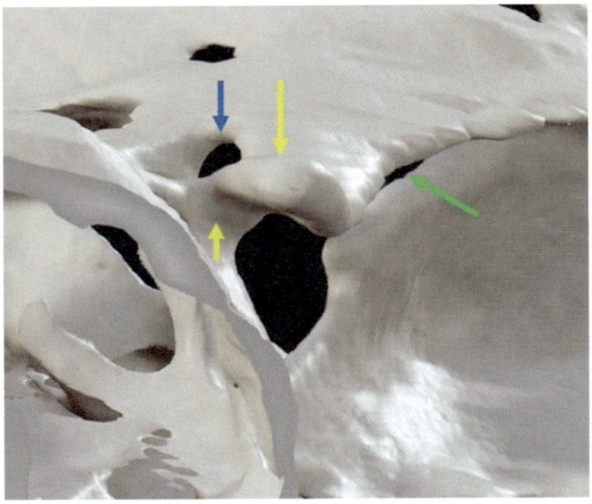

Fig. 1.11 Posterior view of right orbit apex. Three-dimensional CT reconstruction. Posterior lamina and face of sella removed as above. Large yellow arrow, posterior projection of anterior clinoid; small yellow arrow, optic strut; green arrow, superior fissure/superior aspect greater wing of sphenoid; blue arrow, posterior optic canal

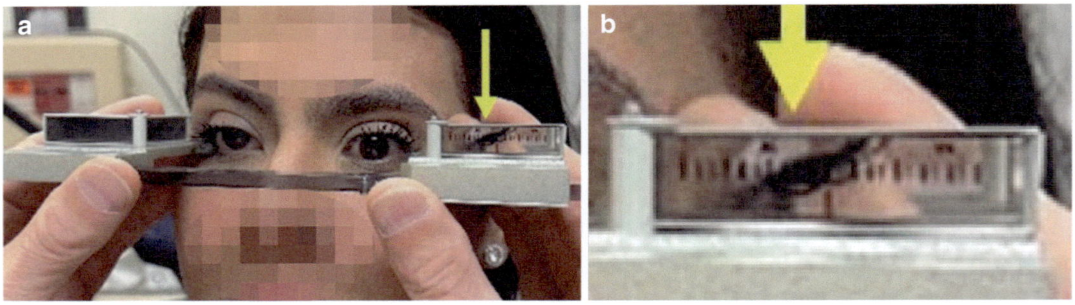

Fig. 1.12 Hertel's exophthalmometry. (**a**) the device rests on the lateral orbital rims. The examiner looks through the prism on the side of the device at the reflection of the cornea (yellow arrow). The superimposed measurement describes the position of the globe. The same procedure is undertaken through the contralateral prism, and the measurements are compared. (**b**) close-up view through prism demonstrating globe projection

Preoperative Patient Evaluation

A complete and comprehensive evaluation is performed as indicated based on the pathology. This typically includes MRI and CT for navigation and angiography with balloon test occlusion and embolization as indicated.

An ophthalmologic history should be taken focusing on any prior surgery or visual disturbances. If there are any concerns, or if the patient has issues such as dry eye, a preoperative ophthalmologic evaluation should be obtained.

The patient should be examined for gross visual field defects, diplopia, eyelid malposition (ptosis or ectropion), and asymmetry in globe position. Exophthalmometry to check for asymmetry in globe position is straightforward to learn and convenient to use in clinic to check for symmetry of globe position (Fig. 1.12).

Surgical Technique

The patient is placed in the supine position. After administration of general anesthesia, the navigation system is applied, registration is performed, and accuracy is confirmed. Antibiotics and steroids are administered. The patient's head may be placed in pins as desired. If head movement is required during surgery, pins are avoided. The navigation system of choice is registered, and accuracy is confirmed. Vector analysis may be performed to finalize and confirm the surgical plan (Fig. 1.8). The optimal surgical portal is marked on the skin for a transcutaneous approach, centered on the primary pathway vector. The patient's face is prepared and draped in sterile fashion, keeping both periorbital regions and any possible additional portals within the field. The eyes are rinsed with balanced salt solution or half-dose povidone mixed with saline, and ophthalmic lubricant is applied. Temporary tarsorrhaphy sutures are placed as desired at the medial or lateral limbus when using transcutaneous incisions, to allow the lids to be opened for monitoring size, shape, and symmetry of the pupils. If tarsorrhaphy sutures are not placed, a clear contact lens or corneal protector may be inserted to prevent inadvertent corneal abrasion. The pupil size should be monitored intermittently during surgery, roughly every 15–20 min depending on the volume and location of the pathway. The surgeons may elect not to place a corneal shield after achieving adequate experience with these techniques. A temporary tarsorrhaphy suture is also placed on the contralateral side for protection and to allow comparison of pupil size and shape.

Surgical Approach

As noted above, the optimal surgical approach is determined by the quadrant of the orbit directly involved with the pathology or transgressed by the approach vector chosen through preoperative planning. The orbit is divided into quadrants due to its relatively square internal shape in the coronal plane. This is important conceptually, as there are numerous anatomic structures and landmarks at the junctions of the four walls. In addition, there are superficial anatomic structures at the border of each quadrant such as the lacrimal gland, trochlea of the superior oblique muscle, and origin of the inferior oblique muscle. By centering portals over each quadrant, these structures are placed at the lateral border of the dissection and less affected by instrument traffic.

The orbital quadrants are V-shaped, narrowing as they converge on the orbital apex (Fig. 1.13). There are large convergence zones where adjacent quadrants can be joined into a single surgical field without damaging structures. The inferior orbital fissure, for example, contains fibrovascular tissue which can be transected without sequelae, in addition to a minor sensory {zygo-

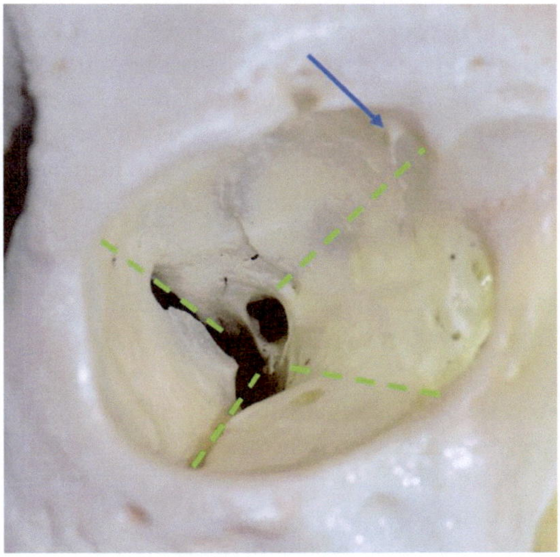

Fig. 1.13 The triangular quadrants of the orbit. Photograph, dry skull, right orbit. Approximate borders between the quadrants are indicated in dashed lines. These borders are not distinct; except for crossing through the superior orbital fissure or optic nerve, the margins of each approach can be transgressed so that, for example, a superior approach can extend somewhat inferiorly down the greater wing of the sphenoid in the lateral orbit. Note that the optic nerve can be accessed through either the medial or superior approaches. While it can also be accessed inferiorly, this may require excessive retraction of the orbital contents. Note the location of the calcified portion of the trochlea of the superior oblique muscle (blue arrow). This structure is not typically calcified and inserts on the periosteum rather than bone; care should be taken to raise the periosteum anterior to this to prevent damage to the trochlea

matic) nerve. A major exception to this, however, is the superior orbital fissure which transmits cranial nerves III, IV, V1, and VI, as well as the ophthalmic vein and sympathetic innervation from the cavernous plexus. Similarly, the optic nerve blocks transition from the apex of the medial quadrant and the superior quadrant.

The apex of the lateral quadrant is bounded by the superior and inferior orbital fissures and consists of the greater wing of the sphenoid bone. The apex of the superior quadrant is bounded by the superior fissure laterally and the optic nerve medially. The apical bone consists of the optic strut, separating the contents of the superior fissure and optic canal and offering access to the anterior clinoid. The apex of the medial quadrant consists of the medial optic canal and, inferiorly, the optic strut. The apex of the inferior quadrant ends at the convergence of the inferior and superior orbital fissures, just above foramen rotundum. From the foramen rotundum, the infraorbital nerve (V2) runs in a thin canal within or below the orbital floor, to pass through a foramen below the inferior orbital fissure and thence to the overlying soft tissue of the cheek.

Superior Quadrant [1, 17, 25–27]

Access: ACF, frontal lobe, frontal sinus, optic nerve, anterior clinoid process (Fig. 1.14).

Boundaries: Medial, frontoethmoidal suture; lateral, greater wing of sphenoid.

Portal: Upper blepharoplasty.

There is one primary approach to the superior orbit, the upper blepharoplasty approach. The incision may be continued laterally over the lateral orbital rim if needed for access to the superior aspect of the lateral orbit. It can be extended medially into the concavity superior to the superior punctum. It should not be continued horizontally onto the lateral nasal wall due to lack of need for that exposure and because it could create an unsightly scar.

Ophthalmic lubricant is placed, and a temporary tarsorrhaphy stitch is placed at the lateral limbus. The incision is made in an upper lid crease. It should be superior to the tarsus, but not high enough to be seen with the eye open. If in

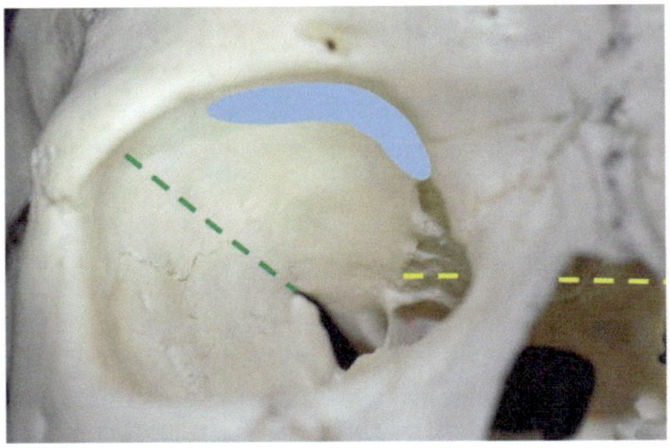

Fig. 1.14 Orbital roof. Photograph right orbit, dry skull. Lamina papyracea removed to demonstrate the interorbital skull base. Blue shading, approximate (but highly variable) position of frontal sinus and frontal outflow tract. Green dashed line, approximate lateral aspect of superior quadrant. Yellow dashed line, plane of interorbital skull base allowing exploration of this region before removal of sinonasal tumor (see section on medial approach below). Face of sella removed. Note the superior orbital fissure, with the base of the anterior clinoid at its medial extent. The optic nerve, though readily accessible from this approach, is actually located at the apex of the medial orbital wall

doubt, this can be marked with the patient awake in the sitting position before surgery. A somewhat more superior incision is advantageous in requiring less dissection and less retraction to access the orbital rim. The skin and orbicularis muscle are transected either with a 15 blade or low-voltage needle-point cautery. Dissection then continues superiorly in the preseptal plane to the orbital rim (Fig. 1.15). As the orbital septum may be diaphanous and difficult to discern, the dissection plane should be the posterior aspect of the orbicularis muscle. Careful dissection will preserve the septum and prevent herniation of prelevator fat. Should fat herniation occur, the fat should not be resected as it provides a layer of protection to the levator muscle and aponeurosis beneath.

As the superior orbital rim is reached, the supraorbital neurovascular bundle will be visible traversing a notch or canal in the orbital rim in the mid-pupillary line. If convenient, the nerve can be preserved. If it obstructs the exposure, it can be transected, and sensation will return to nearly normal in the ensuing months postoperatively. The same is true of the supratrochlear neurovascular bundle located more medially.

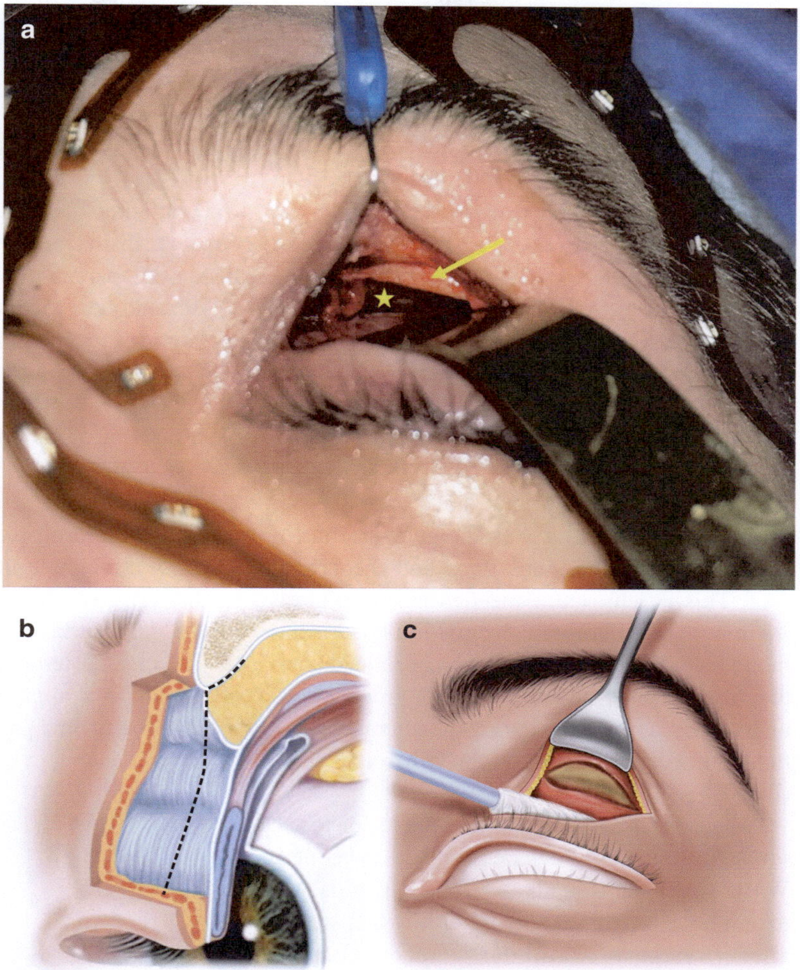

Fig. 1.15 (**a**) Upper blepharoplasty approach to the superior orbit. (**b**) a suborbicularis (preseptal) approach (dotted line) is made to the superior orbital rim. The periosteum is incised and elevated off the orbital roof, where a subperiosteal dissection is undertaken. (**c**) left superior approach showing bone of superior orbital rim, orbital contents displaced inferiorly with malleable retractor. Note the minimal dissection is required to reach this location. Arrow, superior orbital rim; star, orbital roof

The periosteum is then incised on the orbital rim. The trochlea of the superior oblique muscle is a cartilaginous sling that inserts on the trochlear fossa of the medial aspect of the orbital roof several millimeters posterior to the orbital rim. It is thus important to incise the periosteum (periorbita) at rather than behind the orbital rim to avoid damaging the trochlea. The periorbita is then elevated off the orbital rim and orbital roof and the subperiosteal plane is entered. Dissection in the subperiosteal plane will displace the trochlear attachment without damaging it; the trochlea and superior oblique muscle are not exposed as part of the dissection and at the end of the procedure are simply allowed to relax back into position without special attention. We have never had a trochlear injury with a transorbital approach. At the end of the procedure, the portal is closed with 6–0 absorbable sutures to reapproximate the orbicularis muscle, and the skin is closed with 6–0 absorbable or removable sutures. If a CSF leak was encountered, the closure should be watertight with running rather than interrupted technique.

Approach: Superior Quadrant

After exposing the superior orbital rim, the periosteum is dissected from the orbital roof, taking care not to damage the trochlea of the superior oblique as noted above. Dissection continues posteriorly in the subperiosteal plane under endoscopic visualization, using a suction Freer elevator for dissection. The orbital contents are gently retracted with a malleable ribbon retractor. Dissection continues laterally to the lateral orbital wall and medially to the frontoethmoidal suture, immediately superior to where the ethmoid neurovascular bundles are located. The suture often forms a groove, which leads posteriorly to the optic canal and nerve. There are typically three or more ethmoid arteries (Berens), and the vessels can be cauterized with bipolar technique and transected as needed. As dissection continues toward the optic canal and superior orbital fissure, the approach narrows. The superior aspect of the superior orbital fissure is noted and preserved at the lateral field.

For access to the frontal sinus and superior frontal lobe, navigation is used to map the area of bone shared by the sinus floor and the orbital roof. This is removed as needed using an ultrasonic bone aspirator or a drill with a coarse diamond burr. The endoscope is then introduced into the frontal sinus and the desired procedure is undertaken, at times removing the intersinus septum and accessing the contralateral frontal sinus (Fig. 1.16).

To access areas superior and posterior to the orbit, the entire roof can be removed as needed. While this may lead to transient pulsatile exophthalmos, this resolves within 1–2 weeks after surgery without reconstruction. Navigation is then used to choose the site for durotomy as indicated.

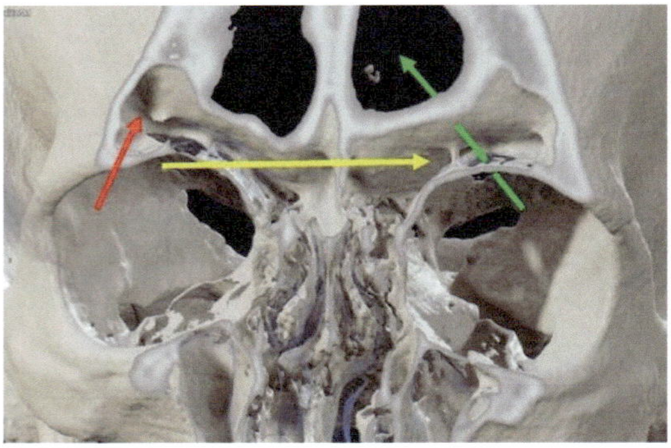

Fig. 1.16 Superior quadrant approach to frontal sinuses and frontal lobes. Red arrow, ipsilateral frontal sinus; yellow arrow, contraportal approach through intersinus septum to opposite frontal sinus; green arrow, ipsilateral approach through posterior wall of frontal sinus to frontal lobe.

Medial Quadrant [1, 28]

Access: Interorbital ACF (intracranial or extracranial); ipsilateral or contraportal optic nerve, ICA, sella, paranasal sinuses (Fig. 1.15).

Boundaries: Medial orbital roof, orbital floor.

Portal: Precaruncular (PC) approach.

The medial orbit also has a single primary portal: it is accessed through the conjunctival precaruncular (PC) approach. A transcutaneous approach medial to this, though possible (a "Lynch" incision), places the approach vector medial to the orbit through the ethmoid sinuses and is of minimal utility. The PC approach to the medial orbit is a largely avascular plane located on the deep surface of the posterior limb of the medial canthal tendon, thus completely sparing all the lacrimal apparatus, and is the most direct route to the lamina papyracea (Fig. 1.17).

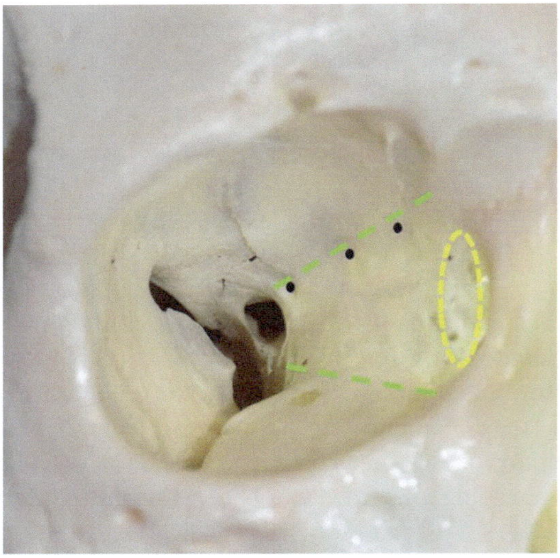

Fig. 1.17 Right orbit, medial quadrant. Photograph, dry skull. Note the lacrimal fossa (dotted yellow ellipse) and foramina of the three ethmoid neurovascular foramina (small black dots). A vector connecting the foramina, immediately inferior to the frontoethmoidal suture (green dashed line), will point posteriorly to the optic canal. The medial (precaruncular) approach is posterior to (and does not expose) the lacrimal sac or lacrimal fossa

Until the surgeon has gained adequate experience, small diameter lacrimal probes can be placed superiorly and inferiorly to demonstrate and protect the lacrimal system. These can be bent and taped to the adjacent skin to use for retraction. The caruncle is grasped with a forceps and placed under gentle lateral traction (Fig. 1.18). A fine scissor (Wescott) is used to make an incision in the small dimple at the medial apex of the caruncle. The scissor is then introduced and gently spread, opening the plane deep to the posterior limb of the medial canthal ten-

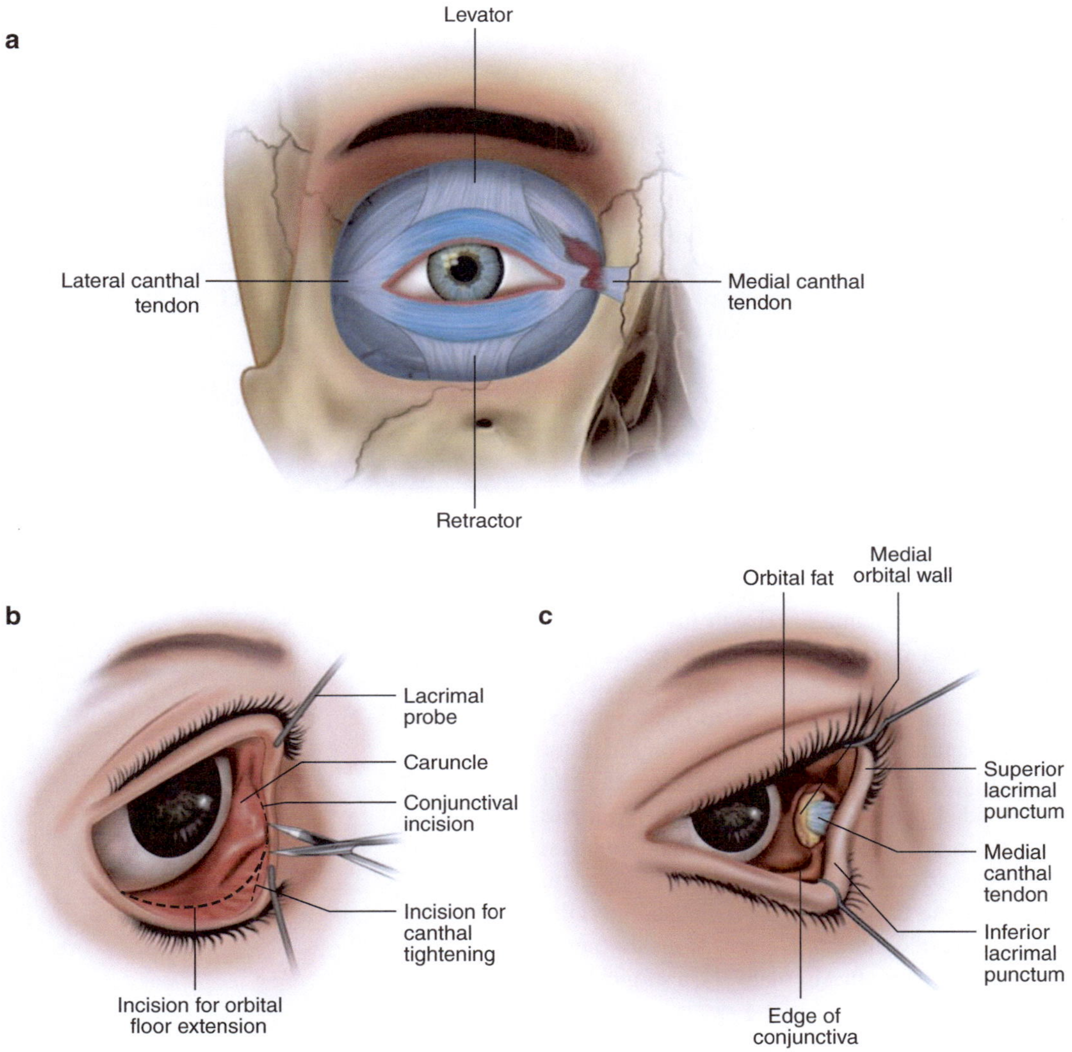

Fig. 1.18 Precaruncular approach to the right medial orbit. (**a**) superficial anatomy demonstrating the location and insertion of the medial and lateral canthal tendons. (**b**) the precaruncular approach. If desired, probes can be placed in the canaliculi to aid in retraction and protection of the canaliculi while learning the procedure. An incision is made with a fine scissor between the caruncle and the medial canthus. This incision is lengthened vertically over a distance of 10–15 mm. Inferiorly, it can be continued to provide access to the orbital floor if necessary. (**c**) this incision opens the relatively avascular preseptal plane posterior to the posterior limb of the medial canthal tendon. This is followed to the posterior lacrimal crest which is posterior to the lacrimal sac and forms the anterior aspect of the lamina papyracea. Here, the periorbita is incised vertically and the subperiosteal plane is entered. This is developed posteriorly, and the ethmoid neurovascular bundles are ligated as needed

don. A small artery is located in this space and is cauterized with bipolar forceps. The incision is widened vertically as needed (typically 1.5 cm). While care should be exercised not to incise superiorly enough to damage the medial horn of the levator aponeurosis, inferior dissection can continue to the orbital floor through the inferior fornix approach described below. The dissection plane is followed medially and posteriorly until the posterior lacrimal crest is reached. The periorbita is then sharply incised in a vertical plane, and a plane is developed between the periorbita and lamina papyracea.

At the procedure's end, the caruncle is restored to its original position. No suturing is required unless edema causes the caruncle to herniate, in which case a 6–0 dissolving suture can be used to fix the caruncle to the medial skin with horizontal mattress technique.

Approach: Medial Quadrant

After creation of the PC portal, the periosteum posterior to the posterior lacrimal crest is incised and elevated. Care is taken not to exert substantial force on the lamina as it will fracture easily, though small fractures in the bone are inconsequential. Dissection continues toward the orbital apex elevating the periosteum to the frontoethmoidal suture superiorly and the orbital floor inferiorly. The ethmoid arteries can be cauterized and divided as needed if dissection is to continue onto the orbital roof. Great care should be taken if the posterior ethmoid artery is to be divided, and the optic nerve must be visualized, and the artery retracted anteriorly away from the nerve before cauterization. Alternatively, a surgical clip may be placed on the vessel.

As the orbital apex is approached, the lamina progresses from a nearly vertical wall to a highly concave shape. Caution should be taken as the posterior ethmoid artery is approached, and the optic nerve is identified posterior to this.

When operating on a sinonasal tumor with this approach, it is possible to enter the cranium superior to the interorbital skull base to investigate involvement of the dura with tumor. Early determination of dural involvement will allow further planning of the procedure. In addition, if the dura is tumor-free, a resorbable layer of 0.25 mm thick polydioxanone (PDS) sheet may be placed between the dura and skull base to protect the brain during transnasal endoscopic resection. A similar technique can be used through a medial transorbital approach to protect the orbital contents from transnasal resection of a tumor.

If the medial periorbita is left intact during the procedure, there is not generally a need for reconstruction of any bone of the medial orbit that might have been removed. If the lamina has been opened and there is significant herniation of orbital fat into the ethmoid sinuses, it is generally adequate to reconstruct the bone with a sheet of thin PDS to span the defect.

Inferior Quadrant [1, 25]

Access: orbital floor, infraorbital nerve, foramen rotundum, MCF, ICA, maxillary sinus (Fig. 1.19).

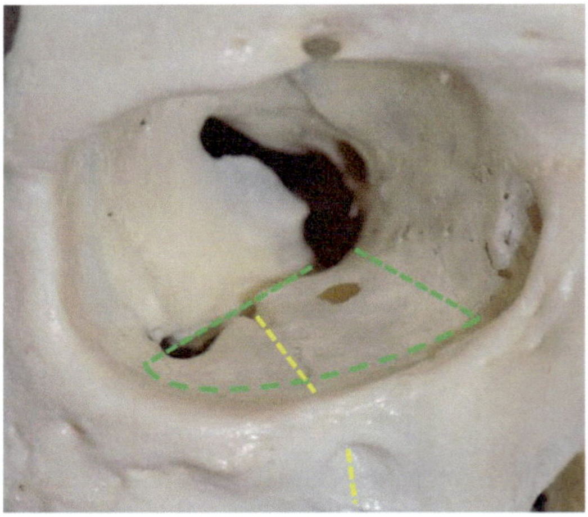

Fig. 1.19 Right orbit, inferior quadrant. Green dashed lines indicate approximate boundaries and region of bone that can be removed. Note the regional course of the infraorbital nerve from the infraorbital foramen to the foramen rotundum. A small area of dehiscence in the bone of the floor is visible posteriorly, a common finding. Yellow dashed line represents the course of the infraorbital nerve from the infraorbital foramen on the face of the maxilla, through the orbital floor and inferior orbital fissure to the foramen rotundum

Boundaries: Inferior orbital fissure and lateral orbital wall; medial orbital wall.

Portal: Inferior transconjunctival.

The access portal to the inferior quadrant is the inferior transconjunctival approach (ITC) (Fig. 1.20). While we originally described this as a preseptal approach, we now prefer the more direct transconjunctival incision directly onto the orbital rim which is more rapid and gives added protection to the lower lid provided by leaving a fat layer deep to the orbital septum. We often perform a lateral canthotomy and inferior cantholysis to increase the laxity of the lower lid and allow increased retraction and exposure. The lower lid is retracted anteriorly with a Ragnell retractor, and the inferior rim is palpated. A 15 blade or monopolar cautery on low voltage is used to incise directly onto the orbital rim. As dissection continues medially toward the caruncle, care should be taken not to use cautery near the inferior lacrimal punctum. Like the superior approach, it is important to incise the periosteum at rather than behind the orbital rim, as the origin of the inferior oblique is near the lateral border of the lacrimal fossa and dissection should be deep to the periosteum at its insertion point to avoid

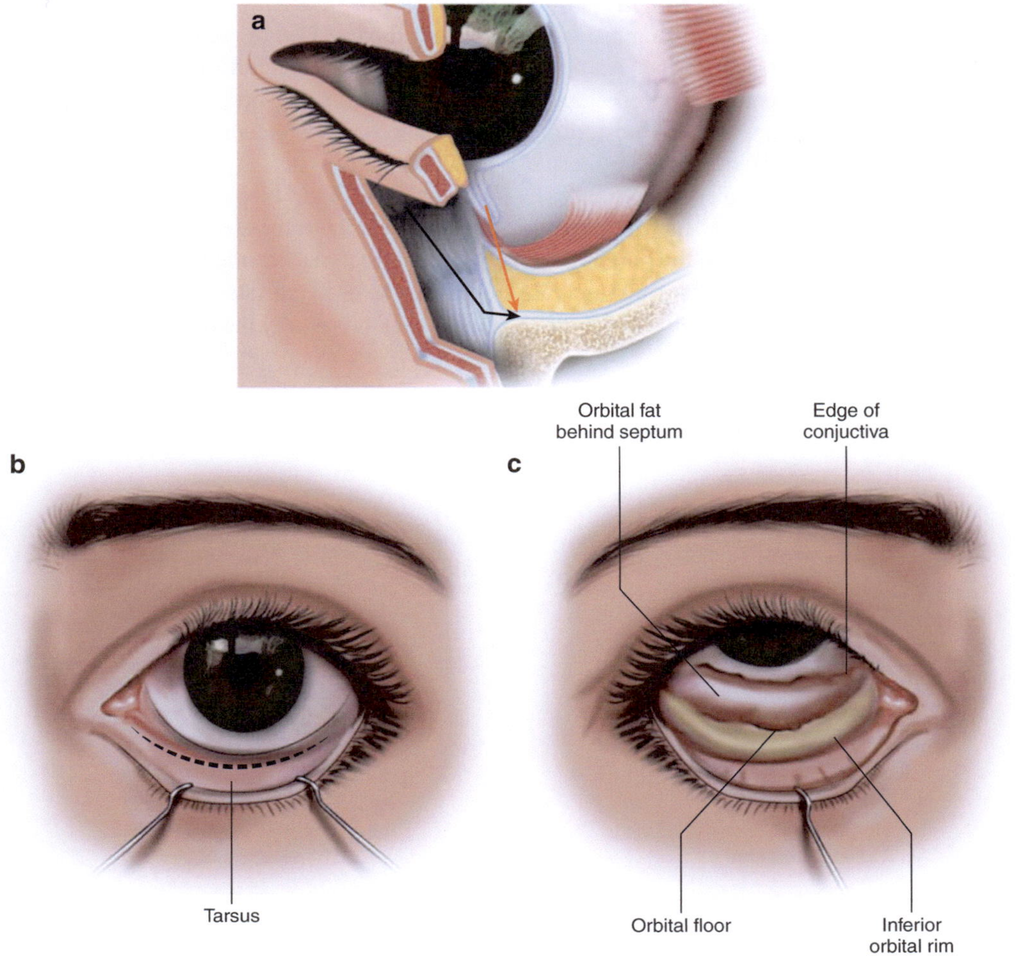

Fig. 1.20 The transconjunctival approach to the inferior orbit. (**a**) a direct transconjunctival approach is created to the inferior orbital rim. This can be done sharply or with low power electrocautery through the conjunctiva (**b**) and orbital fat until the periosteum of the inferior orbital rim is reached (**c**). This is incised and elevated, and a subperiosteal approach is undertaken. The infraorbital nerve runs through the bone of the orbital floor

damage. And similar to the trochlea of the superior oblique, the insertion of the inferior oblique is simply allowed to redrape with its periosteum into its original position at the end of the case.

The inferior transconjunctival approach may be extended medial into a precaruncular approach and laterally into a retrocanthal approach. The ITC does not typically require closure at the end of the case.

Approach: Inferior Quadrant

Upon completing the ITC portal and incising the periosteum of the inferior orbital rim, the periorbita is raised off the orbital floor using a suction Freer under endoscopic visualization. As noted above, care is taken to enter the subperiosteal plane at the orbital rim rather than posteriorly where the origin of the inferior oblique muscle could be damaged. A wide dissection cavity is created from the inferior orbital fissure laterally to the gradual upward slope onto the lamina papyracea medially. The inferior orbital fissure can be followed posteriorly and medially to the foramen rotundum and orbital apex inferior to the optic strut. The orbital floor can be removed as needed to create the pathway to the surgical target. At the end of the procedure, small bone defects can be bridged with a 0.25 mm PDS sheet. Larger defects will require 0.5 mm PDS sheet or titanium mesh lined with thin PDS sheet.

Lateral Quadrant [1, 10, 29, 30]

Access: Infratemporal fossa; foramen rotundum; greater wing of sphenoid; anterior clinoid; Meckel's cave; cavernous sinus; MCF; PCF (Fig. 1.21).

Boundaries: Can be joined with superior and inferior quadrants anteriorly; apex bounded by superior and inferior orbital fissures, but dissection superior and medial to the superior is possible.

Portals: Upper blepharoplasty (see above); LRC +/− canthotomy +/− cantholysis.

The lateral retrocanthal approach (LRC) is one of several portals to the lateral orbit (Fig. 1.22). It is nearly the mirror image of the PC

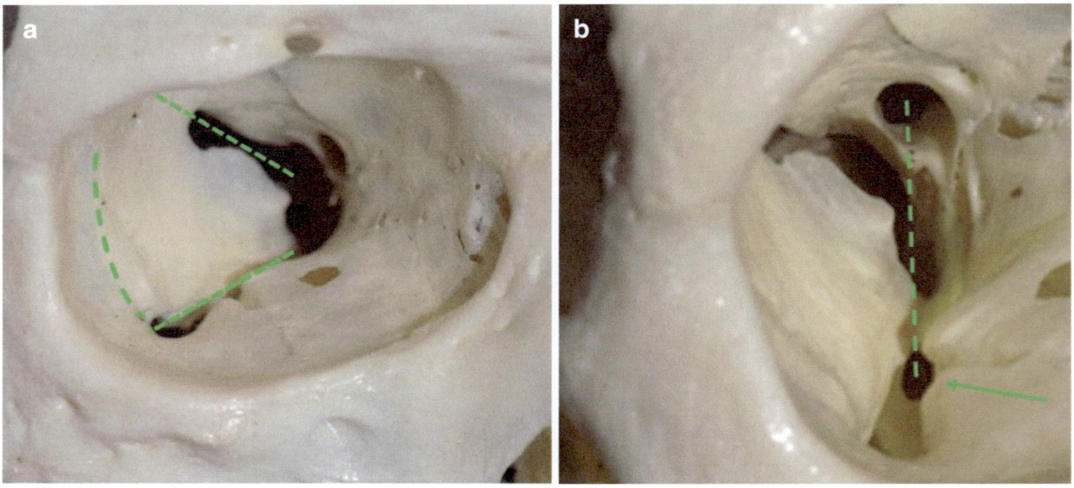

Fig. 1.21 Photographs of dry skull, right orbit, lateral quadrant. (**a**) approximate boundaries of lateral quadrant (dashed green lines), curved line indicates medial border of infratemporal fossa. Note the thick triangular bone of the greater wing of the sphenoid medial to the infratemporal fossa. (**b**) relationship of the optic nerve relative to the superior fissure, inferior fissure, and foramen rotundum. Note view through the inferior fissure into the infratemporal fossa and foramen rotundum at the medial aspect of the fissure (green arrow). The vertical plane passing from the foramen rotundum through the inferior fissure also transgresses the optic canal (dashed green line). For a posterior view of this region, see also Fig. 1.9. Posterior view of right orbit apex above

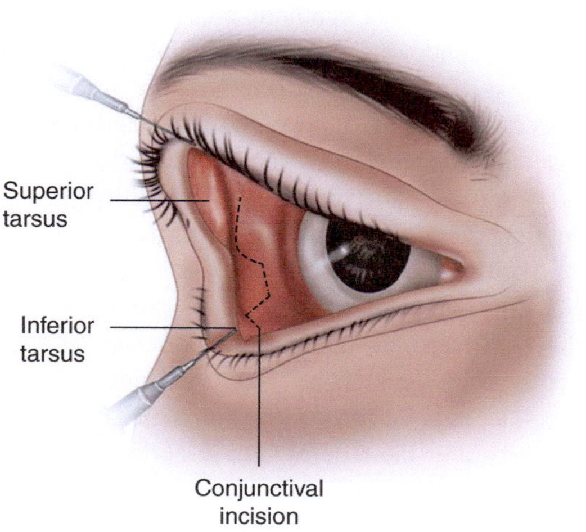

Fig. 1.22 Lateral retrocanthal approach to the lateral orbit. An incision is made through the conjunctiva medial to the anterior aspect of the lateral orbital rim, sweeping approximately 5 mm posteriorly in the region of the lateral canthus to avoid damage to the tendon at its insertion of the medial aspect of the bone. Similar to the precaruncular approach, this approach can be continued inferiorly to the orbital floor. The vertical incision should measure approximately 10–15 mm, taking care superiorly not to damage the lateral horn of the levator aponeurosis. If desired, a lateral canthotomy may be undertaken in addition to or instead of this approach depending on the access desired

approach. The lateral aspect of the upper and lower lids is retracted as demonstrated. Low-voltage cautery or a 15 blade is used to make a direct incision onto the lateral orbital wall. The incision should be 3–4 mm posterior to the rim in the region of the insertion of the lateral canthus to avoid damage to the structure. The subperiosteal plane is elevated directly deep to the incision. The incision can be extended inferiorly into the ITA or superiorly toward the orbit roof. Care must be taken, however, not to damage the lateral horn of the levator aponeurosis.

If further exposure and lid retraction is desired, a lateral canthotomy can be performed to the LRC approach. To do this, a scissor is used to make a full-thickness lid incision at the apex of the lateral canthus to the lateral orbital rim. If still more laxity is required, cantholysis is added (transection of the canthal tendon at the superior and/or inferior aspect of the canthotomy until sufficient laxity of the eyelid has been obtained). If canthotomy is performed, the wound should be closed at the end of the procedure with 5–0 deep monofilament suture to reunite the upper and lower limbs of the lateral canthus. If cantholysis of the upper or lower canthus has been added as well, the detached limb is sutured to the intact limb as with standard canthotomy. If both limbs have been detached, they should be reconstructed with transorbital sutures as described elsewhere to prevent ectropion (KM '00).

Unless the lateral canthal tendon is detached from its insertion, no reconstruction is required. If a CSF leak is encountered, the conjunctiva can be closed with 6–0 absorbable sutures in water-tight fashion. If the canthal tendon is detached, it should be repaired as described elsewhere to prevent ectropion [31].

As an alternative to the LRC approach, a superior blepharoplasty approach (Fig. 1.15) can be used. This may be chosen if a more superior approach vector is desired, such as when approaching the Sylvian fissure or MCA [32], or by surgeon preference.

Approach: Lateral Quadrant

After incising the periosteum of the lateral orbital wall through the portal of choice, the subperiosteal plane is developed. Once a suitable depth is reached, the endoscope is introduced, and the plane is dissected with a suction Freer elevator. The plane is opened as needed anteriorly and, from the inferior fissure below to the superior fissure above to reveal the lateral transorbital triangle, made up of the bone of the greater wing of the sphenoid. As noted earlier, the contents of the inferior fissure can be transected as needed to access the orbital floor, but the contents of the superior fissure, invested in fascia, must be protected unless resection is planned for oncologic reasons. The bone of the temporal fossa is drilled down to the deep periosteum overlying the temporalis muscle, and the greater wing of the sphenoid bone (the triangle) is drilled down to the temporal lobe dura. Medially, a thin rim of bone is left at the superior fissure referred to as the sagittal crest, composing the lateral surface of the superior orbital fissure (Corrivetti X 2). Once the greater wing of the sphenoid is removed, the mid-subtemporal ridge is visible as are the middle meningeal artery and foramen spinosum and the arcuate eminence on the surface of the petrous temporal bone. Dissecting further posteriorly, a segment of the petrous apex can be removed to expose the posterior fossa. Transection of the meningo-orbital band exposes the lateral cavernous sinus and Meckel's cave.

Reconstruction of the bone defect depends on the globe position at the end of the operation. If most of the greater wing of the sphenoid was removed, there is a risk of enophthalmos. This can be corrected with a fat graft or PDS sheet. If a CSF leak was encountered, dural closure is performed in a multilayer fashion with combined inlays and onlays using either autologous, xenograft or synthetic materials, optionally covered with fibrin or other synthetic glues, depending on the preference of the center. Lumbar drainage is optional depending on the size of the leak. Watertight closure of the conjunctiva and skin are mandatory. The skin can be closed with 5–0 dissolving suture and the skin closed with 6–0 dissolving or permanent sutures as indicated.

Multi-quadrant/multiportal approaches [33, 34]. Multiportal approaches are created in the same fashion as their monoportal components. Care should be taken in planning the approaches to be certain that they will be complementary and their convergence zones [35] will overlap in the appropriate positions (Fig. 1.23). They should be separated enough to provide significantly varied viewing aspects of the target, as well as complementary instrumentation angles. When possible, 30–45-° angulation between the pathways is helpful.

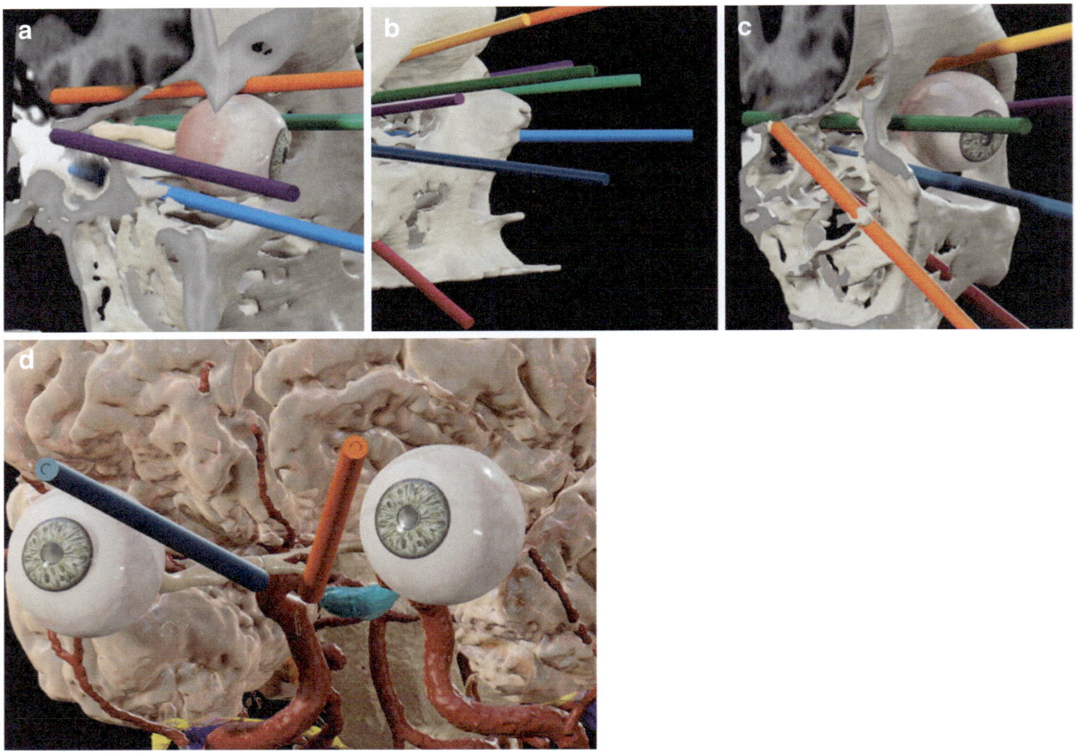

Fig. 1.23 Multiportal approaches to skull base pathology. Three-dimensional reconstruction of fused CT MRI. (**a**) lateral view demonstrating right transorbital approaches from adjacent quadrants approaching a convergence zone. (**b**) lateral view demonstrating combination of right transorbital and paramaxillary (pink) approaches at convergence zone. (**c**) medial view of left transorbital and transnasal (orange) approaches joining at orbital apex. (**d**) left precaruncular contraportal (orange) approach to right cavernous carotid provides additional perspective and viewing/instrumentation space to ipsilateral (blue) approach

Postoperative Care

Standard postoperative imaging is obtained as desired. Visual checks are performed in the recovery room and as indicated during the first 12 h after surgery. Crushed ice may be applied to the surgical site 20 min per hour for 48–72 h. If there is significant conjunctival edema, an ophthalmic ointment containing dexamethasone with polymyxin/neomycin is applied twice daily for 3–5 days. Intravenous steroids may given for 24–48 h or oral steroids if the patient is hospitalized. If the surgical duration is prolonged and there is concern for proptosis with conjunctival exposure and chemosis, a tarsorrhaphy stitch may be left in place for several days. This should be placed at the medial or lateral limbus so that the eyelids can be opened enough to perform visual checks. Additional postoperative care is administered as needed based on the site and type of surgical procedure performed.

Patients are typically seen in clinic 1 week after surgery and at intervals thereafter as indicated by the procedure performed and the patient's recovery. (See Chap. 36 for further details).

Technical Nuances

Gentle Retraction of Orbital Contents

It is critical to gently retract the orbital contents without placing pointed structures or retractor tips into the orbital contents. A thin sheet of silastic may be used to protect the structures. Retraction of orbital contents is performed with a malleable ribbon retractor: it is critical to maintain the retractor parallel to the adjacent orbital wall and avoid angling the retractor tip into the orbital contents where it can compress the globe, ciliary ganglion, or optic nerve (Fig. 1.24).

Monitor Pupil Size and Shape

It is critical to check the pupil regularly, at roughly 15–20-min intervals, particularly when instrumenting posterior to the equator of the globe. This should be done preoperatively to check for preexisting asymmetry and after induction of general anesthesia to check on the effects of the anesthetic agents on pupil size. If asymmetric pupil dilation occurs, the instruments are removed from the orbit until the pupil returns to symmetric shape and size.

Measure Globe Position at the Beginning and End of the Case

This is not critical, but if a significant amount of bone will be removed in creating the approach, the measurement can add precision in the reconstruction. A Hertel's (Fig. 1.12) or Naugle's exophthalmometer can be used to measure the position of the globe at the beginning and end of surgery while the patient is on the operating table.

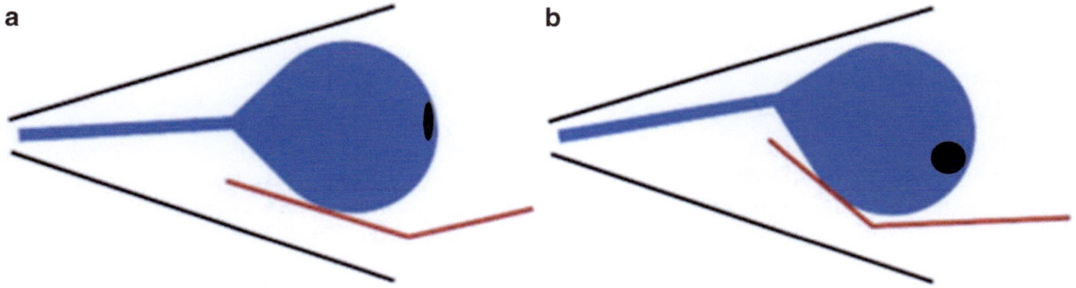

Fig. 1.24 Orbital content retraction technique. (**a**) correct angulation of malleable retractor (red) parallel to the surgical pathway with minimal tissues displacement. (**b**) incorrect retractor position risks damage to the orbital contents such as the ciliary ganglion and optic nerve. Dilation of the pupil is a sign of inappropriate retraction pressure or angulation

We have found that 2–3 mm of proptosis at the end of the case is common due to edema which resolves during the first week after surgery. If a significant amount of bone has been removed during the surgery, exophthalmometry can help in determining adequacy of reconstruction, again aiming for mild proptosis rather than symmetry at the conclusion of the procedure.

Learning Transorbital Endoscopic Surgery

As indicated at the beginning of this chapter, transorbital neuroendoscopic surgery requires a unique set of skills that is not commonly taught within a surgical specialty at the time of this writing. In addition, it (like other forms of endoscopic skull base surgery) is best performed by a multidisciplinary team possessing expertise in all facets of pre- and postoperative care in addition to the surgical procedure itself. For surgeons practicing at an institution where these procedures are not yet being performed, it is best to assemble a team, read fully on the subject, and perform the procedures in a cadaver lab and possibly on training models [36]. In addition, it is strongly recommended that the team attend a hands-on dissection course of the type offered by Endoscopic Transorbital Society or ETOS.

Once a basic education on the techniques has been obtained, it is important to start with simple cases and progress over time. This begins with extraconal orbital and extradural ACF/MCF tumors, progresses to intradural ACF/MC F meningiomas, and eventually moves through to the fifth stage of complexity involving approaches to and through the petrous apex and posterior cranial fossa, as well as the Sylvian fissure and tentorial region [37].

Stage I: extraconal/extradural lesions and posttraumatic CSF leaks of the ACF and MCF.

Stage II: intradural benign tumors of the ACF and MCF, e.g., spheno-orbital meningioma.

Stage III: pathology in Meckel's cave, lateral cavernous sinus, anterior temporal intraparenchymal, and intraconal spaces.

Stage IV: pathology requiring deeper orbital dissection in medial aspect of lesser sphenoid wing, anterior clinoid process, cavernous sinus, and mesial temporal lobe.

Stage V: involvement of petrous apex by tumors such as petroclival meningioma, chordoma, and chondrosarcoma.

The field of transorbital skull base and brain surgery is experiencing a period of rapid growth in research and clinical applications [38], with development progressing from the ACF and MCF to include the petrous apex and posterior cranial fossa [39–41]. The chapters included in this book are intended to provide expert perspectives and experience that will serve as an educational foundation for the novice surgeon, as well as a reference for the experienced surgeon on the journey to master endoscopic transorbital surgery in these technically challenging regions. It is our hope that this book will encourage further international multidisciplinary collaboration, research, and clinical development in this exciting new field.

References

1. Moe KS, Bergeron CM, Ellenbogen RG. Transorbital neuroendoscopic surgery. Neurosurgery. 2010;67(3 Suppl Operative):ons16–28. https://doi.org/10.1227/01.NEU.0000373431.08464.43.
2. Ciporen JN, Moe KS, Lopez S, Ledesma E, Ramanathan D, Rostomily R, Sekhar L. Multiportal endoscopic approaches to the central skull base: a cadaveric study. World Neurosurg. 2010;73(6):705–12. PMID:20934161.
3. Houlihan LM, Belykh E, Zhao X, O'Sullivan MGJ, Preul MC. From Krönlein, through madness, to a useful modern surgery: the journey of the transorbital corridor to enter the neurosurgical armamentarium. J Neurosurg. 2021;5:1–10. https://doi.org/10.3171/2020.8.JNS201251.
4. Houlihan LM, Staudinger Knoll AJ, Kakodkar P, Zhao X, O'Sullivan MGJ, Lawton MT, Preul MC. Transorbital Neuroendoscopic surgery as a mainstream neurosurgical corridor: a systematic review. World Neurosurg. 2021;152:167–179.e4. https://doi.org/10.1016/j.wneu.2021.04.104. Epub 2021 Apr 30.
5. Locatelli D, Pozzi F, Turri-Zanoni M, Battaglia P, Santi L, Dallan I, Castelnuovo P. Transorbital endoscopic approaches to the skull base: current concepts and future perspectives. J Neurosurg Sci. 2016;60(4):514–25. Epub 2016 Jun 9.

6. Vural A, Carobbio ALC, Ferrari M, Rampinelli V, Schreiber A, Mattavelli D, Doglietto F, Buffoli B, Rodella LF, Taboni S, Tomasoni M, Gualtieri T, Deganello A, Hirtler L, Nicolai P. Transorbital endoscopic approaches to the skull base: a systematic literature review and anatomical description. Neurosurg Rev. 2021;44(5):2857–78. https://doi.org/10.1007/s10143-020-01470-5. Epub 2021 Jan 22. Erratum in: Neurosurg Rev. 2021 Aug 14: PMID: 33479806; PMCID: PMC8490260.
7. Pearce E, Bridge H. Is orbital volume associated with eyeball and visual cortex volume in humans? Ann Hum Biol. 2013;40(6):531–40. https://doi.org/10.3109/03014460.2013.815272. Epub 2013 Jul 23. PMID: 23879766; PMCID: PMC3836230.
8. Pearce E, Dunbar R. Latitudinal variation in light levels drives human visual system size. Biol Lett. 2012;8:90–3. [PubMed: 21795263].
9. Bron AJ, Tripathi RC, Tripathi BJ. Wolff's anatomy of the eye & orbit. 8th ed. London: Chapman & Hall Medical; 1997.
10. Bly RA, Ramakrishna R, Ferreira M, Moe KS. Lateral transorbital neuroendoscopic approach to the lateral cavernous sinus. J Neurol Surg B Skull Base. 2014;75(1):11–7. https://doi.org/10.1055/s--0033-1353363. Epub 2013 Sep 9. PMID: 24498584; PMCID: PMC3912142.
11. Balakrishnan K, Moe KS. Applications and outcomes of orbital and transorbital endoscopic surgery. Otolaryngol Head Neck Surg. 2011;144(5):815–20. https://doi.org/10.1177/0194599810397285.
12. Altay T, Patel BC, Couldwell WT. Lateral orbital wall approach to the cavernous sinus. J Neurosurg. 2012;116(4):755–63.
13. Goncalves N, Lubbe DE. Transorbital endoscopic surgery for sphenoid wing meningioma: long-term outcomes and surgical technique. J Neurol Surg B Skull Base. 2020;81(4):357–68. https://doi.org/10.1055/s--0040-1713854. Epub 2020 Aug 20. PMID: 33072477; PMCID: PMC7561457.
14. Lubbe D, Moe KS. Orbital and Transorbital endoscopic surgery. In: Stamm A, editor. Skull base surgery, vol. II. London: Thieme; 2019.
15. Lee WJ, Hong SD, Woo KI, Seol HJ, Choi JW, Lee JI, Nam DH, Kong DS. Combined endoscopic endonasal and transorbital multiportal approach for complex skull base lesions involving multiple compartments. Acta Neurochir. 2022;164(7):1911–22. https://doi.org/10.1007/s00701-022-05203-z. Epub 2022 Apr 29. PMID: 35488013.
16. Dallan I, Castelnuovo P, Locatelli D, Turri-Zanoni M, AlQahtani A, Battaglia P, Hirt B, Sellari-Franceschini S. Multiportal combined transorbital transnasal endoscopic approach for the Management of Selected Skull Base Lesions: preliminary experience. World Neurosurg. 2015;84(1):97–107. https://doi.org/10.1016/j.wneu.2015.02.034. Epub 2015 Mar 5.
17. Ellenbogen RG, Moe KS. Transorbital Neuroendoscopic approaches to the anterior cranial fossa. In: Snyderman C, editor. Master techniques in otolaryngology-head & neck surgery: skull base surgery. Philadelphia: Walters Kluwer; 2015. p. 151–64.
18. Lubbe DE, Douglas-Jones P, Wasl H, Mustak H, Semple PL. Contralateral Precaruncular approach to the lateral sphenoid sinus-A case report detailing a new, multiportal approach to lesions, and defects in the lateral aspect of well-pneumatized sphenoid sinuses. Ear Nose Throat J. 2020;99(1):62–7. https://doi.org/10.1177/0145561319846828. Epub 2019 Apr 24.
19. Hicks K, Moe KS, Humphreys I. Bilateral transorbital and transnasal endoscopic resection of a frontal sinus osteoblastoma and orbital mucocele: a case report and review of the literature. Annal Otol Rhinol Laryngol. 2018;127(11):864–9.
20. Miller C, Rly RA, Moe KS. Endoscopic orbital and periorbital approaches in minimally disruptive skull base surgery. J Neurol Surg Part B Skull Base. 2020;81(4):459–71. PMID: 33072486.
21. Bly R, Hannaford B, Ferreira M, Moe KS. A method of preoperative computerized surgical planning for minimally disruptive skull base surgery. Las Vegas: NASBS annual meeting; 2012.
22. Bly R, Liu J, Cjudekova M, Chang SH, Moe KS. Computer-guided orbital reconstruction improves surgical outcomes. JAMA Facial Plast Surg. 2013;15(2):113–20.
23. Bly RA, Berens AM, Perkins JA, Miller C, Ferreira M, Hauptman JS, Moe KS. Surgical planning in pediatric skull base surgery. Oper Tech Otolaryngol Head Neck Surg. 2019;30(1):9–15.
24. Aghdasi N, Whipple M, Humphreys I, Moe KS, Hannaford B, Bly R. Automated surgical approach planning for complex Skull Base targets: development and validation of a cost function and semantic atlas. Surg Innov. 2018;25:476–84. https://doi.org/10.1177/1553350618782287. PMID: 29947581.
25. Moe KS, Ellenbogen RG. Transorbital Neuroendoscopic approaches to the middle cranial fossa. In: Snyderman C, editor. Master techniques in otolaryngology-head & neck surgery: skull base surgery. Philadelphia: Walters Kluwer; 2015. p. 343–56.
26. Di Somma A, Sanchez España JC, Alobid I, Enseñat J. Endoscopic superior eyelid transorbital approach: how I do it. Acta Neurochir. 2022;164(7):1953–9. https://doi.org/10.1007/s00701-022-05177-y. Epub 2022 Mar 11.
27. Guizzardi G, Mosteiro A, Hoyos J, Ferres A, Topczewski T, Reyes L, Alobid I, Matas J, Cavallo LM, Cappabianca P, Enseñat J, Prats-Galino A, Di Somma A. Endoscopic transorbital approach to the middle Fossa: qualitative and quantitative anatomic study. Oper Neurosurg. 2022;23(4):e267–75. https://doi.org/10.1227/ons.0000000000000308.
28. Moe KS. The precaruncular approach to the medial orbit. Arch Facial Plast Surg. 2003;5(6):483–7. https://doi.org/10.1001/archfaci.5.6.483.
29. Moe KS, Jothi S, Stern R, Gassner HG. Lateral retrocanthal orbitotomy: a minimally invasive, canthus-sparing approach. Arch Facial Plast

Surg. 2007;9(6):419–26. https://doi.org/10.1001/archfaci.9.6.419.
30. Gerges MM, Godil SS, Younus I, Rezk M, Schwartz TH. Endoscopic transorbital approach to the infratemporal fossa and parapharyngeal space: a cadaveric study. J Neurosurg. 2019;133:1–12. https://doi.org/10.3171/2019.7.JNS191743. Epub ahead of print.
31. Moe KS, Linder T. The lateral transorbital canthopexy for correction and prevention of ectropion: report of a procedure, grading system, and outcome study. Arch Facial Plast Surg. 2000;2(1):9–15. https://doi.org/10.1001/archfaci.2.1.9.
32. Almeida JP, Ruiz-Treviño AS, Shetty SR, Omay SB, Anand VK, Schwartz TH. Transorbital endoscopic approach for exposure of the sylvian fissure, middle cerebral artery and crural cistern: an anatomical study. Acta Neurochir. 2017;159(10):1893–907. https://doi.org/10.1007/s00701-017-3296-8. Epub 2017 Aug 14.
33. Di Somma A, Guizzardi G, Valls Cusiné C, Hoyos J, Ferres A, Topczewski TE, Mosteiro A, De Rosa A, Solari D, Cavallo LM, Reyes L, Enseñat J. Combined endoscopic endonasal and transorbital approach to skull base tumors: a systematic literature review. J Neurosurg Sci. 2022;66(5):406–12. https://doi.org/10.23736/S0390-5616.21.05401-1. Epub 2021 Aug 3.
34. Lee WJ, Hong SD, Woo KI, Seol HJ, Choi JW, Lee JI, Nam DH, Kong DS. Combined endoscopic endonasal and transorbital multiportal approach for complex skull base lesions involving multiple compartments. Acta Neurochir. 2022;164(7):1911–22. https://doi.org/10.1007/s00701-022-05203-z. Epub 2022 Apr 29.
35. Guizzardi G, Prats-Galino A, Mosteiro A, Santos C, Topczewski T, Torales J, Roldan P, Reyes L, Di Somma A, Enseñat J. Multiportal combined endoscopic endonasal and transorbital pathways: qualitative and quantitative anatomic studies of the "connection" Skull Base areas. Oper Neurosurg (Hagerstown). 2023;24:e342. https://doi.org/10.1227/ons.0000000000000577. PMID: 36715996.
36. Lee WJ, Kim YH, Hong SD, Rho TH, Kim YH, Dho YS, Hong CK, Kong DS. Development of 3-dimensional printed simulation surgical training models for endoscopic endonasal and transorbital surgery. Front Oncol. 2022;12:966051. https://doi.org/10.3389/fonc.2022.966051. PMID: 35992880; PMCID: PMC9389537.
37. De Rosa A, Di Somma A, Mosteiro A, Ferrés A, Reyes LA, Roldan P, Torné R, Torales J, Solari D, Cavallo LM, Enseñat J, Prats-Galino A. Superior eyelid endoscopic transorbital approach to the tentorial area: A qualitative and quantitative anatomic study. Front Surg. 2022;9:1007447. https://doi.org/10.3389/fsurg.2022.1007447. PMID: 36338650; PMCID: PMC9634414.
38. Schwartz TH, Henderson F Jr, Di Somma A, Kong DS, de Notaris M, Enseñat J, Moe KS. Endoscopic transorbital surgery: another leap of faith? World Neurosurg. 2022;159:54–5. https://doi.org/10.1016/j.wneu.2021.12.081. Epub 2021 Dec 28. PMID: 35007891.
39. Di Somma A, Kong D, de Notaris M, Moe KS, Sánchez España JC, Schwartz TH, Enseñat J. Endoscopic transorbital surgery levels of difficulty. J Neurosurg. 2022;137(4):1187–90.
40. Di Somma A, Andaluz N, Cavallo LM, Topczewski TE, Frio F, Gerardi RM, Pineda J, Solari D, Enseñat J, Prats-Galino A, Cappabianca P. Endoscopic transorbital route to the petrous apex: a feasibility anatomic study. Acta Neurochir. 2018;160(4):707–20. https://doi.org/10.1007/s00701-017-3448-x. Epub 2017 Dec 29.
41. Lee WJ, Hong SD, Woo KI, Seol HJ, Choi JW, Lee JI, Nam DH, Kong DS. Endoscopic endonasal and transorbital approaches to petrous apex lesions. J Neurosurg. 2021;136(2):431–40. https://doi.org/10.3171/2021.2.JNS203867.

Part I

Anatomy and Classification of the Transorbital Approach

2 Superior Eyelid Transorbital Approaches: A Modular Classification System

Matteo de Notaris, Doo-Sik Kong, Alberto di Somma, Joaquim Enseñat, Chang-Ki Hong, Kris S. Moe, and Theodore H. Schwartz

Introduction

Skull base surgery represents a complex and challenging subspecialty within neurosurgery, often requiring innovative approaches to safely access critical anatomical structures. Among the transorbital approaches, also known as TONES (transorbital neuroendoscopic surgery), the superior eyelid transorbital approach stands out as the most versatile from a neurosurgical perspective, offering effective access to the ventral paramedian skull base [1–5]. In an effort to enhance an understanding and promote clinical utilization of this approach, in this perspective piece, we introduce a novel modular classification system for the superolateral transorbital approach that describes its various extensions [6–10]. This framework is grounded in anatomical studies that further solidified the theoretical basis for the classification [11–14].

The classification system, created by an experienced international transorbital multidisciplinary working group (Endoscopic Transorbital Society or ETOS), [8] begins with a simple concept, namely, the division of the transorbital approaches into two primary categories (Figs. 2.1 and 2.2; Table 2.1): standard and extended. Furthermore, the extensions of the superolateral transorbital approach can be further divided into two types: proximal extensions and deep extensions. Together, these extensions can be used to enlarge the surgical corridor, which in turn increases the versatility of the approach.

The standard superolateral transorbital approach involves the drilling of the inner surface of frontal process of the zygomatic bone and then of the greater and lesser sphenoid wings, which provides access to the anterior part of the temporal fossa, the middle fossa, and

M. de Notaris
Unit of Neurosurgery, San Pio Hospital, Benevento, Italy

D.-S. Kong
Department of Neurosurgery, Samsung Medical Center, Seoul, Korea (Republic of)

A. di Somma
Department of Neurological Surgery, Hospital Clínic de Barcelona, Barcelona, Spain

J. Enseñat
Department of Neurosurgery, H. Clinic of Barcelona, University of Barcelona, Barcelona, Spain

C.-K. Hong
Department of Neurosurgery, Asan Medical Center, Ulsan University College of Medicine, Seoul, South Korea

K. S. Moe
Division of Facial Plastic Surgery, Departments of Otolaryngology and Neurological Surgery, University of Washington School of Medicine, Seattle, WA, USA

T. H. Schwartz (✉)
Department of Neurosurgery, Weill Cornell Medicine, NewYork–Presbyterian Hospital, New York, NY, USA

T. H. Schwartz et al. (eds.), *Endoscopic Transorbital Surgery of the Orbit, Skull Base and Brain*,
https://doi.org/10.1007/978-3-031-59504-2_2

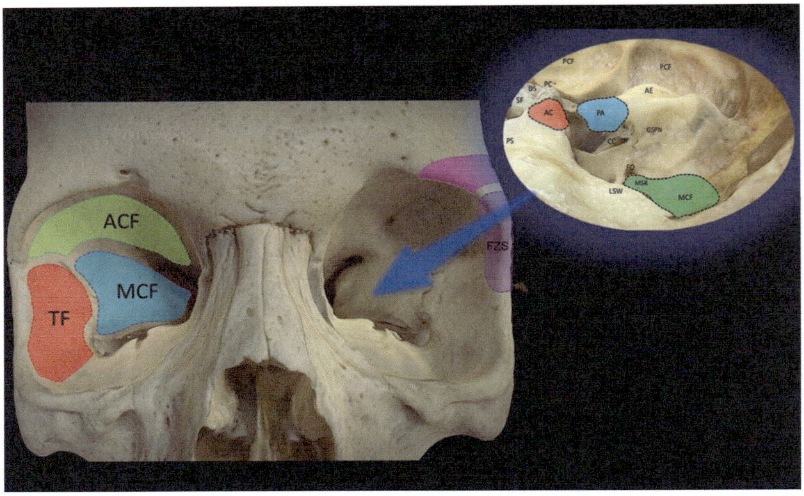

Fig. 2.1 View of the skull showing the (left) standard approach extended approach modules (right). The standard approach includes removal of the bone overlying the temporal fossa (TF; red), middle cranial fossa (MCF; blue), and anterior cranial fossa (ACF; green). The proximal extensions include the lateral orbital rim and superolateral orbital rim (purple). The deep extensions include the anterior clinoid (AC; red), flattening of the mid-subtemporal ridge (MSR; green) and floor of the middle cranial fossa (MCF; green) and petrous apex (PA; blue)

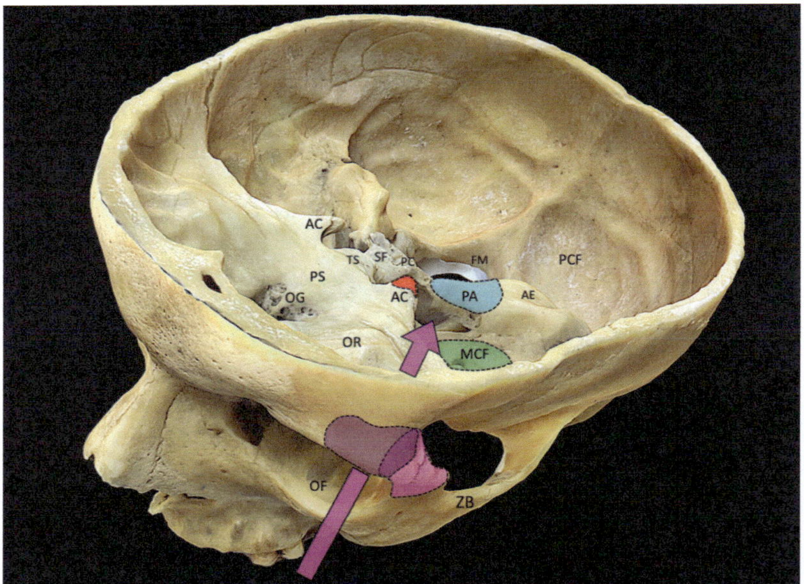

Fig. 2.2 View of the skull showing the anatomy of the proximal extensions (lateral orbitotomy and superolateral orbitotomy; purple) and the deep extensions, including the anterior clinoid (AC; red), flattening of the of the middle cranial fossa (MCF; green) and petrous apex (PA; blue). Also seen are the orbital floor (OF), orbital roof (OF), olfactory groove (OG), planum sphenoidale (PS), tuberculum sella (TS), sellar floor (SF), posterior clinoid (PC), posterior cranial fossa (PCF), foramen magnum (FM), zygomatic bone (ZB)

Table 2.1 Superolateral transorbital

Type of approach	Level of difficulty	Surgical exposure	Proximal extensions	Deep extensions
Standard	1 and 2	Temporal and anterior/middle cranial fossae	Lateral orbitotomy *Adjunct* technique *to* enhance medial and lateral target access as an elective augmentation in the *axial* plane	Drilling of the frontal process of the zygomatic bone to access the temporal fossa
			Superolateral orbitotomy *Adjunct* technique *to* enhance both mediolateral and also cranio-caudal target access as an elective augmentation in the *axial* and *sagittal* planes	Drilling of the greater sphenoid wing to access the middle skull base Drilling of the lesser sphenoid wing: Access the anterior skull base Removal of the sagittal crest Cutting the meningo-orbital band
Extended	3 to 5	Enhancing the deep extension of the surgical targets: Opto-carotid region, middle/infratemporal fossae, posterior fossa	Lateral orbitotomy *Recommended* technique *to* enhance medial and lateral target access as an elective augmentation in the *axial* plane	Anterior clinoidectomy to Access the opto-carotid region Middle fossa floor flattening to access the infratemporal fossa Anterior petrosectomy to access the posterior cranial fossa
			Superolateral orbitotomy *Recommended* technique *to* enhance both mediolateral and also cranio-caudal target access as an elective augmentation in the *axial* and *sagittal* planes	

the paramedian anterior fossa. This approach also includes removal of the sagittal crest and cutting of the meningo-orbital band. Onto this more basic approach can be added two possible proximal extensions, namely, the lateral orbitotomy (LO) and superolateral orbitotomy (SLO), which can be applied at the discretion of the of the operating surgeon, to enlarge the operative corridor. Both of the enlargements to the proximal corridor increase maneuverability. While the LO increases medial-to-lateral reach, the SLO allow the surgeon more freedom to advance a retractor onto the dural overlying the temporal lobe to retract it medially and superiorly, providing increased access to the petrous apex.

The deep extensions, on the other hand, enlarge the distal corridor and expose additional targets. These include maneuvers such as anterior clinoidectomy, middle fossa floor flattening, and anterior petrosectomy. These techniques grant access to the optico-carotid region, posterior fossa, and infratemporal fossa, respectively. Whereas the proximal extensions—LO and SLO—are more optional during the standard approach, depending on the size and extent of the pathology, they are strongly recommended when the deep extensions are being employed.

Finally, we would like to comment on how these maneuvers map onto the five levels of difficulty we introduced in a prior opinion piece [15]. Fundamentally, the lower the level of difficulty, the less one needs either proximal or deep extensions and vice versa. However, there are no absolute recommendations in this regard.

Tailoring the Transorbital Approaches for Surgical Levels of Difficulty

Transorbital approaches, as with any skull base approach, can be applied to a variety of different pathologies with varying degrees of complexity. Acquiring expertise in any new technique often requires a learning curve, and transorbital surgery is no different. Depending on the target one is trying to expose, the approach may require modifications to increase its reach. In a prior publication, we defined five levels of difficulty, ranging from easiest to most difficult [15].

The standard approach—in which the bone of the frontal process of the zygoma and greater and lesser sphenoid wings as well as the sagittal crest are removed, and the meningo-orbital band is cut—is generally suited for a level of difficulty of 1 and 2. These levels, as outlined in our previous article, encompass removal of extraconal lesions, the middle or anterior fossa extradural approach, and the middle or anterior fossa intradural approach for spheno-orbital meningiomas with mostly bony extradural infiltration or limited intradural tumor in the region of the middle compartment of the lesser sphenoid wing. This approach serves as a reliable foundation for addressing less complex cases and generally does not require LO or SLO. However, in some circumstances, if the tumor extends laterally, toward the lateral third of the lesser sphenoid wing, LO may be a useful adjunct.

In contrast, the extended approach modules become more relevant as we ascend to surgical levels of difficulty 3 through 5 (Table 2.1). These advanced levels present formidable challenges, demanding an expanded surgical corridor. The extended approach includes advanced techniques such as anterior clinoidectomy, middle fossa floor flattening, and anterior petrosectomy. These maneuvers unlock access to deeper regions, including the optico-carotid region, the infratemporal and posterior fossae. In these more complex surgical contexts, the LO and SLO proximal extensions are highly recommended. Its incorporation serves a *dual* purpose. Firstly, they substantially increase the lateral-to-medial angle of attack, granting surgeons improved access and visibility to deep target approach-related structures. Secondly, by expanding the superficial corridor of the surgical field, the compression exerted on the orbital content is reduced, thereby safeguarding them from potential complications. Finally, the SLO, and to some extent the LO, can allow the introduction of a retractor, which can support and mobilize the temporal lobe out of the way to expand the surgical corridor and increase maneuverability.

However, depending on the nature of pathology being addressed and its location, some pathologies within levels 3, 4, and 5 may not require LO or SLO. For example, to reach the cavernous sinus (level 4) for a biopsy, LO and SLO are not obligatory. Moreover, some Meckel's cave schwannomas (level 3) can be removed in their entirely, particularly if there is no posterior fossa component, without an osteotomy, using only the standard approach. On the other hand, for intraconal lesions (level 3), such as cavernous hemangiomas, the LO is extremely useful to increase the angle of the lateral-to-medial trajectory. For larger trigeminal schwannomas, particularly those with an intradural posterior fossa extension, LO is recommended as it may aid exposure of the foramen rotundum, dissection of V1 and V2, and visualization over the back of the petrous ridge. Finally, to remove intraparenchymal tumors of the temporal pole (level 3), which involves the dissection and identification of the temporal pole, gyri, sulci, and the temporal horn of the lateral ventricle, LO is highly recommended.

For approaches classified at a level of difficulty 4, such as anterior clinoid meningiomas, full exposure of the optico-carotid region is essential. This requires tasks such as excising the medial portion of the lesser sphenoid wing, performing an anterior clinoidectomy, and exposing the carotid artery. In the context of cavernous sinus (CS) tumors, the technique requires an unveiling Meckel's cave, accessing interdurally the CS and, in some cases, eventually performing the anterior petrosectomy in case of posterior fossa involvement. For the most complex surgeries, like selective amygdalohippocampectomy, LO or SLO aids greatly in increasing exposure.

For cases in level of difficulty 5, an exceptional depth of surgical proficiency and technique are required. For petroclival meningiomas, chordomas, and chondrosarcomas, an approach to the petrous apex and posterior cranial fossa as well as flattening of the middle fossa floor (and mid-subtemporal ridge) to remove lesions extending into infratemporal fossa is critical. Moreover, when addressing intracerebral insular tumors, safety demands extensive intradural exploration combined with the opening of the Sylvian cistern. Finally, for vascular pathology located in the Sylvian fissure, involving vascular microdissection and exposure and management of the middle cerebral artery (MCA) will be greatly facilitated by LO or SLO as well as anterior clinoidectomy.

Conclusion

Our modular classification system not only provides a structured approach to transorbital surgery but also offers a strategic roadmap for tailoring these approaches to distinct surgical levels. By aligning techniques with case management, we aim to streamline surgical decision-making and optimize patient outcomes. This thought piece will hopefully lay the foundation for future research and innovation, promising to advance the practice of transorbital skull base surgery. As we delve into the subtleties of transorbital approaches, we hope to contribute meaningfully to the ongoing evolution of this technique.

References

1. Moe KS, Bergeron CM, Ellenbogen RG. Transorbital neuroendoscopic surgery. Neurosurgery. 2010;67(3 Suppl Operative):ons16–28. https://doi.org/10.1227/01.NEU.0000373431.08464.43.
2. Kong DS, Moe KS. Editorial: endoscopic transorbital surgery for skull base tumors. Front Oncol. 2022;12:1042655. https://doi.org/10.3389/fonc.2022.1042655.
3. Schwartz TH, Henderson F, Di Somma A, et al. Endoscopic Transorbital surgery: another leap of faith? World Neurosurg. 2022;159:54–5. https://doi.org/10.1016/j.wneu.2021.12.081.
4. Zoia C, Mantovani G, Müther M, et al. Through the orbit and beyond: current state and future perspectives in endoscopic orbital surgery on behalf of the EANS frontiers committee in orbital tumors and the EANS skull base section. Brain Spine. 2023;3:102669. https://doi.org/10.1016/j.bas.2023.102669.
5. Mathios D, Bobeff EJ, Longo D, et al. The lateral transorbital approach to the medial sphenoid wing, anterior clinoid, middle fossa, cavernous sinus, and Meckel's cave: target-based classification, approach-related complications, and intermediate-term ocular outcomes. J Neurosurg. 2023;1:1–11. https://doi.org/10.3171/2023.6.JNS23678.
6. Kassam A, Snyderman CH, Mintz A, Gardner P, Carrau RL. Expanded endonasal approach: the rostrocaudal axis. Part I. Crista galli to the Sella turcica. FOC. 2005;19(1):1–12. https://doi.org/10.3171/foc.2005.19.1.4.
7. Kassam A, Snyderman CH, Mintz A, Gardner P, Carrau RL. Expanded endonasal approach: the rostrocaudal axis. Part II. Posterior clinoids to the foramen magnum. FOC. 2005;19(1):1–7. https://doi.org/10.3171/foc.2005.19.1.5.
8. Kassam AB, Gardner P, Snyderman C, Mintz A, Carrau R. Expanded endonasal approach: fully endoscopic, completely transnasal approach to the middle third of the clivus, petrous bone, middle cranial fossa, and infratemporal fossa. Neurosurg Focus. 2005;19(1):E6.
9. Jägersberg M, Brodard J, Qiu J, et al. Quantification of working volumes, exposure, and target-specific maneuverability of the Pterional craniotomy and its minimally invasive variants. World Neurosurg. 2017;101:710–717.e2. https://doi.org/10.1016/j.wneu.2017.02.011.
10. de Notaris M, Kong DS, Di Somma A, Enseñat J, Hong C-K, Moe K, Schwartz TH. Superior eyelid transorbital approaches: a modular classification system (submitted for publication). J Neurosurg. 2024:1–6.
11. Corrivetti F, de Notaris M, Di Somma A, et al. "Sagittal crest": definition, stepwise dissection, and clinical implications from a Transorbital perspective. Oper Neurosurg (Hagerstown). 2022;22(5):e206–12. https://doi.org/10.1227/ons.0000000000000131.
12. Dallan I, Di Somma A, Prats-Galino A, et al. Endoscopic transorbital route to the cavernous sinus through the meningo-orbital band: a descriptive anatomical study. J Neurosurg. 2017;127(3):622–9. https://doi.org/10.3171/2016.8.JNS16465.
13. De Rosa A, Di Somma A, Mosteiro A, et al. Superior eyelid endoscopic transorbital approach to the tentorial area: a qualitative and quantitative anatomic study. Front Surg. 2022;9:1007447. https://doi.org/10.3389/fsurg.2022.1007447.
14. Guizzardi G, Di Somma A, de Notaris M, et al. Endoscopic transorbital avenue to the skull base: four-step conceptual analysis of the anatomic journey. Front Oncol. 2022;12:988131. https://doi.org/10.3389/fonc.2022.988131.
15. Di Somma A, Kong DS, de Notaris M, et al. Endoscopic transorbital surgery levels of difficulty. J Neurosurg. 2022;15:1–4. https://doi.org/10.3171/2022.3.JNS212699.

Anatomy of the Orbit

3

Laura Tiedemann and S. Tonya Stefko

Abbreviations

CN	Cranial nerve
CSF	Cerebral spinal fluid
CCF	Carotid-cavernous fistula
EOM	Extraocular muscle
IOF	Inferior orbital fissure
LPS	Levator palpebrae superioris
NLD	Nasolacrimal duct
SOF	Superior orbital fissure

Introduction

Knowledge of orbital anatomy is critical to any surgery of the face or anterior and middle skull base. The orbit consists of four bony walls, the eye, and ocular adnexa. It is bounded anteriorly by the eyelids and includes seven extraocular muscles (EOMs), nerves, vasculature, lacrimal inflow and outflow systems, and orbital fat existing in a fine web of interconnecting septae [1–3]. The globe itself is approximately 16 mm anterior-to-posterior at birth [4] and, by 20 months of age, is 90% of its adult size, which averages 24 mm (longer for myopic eyes, shorter for hyperopic eyes). Interpupillary and exophthalmometry measurements increase until around 20 years of age [5]. The surrounding paranasal sinuses are rudimentary at birth but pneumatize through childhood and early adolescence and are a source of potential infection into the orbit [6]. Life-changing surgical complications, such as vision loss due to hemorrhage, ischemia, or direct damage to the nerve, dry eye, corneal abrasion, ptosis, diplopia, hypoesthesia, or paresis, may arise from injury to specific structures of orbit during surgery. It is thus critical for surgeons to be aware of the leniency with which various orbit structures can be safely manipulated during orbital and skull-based surgery in order to preserve optimal functionality.

Orbital Osteology and Vasculature

Osteology

Development

Like most of the bones of the skull base and face, the bones of the orbit are derived from neural crest cells. Early in development, the optic vesicle is surrounded by mesenchyme, which eventually becomes the bony orbit. The bones form by

L. Tiedemann
Department of Ophthalmology, University of Pittsburgh Medical Center, Pittsburgh, PA, USA

S. T. Stefko (✉)
Departments of Ophthalmology, Otolaryngology, and Neurological Surgery, University of Pittsburgh Medical Center, Pittsburgh, PA, USA

T. H. Schwartz et al. (eds.), *Endoscopic Transorbital Surgery of the Orbit, Skull Base and Brain*,
https://doi.org/10.1007/978-3-031-59504-2_3

both endochondral and intramembranous ossification [7]. The sphenoid bone contains all important neurovascular structures that enter or leave the orbit.

Facial development is intimately related to orbital development. During week 4–5 of gestation, the orbit bones start to move medially following nasal processes to their final destinations, and the nasolacrimal duct (NLD) begins to form between the lateral nasal process and maxillary prominence with development typically complete by birth [7].

Adult Dimensions

The adult orbit is pear shaped, has a volume of 30 cm^3, and is widest 1 cm posterior to the anterior orbital rim [8]. The orbital rim protects the eye from facial impacts and the superior rim is more prominent in males due to increased development of the frontal sinus [9]. The four walls of the orbit—roof, lateral wall, floor, and medial wall—converge at the orbital apex, where the optic canal (containing the optic nerve and, usually, the ophthalmic artery) and the superior orbital fissure (the anterior extension of the cavernous sinus) (SOF) lie. The medial walls run parallel to each other, with approximately 24–25 mm between them, and both medial and lateral orbital walls have an average length of 40–45 mm. The lateral orbital walls form a 90-degree angle with each other [10].

Orbital Walls

Orbital Roof

Triangular in shape, the orbital roof is composed of mainly the frontal bone, along with a smaller contribution from the lesser wing of the sphenoid bone. Superior to the roof lies the frontal sinus and, posterior to this, the anterior cranial fossa. Two fossae are contained within the orbital roof itself—those of the lacrimal gland and the trochlea of the superior oblique muscle. The orbital lobe of the lacrimal gland sits within the lacrimal fossa superotemporally. The fibrocartilaginous trochlea sits within its fossa 5 mm posterior to the superomedial orbital rim. While the trochlea may be lifted off the adjacent bone intraoperatively, it is important to do this by elevating under its periosteum with the structure itself intact [9].

Lateral Wall

The strongest and thickest of the orbital walls, the lateral wall consists of the zygomatic bone anteriorly and greater wing of the sphenoid bone posteriorly. Anteriorly, the frontozygomatic suture joins the frontal and zygomatic bones. The SOF separates the roof from the lateral orbital wall posteriorly, dividing the lesser and greater wings of the sphenoid bone. The inferior orbital fissure (IOF) separates the lateral wall from the orbital floor. The lateral wall anteriorly extends to the equator of the globe, allowing for peripheral vision while still protecting the posterior half of the globe [11]. The zygomaticosphenoid suture is the thinnest area of the lateral wall and ideal for bone removal during lateral orbitotomy. The temporalis muscle, which lies posterior and lateral to the lateral orbital rim, can be retracted superiorly during a lateral orbitotomy to gain better access to the wall without muscle injury [12].

Located 11 mm inferior to the frontozygomatic suture, the lateral orbital tubercle of Whitnall is the site of attachment for many important suspensory sutures—the lateral rectus check ligaments, Lockwood's ligament (suspensory ligament of the globe), the lateral horn of the levator aponeurosis, lateral canthal tendon, and the orbital septum [13]. Whitnall ligament itself inserts several millimeters superior to the tubercle on the lateral wall and has attachments to the lacrimal gland [14, 15].

Orbital Floor

As part of the other triangular orbital wall, the maxillary bone makes up most of the orbital floor with the palatine bone contributing posteriorly and zygomatic bone anterolaterally. The orbital floor is the roof of the maxillary sinus. The borders of the orbital floor are marked by the IOF laterally and anterior and posterior extensions of the maxilloethmoidal suture medially, running to the posterior edge of the maxillary sinus (approximately 35–40 mm posterior to the orbital rim at the pterygopalatine fossa) [9]. Thus, the floor is the shortest of the four walls [12] and does not reach the orbital apex. During orbital floor fracture repair, care should be taken to avoid dissection posteriorly into the pterygopalatine fossa, which can result in hemorrhage from the internal maxillary artery. The IOF begins approximately 1 cm posterior to the inferior orbital rim [15]. The maxillary bone is thinnest posteromedially, accounting for its dubious distinction as the primary location for orbital floor blowout fractures.

Medial Wall

The ethmoid bone, lacrimal bone, frontal process of the maxillary bone, and lesser wing of the sphenoid bone comprise the medial wall of the orbit, with the majority made up by the lamina papyracea. The wall runs from the anterior lacrimal crest (part of the ascending process of the maxilla) to the optic canal. The posterior lacrimal crest resides in the lacrimal bone, the only orbital bone contained entirely within the orbit and the more structurally and functionally important attachment site of the medial canthal tendon. The lacrimal sac fossa is located between these two crests and varies in size in individuals (women generally have narrower fossae) [12, 16, 17] (Fig. 3.1) [10]. In Asian patients, the lacrimal sac

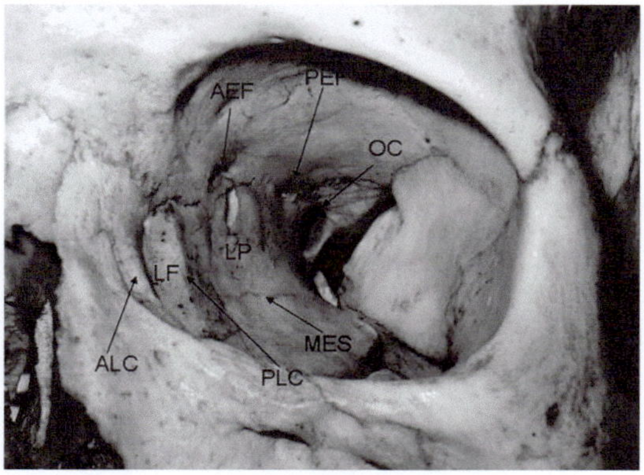

Fig. 3.1 Anatomy of left medial orbital wall, anterior view. Key: *ALC* anterior lacrimal crest, *LF* lacrimal fossa, *PLC* posterior lacrimal crest, *LP* lamina papyracea, *AEF* anterior ethmoidal foramen, *PEF* posterior ethmoidal foramen, *OC* optic canal, *MES* maxilloethmoidal suture (René C. Update on orbital anatomy. Eye (Lond). 2006 Oct;20(10):1119–29. doi: 10.1038/sj.eye.6702376. PubMed PMID: 17019410)

fossa is more frequently predominantly comprised of maxillary bone and is therefore thicker and more difficulty to penetrate during a dacryocystorhinostomy [18, 19]. The bony nasolacrimal canal originates at the lacrimal sac fossa and conveys the NLD from the lacrimal sac via the medial maxillary strut to the inferior meatus of the nose as it runs inferolaterally and slightly posteriorly from its origin [9, 12].

The ethmoid bone is bordered superiorly by the frontoethmoidal suture—a line that also marks the level of the cribriform plate, floor of the anterior cranial fossa, and exit of the ethmoidal arteries [20]—and inferiorly by the maxilloethmoidal suture. Of the bones of the orbit, the ethmoid is the thinnest, specifically in a region called the lamina papyracea, which lies immediately posterior to the thick posterior lacrimal crest. Medial to the lamina papyracea are ethmoidal air cells [12]. In acute bacterial sinusitis, a subperiosteal abscess and/or orbital cellulitis may develop as bacteria migrate from the ethmoid sinus into the orbit via the lamina papyracea or ethmoidal artery foramina.

The lesser wing of the sphenoid comprises the medial aspect of the optic canal. The lateral aspect is formed by the anterior clinoid, which extends from the lesser wing of the sphenoid. The optic strut connects the anterior clinoid and lesser wing to the body of the sphenoid bone, dividing the optic canal from the SOF. It forms the roof of the optic canal as well as part of the floor of the cavernous sinus [9].

Orbital Foramina

Roof

The roof contains the supraorbital notch or foramen, which can be found along the medial third of the superior orbital rim (22–31 mm from midline depending on ethnic variability) [21]. The supraorbital notch transmits the supraorbital neurovascular bundle, which includes the supraorbital nerve (a branch of the frontal nerve, part of V_1) as well as the supraorbital artery and vein. When the neurovascular bundle is injured during surgery, the result is temporary numbness of the forehead and brow.

At the apex of the orbit, between the roof and lateral wall, lies the SOF (Fig. 3.2a) [10]. Located in the sphenoid bone, the SOF separates the orbital apex from the middle cranial fossa. The aperture is further divided by the annulus of Zinn, the common site of origin of the four rectus muscles. Structures traversing the SOF outside of the annulus include the lacrimal nerve and frontal nerve (V_1), the trochlear nerve (IV), the superior ophthalmic vein, and dural veins (Fig. 3.2b) [10]. The orbitomeningeal artery generally travels in its own foramen lateral to this. This region is lined by dura that is continuous with that of the middle cranial fossa and periorbita. Structures lying inside the annulus are located centrally within the SOF and are directed into the intraconal space of the orbit. The superior and inferior division of the oculomotor nerve (III), the nasociliary nerve (branch of V_1), and the abducens nerve (VI) pass through this area. The last and most inferior aspect of the SOF is outside of the annulus and continuous with the IOF inferiorly. The IOF connects the orbital apex with the sphenopalatine fossa and transmits the inferior ophthalmic veins to the cavernous sinus [9], as well as connecting the orbit to the temporal and infratemporal fossae.

Disruption of any of these nerves can result in superior orbital fissure syndrome, orbital apex syndrome, or cavernous sinus syndrome, depending on the area of injury. Superior orbital fissure syndrome is classified by multiple cranial nerve (CN) palsies of CNs III through VI in the absence of optic nerve involvement. In contrast to SOF syndrome which excludes involvement of the optic nerve, orbital apex syndrome is characterized by multiple CN palsies including both the optic nerve of the optic canal and the CNs that transverse the SOF. Symptoms typically include vision loss, proptosis, chemosis, ophthalmoplegia, and V_1 sensory loss. In patients with cavernous sinus syndrome, symptoms may include those of orbital apex syndrome in addition to Horner's syndrome or those related to V_2 involvement [9].

Lateral Wall

Located superiorly along the zygomatic bone is the zygomaticotemporal foramen, containing the zygomaticotemporal canal. This canal transmits

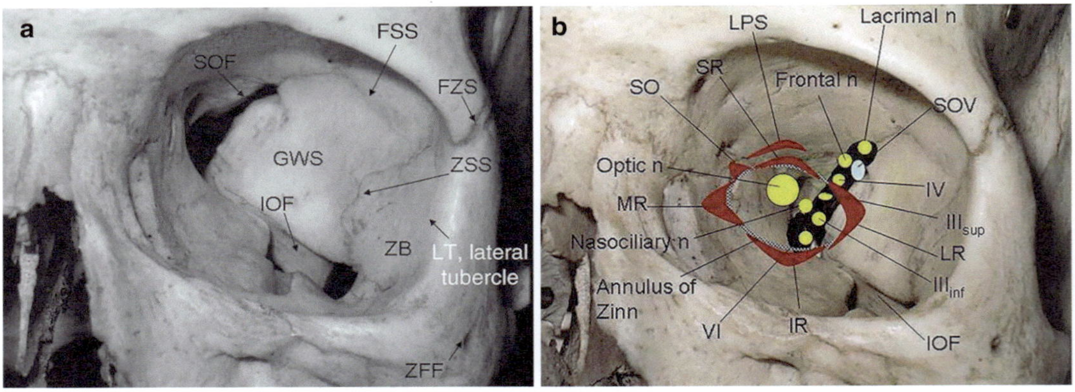

Fig. 3.2 (**a**) Anatomy of the left lateral wall, anterior view. (**b**) Anatomy of the left orbital apex, highlighting the superior orbital fissure, its contents, and the surrounding extraocular muscles. Key: *GWS* greater wing of sphenoid, *SOF* superior orbital fissure, *FZS* frontozygomatic suture, *FSS* frontosphenoidal suture, *ZSS* zygomaticosphenoid suture, *ZB* zygomatic bone, *ZFF* zygomaticofacial foramen, *LT* lateral tubercle, *LPS* levator palpebrae superioris, *SR* superior rectus, *LR* lateral rectus, *IR* inferior rectus, *MR* medial rectus, *SO* superior oblique, *SOV* superior ophthalmic vein, III_{sup} superior division of the oculomotor nerve, III_{inf} inferior division of the oculomotor nerve, *IOF* inferior orbital fissure (René C. Update on orbital anatomy. Eye (Lond). 2006 Oct;20(10):1119–29. doi: 10.1038/sj.eye.6702376. PubMed PMID: 17019410)

zygomaticotemporal vessels and nerve (branch of the zygomatic nerve, part of V_2) to the temporal fossa, supplying sensation to the forehead and temple. The zygomatic nerve enters the orbit through the IOF and runs obliquely along the lateral wall of the orbit [22]. It then supplies a branch to the lacrimal nerve prior to passing through the zygomaticotemporal foramen and the temporal fascia to innervate the skin of the temple. The zygomaticofacial foramen, located more inferiorly along the zygomatic bone, transmits the zygomaticofacial nerve and vessels to the lateral cheek[23] (Fig. 3.3) [10].

Floor

At the apex of the orbit, the IOF lies between the orbital floor and the lateral orbital wall. This juncture is located 24 mm posterior to the orbital rim and joins with the SOF at the apex below the optic canal. Branches of the inferior ophthalmic vein, maxillary branch of the trigeminal nerve, infraorbital artery, and some postganglionic parasympathetic branches from the pterygopalatine ganglion all enter the orbit via the IOF [9, 12]. V_2 exits the skull via the foramen rotundum, gives off its zygomatic branch, and then continues anteriorly as the infraorbital nerve. At a point along the floor of the orbit, this nerve becomes enclosed in its canal, which includes the infraorbital artery, and courses forward to exit on the anterior surface of the maxillary bone at the infraorbital foramen, 1 cm below the inferior orbital rim [12] (Fig. 3.3) [10]. If the infraorbital nerve is damaged during surgery, temporary numbness of the lower eyelid, cheek, upper lip, upper teeth, and gingiva can be expected.

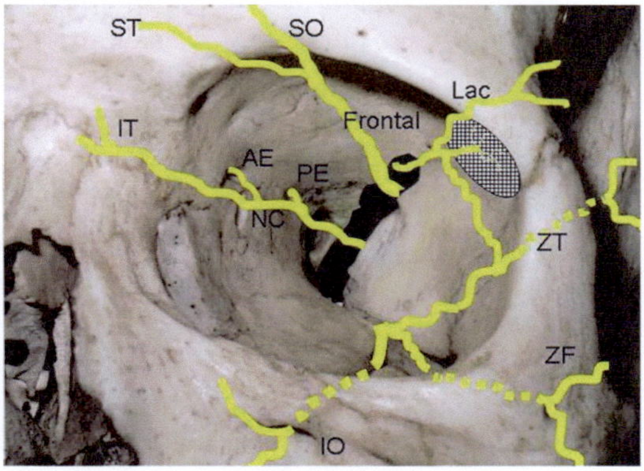

Fig. 3.3 Sensory nerves of the left orbit (excluding the long posterior ciliary nerves and ciliary ganglion sensory fibers). The hatched structure is the lacrimal gland. Key: *ST* – supratrochlear nerve, *SO* supraorbital nerve, *Lac* lacrimal nerve, *ZT* zygomaticotemporal nerve, *ZF* zygomaticofacial nerve, *IO* infraorbital nerve, *NC* nasociliary nerve, *AE* anterior ethmoidal nerve, *PE* posterior ethmoidal nerve, *IT* infratrochlear nerve (René C. Update on orbital anatomy. Eye (Lond). 2006 Oct;20(10):1119–29. doi: 10.1038/sj.eye.6702376. PubMed PMID: 17019410).

Medial Wall

Branches of the ophthalmic artery, the anterior and posterior (and occasional middle) ethmoidal arteries, are transmitted from the orbit via the anterior and posterior ethmoidal foramina. These can be a source of significant bleeding during surgery, which, if unchecked, can cause compartment syndrome. They can be safely cauterized with bipolar cautery during surgery or bone wax may be applied. The arteries also pose a potential route of entry of bacteria, fungi, and neoplasms into the orbit from the sinuses. The location of the arteries is at the level of the frontoethmoidal suture, 24 mm and 36 mm posterior to the anterior lacrimal crest, respectively. When performing orbital surgery or dacryocystorhinostomy, care must be taken to stay below the frontoethmoidal suture in order to avoid inadvertent fracture of the cribriform plate with possible dural tear and leakage of cerebral spinal fluid (CSF) [12, 24, 25].

The optic canal is located in the lesser wing of the sphenoid and connects the orbit to the middle cranial fossa. It transmits the optic nerve, ophthalmic artery, meningeal sheaths, and sympathetic nerve fibers. The canal is approximately 8–10 mm in length, with optic strut separating it from the SOF laterally. The normal diameter of an adult optic canal is 6.5 mm [12], but it may abnormally enlarge in cases of optic nerve gliomas or narrow in the setting of fibrous dysplasia. Dura along the canal is densely adherent to the bone and there is little clearance between the optic nerve and canal.

The entrance to the nasolacrimal canal can be found inferomedially along the medial wall of the orbit.

Orbital Vasculature

Arteries

The major, larger caliber vessels are located centrally at the orbital apex (Fig. 3.4) [10]. The blood supply to the orbit is primarily from the ophthalmic artery, the first intracranial branch of the internal carotid artery, in 96% of patients. However, the middle meningeal artery contributes equally in 3% of individuals and is the only arterial supply to the orbit in 1% of individuals [26]. The ophthalmic artery runs through the dura mater inferior to the intracranial segment of the optic nerve and then within the optic canal to enter the orbit [27, 28]. Branches of the ophthalmic artery supply the EOMs, optic nerve and retina as the central retinal artery, anterior segment as the long posterior ciliary arteries, and the choroid as the short posterior ciliary arteries. The central retinal artery branches from the ophthalmic artery about 1 cm posterior to the globe [29] and then curls into the optic nerve sheath to supply the inner half of the retina. This is a critical watershed zone; damage to the artery in this area will cause immediate and severe, permanent vision loss.

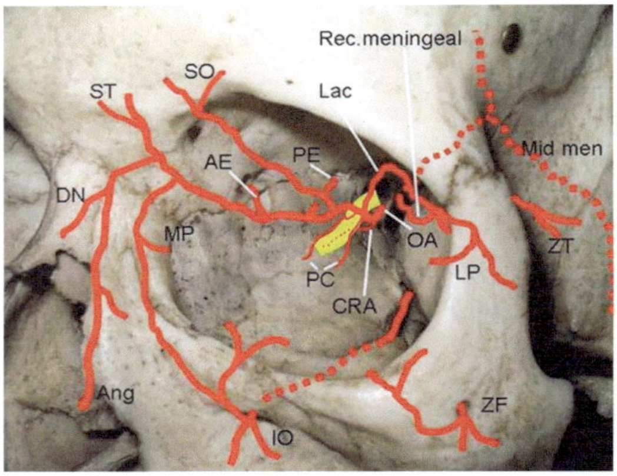

Fig. 3.4 Arteries of the left orbit (excluding the muscular branches, short posterior ciliary, long posterior ciliary, and anterior ciliary arteries). Key: *OA* ophthalmic artery, *CRA* central retinal artery, *PC* posterior ciliary artery, *Lac* lacrimal artery, *LP* lateral palpebral artery, *IO* infraorbital artery, *ZT* zygomaticotemporal artery, *ZF* zygomaticofacial artery, *Mid Men* middle meningeal artery, *Rec Men* recurrent meningeal artery, *Ang* angular artery, *MP* medial palpebral artery, *DN* dorsal nasal artery, *ST* supratrochlear artery, *SO* supraorbital artery, *AE* anterior ethmoidal artery, *PE* posterior ethmoidal artery (René C. Update on orbital anatomy. Eye (Lond). 2006 Oct;20(10):1119–29. doi: 10.1038/sj.eye.6702376. PubMed PMID: 17019410)

There are a rich series of anastomoses in the orbit between the internal and external carotid systems. The four most significant are (1) the anterior deep temporal artery and lacrimal artery through the zygomaticotemporal branch, (2) superficial temporal artery and the supraorbital branch of the frontal artery, (3) infraorbital artery and ophthalmic inferior muscular artery, and (4) angular artery and the dorsal nasal terminal branch of the ophthalmic artery [12]. The internal maxillary artery and facial arteries (branches of the external carotid artery) are smaller contributors to the blood supply of the orbit. Manipulation of the carotid and intracranial ophthalmic arteries should be avoided during surgery to prevent the possibility of vasospasm or significant hemorrhage causing ischemia or stroke.

The supraorbital artery, a branch of the ophthalmic artery, enters the orbit through the supraorbital notch and contributes small muscular branches to the levator, superior rectus, superior oblique, eyebrow, and forehead. The nasofrontal artery becomes the supratrochlear and palpebral arteries. After the external carotid bifurcates into the superficial temporal artery and the internal maxillary artery, the infraorbital artery, the terminal branch of the maxillary artery, passes through the infraorbital fissure to ultimately give muscular branches to the inferior rectus, inferior oblique, and lacrimal gland. The middle meningeal artery is also a branch of the external carotid artery and passes through the SOF to join with the lacrimal artery [9, 12].

Veins

Apart from the lacrimal vein, ethmoidal veins, and superior ophthalmic vein, the veins of the orbit do not follow their respective arteries and have a close relationship with the surrounding fascia [30]. Veins course through fascial planes and are supported by them [9]. This prevents excessive stretching and motility of veins to minimize their risk of collapse. Unfortunately, this same intimate connection to the surrounding fascia makes veins susceptible to changes in flow in instances of orbital fibrosis in Graves disease and venous congestion in orbital tumors [31].

The major sources of outflow from the globe are central retinal vein and retinal vortex veins (typically four to ten total, with at least one exiting from each quadrant of the eye between the rectus muscles) [32, 33]. These veins drain into the main orbital veins—the superior and inferior ophthalmic veins—which then drain into the cavernous sinus. In contrast to the arterial system, these larger orbital veins are found peripherally in the posterior third of the orbit, with only small caliber veins located centrally in the intraconal space [34–36]. In cases of venous arterialization due to carotid-cavernous fistula (CCF), this classically manifests as a dilated superior ophthalmic vein and to a lesser degree its tributaries and inferior ophthalmic vein. The superior and inferior ophthalmic veins can be safely gently retracted or manipulated, if necessary, at the time of orbital surgery or interventional radiology procedure for CCF obliteration. A minority of venous drainage in the orbit travels to the pterygoid venous plexus through the inferior orbital fissure [9].

The superior ophthalmic vein itself runs from medial (starting medial and slightly inferior to the trochlea) to lateral in the orbit (passing between the superior rectus and optic nerve). Most of the venous drainage from the orbit passes through the SOF by way of the superior ophthalmic vein to the cavernous sinus. The many tributaries of the superior ophthalmic vein include the supraorbital and supratrochlear veins that drain the scalp, forehead, eyebrow, and upper eyelid; the medial and inferior ophthalmic veins; the superior vortex veins; the anterior ethmoidal vein; and a vein from the superior rectus [9]. Present in 30–40% of individuals, the medial ophthalmic vein arises from branches of the superior ophthalmic and angular veins [37, 38]. It travels extraconal along the superomedial orbital wall, receiving drainage from the superior and medial rectus muscles. At the SOF, the medial ophthalmic vein rejoins the superior ophthalmic vein. Posterior in the orbit, the superior ophthalmic vein is also joined by the inferior ophthalmic vein, lacrimal vein, and central retinal vein [9]. The lacrimal vein leaves the lacrimal gland and runs along the lateral rectus on its way to the superior ophthalmic vein, while the central retinal vein exits centrally within the optic nerve and branches into smaller vessels in the optic nerve sheath before piercing dura. Once leaving the subdural space, the central retinal vein drains into the superior ophthalmic vein at the orbital apex.

The inferior ophthalmic vein originates as a venous plexus between the globe and inferior rectus. It runs along the lateral border of the inferior rectus and receives tributaries from the inferior vortex veins as well as the inferior, medial, and lateral recti, and the inferior oblique muscle [9, 12]. Extraconal veins collect venous drainage from the lower eyelid and lacrimal sac prior to joining with the inferior ophthalmic vein near the inferior rectus. This dilates inferior to the annulus of Zinn and then passes into the cavernous sinus. Smaller branches of the inferior ophthalmic vein pass through the inferior orbital fissure and join the pterygoid venous plexus. A small middle ophthalmic vein may originate as muscular branch from the medial rectus, running laterally in the extraconal space and draining either into the inferior ophthalmic vein or directly into the cavernous sinus [9].

The Eye, Eyelids, and Adnexa

The Eye

The globe occupies 20–25% of the orbit. Its volume is 6.5–7.0 cm^3 with an average length of 24 mm [8, 39, 40]. The anterior sclera and interior of the eyelids are lined by conjunctiva, mucous membrane that is important in maintaining a proper tear film via mucin-producing goblet cells. The bulbar conjunctiva covers the globe itself (ending at the corneal limbus or junction of clear cornea and opaque, white sclera). The conjunctiva then reflects at the superior and inferior fornices to line the posterior surfaces of both lids, providing a gliding surface.

Eyelids

Figure 3.5 shows the relationship between the eyelids and anterior globe structures [41]. The caruncle is a conical mucosal protuberance that contains sebaceous and sudoriferous glands and is situated at the medial commissure medial to the punctum. The plica semilunaris is a crescent-shaped structure that sits immediately lateral to the caruncle, a remnant of the nictitating membrane or third eyelid [9]. This small pocket of mucosal redundancy allows for free horizontal eye movements. Significant scarring in this area can cause restrictive strabismus with associated double vision. A transcaruncular incision for assess to the medial wall of the orbit is performed by making an incision between the caruncle and the plica and may heal well without sutures.

The palpebral fissure is the area of globe visible when the lids are open. The average horizontal width at the mid-pupil is 27–30 mm [42]. The medial canthus and lateral canthus are the nasal and temporal corners of the eyelids. The canthi are fixed to periosteum inside the orbital rim by their respective canthal tendons, with the lateral canthal angle 1–2 mm superior to the medial [43]. They serve to stabilize the eyelids and are contiguous with the tarsus of the upper and lower eyelids, which provide structure to the eyelids themselves.

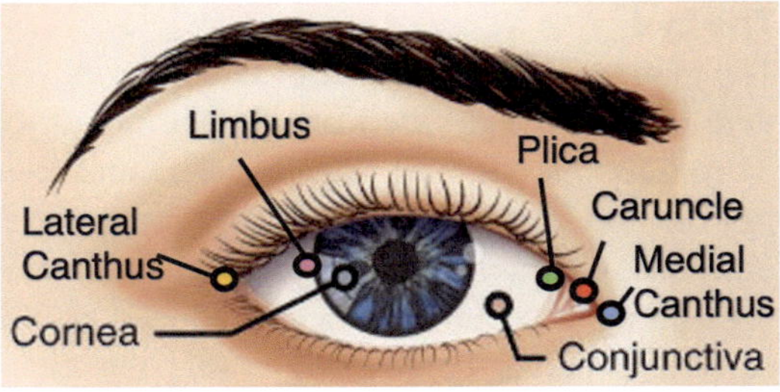

Fig. 3.5 Gross ocular surface anatomy of the right eye (Modified from Seo J, Byun WY, Alisafaei F, Georgescu A, Yi YS, Massaro-Giordano M, Shenoy VB, Lee V, Bunya VY, Huh D. Multiscale reverse engineering of the human ocular surface. Nat Med. 2019 Aug;25(8):1310–1318. doi: 10.1038/s41591-019-0531-2. PubMed PMID: 31384041; Central PMCID: PMC6950645)

A typical upper eyelid should rest 1 mm below the superior limbus [44]. The levator palpebrae superioris (LPS) and Muller muscle are responsible for raising the upper eyelid, while the eyelid retractors and capsulopalpebral fascia maintain retraction of the lower eyelid. Normal LPS function is approximately 15 mm [45], and the muscle is innervated by CNIII. In contrast, Muller muscle, a smooth muscle originating from the undersurface of the LPS at the level of the horizontal suspensory Whitnall ligament [46], raises the upper eyelid 2 mm and is innervated by the sympathetic nervous system [47].

The skin makes up the most superficial layer of the eyelids. It is the thinnest in the body and unique in that there is no underlying connective tissue. The orbicularis oculi muscle closes the eyelids and is innervated by CN VII. The orbital portion is responsible for voluntary blinking, whereas the palpebral portion (pretarsal and preseptal segments) is involved in reflex blink. The pretarsal orbicularis oculi muscle is securely attached to underlying tissues, but the preseptal orbicularis is loosely attached to underlying tissues [12]. The pretarsal orbicularis arises at the medial canthal tendon with the superficial heads surrounding the canaliculi and the deep heads forming the "Horner-Duverney" muscle that attaches to the posterior lacrimal crest [9, 48, 49]. The orbital septum, a thin sheet of fibrous tissue arising from the periosteum of the inferior and superior orbital rims, lies deep to the orbicularis muscle 2–5 mm above the superior border of the tarsus in the upper eyelid and at the level of the inferior tarsus in the lower eyelid [50]. In the upper eyelid, the orbital septum fuses with the levator aponeurosis to form the crease of the eyelid, generally more superior and firmly formed in western eyelids. The orbital septum divides the orbit into preseptal and postseptal (orbital) zones. Preaponeurotic orbital fat lies deep to the orbital septum and anterior to the levator aponeurosis and capsulopalpebral fascia. Orbital fat is globular and generally exuberant in appearance; it serves as an important landmark for the LPS muscle. The septum may serve as an anatomic barrier to infection and hemorrhage; it is responsible for the very sharp demarcation of erythema and swelling at the arcus marginalis in a patient with orbital cellulitis. Orbital cellulitis (in contrast to periorbital cellulits) unsurprisingly carries much greater risk of vision loss, vascular as well as neural injury, and posterior intracranial extension by way of the venous system to the cavernous sinus. A coronal diagram of eyelid anatomy can be found in Fig. 3.6 [51, 52].

Arterial supply to the eyelids comes from the ophthalmic artery (internal carotid system) and the angular and temporal arteries (external carotid system), via the marginal and peripheral arterial arcades of the eyelids. The marginal arterial arcade is situated 2–3 mm from the border of the tarsus margin and is most significant in caliber than the peripheral arcade. The peripheral arterial arcade of the eyelids runs between the levator aponeurosis and Muller muscle at the superior border of the tarsus. The orbital septum guides veinous drainage of the eyelids. Preseptal tissues drain medially into the angular vein and laterally into the superficial temporal vein. Postseptal structures drain into orbital veins, the anterior facial vein, and the pterygoid plexus. Submandibular nodes are responsible for medial lymphatic drainage, whereas lymphatic drainage of the lateral eyelids is carried to the preauricular lymph nodes and then to deep cervical nodes (neck levels II–IV) [9].

Extraocular Muscles

The muscles of the orbit consist of four rectus muscles (superior, inferior, medial, and lateral), two oblique muscles (superior and inferior), and the LPS muscle. The EOMs grow during childhood in conjunction with the growth of the eye and orbit [53]. Any of these muscles can be gently retracted, biopsied, recessed, or resected. However, care should be taken to not exert excessive force as the muscles can be torn from the globe and asystole with cardiac arrest may result due to the oculocardiac reflex.

The muscular branches of the ophthalmic artery provide the main blood supply to the rectus muscles. These branches give rise to the anterior

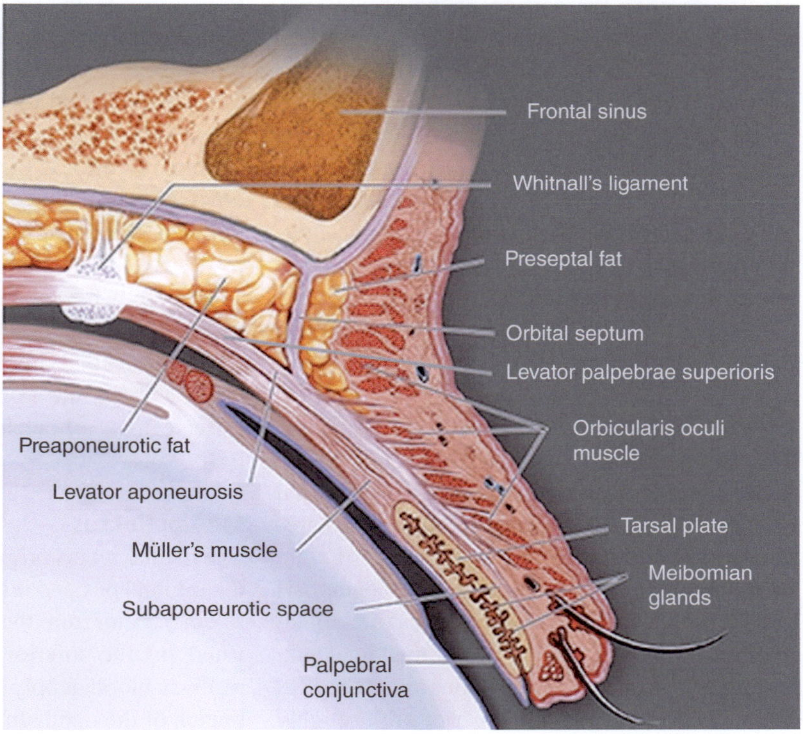

Fig. 3.6 Cross-sectional anatomy of a Western upper eyelid (Bacharach J, Lee WW, Harrison AR, Freddo TF. A review of acquired blepharoptosis: prevalence, diagnosis, and current treatment options. Eye. 2021;35:2468–2481).

ciliary arteries and, ultimately, anastomose with the long posterior ciliary arteries [12]. Each rectus muscle is supplied by 1–4 anterior ciliary arteries. These arteries terminate anteriorly by supplying the anterior segment of the globe. Blood supply and innervation to the rectus muscles and inferior oblique ramifies on the deep surface of the muscles, about 1 cm anterior to the annulus of Zinn. Injury to the EOMs, including disinsertion of more than two EOMs at a time, can result in globe anterior segment ischemia and strabismus. The sclera is thinnest (0.3 mm) immediately posterior to each muscle's insertion on the globe, and accidental penetration in this area may result in a rupture globe and extrusion of the contents of the eye.

Annulus of Zinn

The four rectus muscles originate at the orbital apex at the annulus of Zinn or common tendon. The annulus is a ring of fibrous connective tissue that is centered about the optic canal and central SOF [9]. The "oculomotor foramen" is the term used to describe the portion of the orbital apex that is enclosed by the annulus of Zinn as it transmits both divisions of CN III, the ophthalmic division of CN V, and CN VI. In contrast, CN IV travels through the SOF outside of the annulus, along with the frontal and lacrimal nerves (branches of the ophthalmic division of CN V) [12]. Consequently, after administration of a retrobulbar block (local anesthetic injected into the intraconal space posterior to the globe), akinesia is expected although the superior oblique muscle may remain unaffected.

Levator Palpebrae Superioris

The LPS originates on the periosteum of the lesser wing of the sphenoid in the superomedial orbital apex [9]. The muscle runs from posteromedial to anterior for approximately 40 mm before broadening into its aponeurosis (14–20 mm in length), which attaches to the anterior face of the tarsus [54, 55]. Whitnall ligament, a transverse suspensory ligament around the LPS muscle and running in the superior orbit roughly medial to lateral, aids in translation of the muscle's vector force [56, 57] (Fig. 3.6) [51]. This ligament attaches medially to the connective tissue around the trochlea and laterally passes through the lacrimal gland to attach to the lateral orbital wall slightly above the lateral orbital tubercle [14]. The lateral horn of the levator aponeurosis inserts onto the lateral orbital tubercle and the medial horn inserts onto the posterior lacrimal crest. The medial horn has loose attachments to the posterior limb of the medial canthal tendon [9]. With age and especially with repeated trauma, the levator aponeurosis atrophies and elongates, leading to involutional ptosis. The superior division of CNIII innervates the LPS muscles [12] and is the only EOM to share a common central nucleus [58], producing Hering's phenomenon (elevation/depression of one upper lid decreases/increases the central drive with resultant inverse effect on the opposite upper eyelid height) [59]. The LPS receives blood supply from the lateral muscular branch of the ophthalmic artery [60].

Superior and Inferior Recti

Both superior and inferior rectus muscles originate from the annulus of Zinn, run anterolaterally for approximately 42 and 40 cm, respectively, at a 23-degree angle to the visual axis in primary gaze, and insert onto the sclera 7.7 mm and 6.5 mm posterior to the limbus, respectively [61]. They are both innervated by the third nerve, through the superior and inferior divisions, respectively. The superior rectus receives blood supply from the lateral muscular branch of the ophthalmic artery, while the inferior rectus receives its blood supply from the medial muscular branch of the ophthalmic artery and, to a lesser extent, a branch of the infraorbital artery [60].

Medial Rectus

The medial rectus origin is the annulus of Zinn at the orbital apex and inserts onto the anteromedial sclera 5.5 mm from the medial limbus. It is innervated by the inferior division of CN III and receives blood supply from the medial muscular branch of the ophthalmic artery [61].

Lateral Rectus

The lateral rectus origin is the annulus of Zinn at the orbital apex and inserts onto anterolateral sclera 6.9 mm from the lateral limbus. It is innervated by CN VI and receives blood supply from the lateral muscular branch of the ophthalmic artery and, to a lesser extent, the lacrimal artery [60, 61].

Superior Oblique

The superior oblique originates on the periorbita of the lesser wing of the sphenoid bone medial to the LPS muscle origin (superomedial wall of the orbit) and runs anteriorly outside the EOM cone [62]. After passing through the cartilaginous trochlea at the superomedial orbital rim, the superior oblique changes direction to travel posterolateral. It inserts on the globe inferior to the superior rectus muscle [12]. The muscle forms a 51-degree angle with the visual axis in primary position [63]. The superior oblique is innervated by CN IV, which crosses the superior surface of the LPS muscle. Thus, the superior oblique is the only EOM to have its innervation insert on its superior surface (on the posterior third of the muscle) [9, 12].

Inferior Oblique

The inferior oblique originates on the floor of the orbit immediately lateral to the nasolacrimal groove. The inferior oblique travels inferior to the inferior rectus muscle along its course. The inferior oblique muscle inserts on the posterior inferolateral surface of the globe inferolateral to the macula and immediately inferior to the insertion of the superior oblique muscle. The inferior oblique's insertion on the globe is deep to the lateral rectus muscle and marks the area of the macula responsible for our finest visual discrimination [12]. The muscle forms a 51-degree angle with the visual axis in primary position [64]. The innervation to the inferior oblique comes from the inferior division of CN III, with the nerve traveling on the lateral aspect of the inferior rectus prior to inserting on the underside of the inferior oblique on the posterior third of the muscle [9, 12]. Its blood supply comes from branches off the infraorbital artery [60].

Orbital Fat and Fascia

Orbital Fat

Orbital fat lies posterior to the orbital septum. A membrane known as the intermuscular septum connects the rectus muscles and forms a ring that divides the orbital fat into intraconal fat and extraconal fat [65, 66]. Orbital fat serves to cushion and stabilize the globe as well support the optic nerve and EOMs [12]. Injury to the intermuscular septum, fat, periorbita, or the fibrous septae that further lend support to the orbital structures can result in globe displacement and/or restricted movement.

Preaponeurotic orbital fat is located anterior to the levator aponeurosis in the upper eyelid and the capsulopalpebral fascia in the lower eyelid. Three fat pads are present in each compartment [63]. Though in the upper eyelid the lateral fat pad may be quite small, it is vital not to confuse this with the lacrimal gland. Diaphanous capsules surround each fat pad. These fat pads extend posteriorly as extraconal fat and can be gently elevated and excised during eyelid surgery. Care must be taken to avoid anterior traction on the orbital fat during attempted excision, as doing so may cause retrobulbar hematoma. Of note, the inferior oblique muscle separates the medial and central fat pads of the lower eyelid as it runs from its origin on the medial orbital floor to its insertion on the posterior inferolateral globe [67]. Injury or transection of the inferior oblique should be also avoided during fat excision or inferior forniceal dissection, due to its potential to cause torsional diplopia or substantial retrobulbar hemorrhage.

Orbital Fascia

Periorbita

Periorbita, also called orbital fascia, is the periosteal lining of the bones of the orbit. This dense connective tissue, which originates from the outer endosteal layer of the dura mater and is continuous with it, is also continuous with the orbital septum, the lining of the nasolacrimal canal and that of the lacrimal gland [68]. At the orbital rim, the periosteal lining of the septum and facial bones fuse together—a location termed the "arcus marginalis." The periorbita is loosely attached to the underlying bone except at the orbital rim (arcus marginalis), fissures, foramina, canals, suture lines, and lateral and medial orbital tubercles, where it is firmly attached. The periorbita is vascularized and receives sensory input from the ophthalmic and maxillary divisions of the trigeminal nerve. Vessels and nerves pierce the periorbita on their way into the orbit [12]. At the apex, the periorbita of the optic canal is continuous with the dural sheath covering the intraorbital optic nerve (the optic nerve sheath) and with the intracranial dura mater. Intracranial dura is likewise continuous with the periorbita at the SOF and ethmoidal foramina [68].

Given the loose attachments of the periorbita to the underlying bone, a potential enclosed space may be formed between the two structures where in subperiosteal pus or blood may accumulate. The periosteum can be safely opened and elevated from the bone during orbital surgery to evacuate such fluid.

Tenon's Capsule

This elastic, fibrovascular membrane is the primary intraorbital fascia. It envelops the globe and attaches anteriorly to the intermuscular septum 2–3 mm from the limbus and posteriorly to the optic nerve sheath where it is thinnest. The Tenon's capsule lies under the conjunctiva anteriorly and surrounds the EOMs, separating them from orbital fat and other structures. It is adherent to the episclera more firmly anterior to the recti insertions and more loosely attached posteriorly. These loose posterior attachments allow for sufficient movement of the optic nerve, nerves, and veins while also suspending the globe through connections to periorbital tissues [9, 12].

Extraocular Muscle Capsule and Pulley System

Around each EOM lies a muscle sheath that runs the length of the muscle from origin to insertion [69]. These thicken as they run anteriorly passing through the Tenon's capsule [70]. The capsules themselves are avascular and provide a gliding plane over the surface of the globe. The sheaths of the inferior rectus and inferior oblique are fused [9, 71]. The check ligaments around the rectus muscles are extension of their muscular sheaths and limit EOM movement. For instance, the check ligament of the medial rectus attaches to the medial orbital tubercle of the lacrimal bone to limit adduction. A check ligament also connects the superior rectus with the levator aponeurosis to ensure coordinated elevation of the upper eyelid in upgaze [72]. The fused sheaths of the inferior rectus and inferior oblique expand to become the inferior check ligament, also known as Lockwood's ligament or the suspensory ligament of the globe. It supports globe position, prevents displacement of the globe, and inserts onto the lateral orbital tubercle [12, 73]. The neurofibrovascular bundle attached to the ligament contains the inferior oblique motor nerve [74].

Lymphatic Drainage

Although orbital lymphatics are not easily perceptible in gross dissection, the only tissues that lack lymphatics are the retina, cornea, and epidermis of the eyelids [9]. Lymphatic capillaries contain a single layer of overlapping endothelial cells with discontinuous junctions and no basement membranes or pericytes [9, 75, 76]. This increases permeability of the capillaries, allowing them to absorb a large collection of fluid, plasma, antigens, white blood cells, and red blood cell products, draining them into larger lymphatic trunks prior to junction with the blood circulation [9].

The superficial system of lymphatics of the eyelid drains the anterior lamella, while the deep system drains the posterior lamella. The lateral two-thirds of the upper eyelid, one-third of the lower eyelid, and half the conjunctiva drain into the preauricular nodes. The more medial eyelids and conjunctiva drain into the submandibular nodes. The orbit itself had long been thought to be devoid of lymphatics [77, 78], but, in fact, each orbit drains into bilateral deep cervical lymph nodes (neck levels II–IV), continuing into ipsilateral superficial cervical and mandibular lymph nodes [9].

Of note, the orbitomalar retaining ligament (also known as the inferior arcus marginalis) along the inferior rim of the orbit separates orbital lymphatics from that of the cheek. It is the major suspensory ligament of the infraorbital tissues, and it checks orbital edema/ecchymosis at the orbital rim.

Cranial Nerves and the Autonomic Nervous System

The two critical orbital foramina are the optic canal and SOF, both of which reside in the orbital apex. CNs II–VI traverse these, along with the first intracranial branch of the internal carotid artery (the ophthalmic artery) and the anterior extension of the cavernous sinus.

Cranial Nerves

CN II, the optic nerve, is divided into four segments, specifically intraocular (1 mm), intraorbital (25–30 mm), intracanalicular (5–9 mm), and intracranial (10–16 mm) [9]. There is redundancy in the orbital optic nerve [9], allowing for eye movements without traction from the globe and 1 cm of potential proptosis without optic nerve injury.

Four millimeters in diameter [79], the optic nerve axons are surrounded by CSF and invested by meninges, which are continuous with the pia, arachnoid, and dura mater of the brain. The dural sheath is also termed the "optic nerve sheath." At the apex, this dural lining of the posterior intraorbital optic nerve fuses with the annulus at Zinn anteriorly and the periorbita (periosteum) of the optic canal posteriorly [9]. In the orbit, the sheath protects the nerve, and is tough enough to be grasped by forceps without sequelae, especially in cases where the subarachnoid space is expanded (i.e., during an optic nerve sheath fenestration for papiledema). It is opened during optic nerve sheath fenestration to release CSF and relieve papilledema due to increased intracranial pressure. The axons are also surrounded by myelin produced by oligodendrocytes [9]. The optic nerve leaves/enters the orbit via the optic canal, located superonasally at the apex lateral to the lesser wing of the sphenoid bone.

CNs III, IV, and VI enter the orbit through the SOF and travel anteriorly through the intraconal fat to ramify into the bellies of their respective EOMs. In the cavernous sinus, or as anteriorly as the SOF, CN III divides into superior and inferior divisions. The inferior trunk of CN III is a surgical landmark in the ORBIT classification [80]. The superior division of CN III innervates only those muscles with "superior" in their titles: levator palpebrae superioris and superior rectus. The branch to the LPS travels through the belly of the superior rectus.

The course of the ophthalmic division of CN V starts at the trigeminal ganglion and travels along the lateral wall of the cavernous sinus, prior to dividing into the frontal, lacrimal, and nasociliary branches. As stated above, all enter the orbit through the SOF with the frontal and lacrimal nerves outside of the annulus of Zinn and the nasociliary nerve inside it. The frontal and lacrimal nerves travel through the extraconal fat and branch further to innervate the medial canthus as the supratrochlear nerve, upper eyelid as the lacrimal and supratrochlear nerves, and forehead as the supratrochlear and supraorbital nerves. The nasociliary nerve travels through the intraconal fat and becomes the sensory root of the ciliary ganglion (see below) and long ciliary nerves [9]. The sensory root travels through the ciliary ganglion without synapsing, exiting it as the short ciliary nerves and then piercing the sclera. In contrast, the long ciliary nerves pierce the sclera without passing through the ciliary ganglion. Both short and long ciliary nerves travel anteriorly to give sensory innervation to the iris, cornea, and ciliary muscle [81, 82]. The nasociliary nerve also continues as the anterior ethmoidal nerve, which passes through the anterior ethmoidal canal and later into the nasal cavity with terminal branches innervating the skin of the nasal ala and apex [83]. The posterior ethmoidal nerve, a branch of the nasociliary nerve that is only seen in 15% of cases [84], typically follows the middle meningeal artery and innervates the superior sagittal sinus [23], ethmoid sinuses [85], and part of the dura mater of the anterior cranial fossa [20].

Autonomic Nervous System

In the orbit, parasympathetics provide pupillary constriction, lens accommodation, and secretion from the lacrimal gland. The Edinger-Westphal nucleus in the midbrain sends parasympathetic fibers along with CN III, specifically its inferior division, to synapse in the ciliary ganglion [12]. Innervation to the iris sphincter muscle and ciliary body of the eye is then provided by the short ciliary nerves, causing accommodation and pupillary constriction. The ciliary ganglion sits between the lateral rectus and optic nerve, lateral to the ophthalmic artery, and 1 cm anterior to the annulus of Zinn/15–20 mm posterior to the globe. Parasympathetic secretory fibers to the lacrimal gland start in the pons in the lacrimal nucleus [85, 86]. After originating from the superior salivatory nucleus specifically, these fibers exit the brainstem with CN VII [87]. They pass through the auditory canal without synapsing at the geniculate ganglion to become the greater superficial petrosal nerve [88]. This nerve joins with the deep petrosal nerve (carrying sympathetic fibers) and forms the vidian nerve, which exits the vidian canal in the pterygopalatine fossa. The nerve then joins the zygomatic nerve at the sphenopalatine ganglion. Postganglionic parasympathetic branches from the sphenopalatine ganglion in the form of the zygomatic nerve enter the orbit via the IOF before running superiorly along the lateral wall of the orbit and then entering the lacrimal gland as part of the lacrimal nerve.

The role of the sympathetic system in the orbit is to provide pupillary dilation, vasoconstriction, and innervation to the accessory eyelid retractors, (Muller muscle and the lower eyelid retractors). From their hypothalamic origin, the sympathetic fibers descend along the spinal cord, synapse at the ciliospinal center of Budge-Waller, and then again in the superior cervical ganglion. Second-order neurons leave and run with the common carotid and then the internal carotid artery (as the deep petrosal nerve) through the cavernous sinus where they are adjacent to CN VI for a short distance. The deep petrosal nerve joins the greater superficial petrosal nerve to form the vidian nerve but, in contrast to parasympathetic fibers, sympathetic fibers pass through the sphenopalatine ganglion without synapsing. Sympathetic output then travels anteriorly via the SOF to enter the orbit. These fibers pass through the ciliary ganglion, again without synapsing, and follow short and long posterior ciliary nerves to their end targets of the pupil (resulting in dilation), eyelids (retraction), and orbit. Disruption of this innervation by microvascular occlusion, tumor, or surgery may result in a Horner syndrome (mild ptosis, miosis, anhidrosis).

The Lacrimal System

Secretory System

Lacrimal Gland

The main lacrimal gland is an exocrine gland (considered a minor salivary gland) and is responsible for reflex lacrimation [89]. It contributes to the aqueous component of the tear film and sits in the lacrimal gland fossa of the frontal bone, located superotemporally in the orbit [9]. The lacrimal gland is divided by the lateral horn of the levator aponeurosis into the smaller palpebral lobe inferiorly and the larger orbital lobe superiorly [12]. While both lobes contain secretory ducts, the orbital lobe ducts pass through those of the palpebral lobe before emptying into the upper conjunctival fornix. These ducts, along with those of the accessory lacrimal glands of Krause and Wolfring, produce and secrete the aqueous component of the tear film [12]. The palpebral lobe is visible upon eversion of the upper eyelid, while the orbital lobe is not. Biopsy of part of the palpebral lobe, which can sometimes be mistaken for orbital fat, should be avoided as it can interfere with lacrimal secretion and result in severe dry eye. Thus, the orbital lobe is biopsied when required and always via an external eyelid incision.

The lacrimal artery, a branch of the ophthalmic artery, enters the posterior surface of the lacrimal gland and provides its main blood supply. The recurrent meningeal artery, along with a branch of the infraorbital artery, also contributes. The lacrimal vein drains the gland and empties into the superior ophthalmic vein. Sensory innervation, including pain and temperature, to the lacrimal gland is supplied by the lacrimal nerve, a branch of the ophthalmic division of the trigeminal nerve. The lacrimal nerve exits from the underside of the lacrimal gland, near the entrance of the lacrimal artery, and runs underneath the superotemporal periorbita to the semilunar ganglion and eventually to the spinal nucleus of the trigeminal nerve [12]. Cautery to the underside of the lacrimal gland should be avoided to prevent damage to the lacrimal nerve and arterial supply. The parasympathetic pathway, carried by the greater superficial petrosal nerve, is responsible for the lacrimal gland's main function of reflex lacrimation. Its afferent limb is the corneal nerves (V1), stimulated by ocular surface irritation.

Accessory Lacrimal Glands

The glands of Krause and Wolfring are also exocrine glands and are responsible for basal aqueous tear production, as well as providing a small contribution to reflex tearing. An average of 20 glands of Krause are located in the superior conjunctival fornix, while approximately ten can be found in the inferior fornix. The glands of Wolfring are located at the upper border of the superior tarsus. Neither receives parasympathetic innervation, unlike the main lacrimal gland [12].

Excretory System

Each of the four eyelids contains a lacrimal punctum medially on the margin, rotated slightly posteriorly toward the ocular surface due to the posterior pull of the Horner-Duverney muscle [48]. The puncta lead to a vertical 2 mm segment of the canaliculus called ampulla. The canaliculus in each lid drains tears from each punctum into a common canaliculus at the intersection of the upper and lower eyelid canaliculi in 90% of patients. From the ampulla, the canaliculus makes a 90-degree turn, and tears subsequently flow horizontally into the common canaliculus and then the lacrimal sac, a total distance of approximately 8–10 mm. The valve of Rosenmuller, located at the medial end of the common canaliculus, separates the common canaliculus from the lacrimal sac and prevents reflux of tears. The lacrimal sac sits in the lacrimal sac fossa [12]. The medial canthal tendon wraps around the lacrimal sac with the anterior limb of the tendon anteriorly, attaching to the anterior lacrimal crest and aiding in position of the punctum. The posterior limb of the tendon passes behind the lacrimal sac, inserting on the posterior lacrimal crest [90].

The lacrimal sac transitions to the NLD, which conveys tears from the lacrimal sac to the inferior meatus of the nose. The bony nasolacrimal canal originates at the lacrimal sac fossa and conveys the NLD inferiorly. The duct measures 12–18 mm in length. While the superior part of the NLD is surrounded by the lacrimal bone, the inferior majority of the duct is surrounded by the maxillary bone as the duct runs inferolaterally and posteriorly from its origin [9, 12]. A narrower intercanthal distance or wider nose will result in a greater lateral angulation of an individual's nasolacrimal canal [12]. The valve of Hasner is located at the distal membranous end of the NLD and is imperforate in patients with congenital NLD obstruction. Of note, the lacrimal sac and NLD can be retracted anteriorly in instances of medial wall surgery without damage to either structure. Length measurements for each portion of the lacrimal excretory system can be found in Fig. 3.7 [12].

The palpebral portion of the orbicularis oculi muscle (deep heads), known as "Horner-Duverney muscle," inserts on the posterior lacrimal crest. With each blink, the muscle contracts, resulting in closure of the lacrimal puncti and medial canthi as well as pulling of the tarsus medially and eyelids against the globe. The pressure that is created forces tears into the lacrimal system, allowing of effective drainage of tears [91–93].

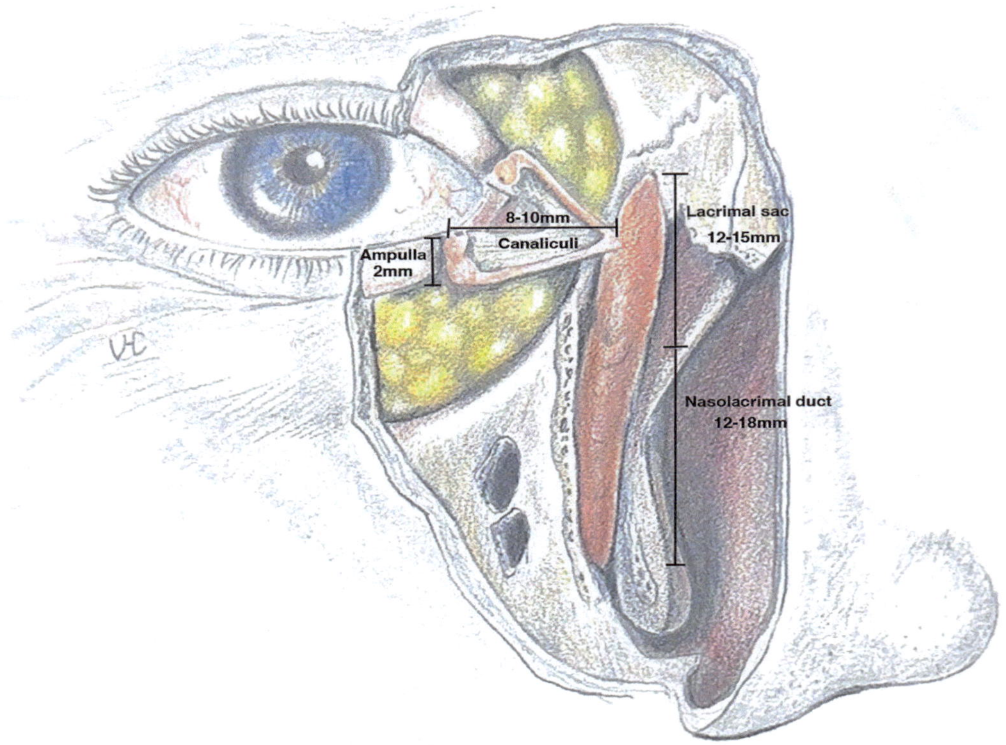

Fig. 3.7 Anatomy of the right lacrimal drainage system, including average adult length measurements for each section (Modified from Servat JJ, Nesi-Eloff F, Baylin E. Anatomy of the ocular adnexa, orbit, and related facial structures. In: Servat JJ, Black EH, Nesi FA, Gladstone GJ, Calvano CJ editors. Smith and Nesi's Ophthalmic Plastic and Reconstructive Surgery. fourth ed. Switzerland: Springer; 2021. p. 3–61)

Practical Surgical Matters

The structures of the orbit, unlike much of the intracranial space or the nose, contain soft tissue structures that are designed to tolerate some degree of displacement/compression. The optic nerve, for example, has approximately 1 cm of redundancy such that it will not be affected when the eye moves. This also, fortunately, allows for some amount of swelling/proptosis that will not harm the eye. Orbital soft tissue, likewise, may be gently moved out of the way with a retractor, especially one that is soft and flexible, such as the SPIWAY® Endonasal Access Guide platform, without damage. The tolerance of the critical neurovascular orbital structures to manipulation becomes less in instances of already-compromised blood supply (e.g., with a sphenoid wing meningioma). When working in the orbit or when it is used as a conduit to the intracranial space, it is possible to remove any wall without rigid reconstruction if the periorbita can remain mostly intact.

When approaching the medial orbit via the conjunctiva (including a transcaruncular approach), the lacrimal system can be retracted anteriorly quite safely. In order to do so, it is critical that the incision angulate posteromedially to land on the posterior lacrimal crest. During surgery, it is important to use dynamic retraction of orbital contents, so that retraction may be relaxed, and the eye may be permitted to reperfuse periodically. It is also vital to know the patient's history of eye surgery—any eye that has undergone surgery is structurally weaker than an eye which has not. This is particularly true of corneal transplant surgery. Retraction of the orbit or eye must proceed extremely cautiously in this instance, and strong consideration of another corridor for surgery should be given.

When beginning any orbital surgery, the surgeon should note the size and reactivity of each pupil. Ideally, they will be equal, making monitoring throughout the case straightforward. Unequal pupils may be due to a neurologic problem (perhaps the one for which the surgery is indicated) or may be mechanical (disruption of the iris sphincter by the same trauma that caused the orbital fracture). If the pupil in the operated orbit changes in size or reactivity, instruments should be removed and the cause for this considered. Pressure on the ciliary ganglion, which is more common when operating laterally and posteriorly in the orbit, can cause the pupil to enlarge and lose reactivity, as can manipulation of the inferior oblique muscle. This change warns the surgeon away from repeated manipulation in these areas. Pressure/damage to the optic nerve will **not** cause an enlarged pupil, but **will** cause the pupil to become less reactive. It may lead to momentary pupillary constriction. Again, instruments should be removed and the nerve allowed to recover, and then a different pattern of surgical movements may be undertaken.

References

1. Koornneef L. Spatial aspects of orbital Musculo-fibrous tissue in man: a new anatomical and histological approach. Amsterdam: Swets and Zeitlinger; 1977.
2. Koornneef L. New insights in the human orbital connective tissue: results of a new anatomic approach. Arch Ophthalmol. 1977;95:1269.
3. Koornneef L. Orbital septa: anatomy and function. Ophthalmology. 1979;86:876.
4. Bhardwaj V, Rajeshbhai GP. Axial length, anterior chamber depth-a study in different age groups and refractive errors. J Clin Diagn Res. 2013;7(10):2211–2. https://doi.org/10.7860/JCDR/2013/7015.3473. PubMed PMID: 24298478; Central PMCID: PMC3843406.
5. Fledelius HC, Stubgaard M. Changes in eye position during growth and adult life based on exophthalmometry. Acta Ophthalmol. 1986;64:481.
6. Scuderi AJ, Harnsberger HR, Boyer RS. Pneumatization of the paranasal sinuses: normal features of importance to the accurate interpretation of CT scans and MR images. AJR Am J Roentgenol. 1993;160(5):1101–4. https://doi.org/10.2214/ajr.160.5.8470585. PubMed PMID: 8470585.
7. Cho RI, Kahana A. Embryology of the orbit. J Neurol Surg B Skull Base. 2021;82(1):2–6. https://doi.org/10.1055/s-0040-1722630. PubMed PMID: 33777615; Central PMCID: PMC7987388.
8. Forbes G, Gehring DG, Gorman CA, Brennan MD, Jackson IT. Volume measurements of normal orbital structures by computed tomographic analysis. AJR Am J Roentgenol. 1985;145(1):149–54. https://doi.org/10.2214/ajr.145.1.149. PubMed PMID: 3873836.
9. Dutton JJ. Atlas of clinical and surgical Orbital anatomy. 2nd ed. Philadelphia: Saunders; 2011.
10. René C. Update on orbital anatomy. Eye (Lond). 2006;20(10):1119–29. https://doi.org/10.1038/sj.eye.6702376. PubMed PMID: 17019410.
11. Fukado Y. Results in 400 cases of surgical decompression of the optic nerve. Mod Prob Ophthalmol. 1975;14:474.
12. Servat JJ, Nesi-Eloff F, Baylin E. Anatomy of the ocular adnexa, orbit, and related facial structures. In: Servat JJ, Black EH, Nesi FA, Gladstone GJ, Calvano CJ, editors. Smith and Nesi's ophthalmic plastic and reconstructive surgery. 4th ed. Cham: Springer; 2021. p. 3–61.
13. Whitnall SE. On a tubercle on the malar bone, and on the lateral attachments of the tarsal plates. J Anat Physiol. 1911;45:426.
14. Lim HW, Paik DJ, Lee YJ. A cadaveric anatomical study of the levator aponeurosis and Whitnall's ligament. Korean J Ophthalmol. 2009;23(3):183–7. https://doi.org/10.3341/kjo.2009.23.3.183. PubMed PMID: 19794945; Central PMCID: PMC2739970.
15. Turvey TA, Golden BA. Orbital anatomy for the surgeon. Oral Maxillofac Surg Clin North Am. 2012;24(4):525–36. https://doi.org/10.1016/j.coms.2012.08.003. PubMed PMID: 23107426; Central PMCID: PMC3566239.
16. Bailey JH. Surgical anatomy of the lacrimal sac. Am J Ophthalmol. 1923;6:665.
17. Groessl SA, Sires BS, Lemke BN. An anatomical basis for primary acquired nasolacrimal duct obstruction. Arch Ophthalmol. 1997;115(1):71–4. https://doi.org/10.1001/archopht.1997.01100150073012. Erratum in: Arch Ophthalmol 1997 May;115(5):655. PubMed PMID: 9006428.
18. Woo KI, Maeng HS, Kim YD. Characteristics of intranasal structures for endonasal dacryocystorhinostomy in Asians. Am J Ophthalmol. 2011;152(3):491–498.e1. https://doi.org/10.1016/j.ajo.2011.02.019. PubMed PMID: 21669403.
19. Patton JM. Regional anatomy of the tear sac. Ann Otol Rhinol Laryngol. 1923;32:58.
20. Seker A, Martins C, Rhoton AL. Meningeal anatomy. In: Pamir MN, Black PN, Fahlbusch R, editors. Meningiomas. Philadelphia: W.B. Saunders; 2010. p. 11–51.
21. Woo SW, Lee HJ, Nahm FS, Lee PB, Choi EJ. Anatomic characteristics of supraorbital foramina in Korean using three-dimensional model. Korean

J Pain. 2013;26(2):130–4. https://doi.org/10.3344/kjp.2013.26.2.130. PubMed PMID: 23614073; Central PMCID: PMC3629338.
22. Jeong SM, Park KJ, Kang SH, Shin HW, Kim H, Lee HK, Chung YG. Anatomical consideration of the anterior and lateral cutaneous nerves in the scalp. J Korean Med Sci. 2010;25(4):517–22. https://doi.org/10.3346/jkms.2010.25.4.517. PubMed PMID: 20357990; Central PMCID: PMC2844612.
23. Spiriev TY, Chowdhury T, Schaller BJ. The trigeminal nerve: anatomical pathways. Trigeminocardiac reflex trigger points. In: Chowdhury T, Schaller BJ, editors. Trigeminocardiac reflex. Cambridge: Academic Press; 2015. p. 9–35.
24. Kurihashi K, Yamashita A. Anatomical consideration for dacryocystorhinostomy. Ophthalmologica. 1991;203(1):1–7. https://doi.org/10.1159/000310217. PubMed PMID: 1766635.
25. Neuhaus RW, Baylis HI. Cerebrospinal fluid leakage after dacryocystorhinostomy. Ophthalmology. 1983;90(9):1091–5. https://doi.org/10.1016/s0161-6420(83)80051-7. PubMed PMID: 6646647.
26. Hayreh SS, Dass R. The ophthalmic artery. I. Origin and intracranial and intracanalicular course. Br J Ophthalmol. 1962;46:65.
27. Bergen MP. A literature review of the vascular system in the human orbit. Acta Morphol Neerl Scand. 1981;19:273.
28. Hayreh SS. The ophthalmic artery. III Branches. Br J Ophthalmol. 1962;46:212.
29. Singh S, Dass R. The central artery of the retina. Br J Ophthalmol. 1960;44:193.
30. Brismar J. Orbital phlebography. III. Topography of the orbital veins. Acta Radiol Diangn (Stockh). 1974;15:577.
31. Bleeker GM. Changes in the orbital tissues and muscles dysthyroid ophthalmopathy. Eye. 1988;2:193.
32. Lim MC, Bateman JB, Glasgow BJ. Vortex vein exit sites: anatomic investigations on human eyes. Clin Anat. 2005;18:269.
33. Takahashi K, Muraoka K, Sutoh N, Ikeda F, Kobayashi H, Yamaguchi Y. Posterior routes of choroidal venous drainage. Jpn J Clin Ophthalmol. 1996;50:161–72.
34. Bergin MP. Relationships between the arteries and veins and the connective tissue system in the human orbit. I. The retrobulbar part of the orbit: apical region. Acta Morphol Neerl Scand. 1982;20:1.
35. Bergin MP. Relationships between the arteries and veins and the connective tissue system in the human orbit. II. The retrobulbar part of the orbit: septal complex region. Acta Morphol Neerl Scand. 1982;20:17.
36. Bergin MP. Some histologic aspects of the structure of the connective tissue system and its relationships with the blood vessels in the human orbit. Acta Morphol Neerl Scand. 1982;20:293.
37. Brismar J. Orbital phlebography. II. Anatomy of the superior ophthalmic vein and its tributaries. Acta Radiol Diangn (Stockh). 1974;15:481.
38. Cheung N, McNab AA. Venus anatomy of the orbit. Invest Ophthalmol Vis Sci. 2003;44:988.
39. Detorakis ET, Drakonaki E, Papadaki E, Pallikaris IG, Tsilimbaris MK. Effective orbital volume and eyeball position: an MRI study. Orbit. 2010;29(5):244–9.
40. Roy A, Kar M, Mandal D, Ray RS, Kar C. Variation of axial ocular dimensions with age, sex, height, BMI-and their relation to refractive status. J Clin Diagn Res. 2015;9(1):AC01–4. https://doi.org/10.7860/JCDR/2015/10555.5445. PubMed PMID: 25737966; Central PMCID: PMC4347057.
41. Seo J, Byun WY, Alisafaei F, Georgescu A, Yi YS, Massaro-Giordano M, Shenoy VB, Lee V, Bunya VY, Huh D. Multiscale reverse engineering of the human ocular surface. Nat Med. 2019;25(8):1310–8. https://doi.org/10.1038/s41591-019-0531-2. PubMed PMID: 31384041; Central PMCID: PMC6950645.
42. Ma H, Chen Y, Cai X, Tang Z, Nie C, Lu R. Effect of aging in periocular appearances by comparison of anthropometry between early and middle adulthoods in Chinese Han population. J Plast Reconstr Aesthet Surg. 2019;72:2002–8.
43. Kakizaki H, Malhotra R, Madge SN, Selva D. Lower eyelid anatomy: an update. Ann Plast Surg. 2009;63(3):344–51.
44. Burch HB, Bahn RS. Graves' Ophthalmopathy. In: Jameson JL, De Groot LJ, de Kretser DM, Giudice LC, Grossman AB, Melmed S, Potts JT, Weir GC, editors. Endocrinology: adult and pediatric. 7th ed. Philadelphia: W.B. Saunders; 2016. p. 1465–77.
45. Anderson RL, Dixon RS. Aponeurotic ptosis surgery. Arch Ophthalmol. 1979;97(6):1123–8. https://doi.org/10.1001/archopht.1979.01020010577015. PubMed PMID: 375893.
46. Ng SK, Chan W, Marcet MM, Kakizaki H, Selva D. Levator palpebrae superioris: an anatomical update. Orbit. 2013;32(1):76–84. https://doi.org/10.3109/01676830.2012.736602. PubMed PMID: 23387464.
47. Jackson TL. Moorsfield manual of ophthalmology. In: Oculoplastics. Philadelphia: Mosby; 2008. p. 1–54.
48. Homer WE. Description of a small muscle at the internal commissure of the eyelids. J Med Phys Sci. 1824;8:70.
49. Duverney J, Article II. De la structure de l'oeil, & de ses usages. In: Jombert C, editor. Oeuvres anatomiques. Paris. C.-A. Jombert.: de M. Duverney; 1761. p. 130.
50. Jones LT. A new concept of the orbital fascia and rectus muscle sheaths and its surgical implications. Trans Am Acad Ophthalmol Otolarygol. 1968;72:755.
51. Bacharach J, Lee WW, Harrison AR, Freddo TF. A review of acquired blepharoptosis: prevalence, diagnosis, and current treatment options. Eye. 2021;35:2468–81.
52. Creative Commons Attribution 4.0 International Public License. Creative Commons, Mountainview. https://creativecommons.org/licenses/by/4.0/legalcode. Accessed 25 May 2023.
53. Eggers HM. Functional anatomy of the extraocular muscles. In: Jakobiec F, editor. Ocular anatomy, embryology, and teratology. New York: Harper & Row; 1982. p. 783.

54. Dunbar KE, Singh R, Lelli GJ. Superior Transverse Ligament. In: Schmidt-Erfurth U, Kohnen T, editors. Encyclopedia of ophthalmology. Berlin: Springer; 2017. p. 1–2.
55. Anderson RL, Beard C. The levator aponeurosis attachments and their clinical significance. Arch Ophthalmol. 1977;95:1437.
56. Goldberg RA, Wu JC, Jesmanowicz A, Hyde JS. Eyelid anatomy revisited. Dynamic high-resolution magnetic resonance images of Whitnall's ligament and upper eyelid structures with the use of a surface coil. Arch Ophthalmol. 1992;110(11):1598–600. https://doi.org/10.1001/archopht.1992.01080230098030. PubMed PMID: 1444919.
57. Soll DB. Evolution and current concepts in the surgical management of the anophthalmic orbit. Ophthalmic Plast Reconstr Surg. 1986;2:163.
58. Liu GT. Disorders of the eyes and eyelids. In: Samuels MA, Feske SK, editors. Office practice of neurology. 2nd ed. Philadelphia: Churchill Livingstone; 2003. p. 35–69.
59. Oberbaum M, Singer SR, Vithoulkas G. The colour of the homeopathic improvement: the multidimensional nature of the response to homeopathic therapy. Homeopathy. 2005;94:196–9.
60. McKeown CA, Cavuoto K, Morris R. Strabismus surgery. In: Hoyt CS, Taylor D, editors. Pediatric ophthalmology and strabismus. 4th ed. Philadelphia: W.B. Saunders; 2013. p. 860–87.
61. McLoon LK, Christiansen SP. Extraocular muscles: extraocular muscle anatomy. In: Dartt DA, editor. Encyclopedia of the eye. Cambridge: Academic Press; 2010. p. 89–98.
62. Kono R, Poukens V, Demer JL. Quantitative analysis of the structure of the human extraocular muscle pulley system. Invest Ophthalmol Vis Sci. 2002;43:2923.
63. Castanares S. Blepharoplasty for herniated intraorbital fat: anatomical basis for a new approach. Plast Reconstr Surg. 1951;8:46.
64. Chowdhury PH, Shah BH, Tiwari N. All about extra ocular muscles: easy to understand. Int J Res Health Sci Nurs. 2020;6(4):7–15. https://doi.org/10.53555/hsn.v6i04.1299.
65. Hu S, Colley P. Surgical orbital anatomy. Semin Plast Surg. 2019;33(2):85–91. https://doi.org/10.1055/s--0039-1685476. PubMed PMID: 31037044; Central PMCID: PMC6486368.
66. Wolfram-Gabel R, Kahn JL. Adipose body of the orbit. Clin Anat. 2002;15:186.
67. Barker DE. Dye injection studies of intraorbital fat components. Plast Reconstr Surg. 1977;59:82.
68. Remington LA. Clinical anatomy and physiology of the visual system. 3rd ed. St. Louis: Butterworth-Heinemann; 2012.
69. Doxanas MJ, Anderson RL. Clinical orbital anatomy. Baltimore: Williams and Williams; 1984. p. 80.
70. Hargiss JL. Surgical anatomy of the eyelids. Trans Pac Coast Otolarygnol Soc. 1963;44:193.
71. Lockwood CB. The anatomy of the muscles, ligaments, and fasciae of the orbit, including an account of the capsule of Tenon, the check ligaments of the recti, and of the suspensory ligament of the eye. J Anat Physiol. 1886;20(1):i2.
72. Fink WH. An anatomical study of the check mechanism of the vertical muscles of the eye. Am J Ophthalmol. 1957;44:800.
73. Hwang K, Choi HG, Nam YS, Kim DJ. Anatomy of arcuate expansion of capsulopalpebral fascia. J Craniofac Surg. 2010;21:239.
74. Stager DR. The neurofibrovascular bundle of the inferior oblique muscle as its ancillary origin. Trans Am Ophthalmol Soc. 1996;94:1073–94. PubMed PMID: 8981719; Central PMCID: PMC1312118.
75. Baluk P, Fuxe J, Hashizume H, Romano T, Lashnits E, Butz S, Vestweber D, Corada M, Molendini C, Dejana E, McDonald DM. Functionally specialized junctions between endothelial cells of lymphatic vessels. J Exp Med. 2007;204(10):2349–62. https://doi.org/10.1084/jem.20062596. PubMed PMID: 17846148; Central PMCID: PMC2118470.
76. Bergin MP. A literature review of the vascular system in the human orbit. Acta Morphol Neerl Scand. 1981;19:273.
77. Warwick R. Eugene Wolff's anatomy of the eye and orbit, vol. 54. 7th ed. Philadelphia: WB Saunders; 1976. p. 496.
78. Duke-Elder S, Wybar KC. System of ophthalmology, volume II: the anatomy of the visual system. St. Louis: CV Mosby; 1961.
79. Cannata G, Pezzato S, Esposito S, Moscatelli A. Optic nerve sheath diameter ultrasound: a non-invasive approach to evaluate increased intracranial pressure in critically ill pediatric patients. Diagnostics. 2022;12:767.
80. Jafari A, Adappa ND, Anagnos VJ, Campbell RG, Castelnuovo P, Chalian A, Chambers CB, Chitguppi C, Dallan I, El Rassi E, Freitag SK, Fernandez Miranda JC, Ferreira M Jr, Gardner PA, Gudis DA, Harvey RJ, Huang Q, Humphreys IM, Kennedy DW, Lee JYK, Lehmann AE, Locatelli D, McKinney KA, Moreau A, Nyquist G, Palmer JN, Prepageran N, Pribitkin EA, Rabinowitz MR, Rosen MR, Sacks R, Sharma D, Snyderman CH, Tonya Stefko S, Stokken JK, Wang EW, Workman AD, Wu AW, Yu JY, Zhang MM, Zhou B, Bleier BS. Orbital resection by intranasal technique (ORBIT): a new classification system for reporting endoscopically resectable primary benign orbital tumors. Int Forum Allergy Rhinol. 2023;13:1852. PubMed PMID: 36808854. https://doi.org/10.1002/alr.23141.
81. Forrester JV, Dick AD, McMenamin PG, Roberts F, Pearlman E. Anatomy of the eye and orbit. In: Forrester JV, Dick AD, McMenamin PG, Roberts F, Pearlman E, editors. The eye. 4th ed. Philadelphia: W.B. Saunders; 2016. p. 1–102.e2.
82. Eggenberger ER, Pula JH. Neuro-ophthalmology in medicine. In: Aminoff MJ, Josephson SA, editors. Aminoff's neurology and general medicine. 5th ed. Cambridge: Academic Press; 2014. p. 479–502.

83. Rea P. Essential clinically applied anatomy of the peripheral nervous system in the head and neck. Cambridge: Academic Press; 2016. p. 21–130.
84. Semmer AE, McLoon LK, Lee MS. Orbital vascular anatomy. In: Dartt DA, editor. Encyclopedia of the eye. Cambridge: Academic Press; 2010. p. 241–51.
85. Barral J, Croibier A. Ophthalmic nerve. In: Barral J, Croibier A, editors. Manual therapy for the cranial nerves. Philadelphia: Churchill Livingstone; 2009. p. 115–28.
86. Kardon R. Anatomy and physiology of the autonomic nervous system. In: Miller NR, Newman NJ, Biousse V, Kerrison JB, editors. Walsh and Hoyt's clinical neuro-ophthalmology. 6th ed. Philadelphia: Lippincott Williams and Wilkins; 2005. p. 673–4.
87. Prasad S, Lee TC, Chiocca EA, Klein JP. Superficial greater petrosal neuropathy. Neurol Clin Pract. 2014;4(6):505–7. https://doi.org/10.1212/CPJ.0000000000000066. PubMed PMID: 29443140; Central PMCID: PMC5759987.
88. Tubbs RS, Menendez J, Loukas M, Shoja MM, Shokouhi G, Salter EG, Cohen-Gadol A. The petrosal nerves: anatomy, pathology, and surgical considerations. Clin Anat. 2009;22(5):537–44. https://doi.org/10.1002/ca.20814. PubMed PMID: 19544297.
89. Jordan A, Baum J, Basic tear Flow. Does it exist? Ophthalmology. 1980;87:920–30.
90. Anderson RL. Medial canthal tendon branches out. Arch Ophthalmol. 1977;95(11):2051–2. https://doi.org/10.1001/archopht.1977.04450110145019. PubMed PMID: 921584.
91. Shinohara H, Kominami R, Yasutaka S, Taniguchi Y. The anatomy of the lacrimal portion of the orbicularis oculi muscle (tensor tarsi or Horner's muscle). Okajimas Folia Anat Jpn. 2001;77(6):225–32. https://doi.org/10.2535/ofaj1936.77.6_225. PubMed PMID:11392011.
92. Becker BB. Tricompartment model of the lacrimal pump mechanism. Ophthalmology. 1992;99:1139.
93. Jones LT. Epiphora: its causes and new surgical procedures of its cure. Am J Ophthalmol. 1954;38:824.

Anatomy of the Skull Base (Through the Transorbital Route)

4

Matteo de Notaris, Francesco Corrivetti, Toma Spiriev, and Lili Laleva

Introduction

During the last 50 years, remarkable advances in cranial base surgery have improved and remodeled the approaches to the skull base [1]. Indeed, traditional microsurgical routes that are used to expose the skull base can be mainly divided into three groups: anterior, anterolateral and posterolateral. Even though, depending on the location and extent of the lesion, these approaches can require extensive soft tissue manipulation, bone disruption, and brain mobilization. However, cranial base surgery has recently been enhanced by a variety of minimally invasive endoscopic procedures to access the midline skull base areas [2]. Anatomic and clinical reports concerning endoscopic approaches have demonstrated the possibility of reaching targeted midline areas [3]. In this scenario, to improve the ventral route to most inaccessible skull base paramedian regions and to "strengthen" and complement the role of the midline endonasal approach to reach "far away" paramedian anatomical regions with poor working angles and areas, the transorbital port has been described to bring the surgeon closer to paramedian targets, i.e., the lateral wall of the cavernous sinus and Meckel's Cave, the parasellar segment of the internal carotid artery, up to the petroclival sincondrosis [4, 5]. As a matter of fact, through the development of transorbital neuroendoscopic surgery (TONES), a new group of transorbital modular pathways to access the skull base ventrally through the orbit have been developed [6]. This was due to the gradual refinement of endoscopic techniques and anatomical research in minimally invasive skull base surgery.

The interests in transorbital surgery rapidly produced a large number of anatomical studies who extensively described skull base anatomy through a transorbital perspective, demonstrating that the entire lateral skull base can be explored through a transorbital access [5, 7–10]. Among TONES corridors, the superior eyelid endoscopic transorbital approach (SETOA) showed to be the most suitable to access the different skull base compartments, especially the middle cranial fossa (MCF) [4, 7].

M. de Notaris (✉)
Laboratory of Neuroanatomy, EBRIS Foundation, European Biomedical Research Institute of Salerno, Salerno, Italy

Unit of Neurosurgery, San Giovanni di Dio and Ruggi D'Aragona Hospital, University of Salerno, Salerno, Italy

F. Corrivetti
Laboratory of Neuroanatomy, EBRIS Foundation, European Biomedical Research Institute of Salerno, Salerno, Italy

Department of Neurosurgery, San Luca Hospital, Salerno, Italy

T. Spiriev · L. Laleva
Department of Neurosurgery, Acibadem City Clinic University Hospital Tokuda, Sofia, Bulgaria

T. H. Schwartz et al. (eds.), *Endoscopic Transorbital Surgery of the Orbit, Skull Base and Brain*,
https://doi.org/10.1007/978-3-031-59504-2_4

More recently, based on this consistent number of anatomical investigations, the SETOA has been demonstrated clinically feasible for different skull base pathologies with encouraging results, and indications are constantly increasing, thanks to the numerous advantages related to this novel minimally invasive route [11–13]. This approach has been rapidly integrated in the neurosurgical armamentarium. Nonetheless, transorbital surgery is challenging and offers a perspective that differs from both transcranial and endonasal views. Therefore, a solid anatomical knowledge is essential to guide surgical procedures based on reliable anatomical landmarks.

At present, the SETOA can be considered a safe and minimally invasive surgical corridor to the anterior and middle cranial fossae as well as in the exposure of the cavernous sinus.

Materials and Methods

Anatomical dissections were performed at the Laboratory of Surgical Neuroanatomy of Barcelona, Spain, and at the Laboratory of Neuroscience EBRIS of Salerno, Italy. Two adult cadaveric embalmed and injected specimens were studied. The head specimens were adequately secured in a rigid three-pin fixation and placed in supine and neutral position, 10° flexed and 5° contralaterally rotated. After the initial skin phase under exoscopic visualization, the SETOA was performed with a rigid endoscope of 4-mm diameter, 18 cm in length, with 0° and 30° rod lenses (Karl Storz, Tuttlingen, Germany), connected to a light source (300 W Xenon, Karl Storz) through a fiberoptic cable and to an HD camera (Endovision Telecam SL; Karl Storz) as an optical device. This allowed the creation of 3D stereoscopic videos and photographs presenting the approach.

To create a representative photorealistic 3D model of the transorbital ventral perspective of the middle fossa and cavernous sinus anatomy, we used 3D perspectives from the database of *3D Atlas of Neurological Surgery project*, as our group is actively involved in the development of it (https://3datlasofneurologicalsurgery.org/).

a b c

Fig. 4.1 QR codes for 3D photorealistic models from the 3D Atlas of Neurological Surgery project and Panum Institute, Department of Cellular and Molecular Medicine University of Copenhagen (published with permission). (**a**) Dry whole skull specimen. (**b**) Sphenoid bone (**c**) dry skull coronal cut

The 3D models of this database represent surface scanning of anatomical specimens using a photogrammetry technique, which allows the extraction of 3D data from 2D photographs. The 3D data were processed using Blender software, and the 3D photorealistic models were uploaded to a dedicated website for 3D visualization. This allows users to see the 3D models from every desktop or mobile device, as well as some of the 3D models that can be displayed in AR mode by scanning the QR next to the Figures (Fig. 4.1a–c).

Another visualization method was portable document format (PDF)-based reconstruction of the CT of the specimens. The procedure allowed to create a three-dimensional (3D) model of the skull base with internal carotid pathway and trigeminal nerve reconstruction obtained from the pre- and post-dissection head CT images and embedded in a PDF file, as already described by our group elsewhere [14].

Anatomic Dissections

Ergonomics: The "Triangle" Method

Each specimen was also used to demonstrate the reproducibility of this technique for simulation and training. The degrees of freedom, angles of visualization, ergonomics, and instrument position represent an important factor to perform a safe and successful surgery. Indeed, it is essential to correctly position the instruments when performing a surgery to avoid instrument collision and inability to perform a correct approach. As a matter of facts, the perspective and maneuverability of the endoscope itself are limited by the unidirectionality of the approach, and a crowded transorbital port entering the site increases risk of interference between instruments. These challenges have led to additional practice in the anatomical lab a clear method to ensure and teach a correct ergonomics.

Following the skin incision followed by soft tissue dissection and the medial orbital retraction, the endoscope is inserted in a "virtual space" that is gradually enlarged by drilling the great sphenoid wing (GSW). During this step, however, due to limited field of view and short focal distances, endoscopes have various limitations, meaning that they must be placed within the surgical field with the shaft reducing the available working space and thereby reducing maneuverability. To overcome this issue, the surgeon must build up a triangled-shaped operative field as follows: *lateral side is represented by the lateral orbital rim, the medial side by the retractor, and the base is the lateral aspect of the upper eyelid crease* (Fig. 4.2a). Once the triangular-shaped operative field is buildup, it must be maintained in order to ensure complete comfort throughout the whole procedure. Furthermore, the instruments have to be inserted and positioned according to specific criteria: the endoscope is in a top-up position (12 o clock), while the two instruments are positioned below, at the base of the triangle (6 o clock) (Fig. 4.2b).

Superior Eyelid Transorbital Approach: Stepwise Dissection

SETOA was performed, as previously described by our group in other publications [4, 15], in this initial step, under exoscopic visualization. The skin incision was placed in the lateral (temporal) half of the superior lid and is designed in a curvilinear fashion (Fig. 4.3a). To expose the lateral orbital rim at the level of the frontozygomatic suture, the skin flap was elevated superolaterally after tarsorrhaphy to identify the suborbicularis plane sparing the orbicularis oculi muscle fibers (Fig. 4.3b). Care should be taken to avoid dissection downwards, directed to the orbital septum, where it was opened to retract the preaponeurotic fat and to expose the levator aponeurosis and to avoid its damage (Fig. 4.3c). Once the lateral orbital rim was exposed, the periosteum was cut, leading the dissection in the subperiosteal plane,

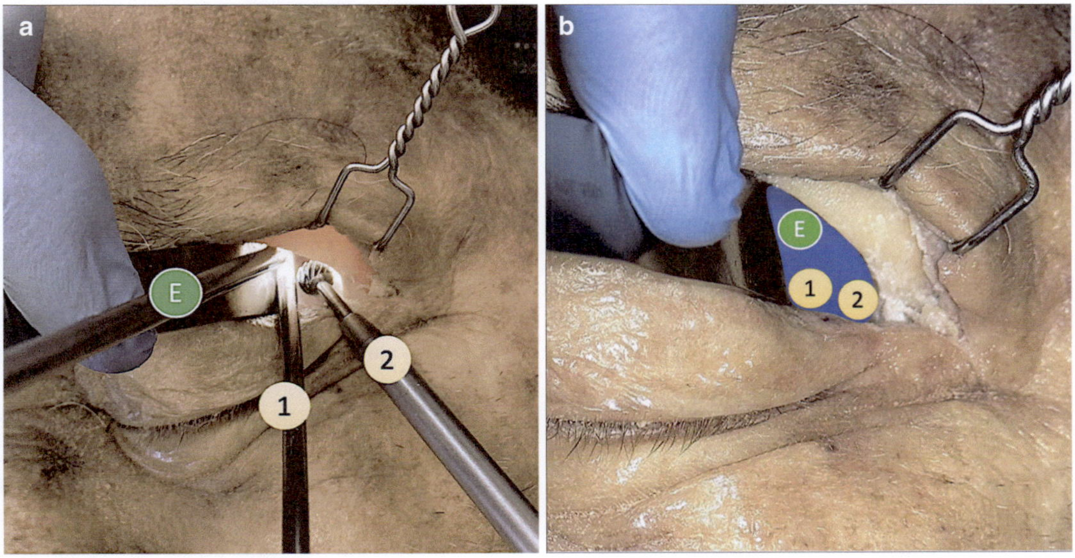

Fig. 4.2 Ergonomics of the transorbital approach, left side (**a**, **b**) triangled-shaped operative field and position of the instruments. E, endoscope; 1, aspirator; 2, drill

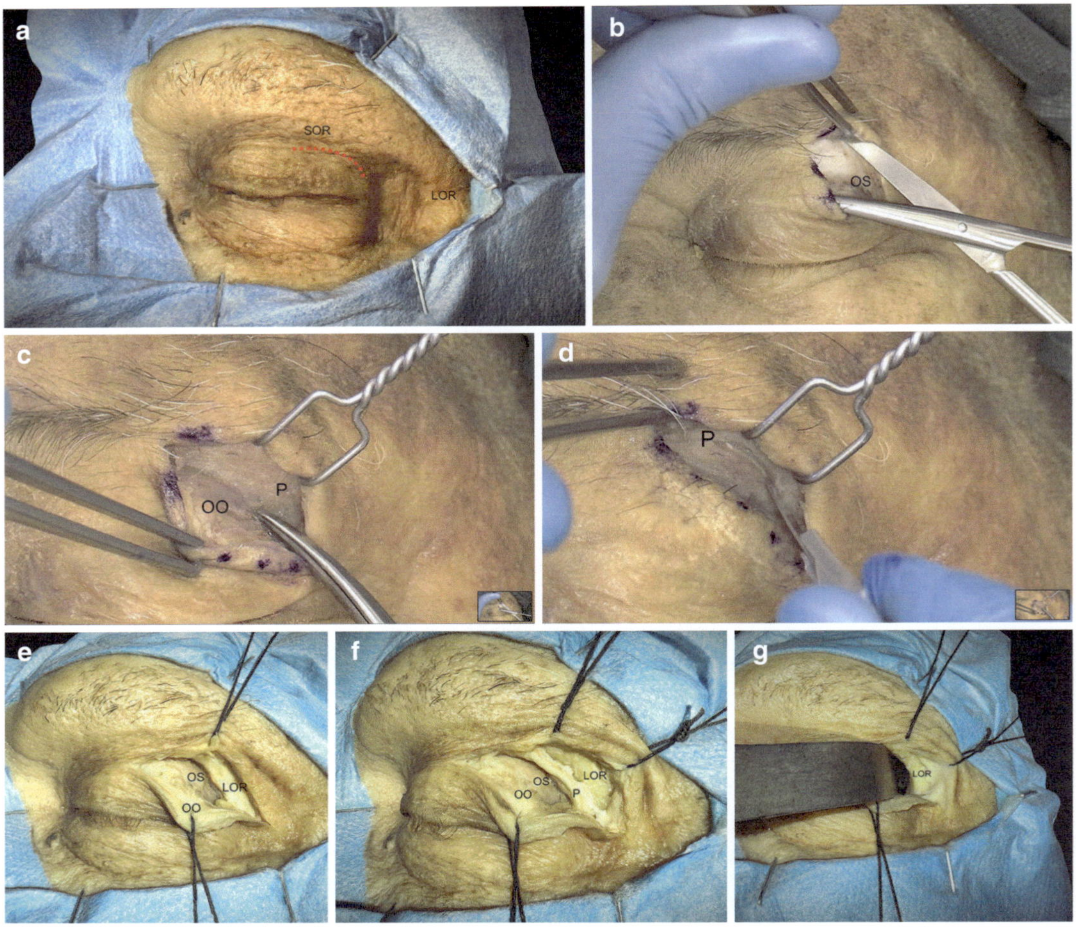

Fig. 4.3 Stepwise soft tissue dissection and presentation of the anatomical layers of the transorbital approach left side (**a**–**g**). *LOR* lateral orbital rim, *OS* optic septum, *OO* orbicularis oculi m., *P* periosteum, *SOR* superior orbital rim

sharply, toward the orbit, exposing the ventral surface of the greater and lesser sphenoid wing and the later part of the orbital roof (Fig. 4.3d–f). A malleable retractor was then inserted to displace the orbital content medially, providing enough space for moving surgical instruments and prevent collision with the endoscope (Fig. 4.3g). From this point, the procedure was performed under endoscopic visualization. Lateral orbital wall is exposed until the lateral edges of the inferior (first) superior and orbital fissures were encountered (Fig. 4.4a).

The lateral orbital wall was widely drilled until the fascia of the temporalis muscle was exposed laterally in the temporal fossa, to gain an adequate working space to proceed the dissection deeply. The ventral aspect of the greater sphenoid wing (GSW) was drilled in a lateral to medial direction until the lateral margin of the superior orbital fissure is recognized. This step of the procedure gives access to the middle cranial fossa and exposes the dura mater of the temporal pole (Fig. 4.4b). Bone drilling proceeded then caudally, until the floor of the MCF is encountered and the midsubtemporal ridge obscure the posterior aspect of the MCF. The medial limit of bone drilling is the most medial portion of the GSW, where the GSW turns from a coronal to a sagittal plane, forming a triangular ridge shaping dorsally, named the "sagittal crest" as we already described in our previous article [15]. This crest separates the medial temporal dura from the pos-

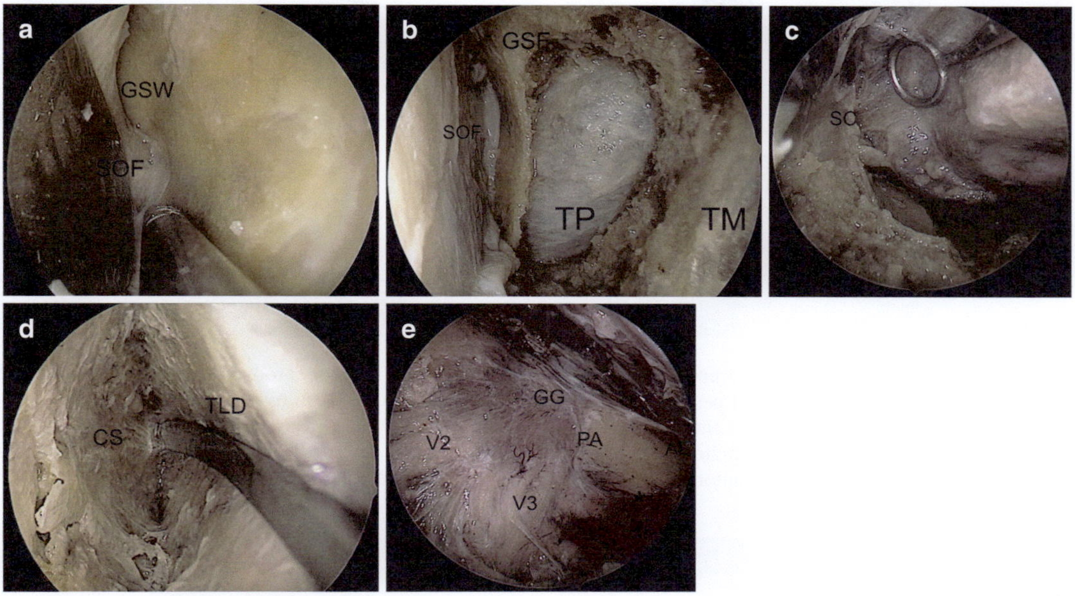

Fig. 4.4 Stepwise endoscopic transorbital dissection of the middle cranial fossa (**a–e**). *AE* arcuate eminence, *CS* cavernous sinus, *GG* Gasserian ganglion, *GSW* greater sphenoid wing, *MSR* midsubtemporal ridge, *PA* petrous apex, *SC* sagittal crest, *SOF* superior orbital fissure, *TM* temporalis muscle, *TLD* temporal lobe dura, *TP* temporal pole, *V2* maxillary nerve, *V3* mandibular nerve, *asterix* greater superficial petrosal nerve (GSPN)

terolateral periorbital (Fig. 4.4c). The sagittal crest was then completely drilled from the base until the anterior aspect of the foramen rotundum is encountered, opening the pathway to perform the interdural dissection of the cavernous sinus (CS) through the meningo-orbital band[14] (MOB). Interdural dissection of the cavernous sinus is performed detaching and peeling the outer layer of *dura propria* (the dura mater of the medial temporal lobe) from the inner dural layer (periosteal layer) made by the epineurium of the cranial nerves and corresponding to the later wall of the CS and more posteriorly the Meckel's cave (Fig. 4.4d).

At this point, the middle cranial fossa floor and the midsubtemporal ridge were then drilled and flattened to obtain a straight working space from the transorbital access. The temporal lobe was then elevated superolaterally, exposing the lateral surface of the Meckel's cave, composed by the third branch of the trigeminal nerve (V3) entering the foramen ovale (Fig. 4.4e). The foramen spinosum, located just lateral to it, gives intracranial access to the middle meningeal artery (MMA) that was cut to gain more surgical exposure along the MCF, until the greater superficial petrosal nerve (GSPN) and the superior edge of the petrous bone were encountered. At this point, the foramen ovale was skeletonized, obtaining space for medial mobilization of the Gasserian ganglion (GG) and the V3 branch to expose the anatomical boundaries of the Kawase's triangle: GSPN, V3, Gasserian ganglion complex, and arcuate eminence (Fig. 4.5).

At this point, dissection can be extended to the anterior or posterior cranial fossa.

Anterior cranial fossa: after drilling the GSW exposing the dura mater of the temporal pole, the drilling can be extended superiorly, resecting the lesser sphenoid wing in order to expose the dura mater of the lateral portion of the anterior cranial fossa (Fig. 4.6).

Posterior cranial fossa extension: bone drilling is performed at the level of the Kawase's triangle, in its inferior portion, under the V3 branch and medially to the GSPN exposes the petrous segment of the ICA (Fig. 4.7a), while proceeding the drilling superiorly, completing the anterior

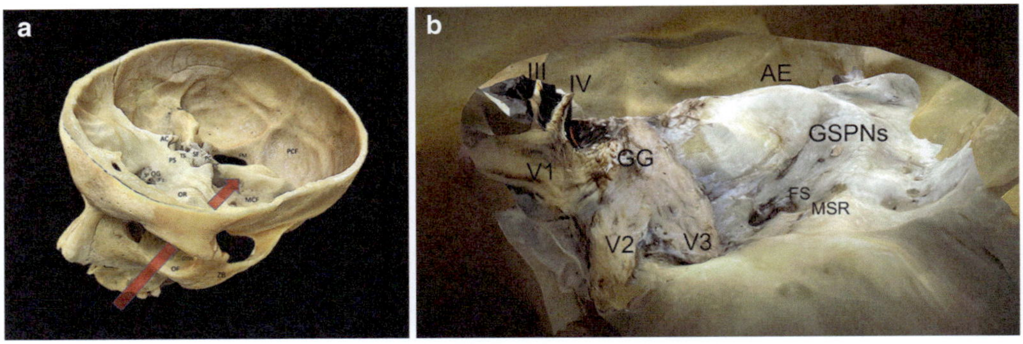

Fig. 4.5 (**a**) Trajectory of the transorbital approach. (**b**) Cavernous sinus, Meckel's cave, and petrous bone exposure from a transorbital perspective. *A* anterior clinoid, *FS* foramen spinosum, *GG* Gasserian ganglion, *GSPN* greater superficial petrosal nerve, *III* oculomotor nerve, *IV* trochlear nerve, *OG* olfactory groove, *PC* posterior clinoid, *FM* foramen magnum, *MCF* middle cranial fossa, *PCF* posterior cranial fossa, *PS* planum sphenoidale, *SF* sellar floor, *TS* tuberculum sellae, *V1* ophthalmic nerve, *V2* maxillary nerve, *V3* mandibular nerve, *ZB* zygomatic bone

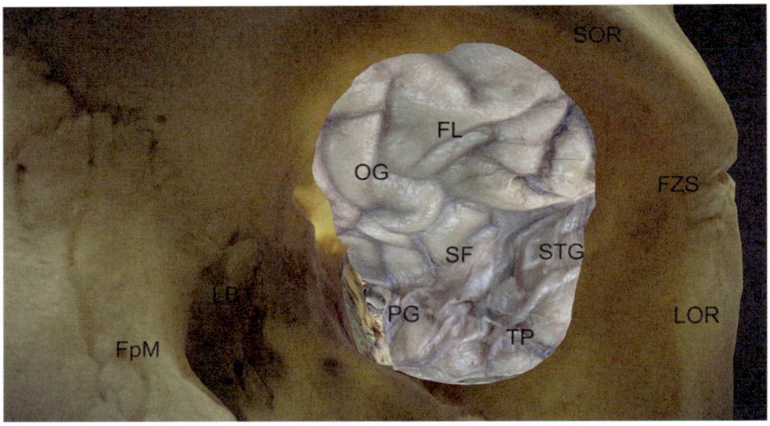

Fig. 4.6 Virtual reconstruction of the anterior and middle cranial fossa intradural exposure from a transorbital perspective. *FL* frontal lobe, *FpM* frontal process of the mandible, *FZS* frontozygomatic suture, *LB* lacrimal bone, *LOR* lateral orbital rim, *OG* orbital gyri, *PG* parahippocampal gyrus, *SF* Sylvian fissure, *SOF* superior orbital fissure, *SOR* superior orbital rim, *STG* superior temporal gyrus, *TM* temporalis muscle, *TP* temporal pole (used with permission of the "3D Atlas of Neurological Surgery Platform")

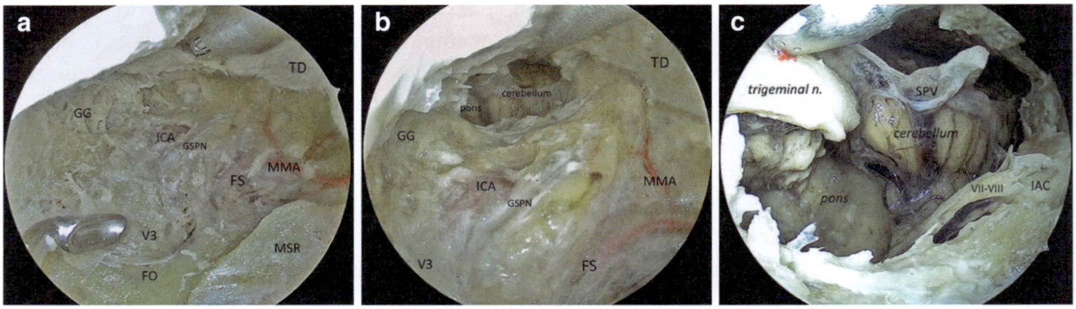

Fig. 4.7 (**a**) Petrous bone exposure; (**b**) anterior petrosectomy; (**c**) posterior cranial fossa access. *FO* foramen ovale, *FS* foramen spinosum, *GG* Gasserian ganglion, *GSPN* greater superficial petrosal nerve, *IAC* internal auditory canal, *ICA* internal carotid artery (petrous segment), *MMA* middle meningeal artery, *MSR* midsubtemporal ridge, *SPV* superior petrosal vein, *TD* temporal dura, *VII–VIII* facial and vestibulocochlear nerve complex, *V3* mandibular nerve (used with permission of the "3D Atlas of Neurological Surgery Platform")

petrosectomy, exposes the dura mater of the posterior fossa (Fig. 4.7b) that must be opened to visualize the cerebellopontine angle, from the trigeminal root medially and the VII–VIII cranial nerve complex laterally (Fig. 4.7c).

Relevant Anatomy

The Orbit

The orbit is a bony quadrangular pyramidal cavity that opens up to the front of the head. It is formed by six bones: frontal, lacrimal, maxilla, zygomatic, ethmoid, palatine, and sphenoid (Fig. 4.8).

Located at the apex of the orbit is the *optic foramen*, which is bounded by the body and the lesser wing of the sphenoid bone. It is located medial to the superior orbital fissure and represent the point at which the optic nerve (CN II) and the ophthalmic artery leave the skull to enter the orbit.

Regarding the orbital anatomy, the SETOA allows to expose:

1. The lateral orbital wall up to the superior orbital fissure.
2. The orbital roof (superior orbital wall) up to the optic canal.

The superior orbital fissure is a relevant landmark that defines the boundaries between these two regions:

1. The lateral orbital wall is formed by the inner surface of the frontal portion of the zygomatic bone and the ventral surface of the greater sphenoid wing (GSW).
2. The anterior portion of the orbital roof is composed of the orbital part of the frontal bone, while the posterior portion is made up of the lesser wing of the sphenoid.

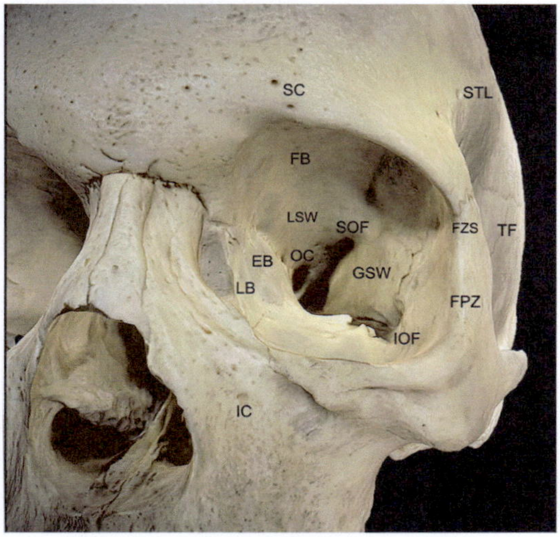

Fig. 4.8 Dry skull specimen presenting the bone anatomy of the left orbit. *SC* supraorbital canal, *FB* frontal bone, *LSW* lesser sphenoid wing, *SOF* superior orbital fissure, *OC* optic canal, *GSW* greater sphenoid wing, *EB* ethmoid bone, *LB* lacrimal bone; *IOC* infraorbital canal, *IOF* inferior orbital fissure, *FPZ* frontal process of the zygomatic bone, *FZS* frontozygomatic suture, *STL* superior temporal line, *TF* temporal fossa (used with permission of the "3D Atlas of Neurological Surgery Platform")

Anterior Cranial Fossa

The superior orbital wall/orbital roof separates the lateral portion of the anterior cranial fossa (ACF) from the orbit. The SETOA allows to expose the entire orbital roof and part of the medial orbital wall. Pushing the orbital content inferiorly allows visualizaction of the superior orbital wall from the SOF to the posterior and anterior ethmoidal arteries. Subperiosteal dissection of the orbital roof can be better accomplished after drilling the lateral orbital wall that comprises the inner surface of the zygoma and the ventral aspect of the GSW, to gain adequate working space.

Then, the lesser sphenoid wing must be drilled. This maneuver exposes the dura mater of the frontal bone in the anterior fossa anteriorly, and then, drilling the LSW allows to skeletonize the superior orbital fissure, mobilizing its contents. The optic canal is located just medially to the superior orbital fissure, in a deeper plane, surrounded by the bone of the medial edge of the

SOF, laterally, and the foramen of the posterior ethmoidal artery medially. Therefore, drilling the medial edge of the SOF opens the optic canal laterally, allowing to perform optic nerve decompression. The bone of the LSW forms the medial edge of the SOF and therefore the lateral portion of the optic canal extends posteromedially to the anterior clinoidal process. Performing an endoscopic anterior clinoidectomy (see Chap. 28, which illustrates the technical nuance for transorbital anterior clinoidectomy) exposes the clinoidal portion of the ICA located between the two dural rings that lie just lateral to the optic nerve.

Temporal Fossa

Drilling the proximal portion of the lateral orbital wall, corresponding to the zygomatic bone, exposes the temporal fossa accommodating the temporalis muscle, exposing the exocranial surface at the level of the pterion, while in the distal portion, the remotion of the GSW exposes the temporal dura and the middle cranial fossa.

Middle Cranial Fossa

The ventral surface of the GSW separates the middle cranial fossa from the orbital space. After complete drilling of the GSW, skeletonization of the lateral edge of the SOF, and remotion of the sagittal crest (see Chap. 29, which provides detailed anatomy of sagittal crest and mid-subtemporal ridge), the limits of the MCF window are the following:

(a) Laterally the lateral surface of the GSW and the temporal fossa.
(b) Superiorly the lateral (horizontal) portion of the meningo-orbital band.
(c) Medially the medial (vertical) portion of the meningo-orbital band.
(d) Inferiorly the floor of the MCF.

Elevating the temporal lobe and detaching the dura mater from the MCF floor exposes from medial to lateral:

(a) The foramen rotundum and the entrance of the maxillary nerve.
(b) The foramen ovale and the entrance of the mandibular nerve.
(c) The foramen spinosum and the exit of the middle meningeal artery (MMA).

Superior Orbital Fissure and Meningo-Orbital Band

The SOF is a cleft between the lesser and greater sphenoid wings. It has an oblique superolateral to inferomedial orientation and gives passage to nerves and vessels running inside the cavernous sinus through the orbit. Skeletonization of the lateral edge of the SOF is obtained after complete drilling of the ventral surface of the GSW and remotion of the sagittal crest. The latter constitutes the most medial portion of the GSW in which the bone orientation changes from coronal to sagittal. The sagittal crest is located in the place where the inner dural layer of the dura propria of the CS is attached to the medial temporal dura that is the transition point between the CS and the posterior aspect of the periorbita, where it becomes contiguous with the periosteum of the lateral orbital wall.

The meningo-orbital band (MOB) is, in fact, a structure located between the medial temporal dura and the lateral aspect of the periorbita. It has a sagittal oriented shape, in its medial portion, and then, it became horizontally oriented, in its lateral extension, where it is constituted only by the juxtaposition of the frontal and temporal dural layers.

Cavernous Sinus and Meckel's Cave

Cutting the MOB in its medial portion allows to detach in an interdural fashion the lateral wall of the cavernous sinus from the medial temporal dura, exposing the nerves running inside the CS, exposing the lateral wall of the CS up to the Meckel's cave. This maneuver, performed starting from the maxillary nerve (V2), progressively exposes, elevating the temporal dura superolaterally the nerves forming the lateral wall of the cavernous sinus, i.e., the ophthalmic branch of the trigeminal nerve and then the trochlear and oculomotor nerves. Extending the dissection posteriorly is possible to expose the Gasserian ganglion inside the Meckel's cave.

Petrous Bone

At this point, an extensive exposure of the MCF extending to the anterior surface of the petrous bone is feasible and necessary to access to the posterior cranial fossa.

Starting from external wall of the Meckel's cave, the MMA must be cut, close to the root of the mandibular nerve in order to detach the portion of the temporal pole covering the greater superficial petrosal nerve (GSPN). GSPN allows the localization of the petrous segment of the ICA just running caudally to it. From there, temporal lobe elevation exposes the ventral petrous surface up to the petrous ridge and the tentorium. Medially, the Kawase's triangle is formed by the root of V3 (medially), the GSPN (laterally), and the petrous ridge (superiorly) and represents a key landmark to entering the posterior cranial fossa.

Posterior Cranial Fossa

The exposure of the anterior aspect of the petrous bone, from the Kawas' triangle medially to the arcuate eminence laterally, allows to accede the posterior cranial fossa through a "partial" anterior petrosectomy. A previous skeletonization of the foramen rotundum can be attempted in order to mobilize the Gasserian ganglion and the mandibular nerve medially, gaining additional exposure of the anterior petrous bone. Hence, this area from the trigeminal ganglion to the internal acoustic canal (IAC) is drilled out; the superior and inferior petrosal sinuses represent the superior and inferior limits, to access the posterior fossa. At this point, neurovascular structures of the posterior fossa can be displayed after cutting the tentorium and the posterior fossa dura. This area of exposure gives access to three main regions:

1. The cerebellopontine angle: between the trigeminal nerve medially and facial and vestibulocochlear nerves laterally. This area is comprised of the anterolateral surface of the pons and the cerebellar hemisphere is between the two nerve roots and the petrosal vein.
2. The middle tentorial incisura: from the origin of the oculomotor nerve to the entrance of the trochlear nerve into the tentorium free edge. This area comprises the anterolateral portion of the mesencephalon and the superior cerebellar artery.
3. Ventral brainstem space: from the basilar artery to the origin of the abducens nerve. This space is hardly accessible and can be visible only through a 30° endoscope.

References

1. de Divitiis O, d'Avella E, de Notaris M, Di Somma A, De Rosa A, Solari D, Cappabianca P. The (R)evolution of anatomy. World Neurosurg. 2019;127:710–35.
2. Cappabianca P, Cavallo LM, Esposito F, De Divitiis O, Messina A, De Divitiis E. Extended endoscopic endonasal approach to the midline skull base: the evolving role of transsphenoidal surgery. Adv Tech Stand Neurosurg. 2008;33:151–99.
3. Castelnuovo P, Dallan I, Battaglia P, Bignami M. Endoscopic endonasal skull base surgery: past, present and future. Eur Arch Otorrinolaringol. 2010;267:649–63.

4. Dallan I, Di Somma A, Prats-Galino A, Solari D, Alobid I, Turri-Zanoni M, Fiacchini G, Castelnuovo P, Catapano G, de Notaris M. Endoscopic transorbital route to the cavernous sinus through the meningo-orbital band: a descriptive anatomical study. J Neurosurg. 2017;127:622–9.
5. Di Somma A, Andaluz N, Cavallo LM, et al. Endoscopic transorbital superior eyelid approach: anatomical study from a neurosurgical perspective. J Neurosurg. 2018;129:1203–16.
6. Moe KS, Bergeron CM, Ellenbogen RG. Transorbital neuroendoscopic surgery. Neurosurgery. 2010;67:ons16–28.
7. Bly RA, Ramakrishna R, Ferreira M, Moe KS. Lateral transorbital neuroendoscopic approach to the lateral cavernous sinus. J Neurol Surg B Skull Base. 2014;75:11–7.
8. Di Somma A, Cavallo LM, de Notaris M, Solari D, Topczewski TE, Bernal-Sprekelsen M, Enseñat J, Prats-Galino A, Cappabianca P. Endoscopic endonasal medial-to-lateral and transorbital lateral-to-medial optic nerve decompression: an anatomical study with surgical implications. J Neurosurg. 2017;127:199–208.
9. Di Somma A, Andaluz N, Cavallo LM, et al. Endoscopic transorbital route to the petrous apex: a feasibility anatomic study. Acta Neurochir. 2018;160:707–20.
10. Gerges MM, Godil SS, Younus I, Rezk M, Schwartz TH. Endoscopic transorbital approach to the infratemporal fossa and parapharyngeal space: a cadaveric study. J Neurosurg. 2019;133:1–12.
11. Jeon C, Hong C-K, Woo KI, Hong SD, Nam D-H, Lee J-I, Choi JW, Seol HJ, Kong D-S. Endoscopic transorbital surgery for Meckel's cave and middle cranial fossa tumors: surgical technique and early results. J Neurosurg. 2018;131:1–10.
12. Almeida JP, Omay SB, Shetty SR, Chen Y-N, Ruiz-Treviño AS, Liang B, Anand VK, Levine B, Schwartz TH. Transorbital endoscopic eyelid approach for resection of sphenoorbital meningiomas with predominant hyperostosis: report of 2 cases. J Neurosurg. 2018;128:1885–95.
13. Jeon C, Hong SD, Woo KI, Seol HJ, Nam D-H, Lee J-I, Kong D-S. Use of endoscopic transorbital and endonasal approaches for 360° circumferential access to orbital tumors. J Neurosurg. 2020;135:1–10.
14. Spiriev T, Mitev A, Stoykov V, Dimitrov N, Maslarski I, Nakov V. Three-dimensional immersive photorealistic layered dissection of superficial and deep back muscles: anatomical study. Cureus. 2022;14:e26727.
15. Corrivetti F, de Notaris M, Di Somma A, Dallan I, Enseñat J, Topczewski T, Solari D, Cavallo LM, Cappabianca P, Prats-Galino A. "Sagittal crest": definition, stepwise dissection, and clinical implications from a Transorbital perspective. Oper Neurosurg (Hagerstown). 2022;22:e206. https://doi.org/10.1227/ONS.0000000000000131.

Part II

Perspectives on Transorbital Surgery

Otolaryngology Perspective

5

Darlene Lubbe and Hamzah Mustak

Introduction: The Learning Curve

At first, it was thought that transorbital surgery would always involve a team approach between an otolaryngologist and ophthalmologist or neurosurgeon. However, the lines quickly became blurred as to which pathology should be managed by which discipline. There was an interest from ENT surgeons to remove orbital tumors, ophthalmologists ventured into the otolaryngology domain, and soon transorbital neuroendoscopic surgery (TONES) was seen as the new kid on the block by interested neurosurgeons, who were until very recently criticized by their peers. There was an expectation that TONES would be performed by a dedicated surgical team, like endoscopic transsphenoidal pituitary surgery (ETSS) and most likely performed by a similar combination of surgeons performing four-handed surgery. Although this has occurred in recent years, the magnitude of the discovery of the transorbital portals and potential of transorbital surgery is only now being understood, more than 13 years after the first transorbital case was performed by Kris Moe [1].

D. Lubbe (✉)
Division of Otolaryngology, Department of Surgery, University of Cape Town, Cape Town, South Africa

H. Mustak
Division of Ophthalmology, University of Cape Town, Cape Town, South Africa
e-mail: hamzah.mustak@uct.ac.za

A sound knowledge of the anatomy and function of the structures of the eye is essential since an orbital portal is created by displacing the soft orbital structures away from the bony orbital walls. Unlike ETSS, the surgical corridor does not remain widely patent once access to the target area has been achieved. Continuous careful retraction of the orbit is required to maintain the surgical pathway and, therefore, the need for four-handed surgery to manipulate the endoscope and instruments through this portal. Multifunctional instruments have made surgery easier by allowing multiple functions at the target area without crowding the surgical portal. Still, the surgical assistant is as important as the primary surgeon, continuously providing space and visualization for the primary surgeon. This teamwork takes considerable time to develop and to master and understanding the principles of each other's specialty is essential.

The Transorbital Journey: Lessons Learned

It is easy to predict which surgeons would gravitate toward endoscopic transorbital surgery. For otolaryngologists, it would be the endoscopic sinus surgeon who is already involved in tumor surgery—those surgeons who perform endoscopic medial maxillectomies or who chase angiofibromas into the pterygopalatine and infra-

T. H. Schwartz et al. (eds.), *Endoscopic Transorbital Surgery of the Orbit, Skull Base and Brain*,
https://doi.org/10.1007/978-3-031-59504-2_5

temporal fossae. It is much easier, much less invasive, and more direct and, frankly, requires less skill to remove a medial orbital tumor through a precaruncular approach than through a transnasal approach. Once you have seen a medial orbital cavernous hemangioma being removed through a medial orbital (precaruncular) approach, you will never contemplate destroying healthy sinus cavities again. Access to these lesions endonasally has been widely described in the otolaryngology literature, with complex sutures being placed around the medial rectus muscle, special retractors used to manipulate instruments through orbital fat at difficult angles, and septal mucoperichondrial flaps used to reconstruct the medial orbital wall where the lamina papyracea has been resected for access. Instead, an incision is made through the caruncle of the eye, two dural retractors are used to dissect onto the tumor, a suture is placed through the lesion, and it is removed en bloc without any collateral damage to uninvolved structures like the sinuses and lamina papyracea without leaving a visible external scar.

Very few ophthalmologists venture outside their field of expertise, whether it is cataract surgery or retinal work. It is the oculoplastic surgeon and/or the orbital tumor surgeon who will see the advantages of transorbital surgery. The traditional orbital surgeon has not been trained to use the endoscope and will not appreciate the advantages of using the endoscope in the posterior orbit. It is only once one witnesses how the endoscope allows perfect visualization of the blowout fracture with the entrapped inferior rectus muscle in the posterior aspect of the orbital floor that the potential of endoscopic transorbital surgery is understood. The fact that navigation is used by some maxillofacial surgeons to ensure a perfect plate position to repair a fracture indicates that this area is not well visualized during traditional open surgery.

Endoscopic transorbital surgery often implies that the periorbital fascia is not breached and that instrumentation occurs in the plane between the periorbita and the bony orbital walls. Transorbital surgery therefore does not mean that an ophthalmologist should always be involved during the surgery—it depends on the indication and the risk to the eye. Traditional anterior ethmoidal artery ligation for epistaxis is a good example of otolaryngologists venturing into the orbit through a Lynch incision without necessarily having "permission" to perform transorbital surgery. Similarly, neurosurgeons don't ask for permission to remove part of the lateral orbital wall during a craniotomy for sphenoid wing meningioma surgery.

The most difficult part of the authors' journey was to convince neurosurgeons that there were benefits and possibly new indications for transorbital surgery. Without visualizing the surgical portal, the width that can be achieved, the superior image provided by a 4 K camera system, the angles and trajectories that can be achieved when compared to a microscope, and, finally and most importantly, the little morbidity caused when compared to some traditional approaches, it is close to impossible to change their surgical preferences. It was only when we brought the neurosurgeon to the table after the surgical corridor to the temporal lobe was created that there was a mindset change and new possibilities were entertained. This was however short-lived due to the time that this new technique took—slow drilling by an otolaryngologist or ophthalmologist who took extreme care not to have a complication. We now know that the portal can be quickly created using surgical loupes and a high-speed drill, navigating safely between the temporalis muscle, dura, and periorbita until the superior orbital fissure and meningo-orbital band are reached. Only then, the endoscope is brought into the surgical field. Younger neurosurgeons are now seeing their peers publish papers on the lateral transorbital approach for sphenoid wing meningiomas, with this new approach threatening to replace the traditional pterional approach for selected cases [2]. Now, an interest has been generated that has placed transorbital surgery on a new trajectory with neurosurgeons taking the lead.

The Otolaryngology Perspective: Separating the Four Portals

Many years of working together with colleagues from neurosurgery and ophthalmology have provided the opportunity to truly understand the role of each surgeon and have allowed us to realize which of the four portals—superior, inferior, lateral, and medial—are most likely to be utilized by the different disciplines. For example, the medial approach will become a standard approach for otolaryngologists to access the ethmoidal arteries and eventually replace the Lynch-Howarth incision. The superior-lateral approach has been adopted by neurosurgeons as a portal to the greater wing of the sphenoid, temporal lobe, and cavernous sinus. In certain centers [3], it has become a very popular approach and is performed without the assistance of an otolaryngologist or ophthalmologist. In other units, the lateral surgical portal is created by the otolaryngologist or oculoplastic surgeon, creating the pathway for the neurosurgeon who can choose to use an endoscope or microscope at the target area. The superior eyelid approach is a useful approach for the otolaryngologist to access lesions that extend from the frontal sinus into the orbit and to drain extradural anterior cranial fossa collections secondary to complicated frontal sinusitis. The superior approach has thus far been underutilized—it provides wide access to the floor of the whole anterior cranial fossa/roof of the orbit and provides access to the optic nerve canal and the anterior clinoid process for a superior and lateral optic nerve decompression. This portal begs to be explored and will most likely follow the same neurosurgical trajectory as the lateral approach. The inferior conjunctival incision is still mainly used by ophthalmologists and oculoplastic surgeons to address orbital tumors and to release entrapped rectus muscles with blowout fractures. It provides good access to the inferior orbital fissure, the infraorbital nerve, and the roof of the maxillary sinus for maxillary sinus lesions that extend into the orbital space (Figs. 5.1 and 5.2).

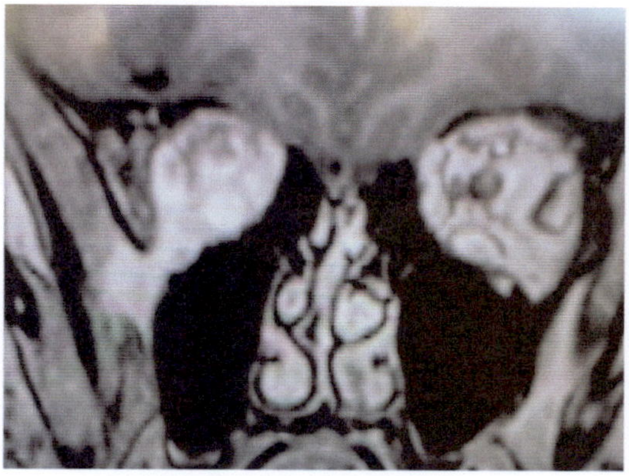

Fig. 5.1 Tumor involving the right inferior orbit, pterygopalatine fossa, lateral wall of maxillary sinus

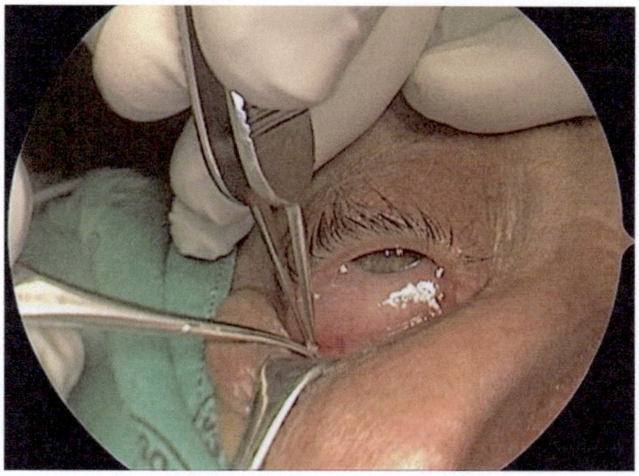

Fig. 5.2 Inferior conjunctival incision to biopsy lesion seen in Fig. 5.1

Otolaryngology Indications for Multiportal Surgery

It has been a unique experience being involved in endoscopic transorbital surgery during the early stages of the development of the different portals. At first, all cases were performed as a combined otolaryngology-ophthalmology team at our unit in Cape Town. Over the last 6 years, we have however come to understand which pathology should be addressed by which specialty. In short, if the periorbital fascia is breached, an ophthalmologist should be the primary surgeon for that part of the surgery. If one remains outside the periorbita and adheres to certain principles with regard to retraction of the orbit, protecting and safeguarding against any damage to the optic nerve or other important neurovascular structures entering the orbit, then the transorbital surgical pathways are a great addition to the armamentarium of the otolaryngologist.

The range of pathology for general otolaryngologists has expanded to include performing balanced decompressions for patients with thyroid eye disease (TED), multiportal optic nerve decompression, managing complicated sinusitis by accessing a subperiosteal abscess through a transcaruncular or lateral approach, draining intracranial abscesses, and creating and maintaining a surgical corridor for the neurosurgeon or ophthalmologist.

Thyroid eye disease is traditionally managed by ophthalmology. Surgical intervention is indicated after very specific criteria are met and medical management has failed. Referral depends on the expertise of the unit, and an otolaryngologist is often primarily asked to perform a medial decompression. A good maximal medial decompression can result in the patient struggling with diplopia postoperatively and may not be the best treatment option. Management should follow a stepwise approach and depends on the severity of the proptosis and visual loss. Transorbital/multiportal surgery allows an otolaryngologist/ophthalmologist to perform a balanced decompression—using a combination of an endonasal and lateral orbital approach:

- Mild proptosis—fat removal only via a lateral/retrocanthal approach.
- Moderate—lateral decompression and fat removal.
- Severe—balanced medial and lateral decompression +/− fat removal.
- Very severe—balanced (medial +lateral) decompression + inferior wall.

It is of the utmost importance that an ophthalmologist should assess the patient with TED. Like ETSS, a multidisciplinary team must be involved in patient care. Decision-making regarding surgical timing and the extent of decompression needed falls within the ophthalmology domain. It makes sense for an otolaryngologist to perform the surgery as the medial component is best managed through an endonasal route to ensure maximal opening of the paranasal sinuses to avoid sinusitis or mucocele formation. The lateral approach can then be performed by either an otolaryngologist or ophthalmologist, but the decision of "how much to do" is an important one and is usually made by the ophthalmologist who will look after the patient in the long term.

The transcaruncular approach for anterior and posterior ethmoid artery ligation should be the standard teaching in otolaryngology units. This medial approach is easy to master and is used for intractable epistaxis, usually related to nasoethmoid fractures [4, 5]. The portal gives excellent access to the whole medial orbit for medial orbital tumors (Fig. 5.3). The optic nerve can be found 6 mm behind the posterior ethmoid artery in the frontoethmoidal suture line which is in line with the nasion—an easy landmark to guide the surgeon about the height of the ethmoidal vessels. Cerebrospinal fluid leaks originating just superior to this line can also be repaired through this minimally invasive portal.

Sinonasal tumors often transgress surgical boundaries, requiring multidisciplinary input. Surgery is often staged if more than one discipline is required to address a specific area that requires an additional surgical incision, extra equipment, and repositioning of the patient or if

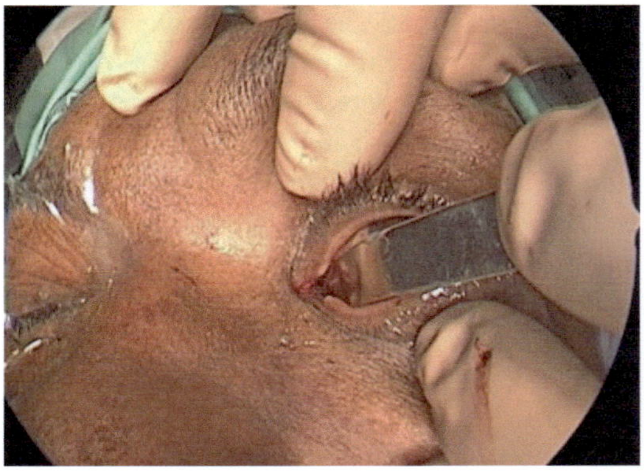

Fig. 5.3 Transcaruncular (medial) approach left eye for ligation of ethmoidal arteries

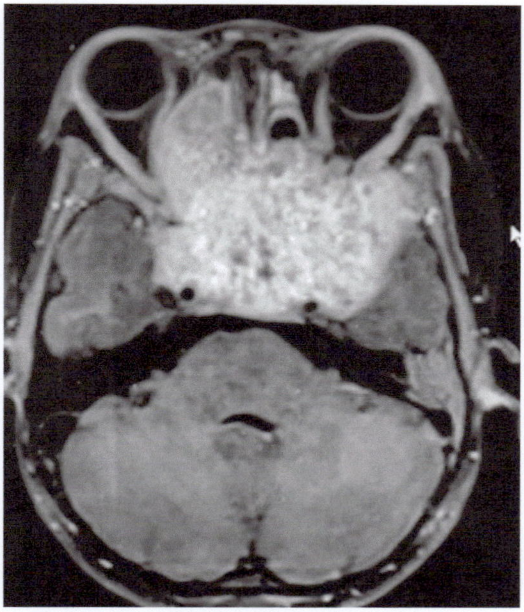

Fig. 5.4 Large angiofibroma crossing surgical boundaries necessitating multiportal surgery

the surgical time is lengthened beyond what is reasonable or safe. Multiportal surgery often allows an otolaryngologist to safely address this interdisciplinary space during a single surgery. Examples of tumors that cross surgical boundaries are a variety of benign and malignant sinonasal tumors that extend from the paranasal sinuses into the orbit, pterygopalatine fossa, infratemporal fossa, temporal fossa, anterior cranial fossa, and greater wing of the sphenoid (Fig. 5.4).

Multiportal Combinations

Certain portals are used by different disciplines for a specific indication. An example would be the **lateral (or superior-lateral/superior eyelid crease) approach**. The lateral portal has now been adapted by all disciplines for different indications, often without the need for interdisciplinary presence. Neurosurgeons now use this portal to address even large sphenoid wing meningiomas involving the temporal lobe, greater wing of the sphenoid, and orbit. There is an advantage to

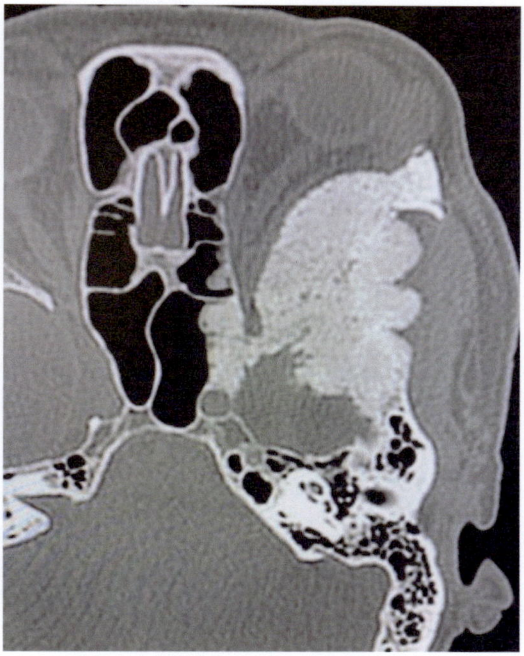

Fig. 5.5 Sphenoid wing meningioma extending to sphenoid sinus with optic nerve decompression

working with colleagues from other disciplines—the most important is sharing knowledge and experience. Small nuances such as placing the incision in the correct eyelid crease, sparing the lateral canthus of the eye, first performing the lateral incision onto the bone before extending the incision medially to avoid damaging the levator muscle, and drilling the lacrimal keyhole area to widen the surgical portal and to serve as a resting place for the endoscope are picked up by working with an oculoplastic surgeon. Sphenoid wing meningiomas often compress the optic nerve and the tumor can extend into the sphenoid sinus (Fig. 5.5). Multiportal surgery combining a binostril endonasal and/or precaruncular approach with the lateral approach allows for the tumor to be addressed through four portals (Fig. 5.6). An optic nerve canal and medial orbital decompression can be safely performed, together with resection of the sphenoid sinus component during the first stage of the procedure. This allows the optic nerve some "space" during the lateral approach when the eye is retracted medially, avoiding damage to the nerve [6].

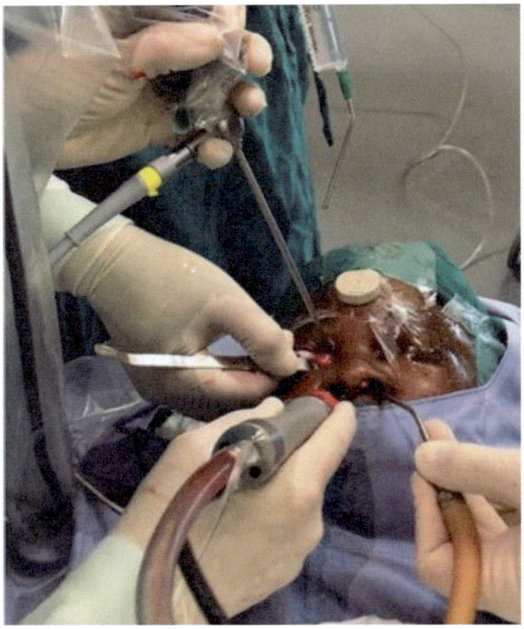

Fig. 5.6 Multiportal surgery and optic nerve decompression during sphenoid wing meningioma surgery

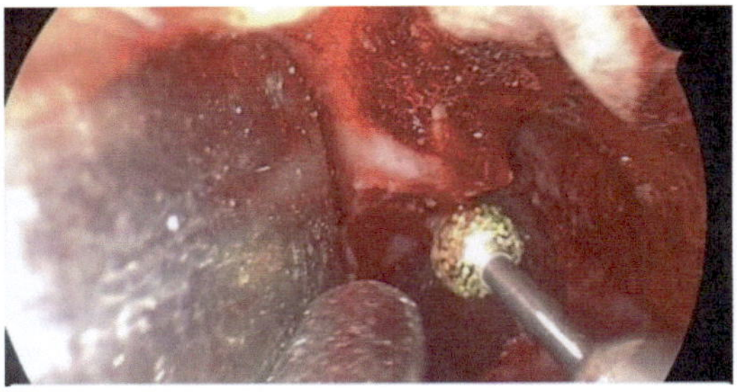

Fig. 5.7 Dural retractor retracting the right orbit laterally to allow for optic nerve decompression

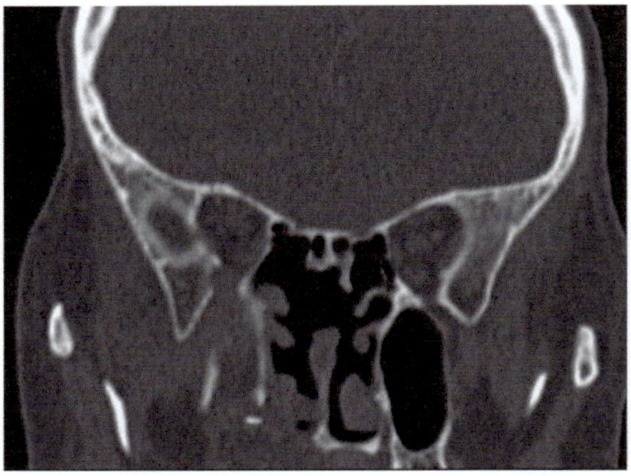

Fig. 5.8 Adenoid cystic carcinoma involving the right infraorbital nerve, maxillary sinus, and orbit

Combining the **transcaruncular approach with a standard ipsilateral or binostril** approach for optic nerve decompression allows retraction of orbital contents out of the ethmoid cavity. This is especially useful when significant proptosis is present. As the posterior 1/3 of the lamina papyracea is removed, orbital fat and medial rectus muscle may herniate into the posterior ethmoids because of the raised intraocular pressure. A dural retractor through a precaruncular incision assists with retraction of this tissue to allow safe drilling of the optic nerve canal (Fig. 5.7).

Tumors involving the maxillary sinus and extending into the inferior orbit or tracking along the infraorbital nerve can now be managed using an **endoscopic Denker's approach with an inferior conjunctival approach** (Fig. 5.8). The infraorbital nerve can be tracked posteriorly to the foramen rotundum. Reconstruction of the orbital floor can be performed through the inferior incision and/or a mucoperichondrial septal flap can be harvested.

The lateral aspect of the frontal sinus is not always fully accessible through an endoscopic Lothrop approach. Although angled scopes allow for full visualization, instrumentation at the target area is not always possible. A superior eyelid approach/eyebrow incision allows one to access the lateral aspect of a well-pneumatized sinus with a zero-degree endoscope and instruments. Pathology that often warrants a more traditional open approach (such as an osteoplastic flap) can be managed using a smaller incision placed in a natural crease line. Examples of pathology involving the lateral aspect of the frontal sinus that can be managed by a combination of an **endonasal and superior approaches** are mucocele, inverting papilloma, cerebrospinal fluid (CSF) leak, and osteomas.

Large angiofibromas can involve areas that are very difficult to access (Fig. 5.4). Once these tumors involve the lateral infratemporal fossa, temporal fossa, and cavernous sinus, alternative surgical strategies need to be entertained.

Multiportal surgery allows combining a binostril and endoscopic Denker's approach with a superior-lateral orbital and paramaxillary approach to allow for a push-pull technique. These techniques have been described in the literature and the only nuance is the use of the endoscope within these surgical portals.

Preoperative Assessment

Any patient undergoing a transorbital approach must have a basic ophthalmological assessment preoperatively. No ophthalmological abnormalities are expected when doing an anterior ethmoid artery ligation, for example, but it is still important to note the size of the pupils, eye movement, and visual acuity. Significant retraction of the globe or pressure on the rectus muscle or neurovascular structures can lead to postoperative complications. It is therefore important to note that no abnormalities are present prior to surgery.

When the periorbital fascia is breached to address extraconal or intraconal tumors, when the eye itself is involved with the disease process, or if any manipulation around the optic nerve or the superior orbital fissure is anticipated, then a full ophthalmological assessment is required—often including visual fields, fundoscopy, and optical coherence tomography (OCT). It is for this reason that it is good practice to always work with an ophthalmologist. Postoperative sequelae can often be difficult to understand and requires the input of a neuro-ophthalmologist to explain and manage transitory diplopia.

Computed tomography (CT) or MRI is essential and is usually performed using navigation protocols. This allows for preoperative planning to ensure the safest, shortest, most direct route to the target area is achieved.

Postoperative Care

Advantages of transorbital surgery are minimally invasive small incisions that often don't require suturing (the inferior and medial portals), minimal swelling at the incision site (managed with ice packs for the first 24 hours after surgery), and early postoperative recovery that allows early assessment of vision and eye movements. Depending on the pathology and extent of multiportal surgery, patients can often be discharged on the same day. Routine intraoperative antibiotics and intravenous dexamethasone are given during the surgery and only continued postoperatively if contamination occurred between the sinonasal cavity and orbit.

Starting a Service and Avoiding Complications

The easiest way to start a transorbital multiportal surgical service is to first identify surgeons who already have endoscopic skills. This would usually involve surgeons doing endoscopic transsphenoidal surgery and could be either an otolaryngology-neurosurgical team or neurosurgeons trained in endoscopy. The next step is to team up with an oculoplastic surgeon/ophthalmologist who is comfortable exploring the orbit and managing potential sequalae related to the surgery. It is important to start with a team that can comfortably work together, learn from each other, and master some of the skills of the other disciplines to perform surgery in the quickest and safest way. The superior-lateral approach for sphenoid wing meningiomas is a perfect example of multidisciplinary input. When starting out, this approach can be frustrating and lengthy because of the amount of hyperostotic bone that requires removal. The authors have learned that to create a surgical portal quickly, it is best that the lateral and superior orbital bony walls are drilled away with a high-speed cutting burr using surgical loupes only. A switch is made to a diamond burr once the temporalis muscle and dura are visualized through a thin layer of egg-shelled bone. At this stage, a zero-degree 4 mm endoscope is used to visualize the finer detail and to help identify the superior orbital fissure (SOF). The SOF is a good landmark for a "change of hands," where the neurosurgeon can expose the meningo-orbital band before incising the middle cranial fossa dura. Interdisciplinary dynamics and endoscopic experience will dictate the composition of the surgical team, but for middle cranial fossa pathology, it will usually consist of a neurosurgical team. The reconstruction, if required, will then be performed by the team performing the resection. This often only requires the placement of fat and fascia to seal the CSF leak.

A good surgical assistant is essential for transorbital surgery. It is not possible to retract the soft orbital tissues, pass the endoscope, and manipulate instruments as a single surgeon. Dural retractors of different widths are used to retract the orbit to create a wider surgical portal. Great care must be taken not to retract too forcefully to achieve a wider corridor, a natural reaction for an assistant trying to provide the primary surgeon with optimal visualization. Traction injuries include superior orbital fissure syndrome with multiple cranial neve palsies with resulting diplopia requiring corrective prisms or surgery.

It is of utmost importance that the transorbital team performs cadaveric dissections to familiarize themselves with the orbital anatomy. The surgical incisions are easy to master, but specific attention should be given to the function of key structures such as the levator muscle, medial and lateral canthal tendons, the insertion point of the trochlea, and the relationship of the orbital periosteum to the attachment of certain rectus muscles and the trochlea. Disregard for the function of these structures and damaging them can cause debilitating visual and cosmetic deformities.

Conclusions

Transorbital surgery can in short be divided into two groups:

1. Surgery on the eye itself—intraconal and extraconal.
2. Transorbital surgery where the periorbital fascia is left intact—used for access to other spaces.

In the first group, an ophthalmologist or neurosurgeon (if trained in orbital surgery) should always be present and involved. In the second group, the composition of the surgical team depends on the pathology that is to be addressed. For tumors/defects of the paranasal sinuses, an otolaryngologist will be the primary surgeon. For intracranial pathology, a neurosurgeon will be the main surgeon. The choice of assistant depends on institutional relationships and experience.

Transorbital surgery is a relatively new field that can be embraced by so many disciplines for their own unique pathology, including maxillofacial surgery, otolaryngology, neurosurgery, and ophthalmology. Each discipline will determine their own team composition, but the potential for novel techniques and instrumentation will increase with multidisciplinary surgery.

References

1. Moe KS, Bergeron CM, Ellenbogen RG. Transorbital neuroendoscopic surgery. Neurosurgery. 2010;67(3 Suppl Operative):ons16–28. https://doi.org/10.1227/01.NEU.0000373431.08464.43. PMID: 20679952.
2. Corvino S, Sacco M, Somma T, Berardinelli J, Ugga L, Colamaria A, Corrivetti F, Iaconetta G, Kong DS, de Notaris M. Functional and clinical outcomes after superior eyelid transorbital endoscopic approach for spheno-orbital meningiomas: illustrative case and literature review. Neurosurg Rev. 2022;46(1):17. https://doi.org/10.1007/s10143-022-01926-w. PMID: 36513789.
3. Kong DS, Moe KS. Editorial: endoscopic transorbital surgery for skull base tumors. Front Oncol. 2022;12:1042655. https://doi.org/10.3389/fonc.2022.1042655. PMID: 36387222; PMCID: PMC9648069.
4. Cornelis MM, Lubbe DE. Pre-caruncular approach to the medial orbit and landmarks for anterior ethmoidal artery ligation: a cadaveric study. Clin Otolaryngol. 2016;41(6):777–81. https://doi.org/10.1111/coa.12648. Epub 2016 Mar 29. PMID: 26987555.
5. Patel TA, Lubbe D. How we do it: using the Nasion as a landmark for identifying the anterior ethmoidal artery. J Laryngol Otol. 2022;137:1054. https://doi.org/10.1017/S0022215122002523.
6. Goncalves N, Lubbe DE. Transorbital endoscopic surgery for sphenoid wing meningioma: long-term outcomes and surgical technique. J Neurol Surg B Skull Base. 2020;81(4):357–68. https://doi.org/10.1055/s--0040-1713854. Epub 2020 Aug 20. PMID: 33072477; PMCID: PMC7561457.

6 Philosophy/Perspectives by Specialty: The Rhinology Perspective

Waleed M. Abuzeid and Dhruv Sharma

A History of Endoscopic Surgery in Rhinology

Innovative surgeons have been attempting to illuminate the dark and complex corridors of the sinonasal cavities for centuries. In 1743, Dr. Andre Levret, a French surgeon, used sunlight directed onto an angled mirror of his own design to visualize and ligate polyps in the nasal cavity [1]. Nearly a century later, in 1841, Dr. Friedrich Hofmann adapted the mirror to allow light to be reflected and focused by creating a concave head mirror with a central hole, which would ultimately come to define the twentieth-century otolaryngologist [2]. The development of the nasal speculum around 1860 by Coakley, in combination with head mirror transillumination, allowed for significantly improved visualization of the nasal cavity [3].

The sinuses continued to evade illumination until the turn of the century and development of endoscopes. Alfred Hirschman is credited with performing the first sinonasal endoscopy in 1901, utilizing a small cystoscope powered by a small electric bulb to visualize the maxillary sinus through an oroantral fistula. These early endoscopes were severely limited in brightness, depth of field, color rendition, and optical quality. A revolutionary technological advancement, which formed the foundation for the subsequent development of the field of rhinology, was the introduction of the rod-lens optical system. Professor Harold Hopkins, Chair in Optics at Reading University in the United Kingdom, developed rigid telescopes in the 1950s and patented his invention in 1959 [4, 5]. The rod-lens system consisted of a series of glass lenses with intervening segments of glass rather than air. This dramatically improved the optical efficiency of the scope by lowering the refractive index and increasing the functional diameter of the lenses culminating in improved light transmission, much improved image quality, an expanded field of view, and a more compact design [6]. Hopkins sold his patent on the rod-lens system to instrument maker Karl Storz of Tubingen, Germany, who produced and disseminated rigid endoscopes for endonasal surgery [4, 5]. In parallel with these advancements, fiber-optic technology was used to develop bright light sources that, coupled with the rod-lens rigid endoscope, finally allowed for superior illumination and excellent color fidelity of the surgical field.

The advantages of rigid nasal endoscopy were initially recognized by Professor Walter

W. M. Abuzeid (✉)
Division of Rhinology & Endoscopic Skull Base Surgery, Department of Otolaryngology: Head and Neck Surgery, University of Washington, Seattle, WA, USA
e-mail: wabuzeid@uw.edu

D. Sharma
Department of Otolaryngology: Head and Neck Surgery, University of Louisville, Louisville, KY, USA

T. H. Schwartz et al. (eds.), *Endoscopic Transorbital Surgery of the Orbit, Skull Base and Brain*,
https://doi.org/10.1007/978-3-031-59504-2_6

Messerklinger of Graz, Austria, a key figure in the development and propagation of endoscopic sinus surgery. Messerklinger had spent much of the 1950s and 1960s elucidating mucus drainage pathways in the sinonasal cavity and, harnessing the endoscope, introduced surgical techniques in 1972 to allow for the diagnosis and treatment of sinus disease in a near bloodless field. These surgical principles continued to be refined culminating in the Messerklinger technique, the basis of which was to open obstructed sinuses by removing anatomic structures compromising their natural ostia to reestablish drainage and ventilation [1, 5, 7]. The Messerklinger technique was propagated by Walter Messerklinger's assistant and eventual Head of Rhinology in Graz, Professor Heinz Stammberger. Based on the Graz experience of over 2500 endoscopic sinus surgeries, Stammberger published several landmark articles on the nascent field of endoscopic endonasal surgery in the 1970s and 1980s [5].

Sinus courses led by Stammberger soon became must-attend events for aspiring rhinologists all over the world and inspired Professor David Kennedy who, at the time, was on the faculty of the Department of Otolaryngology at Johns Hopkins University. Professor Kennedy was instrumental in the propagation of endoscopic endonasal surgery of the sinuses—which he later coined "functional endoscopic sinus surgery" (FESS)—in the United States. With colleagues from around the world, and through countless lectures, courses, and articles, Kennedy further refined the techniques and instruments of FESS, which became the catalyst for an explosion of interest in the expanding subspecialty of rhinology [5]. Over the subsequent 40 years, expertise in the use of transnasal endoscopic surgical techniques, particularly for FESS, became the calling card of the rhinologist.

The Influence of Rhinologists on Endoscopic Endonasal Skull Base Surgery

Neurosurgeons had described various approaches to the skull base but lacked the ability to adequately visualize, instrument, and repair their surgical explorations while minimizing patient morbidity [8]. Indeed, initial efforts in endoscopic endonasal skull base surgery by the neurosurgical community focused on the transsphenoidal approach to pituitary lesions with the endoscope used only as an adjunct to the widely popular microscopic approaches. The experience of rhinologists who, during this nascent phase of endoscopic skull base surgery, were already well versed in endonasal and sinus anatomy—largely through their practice of FESS—proved pivotal to the transition to purely endoscopic approaches, supplanting the microscope for surgical visualization.

In 1992, rhinologist Roger Jankowski, with otolaryngology and neurosurgical colleagues at the Central Hospital, University of Nancy, France, published the first series of purely endoscopic transsphenoidal approaches to pituitary adenomas in the *The Laryngoscope* journal [9]. Jankowski et al. described the use of the endoscope in three cases highlighting the rapidity by which sellar lesions could be accessed, the avoidance of septal dissection with a reduction in potential cosmetic or functional morbidities seen in traditional sublabial transseptal approaches, and the enhanced visualization of the target lesion, particularly those with suprasellar extension, and critical anatomy—including the carotid arteries and optic canals—using a combination of direct and angled endoscopes.

Skull base teams, consisting of otolaryngologists working in tandem with neurosurgeons, subsequently reported their experiences with purely endoscopic endonasal pituitary surgery [10–12]. Jho and Carrau, from the University of Pittsburgh Medical Center, pioneered this approach in the United States, reporting on 50 patients treated via a purely endoscopic approach [12]. These teams drove the development of dedicated endoscopic instrumentation for skull base surgery and heralded the introduction of such advancements as microvascular doppler ultrasonography and CT-and MR-based surgical navigation in pituitary surgery and, eventually, for lesions situated outside the sella [6].

The importance of endoscopic anatomy and the relationship between key anatomic landmarks had always been critical to safe dissection in the sinonasal cavity and skull base. Extended skull base approaches were founded on a detailed understanding of the sphenoid sinus as an anatomic landmark allowing for access to targets from the anterior cranial fossa to the odontoid process [6]. Expanded endonasal approaches have since revolutionized skull base surgery providing access to the entire ventral skull base. Anatomy-based surgical modules oriented in the sagittal plane provide access to median structures from the frontal sinus to the second cervical vertebra. Coronal plane modules are considered at three different depths and allow surgeons to tackle lesions of the paramedian skull base extending laterally to the midline of the orbital roof, from the lateral wall of the nasal cavity and sphenoid to the floor of the middle cranial fossa, and from the paraclival internal carotid artery and occipital condyles to the jugular foramen [13, 14].

Leveraging Advances and Understanding Limitations in Endoscopic Endonasal Surgery

Rhinologists leveraged the expertise gained with the rapid evolution of expanded endonasal approaches in the last 20 years and directly applied techniques and instrumentation to the treatment of rhinologic conditions. For example, the advent of multimodal surgical navigation using fused computed tomography (CT) and magnetic resonance (MR) imaging is seen as a promising alternative to traditional CT-based navigation in the treatment of sinonasal tumors, secondary to superior visualization of critical neurovascular anatomy and lesion boundaries. The principles of skull base reconstruction following skull base tumor resection including the use of vascularized flaps have been applied to the repair of non-iatrogenic skull base defects with cerebrospinal fluid leak including those related to idiopathic intracranial hypertension and other etiologies [15]. Powered drill instrumentation and ultrasonic bone aspirators, a mainstay of modern endoscopic skull base surgery, are now used to efficiently execute extended sinus approaches including the endoscopic modified medial maxillectomy, endoscopic Denker's approach, sphenoid nasalization, and aptly named frontal sinus drill-out (modified Lothrop or Draf III procedure) [5, 16–19]. These extended sinus approaches allow for marked increase in the size of the sinus ostia and are extensively used by rhinologists in the treatment of chronic sinusitis recalcitrant to conventional approaches, extirpation of sinonasal tumors, marsupialization of mucoceles, and repair of cerebrospinal fluid leaks.

Despite these advancements in sinonasal surgical access as understood and practiced by rhinologists over many years, there is a recognition in our field of significant limitations in the endoscopic endonasal approaches. Specifically, access to pathology situated lateral to the median and paramedian endoscopic corridors is challenging. Indeed, the median aspect of the ventral anterior cranial fossa makes up only 20% of the total surface area of the anterior skull base. The remaining area is situated lateral to the orbits, and access to these sites—incorporating the greater wing of the sphenoid, Meckel cave, lateral cavernous sinus, middle cranial fossa, petrous apex, and lateral posterior cranial fossa—via the endoscopic transnasal approach is typically not feasible as critical neurovascular structures such as the optic nerve or paraclival/parasellar internal carotid artery would need to be traversed [8, 20]. The need to mobilize a cranial nerve or major vessel should prompt the surgeon to consider alternative or additional approaches [13]. Pathology in the superior and lateral orbit—including disease secondary to complications of sinusitis such as mucoceles and abscesses—is inaccessible via an endoscopic transnasal route.

Furthermore, the endoscopic transnasal approach is fallible as it relates to accessing challenging locations in the paranasal sinuses. These locations harbor disease that is often the purview of the rhinologist, in contrast to more easily accessible sites that can be tackled by many general otolaryngologists following the democratization of FESS. Specifically, pathology affecting the superior, anterior, and lateral frontal sinus can be difficult if not impossible to instrument via the endoscopic transnasal corridor [21]. Though extended endoscopic approaches such as the frontal sinus drill-out/modified Lothrop procedure/Draf III can optimize visualization of these lesions, instrumentation of the superior, anterior, and lateral frontal sinus may be more limited compromising the ability to tackle benign and malignant tumors, osteomas, ossifying fibromas, allergic fungal sinusitis, mucoceles, and skull base defects, among other pathologies, in these areas. Consequently, rhinologists will often revert to external approaches such as frontal sinus trephination, external frontoethmoidectomy approach (Lynch procedure), or traditional osteoplastic flap [22]. The morbidity associated with external approaches can be significant including compromised cosmesis, postoperative pain, numbness or paresthesias, cerebrospinal fluid leak, and meningitis.

Given these limitations, academic rhinologists have sought to expand their surgical armamentarium with the addition of surgical approaches that would leverage their adeptness with endoscopic surgery while overcoming shortcomings in the endoscopic endonasal approach.

Endoscopic Transorbital Surgery as the Next Frontier

From the perspective of a rhinologist, an ideal surgical approach should allow (1) adequate exposure of the target lesion while minimizing morbidity to structures encountered on approach, (2) identification and protection of critical neurovascular structures, (3) a surgical field that does not constrain instrument excursion thereby preventing instrument collisions and facilitating safe dissection, and (4) the opportunity to address any related surgical complications including cerebrospinal fluid leak or significant hemorrhage. The endoscopic transorbital approach, originally described by Professor Kris Moe, an otolaryngologist, in 2010, meets all of the above criteria [20]. In this publication, a collection of transorbital approaches, grouped under the umbrella term "transorbital neuroendoscopic surgery" (TONES), were used to address diverse skull base pathology including cerebrospinal fluid leak, optic nerve decompression, repair of fractures, and extirpation of tumors. Since this landmark manuscript, the utility of endoscopic transorbital approaches for the management of sinonasal pathology has also been described as discussed below.

The endoscopic transorbital approach provides a direct approach to orbital, frontal sinus, and skull base pathology that is typically shorter than achievable via the endonasal route [8, 20, 23, 24]. The entirety of the orbit including the orbital apex is accessible, as is the width of the frontal sinus including the far lateral, anterior, and superior boundaries. The whole anterior cranial fossa and a significant portion of the middle cranial fossa can be accessed via a unilateral or bilateral transorbital approach that avoids crossing critical neurovascular structures. The skills required are a straightforward extension of the rhinologists' existing transnasal endoscopic techniques and further leverage well-developed psychomotor endoscopic skills. The transorbital approaches have been associated with minimal morbidity including minimally visible scars and temporary ptosis.

There is increased recognition that a combination of endoscopic approaches, so-called multiportal endoscopic surgery, may overcome the limitations associated with use of a single portal. These limitations include a limited working space, collision of instruments that are oriented in a coaxial plane, and an excessive portal entry-to-target distance. The endoscopic transorbital approaches can be used in concert with other portals including the endoscopic transnasal approaches and the recently described endoscopic paramaxillary approach to provide multivector access and instrumentation to a target lesion [24, 25]. Endoscopic transorbital surgery also maintains one of the key advantages of endoscopic expanded endonasal approaches: the two surgeon, four-handed technique. Beyond the technical advantages inherent to four-handed surgery, two or multi-surgeon procedures allow for continuous feedback in real time, harness the inherent expertise of each specialist to optimize operative decision-making, enhance efficiency, maintain motivation, and modulate enthusiasm [13].

Use of Endoscopic Transorbital Surgery in Rhinology

Frontal Sinus Mucoceles

There has been an explosion of reported endoscopic transorbital approaches in the literature over the last decade pertaining to rhinologic pathology. Lim and colleagues report on the use of TONES in a prospective series of 13 patient treated for a variety of sinogenic complications of acute or chronic sinusitis including epidural abscess, orbital and subperiosteal abscess with orbital apex syndrome, and fronto-orbital mucocele [26]. This series highlighted the advantages of the TONES approaches which are coplanar to the target lesion and, therefore, obviate the need for angled endoscopy. The direct access to the target lesion via a short surgical corridor was also aptly demonstrated in this series. All cases made extensive use of stereotactic image-guided surgical navigation, a technology that is now ubiquitous in the practice of rhinology, to plan the most direct transorbital pathway to the target lesion. In two of the reported cases, the endoscopic transorbital approach, via a precaruncular incision, was used to drain an orbital subperiosteal abscess and, because of orbital apex syndrome, to also decompress the entire intracanalicular course of the optic nerve to the dura using either a high-speed diamond drill or an ultrasonic bone aspirator. In another four patients, the abscess was located in the superolateral and posterior orbit—areas that would have been inaccessible via an endoscopic transnasal approach—and all patients underwent successful drainage with concurrent decompression of the infected frontal sinus, all through the endoscopic transorbital approach via a superior lid crease incision. Two patients underwent drainage of an epidural abscess via endoscopic transorbital corridor by creating a small craniotomy in the superior-posterior orbital wall to drain the abscess. The frontal sinus was also decompressed in both patients via the transorbital port by entering the frontal sinus from below through the orbital wall. Patency of the frontal recess demonstrated from "above" through FESS was also performed to address ethmoid sinus disease.

Lim et al. report five cases of chronic rhinosinusitis complicated by frontal sinus mucocele including one case in which frontal sinus obliteration had been performed and another in which endonasal decompression had previously been performed with subsequent recurrent mucocele [26]. Frontal sinus unobliteration and mucocele drainage were achieved transorbitally in all cases. In three of the cases, a unilateral frontal sinus mucocele was drained and the intersinus septum taken down via the transorbital corridor to allow for drainage of the involved sinus through the healthy, contralateral frontal recess. Ipsilateral FESS with frontal sinusotomy was also performed to further reduce the risk of mucocele recurrence. All patients in this case series had resolution of their symptoms with no complications noted.

A subsequent retrospective case series by Miller and colleagues further demonstrated the utility of the transorbital approach for drainage of frontal and fronto-orbital mucoceles arising from sequelae of chronic sinusitis or trauma in 17 patients [27]. This series also demonstrated the utility of a "cross court" approach whereby far lateral frontal sinus pathology—that was not accessible via a previously performed Draf III procedure—was accessed via a transorbital approach through the contralateral orbit via a transpalpebral superior lid crease incision. Indeed, other investigators have reported use of the endoscopic transorbital approach as a salvage procedure to drain mucoceles of the far lateral frontal sinus in cases where extended endonasal surgery involving Draf III sinusotomy has been unsuccessful [28]. The senior author of this chapter (WMA), working with his faculty partner (KSM, coeditor of this textbook), has used this approach in the drainage of unilateral recurrent frontal sinus mucocele as shown in Fig. 6.1.

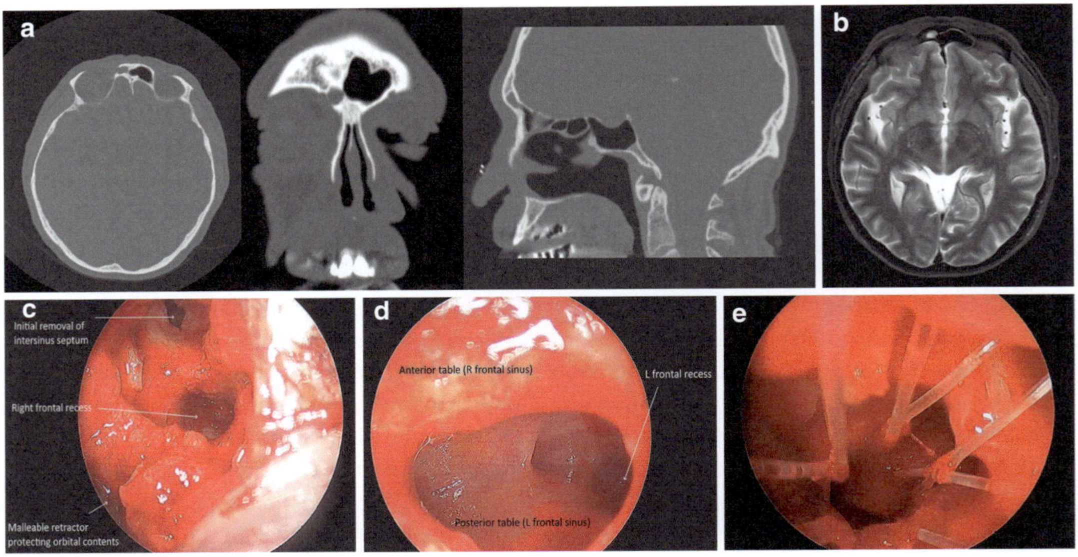

Fig. 6.1 (**a**) Axial, coronal, and sagittal CT views demonstrating recurrent right frontal sinus mucocele and very narrowed right frontal recess with 3 mm anteroposterior diameter. (**b**) MRI T2-weighted confirming right frontal sinus mucocele. (**c**) Right endoscopic transorbital view demonstrating the visualized right frontal recess following endoscopic transnasal frontal sinusotomy, partial removal of the intersinus septum at this stage of the surgery, and inferolateral retraction of orbital contents. (**d**) Right endoscopic transorbital view demonstrating complete removal of the intersinus septum establishing communication between the diseased right and normal left frontal sinuses. (**e**) Right endoscopic transorbital view with a 30-degree endoscope demonstrating the right frontal recess from above following completion of endoscopic transnasal frontal sinusotomy with placement of a drug-eluting dissolvable stent

Sinonasal Tumors

Benign and malignant neoplasms involving the sinonasal cavity and anterior and/or middle cranial fossa have also been addressed using endoscopic transorbital approaches, often in combination with endoscopic transnasal approaches. In one case series, the authors describe a sinonasal melanoma involving the anterior and middle cranial fossa (Fig. 6.2) [23]. The patient underwent surgery using the endoscopic transnasal and transorbital portals allowing for gross total resection of the tumor including the left olfactory nerve and involved periorbita. In this case, the transorbital corridor allowed for resection of the lateral margin of the tumor in the orbit with identification and preservation of key medial orbital structures which are directly visualized and can be dissected free of tumor. The skull base was reconstructed using cadaveric dermis. Final oncologic margins were negative. The patient had no postoperative visual complaints and, at 12 months, had no evidence of local disease recurrence but did have spinal metastases.

A case of frontal sinus osteoblastoma that involved the bilateral floor and the roof of the sinus with an associated fronto-orbital mucocele was addressed through bilateral transorbital approach for tumor resection and mucocele drainage and concurrent endoscopic modified Lothrop procedure to ensure adequate drainage of the entire frontal sinus [29]. The authors postulate that resection of the superior aspect of the tumor would have been a challenge using the modified Lothrop alone and may have necessitated external approaches such as trephination or osteoplastic flap had the transorbital approach not been used.

Juvenile nasopharyngeal angiofibroma (JNA) is a highly vascular benign tumor occurring most commonly in teenage males that is typically addressed by rhinologists through an endoscopic endonasal approach. Encroachment of the dis-

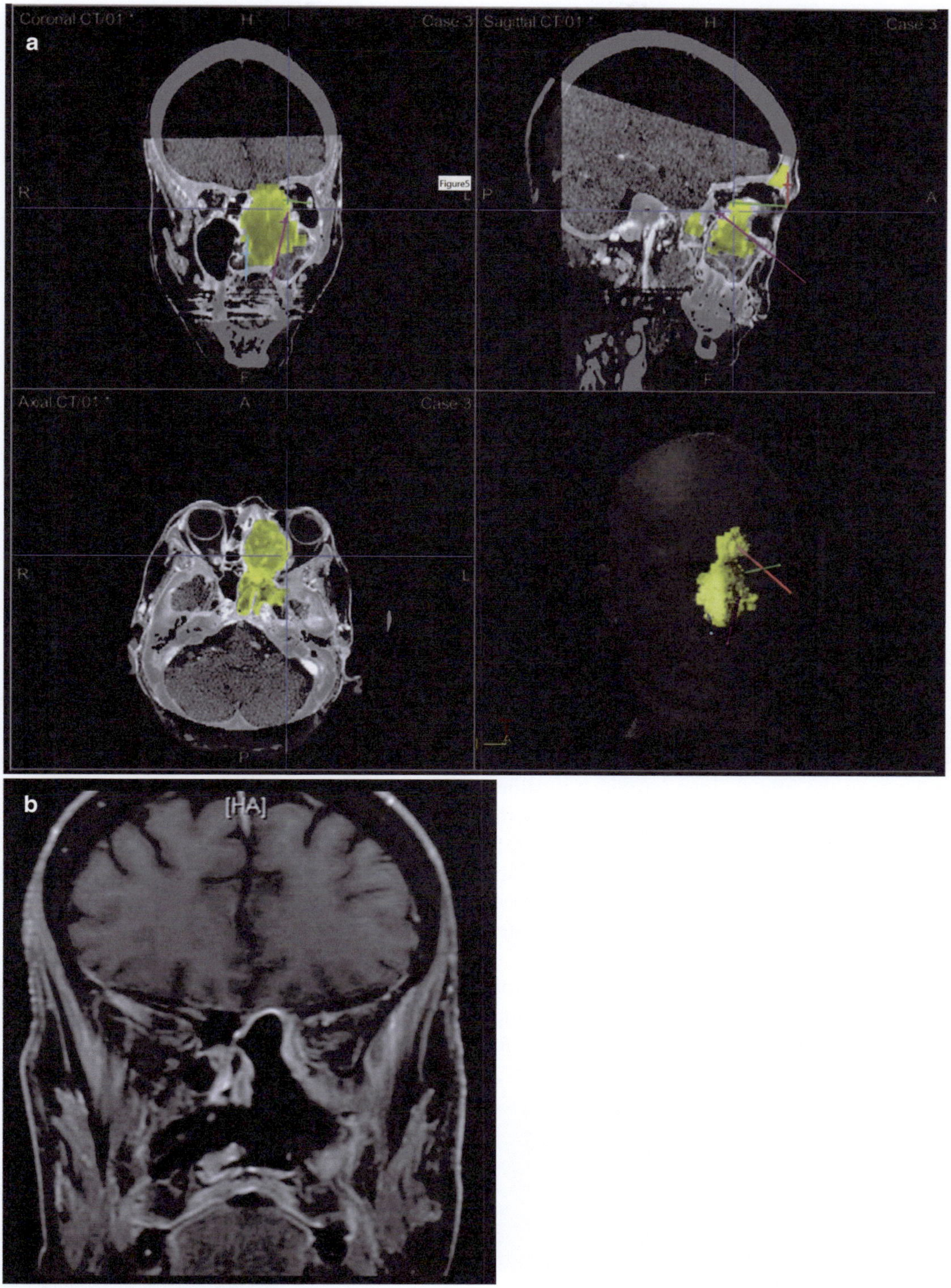

Fig. 6.2 (**a**) Coronal, sagittal, axial, and 3D reconstructed surface view of sinonasal melanoma. The tumor is colorized in yellow. Trajectory planning through the transnasal and transorbital portal is demonstrated. (**b**) Postoperative MRI T1 post-contrast indicating complete resection of the sinonasal melanoma [23]

ease into extrasinus structures such as the orbit or intracranial space often necessitates the use of external approaches. Janakiram and colleagues report the case of a 17-year-old male with an extensive JNA involving the right nasal cavity, sphenoid sinus, pterygopalatine fossa, infratemporal fossa, superior and inferior orbital fissures, cavernous sinus, and anterior temporal fossa [30]. An endoscopic modified Denker's approach and transpterygoid approach were used to resect the sinonasal and inferior orbital fissure components of the tumor. The remainder of the orbital disease at the superior orbital fissure and tumor within the middle cranial fossa was removed via an endoscopic transorbital approach. The surgeons describe a dynamic surgery using both portals in a three surgeon, six-handed fashion to achieve a near total resection with a small 5 mm residual portion of tumor noted on postoperative imaging that was abutting the posterior temporal lobe.

At the University of Washington, we have used the endoscopic transorbital approach extensively to address sinonasal tumors that have one or more components that cannot be addressed through the endoscopic endonasal approach. This includes benign and malignant tumors filling the entirety of the frontal sinus for which modified Lothrop procedure would not allow access to the far lateral or superior most extent of the sinus. In such cases, the endoscopic transorbital approach has allowed for achievement of gross total resection with reconstruction of any disease-related posterior table defect as needed.

The cases above illustrate the adjunctive role of the endoscopic transorbital approaches to augment the endoscopic endonasal approach for maximal operative working space and multivector approaches to the target lesion.

Cerebrospinal Fluid Rhinorrhea

Patients with cerebrospinal fluid rhinorrhea typically present to the office of a rhinologist given the symptom overlap with other rhinogenic causes of nasal drainage. Most skull base defects resulting in CSF rhinorrhea can be repaired via an endoscopic transnasal approach. However, the anatomic location of some defects limits optimal visualization via the endoscopic transnasal corridor. Ramakrishna et al., in their retrospective series of endoscopic transorbital approaches, discuss the treatment of 16 cases of CSF leak [23]. They describe a case of a patient with a Sternberg canal encephalocele causing erosion of the skull base (Fig. 6.3). A combined endoscopic transnasal and transorbital approach was used to visualize and reduce the encephalocele followed by placement of a cadaveric dermis underlay graft and a vascularized nasoseptal flap as an overlay graft. The repair proved durable and there were no visual complications.

In a reported case, a 65-year-old male with a history of orbital exenteration and radiotherapy for squamous cell carcinoma developed a high-flow orbital apex/middle cranial fossa CSF leak complicated by meningitis and pneumocephalus [31]. The patient underwent emergent surgery using a combined endoscopic transorbital and endonasal approach to reconstruct the temporal lobe and orbital defect using abdominal dermis fat and a pedicled nasoseptal flap. The transorbital port was critical for flap placement. The patient eventually recovered with resolution of the meningitis, pneumocephalus, and CSF leak.

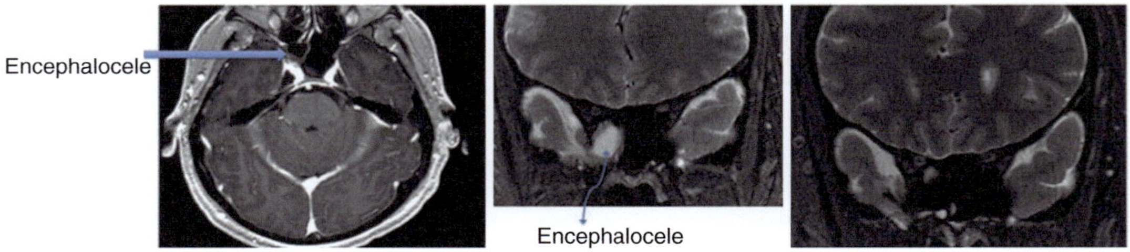

Fig. 6.3 (provisional approval obtained from publisher, formal approval pending) Left and center panel: Axial and coronal MRI T1 with contrast demonstrating encephalocele arising from Sternberg canal. Right panel: Postoperative coronal MRI T2 following resection of the encephalocele and skull base repair [23]

This dual port approach has also been used by rhinologists to reconstruct skull base defects associated with large meningoencephaloceles that impinge on the orbital contents, including in one case of iatrogenic skull base injury after orbital decompression surgery with an absent lamina papyracea, allowing for controlled dissection that protects the orbital contents and instrumentation from multiple angles that facilitate the placement and stabilization of the reconstruction construct [32].

The utility of the endoscopic transorbital approach, often as an adjunct to the traditional endoscopic endonasal approach, in repairing complex skull base defects will continue to be explored—and the boundaries of what can be achieved defined by rhinologists and their multidisciplinary colleagues in neurosurgery and ophthalmology.

Conclusion

Over the last 50 years, rhinologists have helped define the boundaries of what is achievable in endoscopic transnasal surgery. As minimization of functional and cosmetic morbidity and maximization of quality of life becomes increasingly important, the drive to expand beyond the transnasal route will only grow. A future in which a multidisciplinary team can safely and effectively address disease pathology using any number of endoscopic portals—be it transnasal, transorbital, paramaxillary, and/or other yet to be defined routes—edges closer to reality. Only through close collaboration with colleagues in neurosurgery, ophthalmology, radiology, and other related fields, iterative learning, and critical appraisal can the rhinologist continue to help define the state of the art.

References

1. Berryhill McCarty E, Frost A. Shedding light in otolaryngology: a brief history on the surgical tools of visualization and access. World J Otorhinolaryngol Head Neck Surg. 2022;8(3):245–8.
2. Lapena JF. Mirrors and reflections: the evolution of indirect laryngoscopy. Ann Saudi Med. 2013;33(2):177–81.
3. Leopold D. A history of rhinology in North America. Otolaryngol Head Neck Surg. 1996;115(4):283–97.
4. Linder TE, Simmen D, Stool SE. Revolutionary inventions in the 20th century. The history of endoscopy. Arch Otolaryngol Head Neck Surg. 1997;123(11):1161–3.
5. Kane KJ. The early history and development of functional endoscopic sinus surgery. J Laryngol Otol. 2020;134(1):8–13.
6. Prevedello DM, Doglietto F, Jane JA Jr, Jagannathan J, Han J, Laws ER Jr. History of endoscopic skull base surgery: its evolution and current reality. J Neurosurg. 2007;107(1):206–13.
7. Tajudeen BA, Kennedy DW. Thirty years of endoscopic sinus surgery: what have we learned? World J Otorhinolaryngol Head Neck Surg. 2017;3(2):115–21.
8. Schwartz TH, Henderson F Jr, Di Somma A, Kong DS, de Notaris M, Ensenat J, et al. Endoscopic Transorbital surgery: another leap of faith? World Neurosurg. 2022;159:54–5.
9. Jankowski R, Auque J, Simon C, Marchal JC, Hepner H, Wayoff M. Endoscopic pituitary tumor surgery. Laryngoscope. 1992;102(2):198–202.
10. Carrau RL, Jho HD, Ko Y. Transnasal-transsphenoidal endoscopic surgery of the pituitary gland. Laryngoscope. 1996;106(7):914–8.
11. Cappabianca P, Alfieri A, de Divitiis E. Endoscopic endonasal transsphenoidal approach to the Sella: towards functional endoscopic pituitary surgery (FEPS). Minim Invasive Neurosurg. 1998;41(2):66–73.
12. Jho HD, Carrau RL. Endoscopic endonasal transsphenoidal surgery: experience with 50 patients. J Neurosurg. 1997;87(1):44–51.
13. Kasemsiri P, Carrau RL, Ditzel Filho LF, Prevedello DM, Otto BA, Old M, et al. Advantages and limitations of endoscopic endonasal approaches to the skull base. World Neurosurg. 2014;82(6 Suppl):S12–21.
14. Martinez-Perez R, Requena LC, Carrau RL, Prevedello DM. Modern endoscopic skull base neurosurgery. J Neuro-Oncol. 2021;151(3):461–75.
15. Campbell RG, Farquhar D, Zhao N, Chiu AG, Adappa ND, Palmer JN. Cerebrospinal fluid rhinorrhea secondary to idiopathic intracranial hypertension: long-term outcomes of endoscopic repairs. Am J Rhinol Allergy. 2016;30(4):294–300.
16. Takakura H, Tachino H, Oi Y, Do TA, Shojaku H. Novel application of an ultrasonic bone aspirator for endoscopic modified medial Maxillectomy. Front Surg. 2022;9:870380.
17. Massey CJ, Bury S, Diamond J, Singh A. Novel use of an ultrasonic bone aspirator for extended endoscopic frontal sinusotomy: a feasibility study. Am J Rhinol Allergy. 2016;30(6):443–7.
18. Chin D, Snidvongs K, Kalish L, Sacks R, Harvey RJ. The outside-in approach to the modified

endoscopic Lothrop procedure. Laryngoscope. 2012;122(8):1661–9.
19. McCormick JP, Suh JD, Wang EW, DeConde AS, Wang MB, Yang HH, et al. Modified endoscopic Denker's approach for Management of anterior maxillary sinus tumors: multicenter series of 58 cases. Am J Rhinol Allergy. 2022;36(6):763–72.
20. Moe KS, Bergeron CM, Ellenbogen RG. Transorbital neuroendoscopic surgery. Neurosurgery. 2010;67(3 Suppl Operative):ons16–28.
21. Becker SS, Bomeli SR, Gross CW, Han JK. Limits of endoscopic visualization and instrumentation in the frontal sinus. Otolaryngol Head Neck Surg. 2006;135(6):917–21.
22. Georgalas C, Goudakos J, Fokkens WJ. Osteoma of the skull base and sinuses. Otolaryngol Clin N Am. 2011;44(4):875–90. vii
23. Ramakrishna R, Kim LJ, Bly RA, Moe K, Ferreira M Jr. Transorbital neuroendoscopic surgery for the treatment of skull base lesions. J Clin Neurosci. 2016;24:99–104.
24. Ciporen JN, Moe KS, Ramanathan D, Lopez S, Ledesma E, Rostomily R, et al. Multiportal endoscopic approaches to the central skull base: a cadaveric study. World Neurosurg. 2010;73(6):705–12.
25. Konuthula N, Abuzeid WM, Humphreys IM, Bly RA, Moe K. Endoscopic paramaxillary approach to the infratemporal fossa and pterygomaxillary space: computer modeling analysis and clinical series. J Neurol Surg B Skull Base. 2022;83(Suppl 2):e514–e20.
26. Lim JH, Sardesai MG, Ferreira M Jr, Moe KS. Transorbital neuroendoscopic management of sinogenic complications involving the frontal sinus, orbit, and anterior cranial fossa. J Neurol Surg B Skull Base. 2012;73(6):394–400.
27. Miller C, Berens A, Patel SA, Humphreys IM, Moe KS. Transorbital approach for improved access in the management of paranasal sinus Mucoceles. J Neurol Surg B Skull Base. 2019;80(6):593–8.
28. Arosio AD, Coden E, Valentini M, Czaczkes C, Battaglia P, Bignami M, et al. Combined endonasal-transorbital approach to manage the far lateral frontal sinus: surgical technique. World Neurosurg. 2021;151:5.
29. Hicks KL, Moe KS, Humphreys IM. Bilateral transorbital and transnasal endoscopic resection of a frontal sinus Osteoblastoma and orbital Mucocele: a case report and review of the literature. Ann Otol Rhinol Laryngol. 2018;127(11):864–9.
30. Janakiram TN, Parekh P, Haneefa H, Prasad SK. Endoscopic three-surgeon six-handed transorbital transnasal technique for excision of juvenile nasopharygeal angiofibroma: new frontier explored. Asian J Neurosurg. 2017;12(4):790–3.
31. Lucke-Wold B, Mendez G, Cua D, Akins P, Gillham H, Ciporen J. Combined endoscopic Transorbital and Endonasal repair of high flow orbital apex/ middle fossa cerebrospinal fluid leak with a Nasoseptal flap. J Neuroinflamm Neurodegener Dis. 2018;2(1):100005.
32. Schaberg M, Murchison AP, Rosen MR, Evans JJ, Bilyk JR. Transorbital and transnasal endoscopic repair of a meningoencephalocele. Orbit. 2011;30(5):221–5.

7 The Orbital and Oculoplastic Surgery Perspective

Sayyada Hyder, Allison Coombs, and Kyle J. Godfrey

Introduction

Transorbital approaches to the brain and skull base may offer patients and surgeons certain advantages in judiciously selected cases but also carry inherent risks to the visual system. Mitigation of these risks is aided by strategic, multidisciplinary collaboration between orbital surgeons and neurological surgeons. Depending on the patient's pathology, provider practice patterns, and resources in each institution, the clinical care team may also include otorhinolaryngologists and nonsurgical neuro-ophthalmologists. This collaboration extends from preoperative patient selection and evaluation, shared intraoperative perspective, and critical evaluation and optimization of postoperative outcomes.

Orbital surgeons, also called oculoplastic or oculofacial surgeons, are fellowship-trained ophthalmologists subspecialized in surgery of the delicate and anatomically complex soft tissues surrounding the eyes, including the eyelids, orbital contents, globes, and bony orbit. The orbital surgeon's experience operating within the orbit enhances neurosurgical access through various minimally invasive approaches to the orbit and concurrently enhances safety when utilizing an orbital corridor. In fact, transorbital approaches to the anterior and middle crania fossae are a natural evolution and extension of minimally invasive orbital decompression surgery performed commonly by oculoplastic and orbital surgeons. This highly relevant experience in orbital surgical approach and deep orbital surgery can be leveraged by neurosurgeons utilizing transorbital approaches. The orbital surgeon's skill set augments the neurosurgical and skull-base surgery team approach through detailed preoperative ophthalmologic analysis of the visual system including appropriate patient selection and risk stratification, intraoperative experience with orbital anatomy and tissue handling, and postoperative monitoring of the visual system and orbit to appropriately identify and treat complications and facilitate comprehensive, critical evaluation of surgical outcomes. Through collegial and patient-focused collaboration, orbital surgeons, otorhinolaryngologists, and neurological surgeons can ensure individual patient outcomes are optimized and the broader scientific study of this surgical corridor will allow surgeons to select the least morbid, most effective approach to their patient's pathology.

S. Hyder · A. Coombs
Department of Ophthalmology, Weill Cornell Medical College, New York, NY, USA
e-mail: sah4015@nyp.org; alc2053@med.cornell.edu

K. J. Godfrey (✉)
Department of Ophthalmology, Weill Cornell Medical College, New York, NY, USA

Department of Neurological Surgery, Weill Cornell Medical College, New York, NY, USA
e-mail: kyg9004@med.cornell.edu

T. H. Schwartz et al. (eds.), *Endoscopic Transorbital Surgery of the Orbit, Skull Base and Brain*,
https://doi.org/10.1007/978-3-031-59504-2_7

Preoperative Considerations: Patient Selection, Evaluation of the Visual System and Ocular Adnexae, and Patient Counseling

Careful preoperative evaluation, including consultation with an orbital surgeon, helps optimize the success and safety of transorbital neurological surgery. The ophthalmologic assessment ensures appropriate surgical candidacy, documents the baseline status of the visual system, and enables appropriate counseling of vision-related risks, benefits, and expectations for deep orbital surgery. Through thoughtful discussion between the patient and the surgical team, an optimal approach can be selected for each patient.

When considering a transorbital approach, the afferent and efferent visual system is assessed by the orbital surgeon. Identification of subtle cranial neuropathies and visual dysfunction preoperatively helps distinguish disease-related findings from iatrogenic or surgically induced sequalae during postoperative evaluation. This comprehensive visual, orbital, and ophthalmologic assessment often includes, but is not always limited to, best corrected visual acuity, pupillary examination, extraocular motility, intraocular pressure, color vision testing, automated perimetry, and optical coherence tomography of the optic nerve and ganglion cell layer. Globe position, including quantitative exophthalmometry (e.g., Hertel or Naugle), is assessed, as well as eyelid position and function; related measurements include levator palpebrae superior function, margin-reflex distance 1, and margin-reflex distance 2. The patient should be evaluated for any risk factors for postoperative lagophthalmos, abnormal periorbital sensation, and ocular alignment. Additionally, a comprehensive eye examination, including evaluation of the cornea, anterior chamber, lens, vitreous, retina, and optic nerve, is performed to identify any underlying pathology which may warrant treatment or that may place the visual system at higher risk for damage during transorbital surgery. Relative contraindications to deep orbital surgery include, but are not limited to, recent intraocular surgery or destabilizing globe injury, inflammatory conditions of the orbit, and prior orbital surgery which may have compromised surgical planes or distorted anatomy [1, 2]. Care should be taken with preoperative counseling of patients on anticoagulants or with bleeding dyscrasias, as orbital hemorrhage may result in vision loss (detailed later in this chapter). Diseases of the optic nerve which may be exacerbated by fluctuation in intraocular pressure or optic nerve retraction, such as glaucoma, should be identified and optimized, as manipulation during transorbital surgery can create catastrophic visual compromise [3]. When appropriate, alternative approaches (e.g., transnasal, pterional craniotomy, or frontotemporal craniotomy) should be selected in patients who are deemed high-risk transorbital patients after appropriate discussion between the patient, orbital surgeon and ophthalmology specialists, and neurological surgery team.

Patients should be thoroughly counseled regarding risks associated with extended deep orbital surgery and the retraction required to facilitate adequate surgical exposure in these cases. All patients will have some degree of postoperative edema and ecchymosis, which may persist beyond 2 weeks. Patients should additionally be counseled about potential postoperative changes in globe position, such as exophthalmos or hypoglobus, which may influence the perceived esthetic outcome. Additionally, eyelid height and function may be altered transiently or permanently (e.g., ptosis). Risks of visual dysfunction, including, but not limited to, transient or permanent decrease in vision, loss of vision, or double vision, should be discussed.

Of additional preoperative consideration is the route of access to the orbit and the specific risks associated with each approach. Access to the deep orbit for transorbital endoscopic surgery can be accomplished via eyelid crease-based approaches, conjunctival-based approaches, and canthal-based approaches (discussed in additional detail elsewhere in this chapter and book), which have infrequent risks of functional changes, cosmetically significant scarring, or eyelid malposition, and should be discussed thoroughly. Finally, a discussion regarding alterations in facial nerve sensation, commonly hypoesthesia around the orbit, should be noted as a possible adverse effect from the transorbital approach. This is most common in the distribution of cranial nerves V1 and V2, particularly in the distribution of the perforating zygomaticofacial and zygomaticotemporal branches in the lateral wall of the orbit which may require sacrifice during the approach to facilitate adequate exposure.

Through comprehensive preoperative ophthalmologic evaluation with the operating orbital surgeon, patients can be appropriately selected, counseled, and risk stratified for transorbital neurosurgical approaches. Identifying the baseline functionality and health of the visual system prior to surgical intervention is imperative to identify appropriate candidates for this surgical approach and to establish baseline characteristics to facilitate the critical assessment of postoperative surgical outcomes.

Intraoperative Considerations: Surgical Approach, Navigating the Orbit, Intraoperative Monitoring of the Visual System, and Managing Intraoperative Adverse Events

Traditional craniotomy-based approaches to the brain and skull base have well-established morbidities. In appropriately selected patients, and with experienced surgical teams, the risk profile of a transorbital approach may be favorable. The orbital surgeon can offer an armamentarium of minimally invasive surgical approaches to the orbital corridor that can broadly be categorized as eyelid crease based, canthal based, or conjunctival based.

The surgical approach is selected based on several factors, although the preeminent consideration is the location of the pathology relative to the optic nerve. An extended discussion on surgical approaches to the orbit is beyond the scope of this book. However, selected surgical approaches relevant to transorbital neurosurgery will be detailed in other chapters, and a few relevant considerations are discussed here from an orbital surgeon's perspective.

Eyelid crease-based approaches have become the workhorse transorbital approach to the anterior and middle cranial fossae at the authors' institution. The preoperative marking of the eyelid crease is critical and should be approached with consideration to the patient's gender, ethnicity, age, and the height and shape of the contralateral eyelid crease. To this end, dynamic assessment with the patient awake and seated in an upright position and marking with a fine-tipped pen may facilitate the most anatomically and esthetically optimal incision. In younger patients, the marking should not extend past the lateral canthus whenever possible due to the increased risks of cosmetically significant scarring beyond the lateral canthus. However, when properly marked and closed, the morbidity of this incision is minimal, and adequate exposure should be prioritized to minimize the force of necessary retraction of the orbital contents, including the levator palpebrae superioris aponeurosis anteriorly and the superior orbital fissure and optic canal contents posteriorly.

After the skin is incised and the orbicularis oculi is divided, the orbital surgeon follows a preseptal course to the orbital rim to avoid herniation of orbital fat and iatrogenic damage to the levator palpebrae superioris and other post-septal orbital structures. Similarly, after the periosteum is incised at the arcus marginalis, a subperiosteal plane is then carried posteriorly into the deep orbit to expose the superior and inferior orbital fissures. This approach allows wide access to the superior and lateral orbit and can be further extended to provide access to the superomedial aspect of the orbit. With the exposure facilitated by this approach, targeted osteotomies in the frontal and sphenoid bones can be created, allowing the endoscope-assisted surgeon to access much of the skull base, including the anterior and middle cranial fossae, the lateral cavernous sinus, Meckel's cave, and the lateral posterior fossa [4].

Given the subperiosteal plane utilized in the eyelid crease-based approach and that the orbital contents are largely bypassed in the orbital corridor used to access the orbital apex and transorbital osteotomy sites, the primary surgical morbidity to the eyelid and orbit relates to the necessary retraction of the orbital soft tissues, particularly, the delicate neurovascular structures passing through the superior orbital fissure and optic canal at the orbital apex. To minimize neuropraxia, or more significant injury, retraction must be exquisitely delicate and dynamic as the case progresses, utilizing the minimal necessary amount of retraction in each moment to facilitate adequate exposure. Rigid fixation of instruments and retractors is avoided. During the dissection of the superior orbital fissure, often referred to surgically as the sagittal crest, frequent retraction breaks should be taken to relieve pressure from the optic nerve, superior ophthalmic vein, the tightly clustered cranial nerves 3, 4, 5, and 6, and the sympathetic fibers in the superior orbital fissure [5]. To this end, in certain cases, removal and replacement of the lateral orbital rim may improve the angle of approach to selected pathology. There is minimal postoperative morbidity to lateral marginotomy, and when a more oblique angle of approach is required, careful consideration should be considered to incorporating this adjunctive step.

Additionally, to avoid iatrogenic damage to these nerves, monopolar cautery should always be avoided within the orbit in favor of bipolar cautery [6]. During retraction breaks, the pupil can be assessed. Frequent pupillary assessment intraoperatively aids in monitoring the optic nerve and visual system to ensure that excess force is not being applied to the orbital apex during retraction. Although the presence of stable pupil does not ensure retraction is appropriate, evidence of pupillary dilation suggests direct optic nerve compression or may indicate compression of the lateral ciliary ganglion at the orbital apex through which the parasympathetic pupillary fibers pass. Additionally, proper technique and positioning while retracting orbital tissues minimizes pressure on the globe and torque on the optic nerve and muscles.

More anteriorly, the cornea and anterior aspect of the globe are protected with corneal shields lubricated with ophthalmic lubricant. It is often helpful to drape the patients in a manner that enables visualization of both eyes during surgery to facilitate intraoperative assessment of relative globe position. To avoid damage to the ocular surface, Betadine can be used to prep the eyelids, but chlorhexidine should not be used.

Following any intradural work by the neurological surgery team, at the conclusion of the case, attention is directed to reconstruction of the orbit. When approaching reconstruction of the orbit, decisions are made collaboratively between the orbital surgeon and the neurosurgeon incorporating all factors related to the surgical pathology, location, osteotomy size, and presence and size of any dura mater defect. While symmetry in postoperative exophthalmometry and globe position is the gold standard, priority is given to minimizing iatrogenic risks to visual function from compression of soft tissues at the orbital apex with anticipated postoperative edema and to minimizing the risks of other surgical complications such as cerebrospinal fluid leak and infection. In cases of small surgical osteotomies, following any necessary dural reconstruction by the neurosurgery team, more extensive orbital reconstruction may be deferred. In cases of larger osteotomies, consideration can be given to the placement of free fat grafts, customized absorbable sheets (e.g., polydioxanone), or nonabsorbable orbital implants (e.g., porous polyethylene). Orbital reconstruction may be deferred in hyperostotic meningioma in cases of anticipated recurrence or subtotal resection. Soft tissue closure is performed in a layered, esthetically optimal fashion standard for orbital surgery. An ophthalmic pressure patch is typically placed for extubation and removed in the recovery area at which time vision and ocular motility are assessed.

Postoperative Assessment

Patients undergoing transorbital neurological surgery require close postoperative monitoring to identify and manage any complications and are typically admitted to the hospital for postoperative observation for one to two days. Immediately postoperatively, the patient is monitored closely for the development of retrobulbar hemorrhage and orbital compartment syndrome or orbital apex syndrome. The risk of orbital compartment syndrome and orbital apex syndrome is greater with longer duration surgeries, in the management of vascular lesions and in patients taking preoperative anticoagulation [7]. This risk can be minimized by achieving successful hemostasis intraoperatively, followed by the placement of a pressure patch over the surgical orbit during extubation. Deep extubation from general anesthesia is preferable, and communication with the anesthesia team is critical to avoid Valsalva during extubation, when possible. In the event of a retrobulbar orbital hemorrhage, the ophthalmologist's skill set can be utilized for management of this emergent complication, necessitating emergent lateral canthotomy and cantholysis or reopening of the surgical wound to relieve the resultant orbital compartment syndrome. Vision loss from optic nerve ischemia can occur rapidly in orbital compartment syndrome and must be monitored for, and addressed, immediately [8].

Postoperatively, patients are typically prescribed a systemic steroid taper, topical steroid-antibiotic ophthalmic ointment to the incision, and a frequent icing regimen. Following discharge, ophthalmologic follow-up is typically coordinated for one-week and three-month intervals. The outpatient postoperative assessment includes the same detailed ophthalmologic examination that was performed preoperatively.

In the authors' experience, postoperative ophthalmologic complications are typically transient neuropraxias presumed to be secondary to retraction at the orbital apex (e.g., ptosis, motility deficits, hypoesthesia). However ophthalmologic assessment is critical to differentiate transient complications from those requiring time-sensitive intervention to prevent long-term visual sequelae [9]. Given that the periorbita is not violated during these approaches, and osteotomy volumes are small, cosmetically significant enophthalmos and the need for extensive orbital reconstruction are rare in the authors' experience.

Conclusion

Transorbital approaches to select intracranial pathology may have favorable risk profiles and outcomes when compared with traditional craniotomy approaches in appropriately selected patients cared for by experienced multidisciplinary teams. As these approaches disseminate in the neurosurgical community, it will be advantageous to leverage the collective experience of orbital surgeons and approach such cases in a collaborative, multidisciplinary fashion whenever possible. Morbidity to the visual system, in experienced hands, will primarily be related to retraction at the orbital apex. Accordingly, adequate exposure while minimizing orbital soft-tissue retraction at the apex should be prioritized, regardless of the specific approach utilized. Decisions regarding orbital reconstruction should be tailored to the individual patient and case, with priority given to minimizing risks to visual function. Critical evaluation of ophthalmologic outcomes enabling multidisciplinary collaboration will help optimize case selection and surgical techniques and advance this innovative field safely.

References

1. Dallan I, Cristofani-Mencacci L, Fiacchini G, Caniglia M, Sellari-Franceschini S, Berrettini S. When multidisciplinary surgical trans-orbital approaches should be considered to reach the skull base. Acta Otorhinolaryngol Ital. 2021;41(Suppl. 1):S59–66. https://doi.org/10.14639/0392-100X-suppl.1-41-2021-06. PMID: 34060521; PMCID: PMC8172113.
2. Locatelli D, Dallan I, Castelnuovo P. Surgery around the orbit: how to select an approach. J Neurol Surg B Skull Base. 2020;81(4):409–21. https://doi.org/10.1055/s-0040-1713893. Epub 2020 Sep 21. PMID: 33072481; PMCID: PMC7561455.
3. Holländer H, Makarov F, et al. Evidence of constriction of optic nerve axons at the lamina cribrosa in the normotensive eye in humans and other mammals. Ophthalmic Res. 1995;27(5):296–309.
4. Schwartz TH, Henderson F, et al. Endoscopic transorbital surgery: another leap of faith? World Neurosurg. 2022;159:54–5.
5. Corrivetti F, de Notaris M, Di Somma A, Dallan I, Enseñat J, Topczewski T, Solari D, Cavallo LM, Cappabianca P, Prats-Galino A. "Sagittal crest":

definition, stepwise dissection, and clinical implications from a transorbital perspective. Oper Neurosurg (Hagerstown). 2022;22(5):e206–12. https://doi.org/10.1227/ons.0000000000000131.
6. Schietroma JJ, Tenzel RR. The effects of cautery on the optic nerve. Ophthalmic Plast Reconstr Surg. 1990;6(2):102–7. https://doi.org/10.1097/00002341-199006000-00004.
7. Saul N. Rajak, Richard G. Douglas. et al. Postoperative care and complications following open and endoscopic orbital surgery.
8. McCallum E, Keren S, Lapira M, Norris JH. Orbital compartment syndrome: an update with review of the literature. Clin Ophthalmol. 2019;13:2189–94. https://doi.org/10.2147/OPTH.S180058. PMID: 31806931; PMCID: PMC6844234.
9. Foulsham W, North VS, Botsford BW, Dinkin MJ, Henderson F Jr, Godfrey KJ, D'Amico DJ, Schwartz TH, Orlin A. Multilayered macular hemorrhages as an unusual complication of transorbital neuroendoscopic surgery. Am J Ophthalmol Case Rep. 2022;26:101556. https://doi.org/10.1016/j.ajoc.2022.101556. PMID: 35514795; PMCID: PMC9062224.

Lateral Transorbital Surgery: The Neurosurgeon's Perspective

8

Theodore H. Schwartz

Introduction

Twenty years ago, if you had told the neurosurgery community that in a mere two decades, skull base surgeons would be working through the nostrils using endoscopes to remove not merely pituitary tumors but also craniopharyngiomas, chordomas, chondrosarcomas, and tuberculum sella meningiomas, your remarks would have been met with raised eyebrows and a few polite chuckles. From our current perspective, it's now difficult to imagine *not* removing these tumors using an extended endoscopic endonasal approach (EEA). EEA provides a unique perspective to an area of the brain that is difficult to expose without manipulating, and possibly damaging, the very anatomy we are trying so desperately to preserve. Whether outcomes have improved compared with more traditional transcranial approaches is still a matter of debate, but one would certainly never be faulted for choosing an EEA, which has now become a widely accepted neurosurgical technique.

To some of us in the skull base community, it has become more and more apparent that lateral transorbital approach (TOA) (and I am limiting this discussion to the lateral approach since it is the one most employed by neurosurgeons) is poised to explode into our collective neurosurgical consciousness as a similarly powerful minimal access approach that can expose specific areas of the skull base that have vexed neurosurgeons for decades [1–3]. The idea of using the orbit, already crowded with our most precious sensory organ, as a corridor for surgery, seems counterintuitive and even in direct conflict to our primary maxim, *primum non nocere.* The purpose of this chapter is to understand the philosophical basis of TOA and how it arose from EEA and then provide an overview of some of the targets for TOA to assist the neurosurgeon with case selection. As with any minimally invasive keyhole skull base approach, the key to success is case selection.

Philosophy

The development and successful implementation of EEA rested on a collaboration between two surgical subspecialties: otorhinolaryngology and neurosurgery. Neurosurgeons had previously attempted a ventral approach, transsphenoidal or transoral, to reach the midline skull base but lacked the instrumentation, ability to visualize, and skill to repair their surgical explorations with

T. H. Schwartz (✉)
Department of Neurosurgery, Weill Cornell Medicine, New York–Presbyterian Hospital, New York, NY, USA
e-mail: schwarh@med.cornell.edu

T. H. Schwartz et al. (eds.), *Endoscopic Transorbital Surgery of the Orbit, Skull Base and Brain*,
https://doi.org/10.1007/978-3-031-59504-2_8

acceptable morbidity. Leveraging the expertise of the rhinology community and their facility with endoscopic sinus surgery provided the required innovative perspective to overcome these limitations.

Likewise, the TOA emerged from the work of forward-thinking otorhinolaryngology and oculoplastic surgeons who provided the initial impetus, using their viewpoint to look past its conventional boundaries [1–3]. Just as the EEA allows the surgeon access to the suprasellar cistern, medial cavernous sinus, and clivus from a new point of view, so, too, does the TOA expose the greater wing of the sphenoid, Meckel's cave, lateral cavernous sinus, and temporal pole together with the middle cranial fossa, petrous apex, and lateral aspects of the posterior fossa. The TOA provides exposure on the far side of the paraclival and parasellar internal carotid artery, generally considered the lateral limit of the EEA. Both approaches leverage natural corridors that require removal of normal anatomy, for the EEA the nasal sinuses and for the lateral TOA the bone of the orbit, mostly the greater wing of the sphenoid bone. What is lost in "nonessential" anatomy is gained in exposure, a trade-off made to reduce potential risk to more vital structures.

From the neurosurgeon's perspective, the lateral TOA provides access to some of the same locations of the skull base that can be reached with other approaches and thus can be used as a minimal access substitute. For example, the pterional, minipterional, and orbitozygomatic can be used to reach the mid- and inner portions of the lesser wing of the sphenoid as well as the anterior clinoid process. The lateral TOA also exposes these areas, but the TOA cannot access the lateral portion of the lesser sphenoid wing. Pathologies in these locations would be better suited to an open approach. Likewise, the medial aspect of the greater wing of the sphenoid, bordered by foramen rotundum, ovale, and spinosum, can all be exposed via the TOA. Regions including the floor of the middle fossa, the cavernous sinus, and Meckel's cave, which might require a Dolenc approach or a subtemporal approach with or without a zygomatic osteotomy, can all be reached with the TOA. Once again, the lateral aspects of these approaches, on the other hand, cannot be exposed. Case selection is critical. Of note, lateral sphenoid encephaloceles, often repaired using the EEA transpterygoid approach, may also be repaired through the lateral TOA, and there is evidence that the lateral TOA may offer less morbidity, since endonasal mobilization of the contents of the pterygopalatine fossa may cause damage to V2 and the Vidian nerve.

Other neurosurgical targets exposed by the lateral TOA include the petrous apex, which can also be exposed with a subtemporal approach, and the anterior fossa, as might be exposed by the subfrontal, orbitofrontal, and supraorbital approaches. However, for removing pathology of the anterior fossa, the lateral TOA will be suitable only for pathology that is uniquely lateral to the cribriform plate and behind the frontal sinus. It's not that these areas are impossible to reach via TOA, just that they might be more easily reached with a different approach. In Fig. 8.1, we summarize the most suitable targets for the lateral TOA.

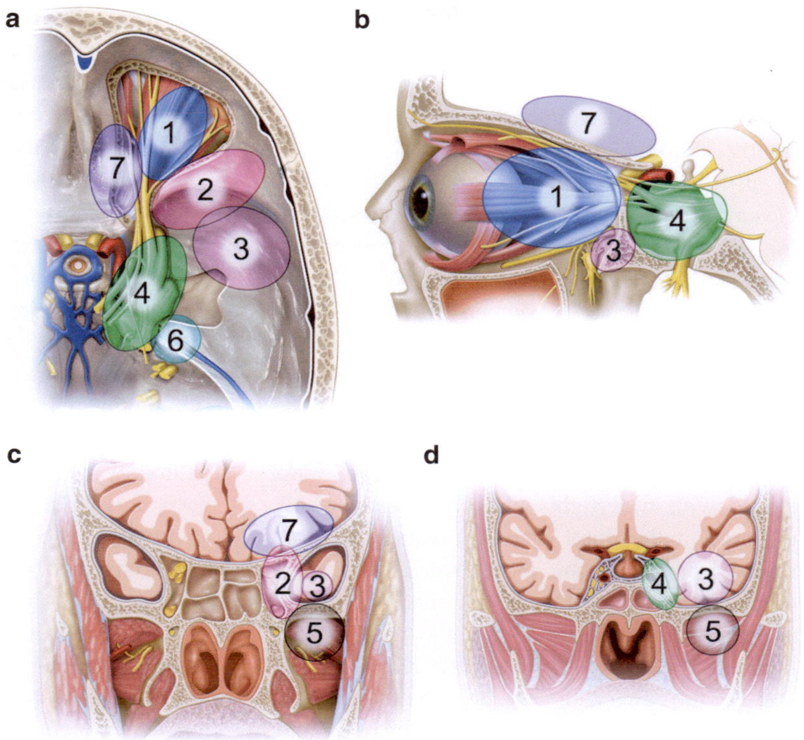

Fig. 8.1 Lateral TOA skull base targets. Illustration of four views (**a–d**) of the ventral anterior and middle fossae of the skull base. Each target is numbered and color coded. (1) The orbit. (2) The lesser sphenoid wing and anterior clinoid. (3) The middle fossa. (4) The lateral wall of the cavernous sinus and Meckel's cave. (5) The infratemporal fossa. (6) The petrous apex. (7) The anterior fossa

Technique

The equipment and ergonomics of the TOA are derived directly from EEA. For this reason, any surgeon whose operating room is equipped for EEA and who has a working knowledge and access to EEA tools will not need to purchase and learn to use any new equipment to pivot to TOA. Both rely on the endoscope for visualization because the corridor is long and narrow, and the scope can be held by a second surgeon or mechanical arm. The skills of endoscope-assisted microsurgery and the instruments employed are identical. The surgeon must be comfortable looking at a two-dimensional screen, away from the operative field. However, there are also several differences between the two approaches. Whereas EEA can be performed by one or two surgeons, transorbital surgery may require three. In addition to manipulating the instruments, holding, and cleaning the scope, someone must retract the orbit for a significant portion of the operation. Understanding the degree of retraction and insisting on intermittent relaxation to check the pupil are critical aspects to ensure the safety of the approach. For this reason, at our center, we work closely with oculoplastic surgery. They not only perform the approach and the closure, but we rely on them to retract the orbit as well. This is not required, by any means, but involving oculoplastics only leads to greater care with exopthalmometry measurements, acuity testing, diplopia assessment, and orbital reconstruction and probably improves the cosmetic outcome. In addition, should one of the other three TOA corridors be required (superior, medial, or inferior), the oculoplastic surgeons will have more experience and comfort in creating these corridors. As with EEA, using oculoplastics for all cases makes the relationship and surgery more fluid in those cases where they are more desperately needed. Hopefully, referrals soon run in both directions and both practices benefit.In its infancy, the EEA was plagued with one major barrier to widespread acceptance: cerebrospinal fluid leaks and the associated risk of pneumocephalus and meningitis. Although mostly overcome, the proximity of air-filled sinuses to CSF breech still makes closure of the skull base a critical and challenging aspect of the operation. The transorbital approach, on the other hand, temporarily displaces the orbit and its contents, which fall back into place at the end of the operation. This eliminates any dead space and provides a natural tamponade to prevent cerebrospinal fluid egress. Moreover, the periosteum/periorbital layer over the lateral orbital rim and skin of the eyelid are closed with watertight sutures. Multilayer soft closures of the dural opening, maneuvers borrowed from EEA, are more than adequate, in combination with the barriers inherent in the approach, to markedly reduce the risk of CSF leak and its associated morbidity. That said, for some of the cases with very large dural openings, we have placed an occasional lumbar drain and kept it open for a few days so we can sleep better at night.

Lateral TOA Skull Base Targets

Although not a comprehensive list, we have identified at this time seven potential targets of the transorbital approach. We will review and discuss each one in turn (Fig. 8.1):

1. *The Orbit*: The lateral TOA provides access to pathology of the lateral and superior orbit; however, pathology *limited* to the orbit is often removed by the oculoplastic surgeons by themselves. As neurosurgeons, we mostly encounter tumors that extend *into* the orbit from another location or extend *from* the orbit to the skull base. The lateral TOA is then only applicable to pathology lateral to the optic nerve, in which the approach is suitable for removing the rest of the pathology, namely, those parts of the tumor that extent out of the orbit.
2. *The Lesser Sphenoid Wing and Anterior Clinoid*: The lateral TOA is suitable to pathology in the mid- and inner portions of the lesser wing, as well as the anterior clinoid. The lateral aspects of the wing cannot be reached. The anterior clinoid is challenging to remove, since one must work above and around the superior orbital fissure. Taking a more superior to inferior trajectory makes this easier. Also, in some circumstances, to decompress the optic nerve, it may not be required to remove the entire clinoid, but rather the inferior and medial aspect of it, which is easier to remove via the TOA. The most common pathology here is the meningiomas, but we have encountered metastases here as well. Just beyond the less wing is the Sylvian fissure. One could, in theory, clip an MCA aneurysm with this approach.
3. *The Middle Fossa*: This includes the anterior part of the temporal lobe as well as the floor of the middle fossa. Included here are intraparenchymal pathologies within the temporal lobe, including the amygdala and hippocampus, as well as extra-axial pathology on the floor of the middle fossa bordering on the foramina rotundum, ovale, and spinosum. The most common pathologies encountered here are gliomas, mesial temporal sclerosis, meningiomas, and lateral sphenoid encephaloceles.
4. *The Lateral Wall of the Cavernous Sinus and Meckel's Cave*: Once the meningo-orbital band is cut and the medial temporal lobe is lateralized, the lateral TOA provides excellent exposure of the lateral cavernous sinus and Meckel's cave. Pathology here are trigeminal schwannomas, meningiomas, pituitary adenomas, and lymphomas.
5. *The Infratemporal Fossa*: The lateral TOA can access a limited amount of the very superior aspect of the infratemporal fossa. We have used this approach mainly to biopsy pathology in this area such as metastases, malignant head and neck cancers, lymphomas, etc.
6. *The Petrous Apex*: The same corridor that can be used to expose the floor of the middle fossa and the lateral aspect of Meckel's cave can be

followed back to reach the petrous apex. The exposure is quite similar to that provided by the subtemporal approach, although the angle of attack is slightly different, coming in from a more anterior trajectory. Pathology here includes meningiomas and acoustic neuromas, should one drill out the porus acusticus.

7. *The Anterior Fossa*: By drilling through the roof of the orbit, one can easily reach certain areas within the anterior fossa. The easiest areas to expose lie just above the midportion of the orbit, lateral to the cribriform plate and medial to lateral extent of the lesser sphenoid wing. While it is possible to expose more of the anterior fossa, one might have to extend the lateral TOA by removing more of the orbital rim. Here, we are limiting our discussion to the standard TOA, without any additional rim removal, which might be considered an "extended" TOA.

Conclusions

The natural evolution of neurosurgery toward less invasiveness, found in all its subspecialties, relies on technical innovations, as well as alterations in philosophy and perspective. The TOA follows in this long line of neurosurgical innovations and is the natural evolution of our field. The TOA is now poised to become a new arrow in the skull base surgeon's quiver. The technical leap is only a small step away from EEA. The philosophical chasm is the more daunting hurdle. For those of us who have already taken this first step, while the path forward may seem unnerving, the advantages are clear. As with EEA, it's critical that one understands the anatomy, spends time in the cadaver laboratory, and not progresses too rapidly. The key to success is case selection and understanding one's ability and the limitations of the approach. Early poor results will create negative bias. Slow progression of skills in a stepwise fashion, from extradural to intradural pathology, is recommended. Attendance in transorbital courses with hands-on components is also strongly suggested.

References

1. Di Somma A, Kong DS, de Notaris M, Moe KS, Sánchez España JC, Schwartz TH, Enseñat J. Endoscopic transorbital surgery levels of difficulty. J Neurosurg. 2022;15:1–4. https://doi.org/10.3171/2022.3.JNS212699.
2. Moe KS, Bergeron CM, Ellenbogen RG. Transorbital neuroendoscopic surgery. Neurosurgery. 2010;67(suppl 3):pns16–28.
3. Schwartz TH, Henderson F Jr, Di Somma A, Kong DS, de Notaris M, Enseñat J, Moe KS. Endoscopic transorbital surgery: another leap of faith? World Neurosurg. 2022;159:54–5.

9 Transorbital Neuroendoscopic Surgery in the Pediatric Population

J. Nathaniel Perkins, Kris S. Moe, Jacob Ruzevick, and Randall A. Bly

Introduction

Treating pediatric skull base lesions is complex and requires multidisciplinary discussion and careful planning. The recently developed transorbital endoscopic approaches are being used with increasing frequency in the adult population. For more than a decade, we have also been using these approaches in the pediatric population for multiple indications. Similar to the adult population, the goal has been to improve surgical access to anatomically challenging regions while decreasing surgical morbidity. In our experience, a transorbital approach either in isolation or combined with another surgical approach can offer improved visualization and instrumentation capability. It may reduce the need for incisions on the face. The specific surgical approaches are similar in children as described previously for adults [1].

The pathology seen in pediatric skull base are more likely to be congenital and benign in comparison to adults (Table 9.1).

Based on the location of the lesion, any of the pathology listed above could be considered for a transorbital endoscopic approach. In cases where there is invasion into the orbit such as JNA, neuroblastoma, and fibrous dysplasia, an additional surgical portal through the orbit can provide early identification of normal structures within the orbit. In this way, the lesion can be dissected off the normal structures, as opposed to a transnasal approach in which the critical orbital structures are not visualized until after significant lesion resection has already occurred. In addition to the pathology listed, other potential indications for transorbital surgery in children include epistaxis and orbital abscess (Fig. 9.1). In our experience, a medial transorbital approach has been utilized

Table 9.1 Pediatric skull base pathology

Juvenile nasopharyngeal angiofibroma (JNA)
Cerebral spinal fluid (CSF) leak, meningoencephalocele
Pituitary adenoma
Osteoma
Inverted papilloma
Fibrous dysplasia
Craniopharyngioma
Nasal dermoid
Neuroblastoma
Rhabdomyosarcoma
Chondrosarcoma

J. N. Perkins · R. A. Bly (✉)
Department of Otolaryngology-Head and Neck Surgery, University of Washington, Seattle Children's Hospital, Seattle, WA, USA
e-mail: randbly@uw.edu

K. S. Moe
Division of Facial Plastic Surgery, Departments of Otolaryngology and Neurological Surgery, University of Washington School of Medicine, Seattle, WA, USA
e-mail: krismoe@uw.edu

J. Ruzevick
Department of Neurological Surgery, University of Washington, Seattle Children's Hospital, Seattle, WA, USA

T. H. Schwartz et al. (eds.), *Endoscopic Transorbital Surgery of the Orbit, Skull Base and Brain*, https://doi.org/10.1007/978-3-031-59504-2_9

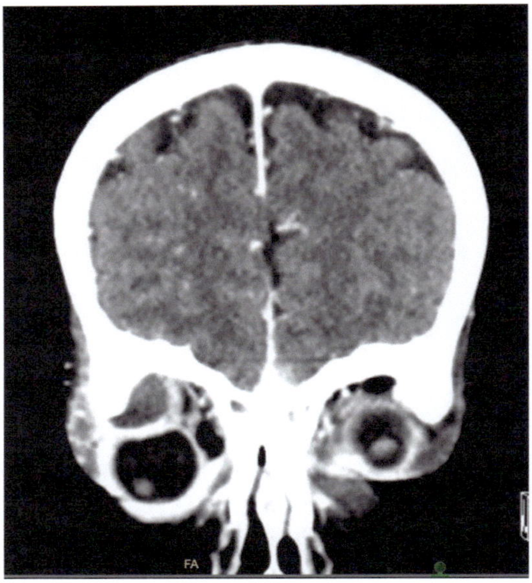

Fig. 9.1 Coronal CT showing a right superior subperiosteal abscess in an 8-year-old boy that was treated with a superior transorbital endoscopic approach

to ligate anterior and posterior ethmoid arteries. For young patients with refractory epistaxis, this is an option to be considered along with embolization and transnasal vessel ligation.

An obvious concern when considering pediatric transorbital surgery is the size of the orbit. The globe is proportionally larger within the orbit in children (under age 8 years) compared to adults. Although the growth rate of the globe is proportional to orbit growth, the ratio of globe volume to orbit volume reduces over time. For the globe and orbit, there is rapid growth in the first 12 months of age, then slower from 12 to 35 months of age, followed by slow growth until age 8 years when the globe is >95% of adult size [2]. Prior publications have shown endoscopic transorbital approaches to be safe and effective down to age 6 years [3]. While this age corresponds to a point of fairly mature orbital volume, we believe there is no specific lower limit for age to consider for transorbital approaches, but the relative size of the globe within the orbit must be considered.

There is often a concern raised about the impact on facial growth with surgery on the craniofacial skeleton in young children. Although animal studies showed some asymmetric growth after septal surgery, those effects are not observed in recent clinical studies [4, 5]. Similarly, we would not expect to see an impact on facial growth after performing transorbital endoscopic surgery; however, these outcomes should be reported when data is available. We have not noted an alteration of orbital growth postoperatively in our patient population to date.

The smaller anatomy of younger children may translate to more constrained surgical pathways. There can be increased frequency of instrument collision and reduced instrument range of motion. This smaller corridor presents a similar challenge for transnasal endoscopy in young children. As such, the addition of a transorbital portal to another approach can improve the working space and offer a significantly wider range of approach angles through which to work [6].This provides both improved visualization and instrumentation capabilities. In this regard, the opportunity to access skull base lesions through a multiportal approach is especially important to consider in pediatric patients. Transorbital endoscopic approach in children to surgically treat osteomas was found to be effective while also reducing the need for facial incisions [7].

Preoperative Considerations

Surgical planning begins with an in-depth analysis of the imaging. Our practice is to incorporate the data into a segmentation software such as Slicer and segment the target lesion and relevant anatomy [8]. By using 3D reconstruction and virtual endoscopy, measurements can be made as needed, which allows for improved presurgical planning and counseling (Figs. 9.2 and 9.3).

Preoperative counseling is critical in the pediatric population so that expectations can be established with the family and caregivers. The postoperative period can be very stressful for families and caregivers of the pediatric patient.

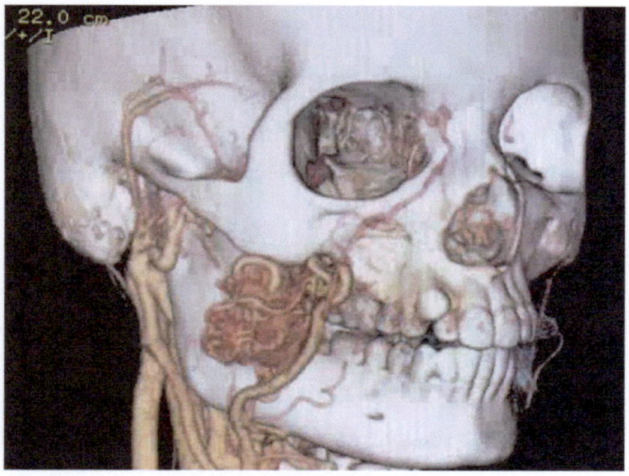

Fig. 9.2 Segmentation example of the bone and vasculature (including the lesion) for an 11-year-old patient with arteriovenous malformation of the right inferior orbit, infratemporal fossa, and maxilla

Understanding basic components of postoperative care includes the following: (1) the number of family members or caregivers who are allowed to stay overnight with the child in the ICU and ward (many hospitals have limits), (2) anticipated duration of sedation postoperatively, (3) expected duration of endotracheal tube required after the surgery, (4) use of an external ventricular drain (EVD) or lumbar drain (LD) and what the mobility restrictions will be in place, including if hair will need to be shaved, (5) use of nasal packing (absorbable/nonabsorbable) and how it will be removed if necessary, and (6) need for postoperative imaging studies that require sedation to obtain (e.g., MRI in young children typically requires sedation). All these seemingly simple and routine aspects of postoperative care can take center stage in pediatric patients, especially if there are surprises for the families and caregivers.

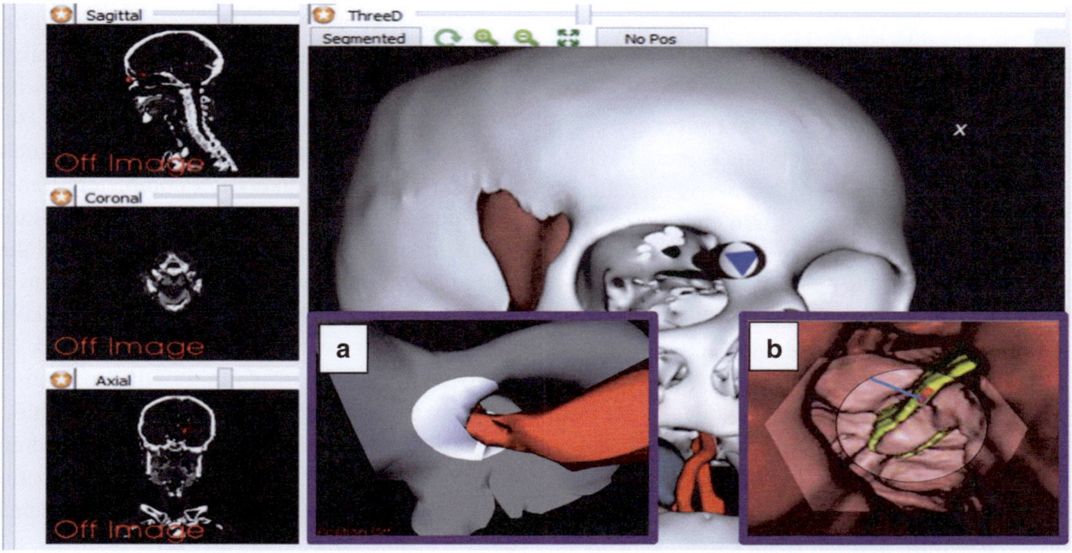

Fig. 9.3 Screenshot from custom surgical planning software for a superior-medial transorbital approach to a suprasellar lesion, with highlighted virtual endoscopy images with (**a**) bone and (**b**) soft tissue segmentations showing critical neurovascular structures

Intraoperative Considerations

Image navigation has been shown to be equally effective and accurate in the pediatric population as in adults [9, 10]. Placement of the patient tracker should be planned appropriately around other surgical sites, including possible EVD placement.

In prior work, the acceptable amount of globe retraction away from the orbital wall was 1 cm using a malleable retractor [11]. Sustained retraction could lead to globe injury, so there are multiple times during which the globe is not subjected to the 1 cm displacement. Dynamic (intermittent) retraction may be an important aspect to maintaining globe health. Therefore, we do not recommend the use a self-retaining retractor apparatus for transorbital surgery. Due to the smaller anatomy within the pediatric population, it is important to avoid continuous retraction throughout the operation.

Smaller-sized instrumentation should be considered. The option to use a 2.7 mm endoscope instead of the standard 4 mm offers the advantage of size at the compromise of resolution. Irrigation sheaths are available for 2.7 mm endoscopes. The image from a smaller endoscope is more likely to become obscured, even with the irrigation sheath in place, compared to the 4 mm endoscope. This typically requires more frequent removal and manual cleaning. There are smaller-sized microdebriders, and certain types of drills are smaller than others at the proximal portion that resides at the nasal vestibule during skull base drilling. Ultrasonic bone aspirators have been used with good success in pediatric transorbital cases. Otologic instruments such as cupped forceps and size 3 and 5 French Frazier suctions can sometimes be helpful in these small surgical corridors. These factors related to instrumentation should be evaluated before the surgery so that they are available when needed.

Relevant anatomic differences from adults are observed, especially at the frontal sinus. For children aged 5 years and younger, the frontal sinus is absent. Pneumatization begins at 5 years of age, and a sinus cavity is not typically observed until after age 10 years [12, 13]. The maxillary sinus is present at birth, and there is rapid growth within the first 12 months of age and then subsequent slower growth rate. The ethmoid sinuses are the first of the paranasal sinuses to be fully formed. The sphenoid sinuses are typically not present at birth, and they begin as two very small spaces with a thick osseus septum as early as 9 months of age.

The smaller blood volume in pediatric patients must be considered during skull base surgery. Depending on the pathology and other factors, blood products should be available and the bleeding risks discussed with the multidisciplinary team. Due to the paucity of literature on pediatric transorbital approaches, risk factors for transfusion can be transferred from the experience of pediatric craniofacial and transnasal endoscopic surgery. In this literature that includes an open approach such as coronal incision, the following risk factors were noted to be associated with need for transfusion: weight < 10 kg, age < 18 months, presence of craniofacial syndrome, operative time > 5 h, revision operations, and patients with known elevated intracranial pressure [14]. However, these cases involved large skin incisions, so the data is likely not completely transferrable. Transnasal endoscopic pediatric skull base surgery is reported in the literature, and the risk of blood transfusion is overall low, primarily a function of the pathology [15–17]. It is likely that one of the best ways to reduce the risk of transfusion is by performing the operation through an endoscopic approach when possible.

Furthermore, the majority of young children will not participate in suture removal postoperatively, so the use of absorbable sutures when needed can be beneficial.

Postoperative Considerations

Postoperative care related to transorbital incisions is similar to adults. However, many key aspects of the care need to be carefully planned for pediatric skull base surgery. If there is concern for a CSF leak or if there was a CSF leak repair, sedation should be considered as an option postoperatively. In our practice, perioperative management is individualized for each unique case and lesion pathology. If the patient is under age 4, and if there was a repair at the skull base, we may plan for 3 days of sedation. Postoperative sedation permits a postoperative MRI to occur if indicated. Further, if an EVD or LD is in place, this sedation plan allows for safe titration of CSF without the patient moving significantly. If there is nasal packing, the duration of that should be considered. If nonabsorbable, our group will typically remove this on postoperative day 7. We have observed that for patients aged 7 years and older, we can typically remove a nasal sponge at bedside without sedation. We often place the sponge within a surgical glove finger to make it easier to remove. For younger patients, we plan for a brief sedation at bedside in order to safely remove the packing.

In contrast to transnasal endoscopic surgery where debris can build up postoperatively that may require debridement, the transorbital surgical approach generally does not require any specific maintenance. We apply topical antibiotic-containing ophthalmic ointment to the incision postoperatively for 5 days and monitor clinically. If a transnasal endoscopic approach was also used, we do not routinely perform debridement at a specified time frame in the first few weeks. Depending on the surgery performed, age, and cooperation of the child, we perform routine examinations and begin endoscopic assessment with possible debridement at 1 month postoperatively. For young children of any age, we typically can perform flexible endoscopy in the clinic to assess the intranasal cavity. Based on those findings, we rarely would elect to sedate the child specifically for debridement purposes. Instead, we continue with saline spray and irrigation if tolerated and monitor clinically with flexible endoscopy.

The pediatric endoscopic transorbital cases below highlight some of the principles discussed that apply to pediatric transorbital endoscopic skull base surgery:

Case 1

A 13-year-old female presented with left-sided nasal obstruction and epiphora. Imaging showed a left-sided expansile maxillary mass with extension into the orbit (Fig. 9.4). It was hypointense on T1 with hyperintense STIR signal, and it avidly enhanced with contrast. Endoscopic biopsy revealed esthesioneuroblastoma. Multidisciplinary conference discussion resulted in the plan for surgical excision through a multiportal endoscopic approach. A precaruncular transconjunctival incision was made on the left side to gain access to the medial and inferior orbit. The anterior and posterior ethmoid arteries were ligated and divided. The mass was visible immediately, and there was absent bone in the majority of the orbit floor and medial wall. Normal bone was identified circumferentially around the defect. The orbital structures were well visualized at this point, and the tumor was then dissected free. The remainder of the mass was resected through transnasal and transmaxillary surgical portals. Gross total resection was performed, and the orbital walls were reconstructed using titanium mesh (Fig. 9.5). Her tumor was Kadish stage C; she was treated with proton beam therapy and chemotherapy postoperatively, and she is free of disease at greater than 10 years. Approximately 5 years after completing proton therapy, she developed exposure of her titanium mesh which required removal and reconstruction.

Case 2

A 14-year-old boy presented with eye pain and discomfort. He underwent imaging that showed an osseus mass arising from the left frontal sinus with extension intracranially as well as into the superior medial orbit (Fig. 9.6). He underwent a superior orbital endoscopic approach using a superior lid crease incision to resect the extradural tumor (Fig. 9.7). The skull base and orbital roof were reconstructed with PDS (polydioxanone) sheets.

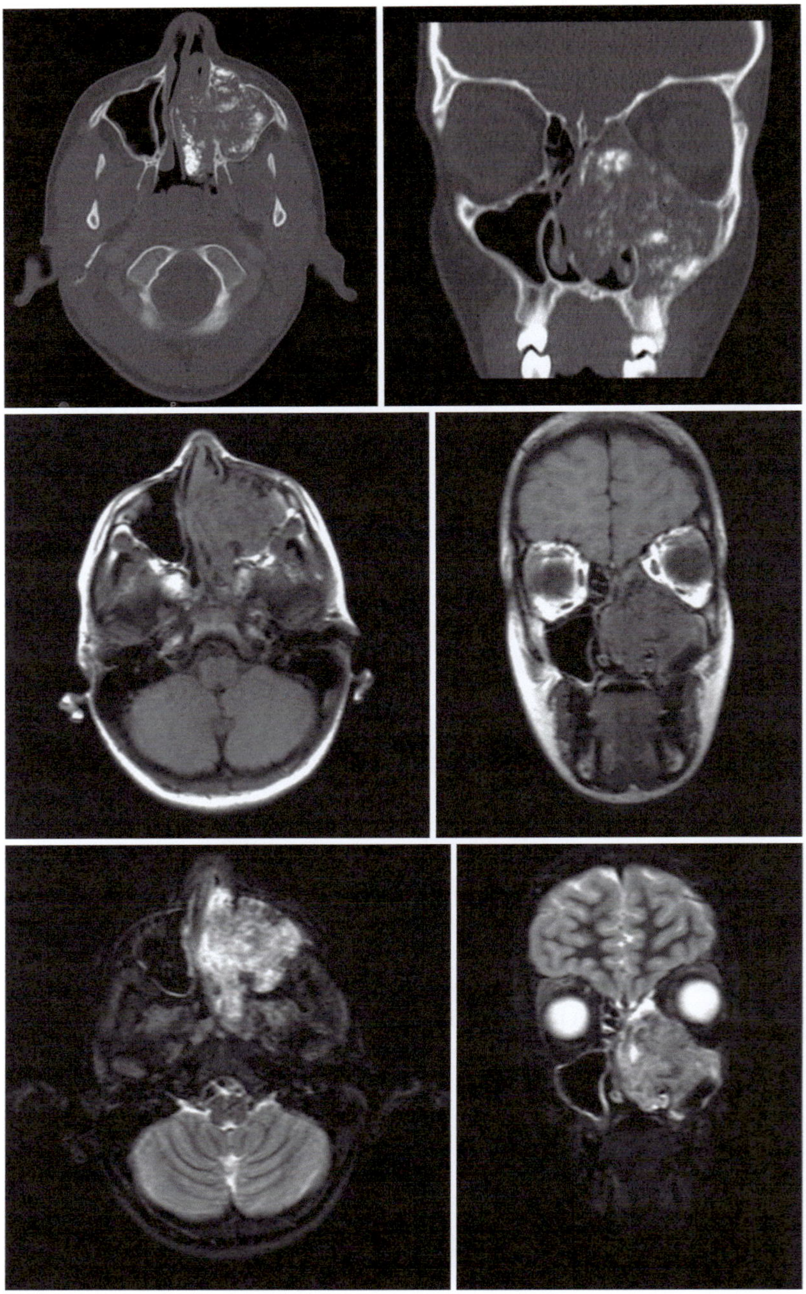

Fig. 9.4 Preoperative esthesioneuroblastoma CT (top row), T1 MRI (middle row), and STIR MRI (bottom row), which demonstrate an expansile left maxillary sinus mass extending into the nasal cavity with erosion of the orbital floor and anterior maxillary sinus wall

Fig. 9.5 Postoperative T1 (top row) and STIR MRI (bottom row) approximately 6 years after resection, proton therapy, and chemotherapy

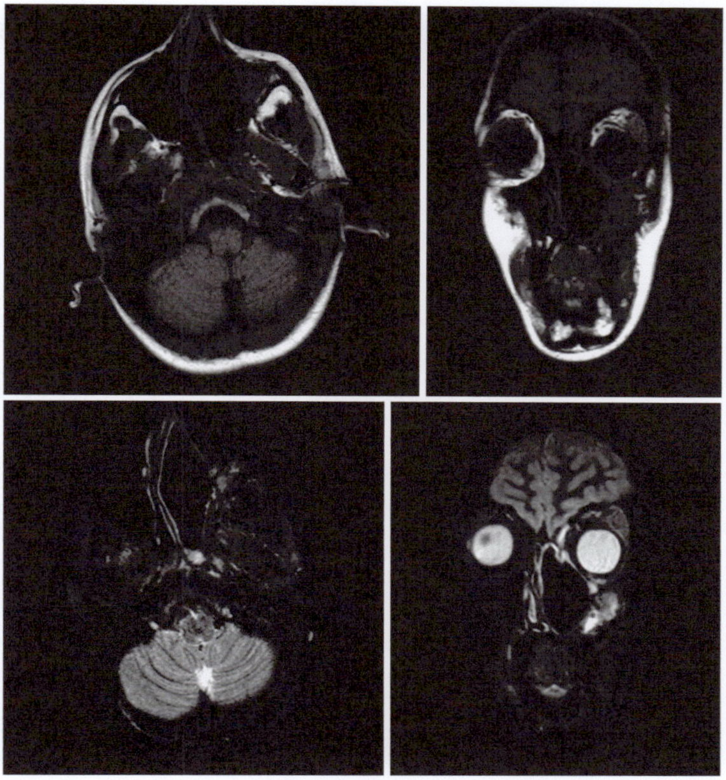

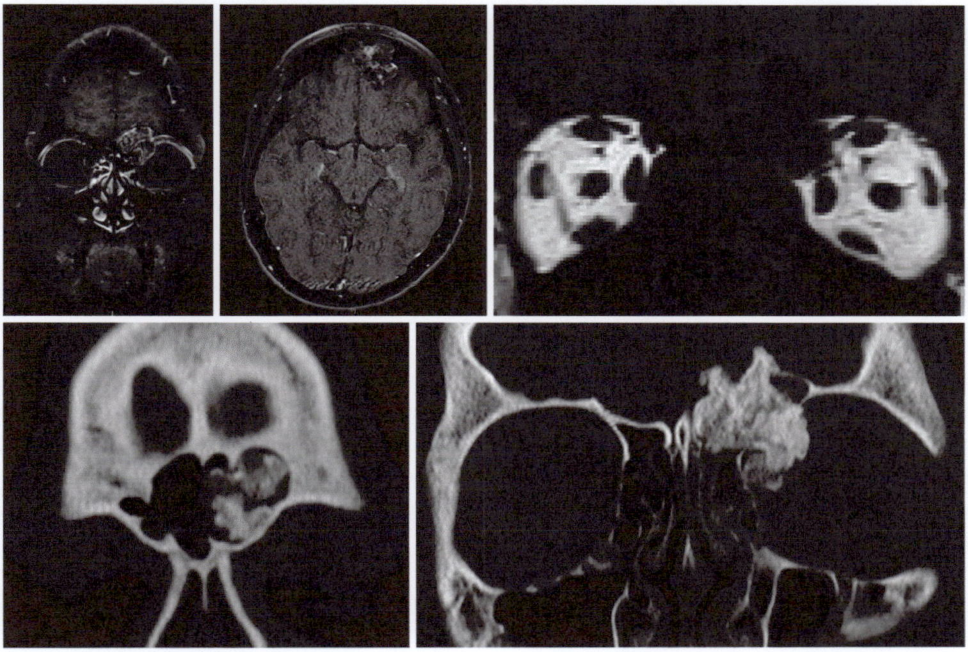

Fig. 9.6 Preoperative STIR and T1 MRI images (top row) and coronal CT images at two locations (bottom row)

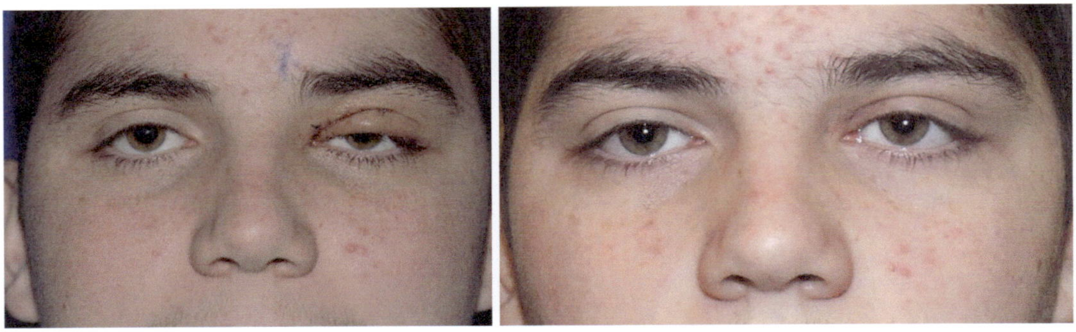

Fig. 9.7 Clinical photographs taken at 5 days (left) and 3 weeks (right) postoperatively after undergoing endoscopic superior transorbital resection of the osteoma through a left superior lid crease incision

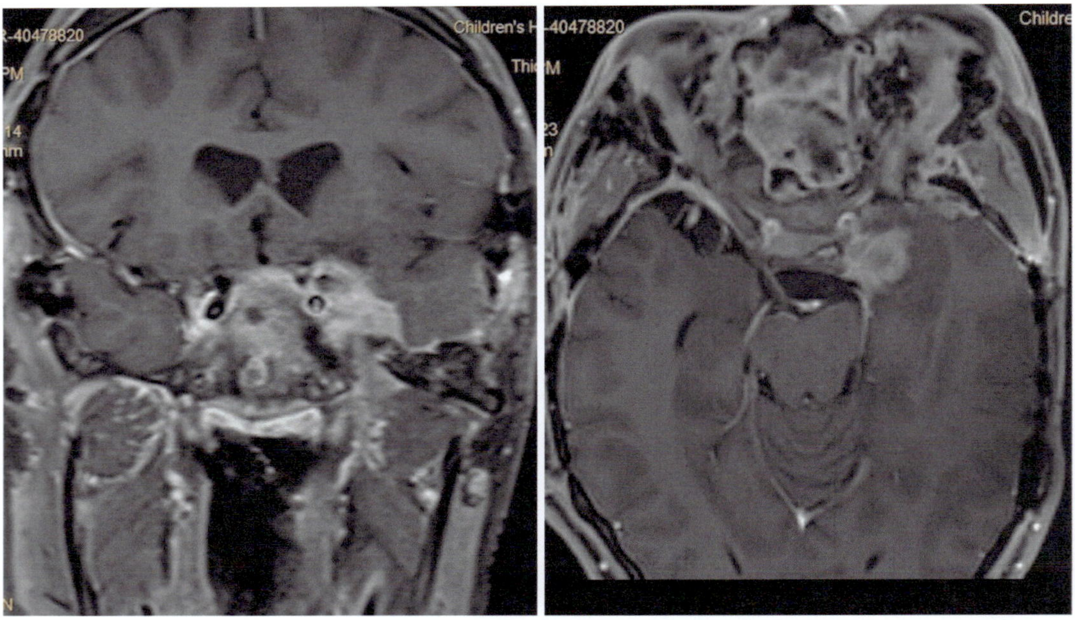

Fig. 9.8 Preoperative coronal and axial MRI images showing meningioma in a patient with compressive optic neuropathy

Case 3

A 15-year-old boy with a history of neurofibromatosis type 2, multiple prior surgeries of the anterior cranial fossa for meningioma resection, presented with a decline in vision over 1 year. Ophthalmologic exam revealed compressive optic neuropathy. Imaging revealed meningioma tumor compressing orbital apex (Fig. 9.8). He underwent a combined endoscopic transnasal approach and a medial transorbital approach for tumor resection and optic canal decompression. The patient had improved vision postoperatively (Fig. 9.9).

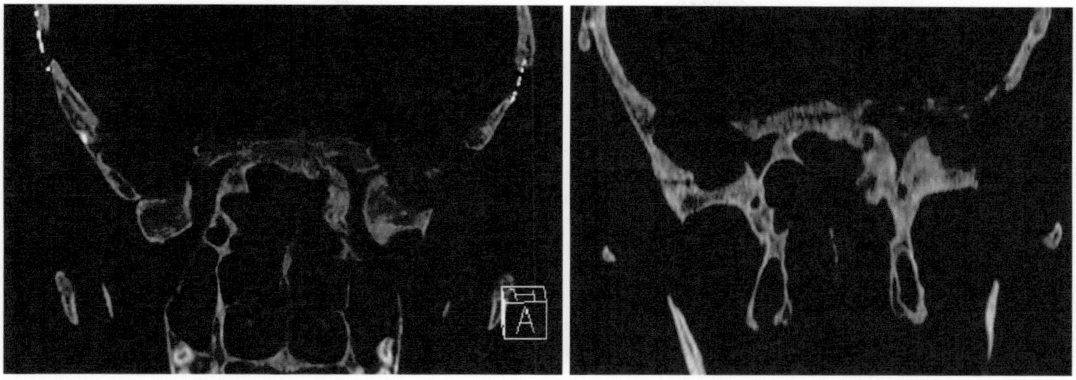

Fig. 9.9 Preoperative CT (left) of compressive optic neuropathy due to meningioma and postoperative CT (right) showing superior/lateral optic canal decompression

Conclusion

Transorbital neuroendoscopic surgery is a relatively new field, particularly as applied to the pediatric population. However, with over 10 years of clinical and research experience, we believe that these approaches are safe and highly effective. Reports in the literature describe procedures performed mostly on children aged 6 and older, which corresponds to the point when the orbit has attained nearly adult size—while these techniques may be used on younger children, appropriate pathology is not commonly encountered.

Surgical planning is particularly important in this population, given the tighter anatomic constraints. Likewise, meticulous surgical technique is critical, with dynamic retraction of the orbital contents, frequent relaxation periods when retractors are removed, and maintenance of a pathway diameter of 1 cm or less.

Transorbital endoscopic procedures, particularly when combined with other approaches in a multiportal technique, may improve the ability to access, visualize, and instrument pathology in highly challenging areas of the skull base. The techniques are minimally disruptive, leading to rapid recovery with minimal morbidity. We look forward to further contributions to the international literature as these procedures enter the mainstream surgical armamentarium.

References

1. Moe KS, Bergeron CM, Ellenbogen RG. Transorbital neuroendoscopic surgery. Neurosurgery. 2010;67(3):ons16–28.
2. Escaravage GK Jr, Dutton JJ. Age-related changes in the pediatric human orbit on CT. Ophthalmic Plast Reconstr Surg. 2013;29(3):150–6.
3. Balakrishnan K, Moe KS. Applications and outcomes of orbital and transorbital endoscopic surgery. Otolaryngol Head Neck Surg. 2011;144(5):815–20.
4. Copray JC. Growth of the nasal Septal cartilage of the rat in vitro. J Anat. 1986;144:99.
5. Tasca I, Compadretti GC. Nasal growth after pediatric Septoplasty at long-term follow-up. Am J Rhinol Allergy. 2011;25(1):e7–12.
6. Bly RA, Su D, Ferreira M, Moe KS. Computer modeled multiportal approaches to the Skull Base. Journal of neurological surgery part B. Skull Base. 2012;73(S01):A112.
7. Badran KW, Suh JD, Namiri N, Wrobel B, Ference EH. Pediatric benign Paranasal sinus Osteoneogenic tumors: a case series and systematic review of outcomes, techniques, and a multiportal approach. Am J Rhinol Allergy. 2018;32(6):465–72.
8. Kikinis R, Pieper SD, Vosburgh K. 3D slicer: a platform for subject-specific image analysis, visualization, and clinical support. In: Jolesz FA, editor. Intraoperative imaging image-guided therapy, vol. 3. New York: Springer; 2014. p. 277–89.
9. Benoit MM, Silvera VM, Nichollas R, Jones D, McGill T, Rahbar R. Image guidance systems for minimally invasive sinus and skull base surgery in children. Int J Pediatr Otorhinolaryngol. 2009;73(10):1452–7.
10. Bergeron M, Leclerc JE. Is image guidance accurate in children sinus surgery? Int J Pediatr Otorhinolaryngol. 2015;79(4):469–73.

11. Bly RA, Ramakrishna R, Ferreira M, Moe KS. Lateral transorbital neuroendoscopic approach to the lateral cavernous sinus. J Neurol Surg B Skull Base. 2013;9:011–7.
12. Adibelli ZH, Songu M, Adibelli H. Paranasal sinus development in children: a magnetic resonance imaging analysis. Am J Rhinol Allergy. 2011;25(1):30–5.
13. Barghouth G, Prior J, Lepori D, Duvoisin B, Schnyder P, Gudinchet F. Paranasal sinuses in children: size evaluation of maxillary, sphenoid, and frontal sinuses by magnetic resonance imaging and proposal of volume index percentile curves. Eur Radiol. 2002;12:1451–8.
14. Goobie SM, Haas T. Bleeding Management for pediatric craniotomies and craniofacial surgery. Pediatr Anesth. 2014;24(7):678–89.
15. Munson PD, Moore EJ. Pediatric endoscopic skull base surgery. Curr Opin Otolaryngol Head Neck Surg. 2010;18(6):571–6.
16. Yang J, Kim YH, Phi JH, Kim SK, Wang KC. Complications of endoscopic skull base surgery for sellar and parasellar tumors in pediatric population; neurosurgical perspectives. Front Oncol. 2022;12:769576.
17. Chivukula S, Koutourousiou M, Snyderman CH, Gardner PA, Tyler-Kabara EC. Endoscopic endonasal skull base surgery in the pediatric population. J Neurol Surg B Skull Base. 2012;73(S01):A082.

Part III

Sinonasal Pathology

Sinonasal Tumors

10

Patricia G. Johnson and Ian M. Humphreys

In 2010, transorbital neuroendoscopic surgery (TONES) was described as a coplanar portal to the skull base that affords spatial freedom to maneuver using three- and four-handed surgery via simultaneous use of multiple portals (e.g., transnasal and transorbital portal) [1, 2]. These portals can be used singularly or in a multiportal strategy separated by anatomic regions (e.g., nose and orbit). It is important to note that these portals are vector-based pathways that in and of themselves are not solutions to any given tumor (malignant or benign) but rather represent a portal for visualization and instrumentation of a given target. Any lesion may benefit from a transorbital, transnasal, or multiportal strategy. As described in earlier chapters, there are four major transorbital approaches: superior eyelid crease (SLC), precaruncular (PC), inferior transconjunctival lower eyelid (ITCs), and lateral retrocanthal (LRC). Each approach affords access to a different portion of the skull base and its adjacent paranasal sinuses [1, 3].

Sinonasal tumors currently represent a minority of the reported pathology wherein the TONES approach is utilized [3]. Despite its published rarity compared to cerebrospinal fluid (CSF) leaks and meningiomas, the TONES cases reported for sinonasal tumors have been feasible, successful, and oncologically sound [3–8]. Resection of amenable lesions via a transnasal and transorbital approach is associated with minimal local morbidity and improvement in neurologic and visual deficits due to sinonasal tumors including vision disturbance, diplopia, gaze restriction, and proptosis [2, 3, 5, 6, 9]. The transorbital portal does allow for adequate repair of both dural and bone defects, including multilayer dural repairs as indicated [2–4, 9].

There are three main instances where TONES may be considered in addition to a transnasal approach of a sinonasal tumor: (1) when the transnasal route alone affords inadequate access, visualization and/or instrumentation of the target (e.g., lateral or superior aspect of frontal sinus, lateral sphenoid sinus, etc.), (2) when challenging working angles are required for appropriate resection (e.g., around the orbit for lateral frontal sinus pathology), and (3) when tumor characteristics are complex and there is an anticipated benefit for multiple spatially separated instruments used simultaneously to manipulate the target of interest (e.g., fibro-osseous lesions of the sinuses or skull base).

P. G. Johnson
Division of Otolaryngology—Head and Neck Surgery, Allegheny Health Network, Pittsburgh, PA, USA

I. M. Humphreys (✉)
Department of Otolaryngology—Head and Neck Surgery, University of Washington School of Medicine, Seattle, WA, USA
e-mail: ihumphre@uw.edu

T. H. Schwartz et al. (eds.), *Endoscopic Transorbital Surgery of the Orbit, Skull Base and Brain*,
https://doi.org/10.1007/978-3-031-59504-2_10

Unique to the management of sinonasal tumors is the consideration of how and where the tumor is attached to the surrounding sinus, skull base, and/or neurovascular structures. In sinus tumor surgery, proper management of the attachment site is critical to optimizing outcomes. At times, the site of tumor attachment is in a favorable location such as the inferior nasal septum, wherein there are no critical functional or structural implications of attachment site removal. However, when the attachment site involves an area with underlying critical neurovascular structures such as the olfactory and optic nerves, carotid artery, or dura surgical complexity and risk is much greater. For some sinus tumors, attachment site removal may mandate mucosal removal only, whereas in others (e.g., sinus cancers), the bone under the mucosal attachment site may need to be resected (e.g., melanoma), thus placing the deepest structures at risk for injury (e.g., dura). In summation, complete and thorough management of the tumor's attachment site must be aligned with best practices in management for any given histology, and the operating surgeon must account for these factors in both the preoperative planning and intraoperative management of sinus tumors. It should be stated that often the attachment site, or sites, of sinus tumors may not be fully identifiable until the intraoperative exploration of the lesion, and therefore, a thorough and thoughtful operative plan will include contingencies (e.g., additional surgical approaches) to the extent possible.

In addition to the contributions that sinus tumor attachment has on surgical decision-making, the operative surgeon must also consider the physiologic function of the sinuses. Important physiologic functions of the sinuses include mucus production, olfaction (e.g., ethmoid skull base and superior septum), mucociliary clearance, nasal airflow, and immunity. Therefore, when considering a surgical strategy for any given lesion within the sinuses, the operating surgeon must consider all of these factors. It is important to consider both goals of complete and thorough resection of the tumor commensurate with the known histology and the future healing and physiologic function of the sinuses. For example, it is possible that a TONES approach alone may be sufficient to resect a given tumor (e.g., frontal sinus inverted papilloma); however, surgical resection via this approach alone may leave the frontal sinus outflow at risk for postoperative stenosis (and consequent chronic sinusitis), and therefore, a concurrent transnasal frontal sinus exploration may also be indicated to prevent these predictable future complications.

In the authors' experience, a useful framework to consider when deciding a surgical approach strategy for sinonasal tumors includes the following concepts: (1) obtaining surgical access to confidently visualize a given target, (2) affording an ability to instrument and manage the surgical target in a way that permits free mobility of the surgical instruments while maintaining optimal visualization to ensure optimal attachment site management, and (3) performance of reconstruction or further exploration of the sinuses to permit optimal wound healing and prevent postoperative sinus disorders (e.g., sinus stenosis, sinusitis, etc.). With these technical considerations in mind, the surgeon should also consider the histologic context of a given target wherein a sinus malignancy would more commonly be expected to have advanced resection considerations (e.g., margins) than a benign entity. Sinus malignancies may require adjuvant therapies (e.g., radiation) that could influence wound healing in the postoperative period, surgical repair options, and by extension selection of multiportal approach considerations in the surgical plan. Lastly, in both benign and malignant tumor management, the need for future endoscopic disease surveillance should be considered.

Ultimately, if a TONES approach is selected, the transorbital quadrant chosen should allow for the most coplanar view of the pathology. While its addition can greatly simplify the mechanics of the operation, TONES is intended to complement the transnasal corridor, not replace it [2, 3]. Further, transorbital retraction of the orbital contents allows both for improved visualization of the ethmoid and supraorbital anterior cranial fossa (ACF) and for the traction and countertraction often needed to safely dissect tumor off the periorbita, orbital fat, or extraocular muscles.

The following four cases highlight the considerations for TONES as an adjunct portal for sinonasal tumor management:

Case 1: Right Frontal Sinus Osteoma (Fig. 10.1)

With respect to accessing and manipulating tumors within the frontal sinus, the SLC is the preferred approach providing a wide portal that is close in proximity to both the posterior table and the superior-lateral frontal recess [4, 9]. However, frontal sinus pneumatization varies, and therefore, preoperative imaging and vector planning need to confirm these relationships. Figure 10.1a, b demonstrates a large right centered frontal sinus osteoma that extends nearly to the top of the frontal sinus both midline and laterally as well as displacing the intersinus septum and tumor contents into the left frontal sinus. The entire anterior-posterior diameter of the sinus contains osteoma. The osteoma closely abuts nearly the entire posterior table. The SLC approach was chosen to aid in resection of this mass to allow for dissection of osteoma off of both frontal sinus tables and the lateral recess of the frontal sinus. Endoscopic view through the SLC portal offers coplanar views with the posterior and anterior tables of the frontal sinus and allowed for gross total resection of the tumor (Fig. 10.2a–c). Excellent access and visualization of the AEA is accomplished, and the AEA can be successfully and safely ligated as was required in the case (Fig. 10.3).

As noted previously, the paranasal sinuses are anatomically and physiologically complex spaces. In some cases, concomitant endonasal approaches can be used to create an extended frontal sinusotomy (endoscopic modified Lothrop procedure (EMLP)) that permits an additional portal for target visualization and instrumentation during tumor removal. Further, in this situation, multiportal techniques ensure postoperative adequate frontal sinus drainage and ventilation as well as monitoring for tumor recurrence while respecting physiologic function of the frontal sinus itself [2]. Lastly, reconstruction of bony defects of the orbital roof or skull base due to post-obstructive disease, destruction by a tumor, or removal by the approach itself can be accomplished via the SLC [2]. For example, in the frontal sinus osteoma (Fig. 10.1a), the majority of the osteoma was accessible and resected through the SLC portal alone. However, an endonasal portal was added which permitted further frontal sinus surgery to preserve sinonasal function and ensure

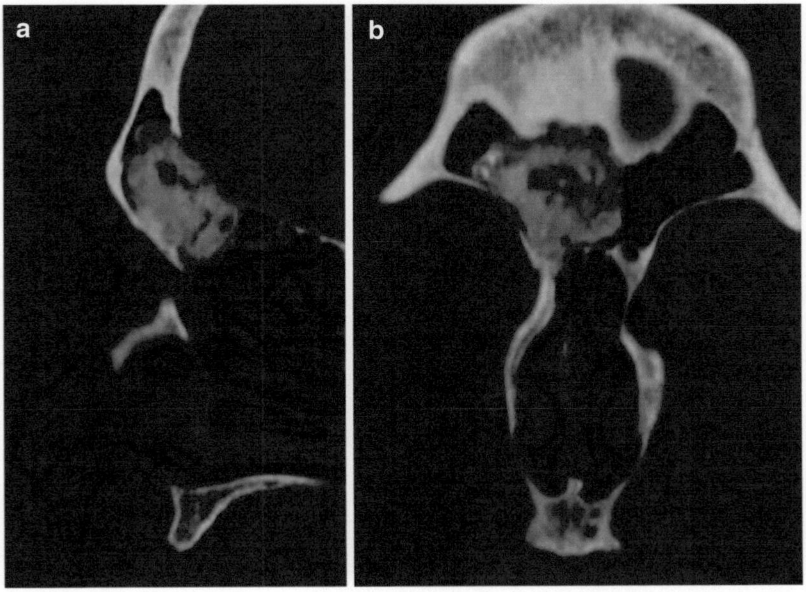

Fig. 10.1 Preoperative sagittal (**a**) and coronal (**b**) CT showing large right frontal sinus osteoma

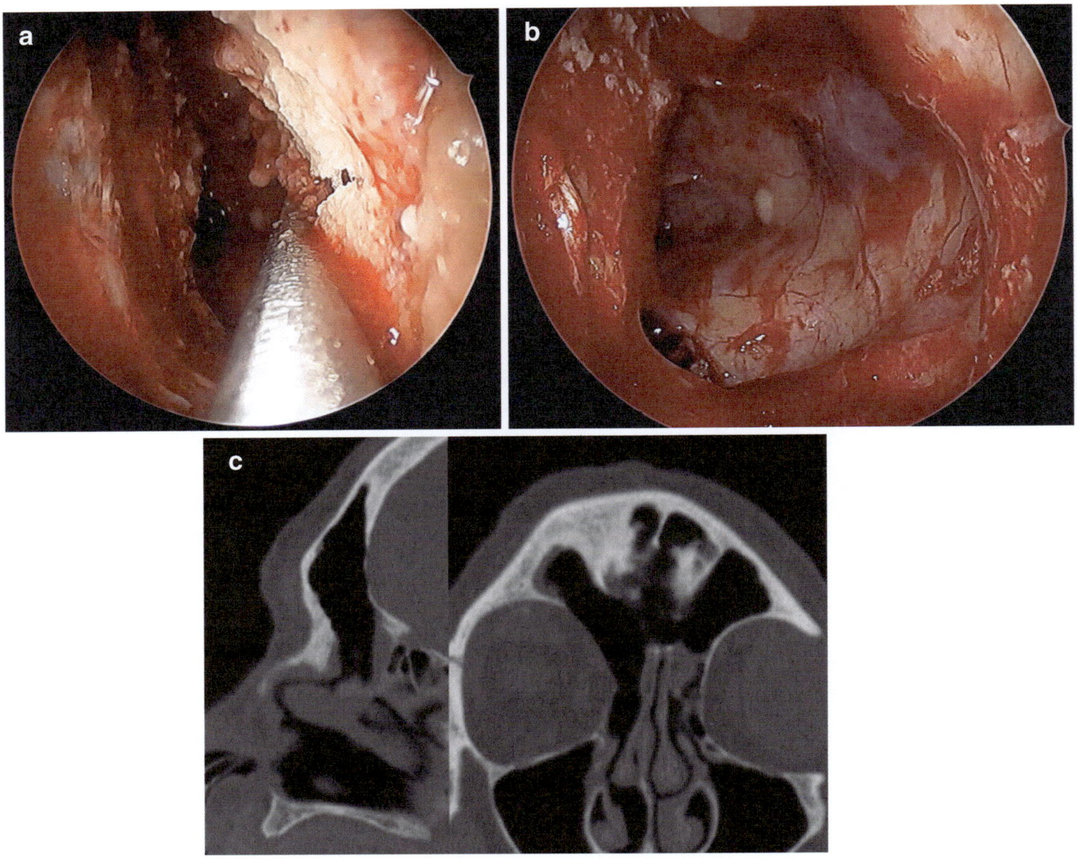

Fig. 10.2 (**a**) Intraoperative view through right SLC approach. Coplanar view of anterior and posterior tables as a Cottle elevator is used to dissect osteoma off the anterior table. (**b**) Intraoperative view through right SLC approach. View across to the left frontal sinus. Frontal osteoma completely resected off both the anterior and posterior tables. (**c**) Postoperative sagittal and coronal CT showing complete resection of right frontal sinus osteoma

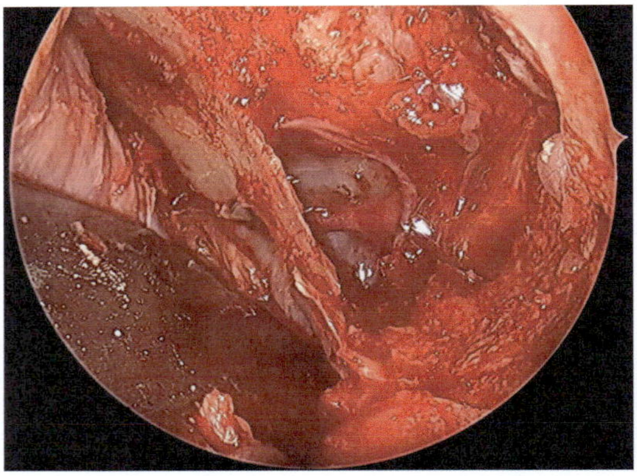

Fig. 10.3 Malleable retractor gently introduced through right SLC approach to retract orbital contents. Anterior ethmoid artery (AEA) seen traversing the lamina papyracea from the orbit into the ethmoid sinuses. AEA successfully ligated on the orbit side of the lamina papyracea

patency of the frontal sinus and outflow and for postoperative surveillance. In this case, a Draf IIb was deemed appropriate and an EMLP (or Draf III) was not required. Once the osteoma was resected, a polydioxanone (PDS) sheet was introduced through the SLC portal to reconstruct the bony orbit defect.

Case 2: Right Ethmoid Skull Base Inverted Papilloma with Supraorbital Extension

Beyond the frontal sinus, the SLC approach can provide additional access to the supraorbital ACF, the orbital apex, and around the optic chiasm [1, 4]. The second case in Fig. 10.4a, b dem-

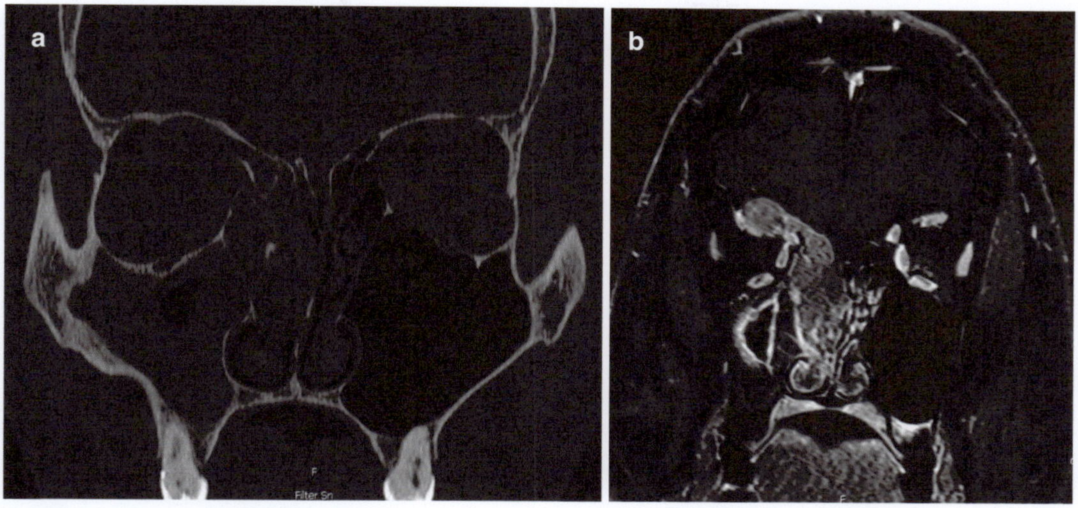

Fig. 10.4 (**a**) Preoperative CT of inverted papilloma (IP) of the right ethmoid skull base extending through supraorbital ethmoid (SOE) air cell into the superior orbit. (**b**) Preoperative T1 post-contrast MRI showing extension of the IP into the superior orbit with post-obstructive mucocele

onstrates a large ethmoid skull base inverted papilloma (IP). Inverted papilloma, while benign, has an approximately 15% risk of malignant transformation and is therefore considered a premalignant neoplasm. Further, it is known that IP may involve adjacent bone and therefore requires partial thickness resection of the bony attachment site. Additional bone removal has significantly reduced recurrence risk of inverted papilloma and is an important step in the management of this pathology. In the present case, there was supraorbital extension and expansion through a supraorbital ethmoid air (SOE) cell causing significant displacement of the sinonasal portion of the AEA. The supraorbital extension and post-obstructive mucus collection extended lateral to the superior rectus. Therefore, the SLC approach was chosen as an adjunct portal as it can allow for improved visualization and access to tumors and obstructive pathology that have extended into the superior orbit and are too lateral to be accessed via a transnasal portal alone [6]. This portal can be further leveraged to retract the orbital contents and allow for adequate clearance of the ethmoid skull base and orbital roof (Fig. 10.5a–d) [2]. The use of the SLC portal allowed for clearance of the post-obstructive component lateral to the superior rectus and for the excision of bony attachment sites and microscopic clearance of tumor at the supraorbital ACF in a way that would not have been possible with transnasal access alone.

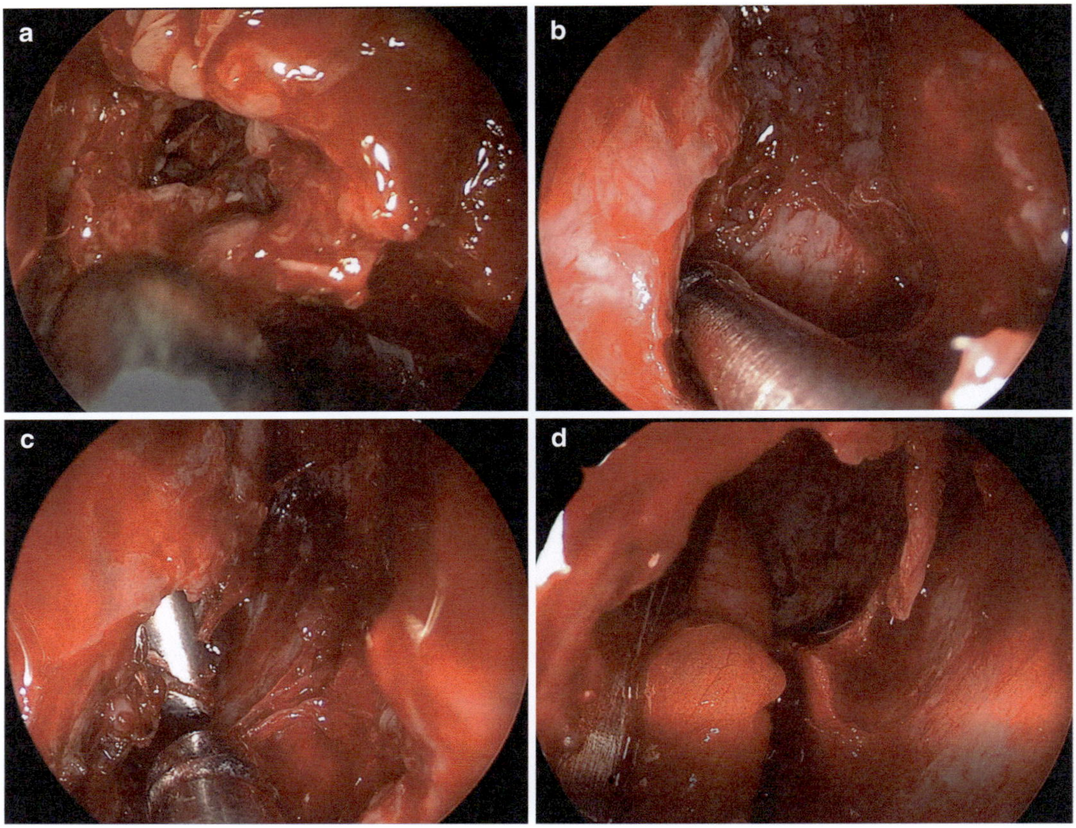

Fig. 10.5 (**a**) Transnasal view of orbital contents and IP without a clear plane of dissection. (**b**) Orbital contents retracted laterally using a malleable retractor through the SLC approach. This enabled a clear dissection plane between orbital contents and IP for safe resection and preservation of the orbital contents. (**c**) Resecting bony attachments with instruments introduced through the SLC portal viewed transnasally. (**d**) IP has been cleared from supraorbital ACF

Case 3: Left Ethmoid Aneurysmal Bone Cyst

TONES approaches can also be combined with transcranial techniques. For example, Fig. 10.6a, b demonstrates an aneurysmal bone cyst (ABC), a benign but locally aggressive sinonasal tumor. The tumor extends medially along the floor of the orbit to the lateral maxillary wall and posteriorly to the orbital apex, displacing the orbital contents. Not demonstrated in these images is intracranial extension for which a craniotomy approach was utilized in conjunction with the transnasal and transorbital approaches. To access the sinonasal and orbital components, a PC approach was selected. The PC approach is ideal for accessing the interorbital ACF (fovea ethmoidalis and cribriform) and is used frequently as transnasal adjunct for sinonasal tumors [1, 3, 5]. The AEA, posterior ethmoid artery (PEA), optic nerve, and orbital apex can all be directly accessed at an ideal angle with a coplanar view using a 0° endoscope [1] (Fig. 10.7). The PC incision may be extended inferiorly to leverage the ITC approach to access the orbital floor, maxillary sinus, and infraorbital nerve [1, 3, 5, 7, 8]. The ITC approach can be used alone or as an extension of both the LRC and PC approaches as

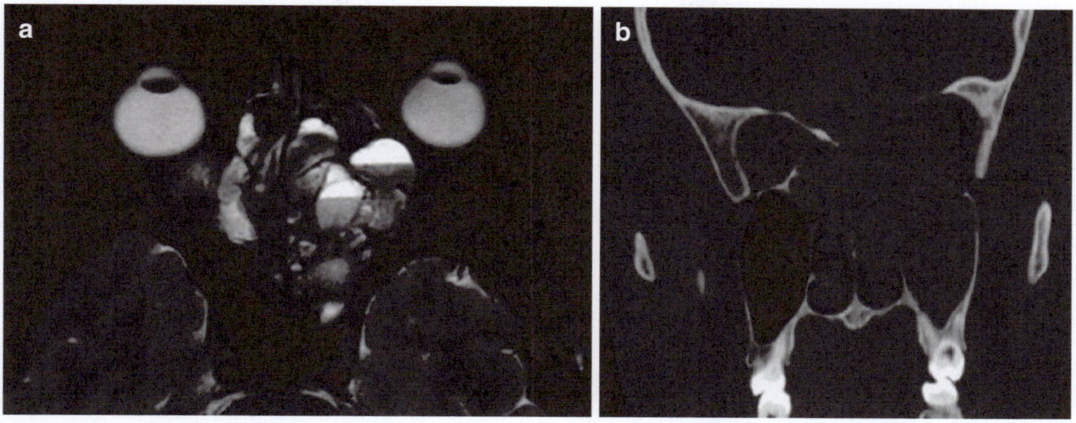

Fig. 10.6 (**a**) Extensive ABC on T2 MRI. (**b**) CT demonstrating medial extent of ABC and involvement of the orbital floor out laterally to V2/infraorbital foramen

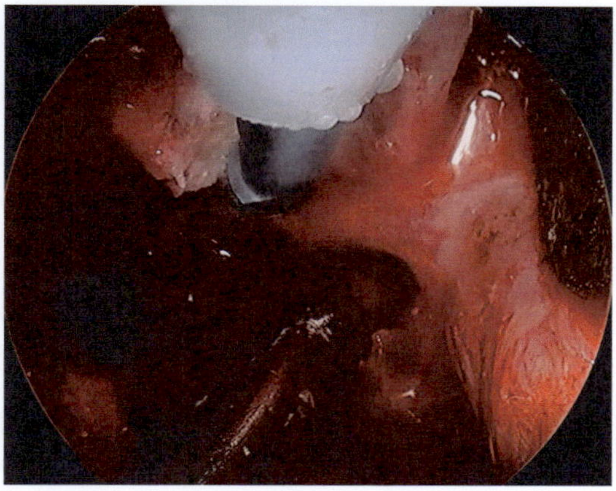

Fig. 10.7 Left PC approach to the ABC seen in Fig. 10.6a, b. Malleable retractor through the PC portal retracting orbital contents. View is coplanar with the orbital apex and optic nerve allowing safe resection of ABC with ultrasonic bone aspirator

the incisions are all transconjunctival [1, 3, 8]. Whether used independently or in conjunction with LRC and PC approaches, preservation of the infraorbital nerve when appropriate and reconstruction of the orbit is aided by the coplanar view afforded by the PS approach. The addition of the ITC portal to the PC portal allowed for gross total resection of the ABC, identification and preservation of the infraorbital nerve, as well as adequate reconstruction of the orbit spanning the defect across the orbital floor.

The LRC approach is used less commonly for sinonasal pathology. However, it may be considered for lesions with extension into the middle fossa and infratemporal fossa, as the LRC approach allows coplanar access to these locations without the need to cross over major neurovascular structures [1, 3]. The deep orbit, lateral recess of the sphenoid, and cavernous sinus are accessible through this approach as well with the advantage that the optic nerve is anatomically protected by the contents of the superior orbital fissure and the optic strut [1, 3].

Case 4: Left Sinonasal Ameloblastoma

Ameloblastoma is a rare benign neoplasm of odontogenic origin that has malignant potential and most commonly involves the mandibular teeth. Rarely, these tumors can involve the maxillary dentition and therefore the paranasal sinuses. They often present at an advanced local stage of disease. Historically, these have most commonly been managed with open techniques (e.g., lateral rhinotomy or sublabial approaches). In this case, the patient presented with a large soft tissue mass filling the entirety of the left paranasal sinuses (Fig. 10.8a, b). Notice in the preoperative MRI that the tumor fills the frontal sinus but the attach-

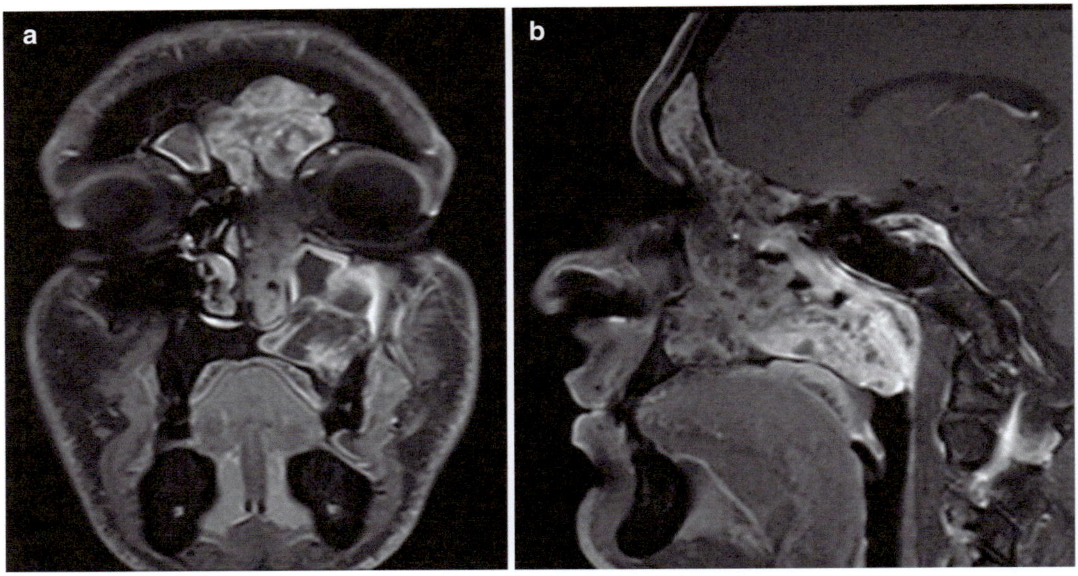

Fig. 10.8 Preoperative MRI, coronal (**a**) and sagittal (**b**) views, demonstrating extensive left frontal sinus and skull base extension of the ameloblastoma

ment point of the tumor within the frontal sinus (if any) was unknown. Intraoperatively, the tumor had attachments to the ethmoid skull base and within the frontal sinus (e.g., recess) such that a transnasal technique alone was insufficient to confirm an oncologically appropriate resection. Therefore, a combination of a transnasal and left SLC approach was utilized. A PC approach could have been considered, and this would have provided both visualization and instrumentation of the ethmoid skull base and inferior aspect of the frontal outflow. However, visualization and instrumentation of the frontal sinus proper would not have been feasible, and additional attachment sites within the frontal sinus itself could have been missed. Also, in this case, the PC approach would have added little to what a transnasal approach alone could afford. Therefore, the SLC approach was chosen and which afforded an opportunity to thoroughly manage this lesion regardless of the number or location of the attachment point(s) within the frontal sinus. A frontal trephine would have provided less optimal visualization of the frontal sinus outflow, and the SLC approach provides greater maneuverability. Through a combination of both SLC and transnasal working corridors, a gross total resection was achieved, and the patient has now been observed for 3 years without evidence of disease recurrence (Fig. 10.9a, b).

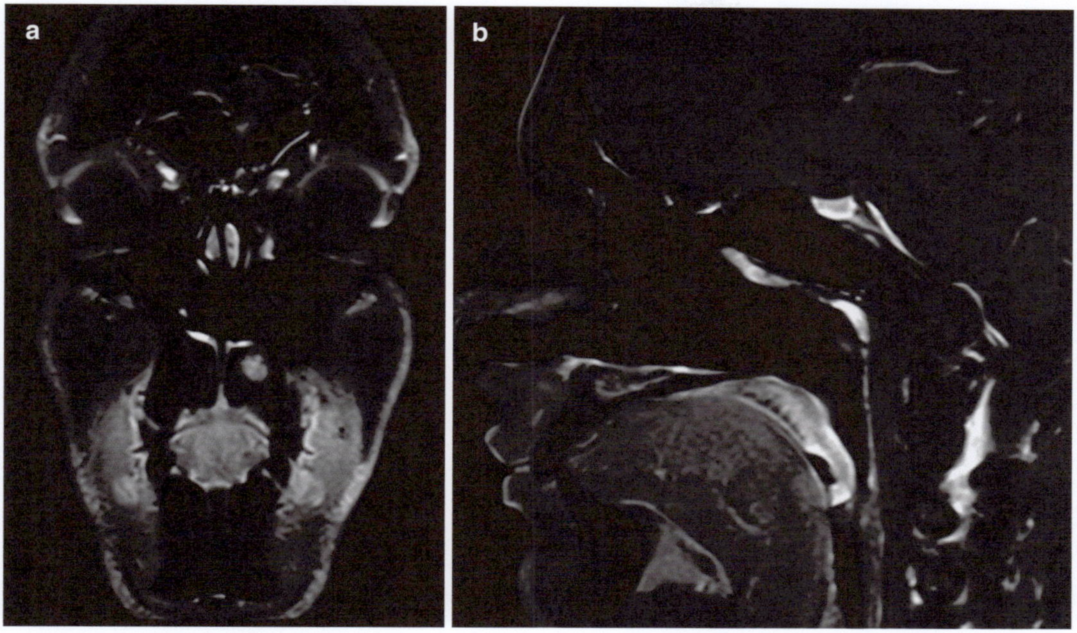

Fig. 10.9 Postoperative MRI, coronal (**a**) and sagittal (**b**) views, demonstrating gross total resection of the ameloblastoma

References

1. Moe KS, Bergeron CM, Ellenbogen RG. Transorbital neuroendoscopic surgery. Neurosurgery. 2010;67:16–28.
2. Balakrishnan K, Moe KS. Applications and outcomes of orbital and transorbital endoscopic surgery. Otolaryngol Head Neck Surg. 2011;144(5):815–20.
3. Ramakrishna R, Kim LJ, Bly RA, Moe KS, Ferreira M. Transorbital neuroendoscopic surgery for the treatment of skull base lesions. J Clin Neurosci. 2016;24:99–104.
4. Moe KS, Kim LJ, Bergeron CM. Transorbital endoscopic repair of CSF leaks. Laryngoscope. 2011;121:13–30.
5. Houlihan LM, Knoll AJS, Kakodkar P, Zhao X, O'Sullivan MGJ, Lawton MT, et al. Transorbital neuroendoscopic surgery as a mainstream neurosurgical corridor: a systematic review. World Neurosurg. 2021;152:167–79.
6. Tham T, Costantino P, Bruni M, Langer D, Boockvar J, Singh P. Multiportal combined transorbital and transnasal endoscopic resection of fibrous dysplasia. J Neurol Surg Rep. 2015;76(2):e291–6.
7. Dallan I, Castelnuovo P, Locatelli D, Turri-Zanoni M, AlQahtani A, Battaglia P, et al. Multiportal combined transorbital transnasal endoscopic approach for the management of selected skull base lesions: preliminary experience. World Neurosurg. 2015;84(1):97–107.
8. Raza SM, Quinones-Hinojosa A, Lim M, Boahene KDO. The transconjunctival transorbital approach: a keyhole approach to the midline anterior skull base. World Neurosurg. 2013;80(6):864–71.
9. Hicks KL, Moe KS, Humphreys IM. Bilateral transorbital and transnasal endoscopic resection of a frontal sinus osteoblastoma and orbital mucocele: a case report and review of the literature. Ann Otol Rhinol Laryngol. 2018;127(11):864–9.

Part IV

Orbital Pathology

11 Extraconal Tumours

Hamzah Mustak and Darlene Lubbe

Introduction

The orbit can be divided into well-defined anatomical compartments [1]. The four recti muscles attaching to the globe divide the orbit into the intraconal and extraconal compartments [2, 3]. The intraconal compartment contains the globe, optic nerve complex, orbital vessels and nerves [2, 3]. The extraconal compartment consists of the bony orbital walls, peri-orbita, fat and the lacrimal gland [1–3]. The orbital septum divides the preseptal eyelid and adnexal structures from the post-septal compartment [3]. Localizing orbital lesions to these anatomical compartments aids in the diagnostic approach and guides the surgical approach to managing these lesions. This chapter deals with the evaluation and surgical approach to extraconal lesions [2, 3].

Pertinent Anatomy

The **extraconal compartment** is the space within the orbit outside the muscular cone formed by the recti muscles (Fig. 11.1). The orbital septum forms the base of the extraconal compartment, the external borders are formed by the bones of the orbit and their periosteum and the internal borders are formed by the extraocular muscles and their surrounding fascia which pass posteriorly and converge on the tendinous ring known as the annulus of Zinn at the orbital apex [2–4]. Several nerves pass outside the annulus of Zinn in the extraconal compartment, whilst oth-

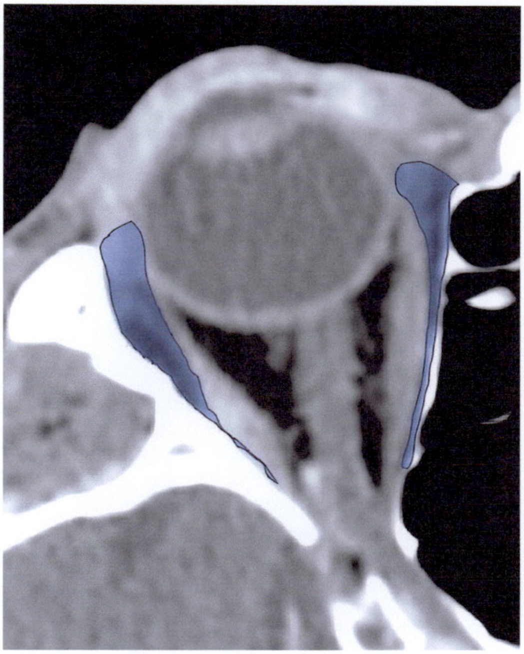

Fig. 11.1 CT scan of the orbit showing the extraconal compartment highlighted in blue

H. Mustak
Division of Ophthalmology, Groote Schuur Hospital, University of Cape Town, Cape Town, South Africa

D. Lubbe (✉)
Division of Otorhinolaryngology, Groote Schuur Hospital, University of Cape Town, Cape Town, South Africa

T. H. Schwartz et al. (eds.), *Endoscopic Transorbital Surgery of the Orbit, Skull Base and Brain*,
https://doi.org/10.1007/978-3-031-59504-2_11

ers arise in the intraconal space but traverse through the extraconal space [3, 4]. Several branches of the ophthalmic artery also take origin in the intraconal space but pass into the extraconal compartment [3, 4]. The various nerves and vessels that pass through the extraconal space are shown in Table 11.1.

Table 11.1 Nerves and vessels of the extraconal space

Nerves and vessels of the extraconal compartment	
Nerves	• Trochlear nerve (CN IV) • Branches of the ophthalmic division of the trigeminal nerve – Frontal nerve – Supraorbital nerve – Supratrochlear nerve – Lacrimal nerve – Infratrochlear nerve • Branches of the maxillary division of the trigeminal nerve – Zygomatic nerve – Zygomaticotemporal nerve – Zygomaticofacial nerve – Infraorbital nerve
Arteries	• Extraconal branches of the ophthalmic artery – Lacrimal artery – Supraorbital artery – Posterior ethmoidal artery – Anterior ethmoidal artery – Internal palpebral artery – Supratrochlear artery (frontal artery) – Dorsal nasal artery • Infraorbital artery
Veins	• Superior ophthalmic vein • Inferior ophthalmic vein • Infraorbital vein

The lacrimal gland and extraconal fat make up the other tissue structures of the extraconal space. The lacrimal gland comprises two lobes, the palpebral and the orbital, which are separated by the orbital septum.

Aetiology of Extraconal Tumours

The extraconal compartment is often involved in orbital pathology but is usually not the primary source of pathology [4, 5]. Extraconal orbital lesions may arise between the recti muscles and the peri-orbita (Fig. 11.2a), in the subperiosteal space (Fig. 11.2b) and within bones comprising the orbital wall (Fig. 11.2c) [2–4]. The subperiosteal space within the extraconal compartment lies between the cortical bone and its adjacent periosteum [5]. The extraconal space between the periosteum and muscle cone contains fat as well as small nerves and vessels [3].

Superior, medial wall and orbital floor lesions tend to originate from sinonasal pathology [4]. Superior and lateral lesions are often of lacrimal gland origin [3, 4]. Involvement of the extraconal fat compartment usually involves the adjacent boundary tissue structures such as the peri-orbita, recti muscles or bone [4]. Examples of this are metastatic lesions to the bone, rhabdomyosarcoma and lymphoma [4]. These masses may have an ill-defined infiltrating mor-

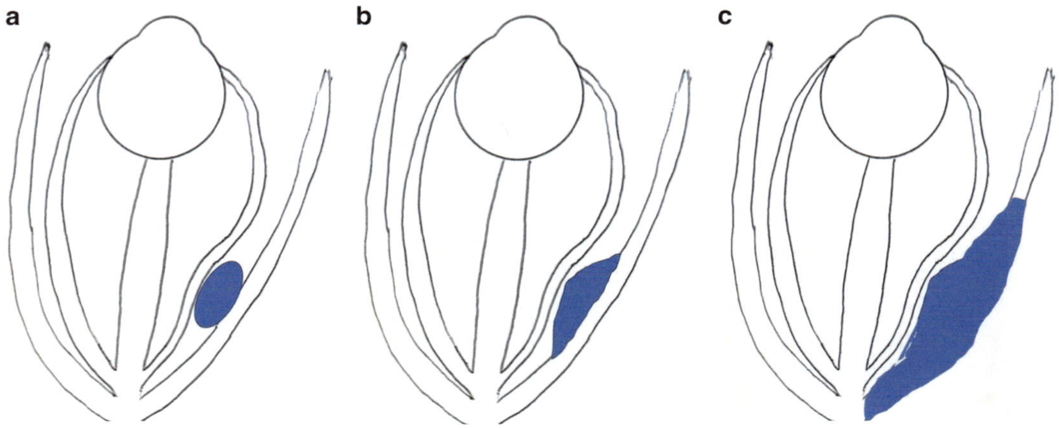

Fig. 11.2 Topographical classification of extraconal tumours. (**a**) Tumour between the recti muscles and the peri-orbita. (**b**) Tumour in the subperiosteal space. (**c**) Tumour within bones comprising the orbital wall

Table 11.2 Involved tissue structures

Adnexal structures (lacrimal gland and sac)	Other extraconal structures and adjacent structures (nerves, vessels, bones, sinuses)
Epithelial lacrimal gland tumours • Benign mixed tumour • Adenoid cystic carcinoma • Adenocarcinoma • Undifferentiated *Non-epithelial lacrimal gland tumours* • Lymphoma • Reactive lymphoid hyperplasia • Plasmacytoma *Lacrimal sac tumours* • Inverting papilloma • Squamous cell carcinoma	• Dermoid/epidermoid • Rhabdomyosarcoma • Schwannoma • Neurofibroma • Fibrous dysplasia • Osteoma • Metastases • Myeloma • Meningioma • Venolymphatic malformations • IgG4 disease • Idiopathic orbital inflammatory disease/orbital pseudo-tumour

phology and tend to involve both the intra- and extraconal compartments [1, 4].

Lesions involving the peri-orbita as well as the orbital bone may also arise from contiguous spread along the dura or meninges, invading the orbit via the cranial foramina as well as the superior and inferior orbital fissures [1]. An example of this is spheno-orbital meningiomas.

Perineural spread of cancer along the first and second divisions of the trigeminal nerve often due to skin cancers can also present with masses of the extraconal space [4]. Table 11.2 lists the commonly seen pathologies of the extraconal space based on the involved tissue structures.

Clinical Presentation and Physical Exam

The most common presentations of extraconal tumours are proptosis, globe displacement (dystopia) with diplopia or distortion of vision and pain [4]. The physical examination should include general inspection for proptosis and dystopia as well as adnexal features such as oedema, ptosis, chemosis and temporal fullness [4]. A thorough ophthalmic examination should be conducted including visual acuity and optic nerve function tests, as well as extraocular motility. In cases of proptosis, the orbit should be palpated for obvious masses and note taken of the consistency, borders and extent of involvement of the mass [4].

Examination should include inspection of the facial skin for skin cancers as well as palpation of the pre-auricular, submental and submandibular glands [4].

A systemic enquiry for symptoms of common sites of primary malignancy such as lung, breast and prostate should be performed.

Diagnostic Work-Up

Imaging

Diseases of extraconal space are best evaluated with CT and magnetic resonance imaging (MRI) [1]. CT is more useful for assessment of bony changes such as erosion, remodelling and hyperostosis which informs on the underlying pathophysiology and differential diagnosis. MRI is likely to be more sensitive than CT for evaluation of the soft tissue structures such as the marrow space changes within the bone, fat compartment, perineural spread and related intracranial abnormalities such as dural involvement [1].

Laboratory Tests

Serology

Serological tests are usually guided by the clinical features as well as the radiographic features of the tumour/lesion [4]. In cases of inflammatory features, a full blood count as well as inflammatory markers such as CRP and ESR may be helpful. Serum IgG4 levels should be considered in cases of inflammatory or sclerosing-type lesions [4]. Features suggestive of metastatic disease may warrant certain tumour marker serology such as prostate-specific antigen levels in men. This should however be guided by the clinical presentation, morphology and behaviour of tumour on imaging and the systemic enquiry and examination.

Definitive diagnosis of orbital tumours, however, is usually made on histopathology.

Surgical Approaches and Decision-Making

The surgical approach is dictated by two factors: tumour location and tumour biology [5].

Topographic Location

The location of lesions can be divided into:

1. Anterior, mid and posterior third of the orbit
2. Superior or inferior
3. Medial or lateral

Extraconal lesions tend to be more accessible than intraconal lesions due to the ability to stay within the subperiosteal space which provides direct access to the lesion or only requires the peri-orbita to be opened once the lesion is reached [2, 5]. This allows for the avoidance of orbital fat herniation which may impede visualization particularly when using transorbital endoscopic approaches.

Tumour Biology

1. Benign morphology
2. Infiltrative
3. Malignant morphology

Benign lesions tend to be slowly progressive in nature and are usually well circumscribed on imaging [4]. These lesions either mould to the adjacent structures or cause a pressure effect such as indentation of the globe or scalloping of the bone in the case of a pleomorphic adenoma/benign mixed tumour of the lacrimal gland [4]. Several benign lesions can be removed via minimal access approaches as they can either be removed piecemeal or decompressed to reduce their bulk. Venolymphatic malformations and dermoid/epidermoid cysts are examples of this approach [4, 5].

Infiltrative lesions such as lymphoma, IgG4 disease and myeloma do not require complete excision but simply a diagnostic biopsy as their management is usually nonsurgical. Malignant lesions arising primarily in the orbit such as adenoid and adenoid cystic carcinoma of the lacrimal gland warrant complete excision and may require a bony orbitotomy in cases of invasive disease of the orbital wall [4, 5].

Lesions of the superior and lateral extraconal space are best approached through a superolateral eyelid skin crease approach. Lesions of the inferior orbit can be approached either through a transconjunctival or lower eyelid skin approach such as the subciliary or direct orbital rim approach [2, 5].

Lesions of the mid and posterior orbit may require a bony orbitotomy such as a lateral orbitotomy in the case of lateral lesions or an endonasal translaminar approach in the case of medial lesions.

Surgical Technique

Superior and Lateral Approach

The skin incision is usually made in the crease of the upper eyelid and can be extended over the lateral orbital rim depending on the degree of access required (Fig. 11.3). Dissection is continued in the suborbicularis plane towards the superolateral bony rim exposing the periosteum. The periosteum is then incised in a C shape over the superolateral aspect of the orbit using a scalpel or needle cautery. A sharp periosteal elevator is then used to develop the subperiosteal dissection plane. The subperiosteal dissection is continued to follow the reflection of the periosteum. The dissection is then carried posteriorly to expose the reflection of the superior and inferior orbital fissures. Perforating neurovascular bundles can either be preserved or cauterized and dissected depending on the pathology, target site and the exposure required.

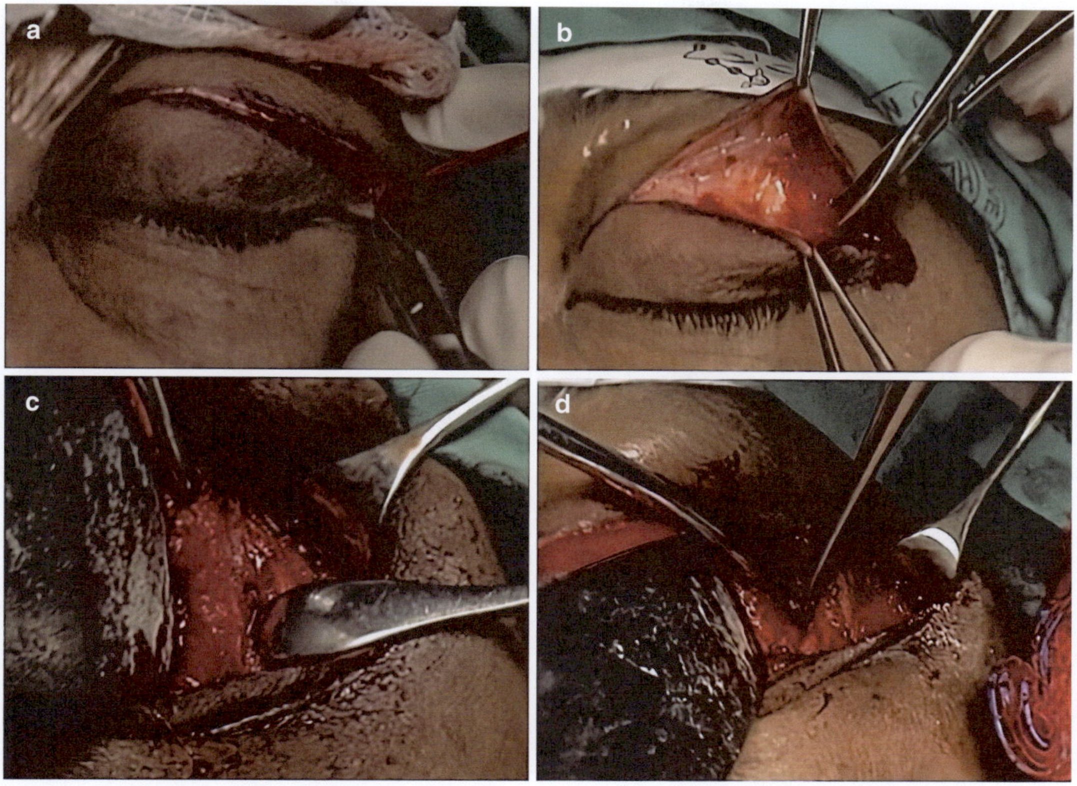

Fig. 11.3 The superior lateral approach. (**a**) Lid crease incision extended over the lateral orbital rim. (**b**) Suborbicularis dissection preserving the orbital septum. (**c**) Exposure of the periosteum over the lateral orbital rim. (**d**) Subperiosteal dissection following curvature of the lateral orbital wall maintaining the intact periosteum

Inferior Corridor

This approach utilizes either the transconjunctival incision with development of a pre-septal dissection plane over the inferior rim or a transcutaneous approach such as a subciliary or direct orbital rim approach. The transconjunctival approach is described (Fig. 11.4). The lower eyelid is retracted anteriorly with a Desmarres lid retractor, and a transconjunctival incision is made, using Stevens scissors, at the inferior border of the tarsus, approximately 4 mm from the eyelid margin. The incision is then extended across the horizontal length of the eyelid and can be incorporated with the transcaruncular approach for increased exposure if needed. Dissection is carried inferiorly to expose the periosteum of the inferior orbital rim. The periosteum is then incised with a #15 blade or the monopolar cautery along the inferior orbital rim. A subperiosteal dissection plane is then created with the periosteal elevator. The subperiosteal dissection is then carried posteriorly over the inferior orbital rim. A malleable retractor can then be placed to retract the orbital soft tissue allowing development of the subperiosteal dissection towards the orbital apex.

Medial Corridor: The Transcaruncular Approach

Stevens or sharp iris scissors are used to create a vertical incision through the midportion of the caruncle (Fig. 11.5). The incision can be extended both superiorly and inferiorly through the conjunctiva to create a wide window of exposure. The condensed fibrous layer just deep to the

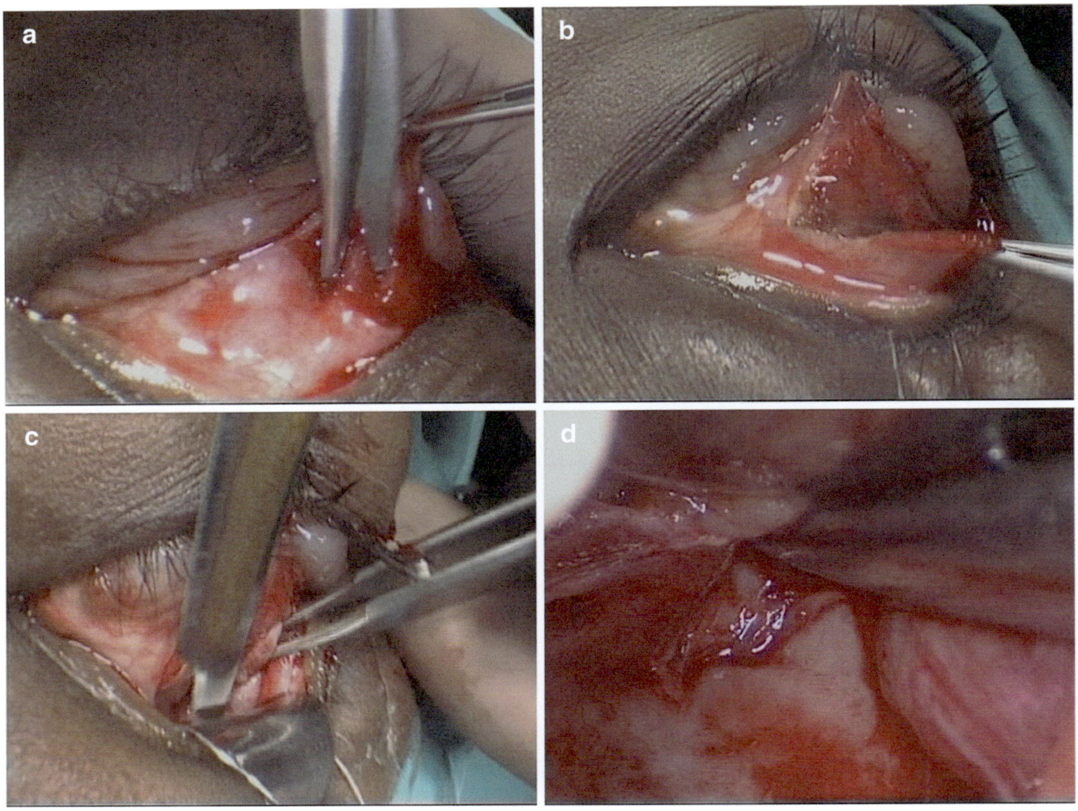

Fig. 11.4 The inferior orbital approach. (**a**) Incision through the conjunctiva 1–2 mm below the lower end of the tarsal plate. (**b**) Pre-septal dissection down towards the inferior orbital rim. (**c**) The periosteum over the inferior rim is excised. (**d**) Subperiosteal dissection over the inferior rim exposing the inferior orbit

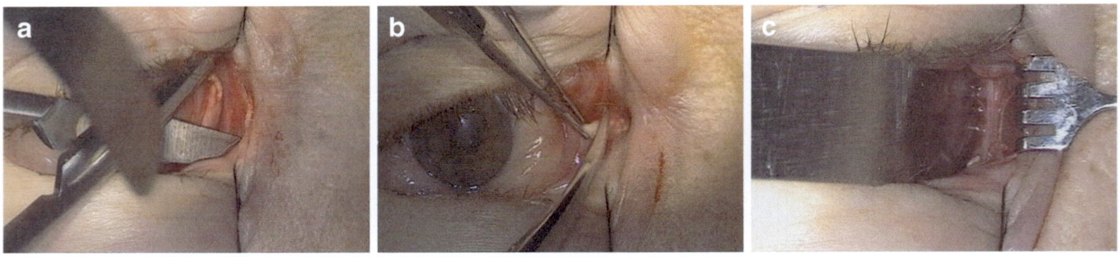

Fig. 11.5 Transcaruncular approach to the medial corridor. (**a**) The caruncle is grasped with a toothed forceps and incised. (**b**) The dissecting scissors are then directed in a posterior-medial direction towards the posterior lacrimal crest on the medial orbital wall. (**c**) The periosteum of the medial orbital wall is exposed and can then be incised allowing for subperiosteal dissection along the medial orbit

caruncle is incised in the direction of the posterior lacrimal crest using sharp scissors. Spreading of the scissor tips against the medial orbital wall will then expose the periosteum overlying the lamina papyracea. The periosteum is then incised and a subperiosteal dissection plane is developed. Dissection should continue posteriorly in the subperiosteal plane. The anterior and posterior ethmoidal arteries are identified and can either be spared or cauterized with bipolar cautery, depending on the extent of dissection needed.

Summary Points

The extraconal space consists of orbital fat, nerves, vessels, the lacrimal gland, peri-orbita, periosteum and the bony walls of the orbit. Although commonly involved in orbital pathology, it is seldom the primary site of pathology. Tumours of the extraconal space are accessible through approaches that utilize the subperiosteal dissection plane thus avoiding the herniation of orbital fat until incision of the peri-orbita is required.

Topographical classification as well as biomorphological characteristics of the lesions aids in formulation of a differential diagnosis as well as planning the surgical approach to accessing these lesions.

References

1. Purohit BS, Vargas MI, Ailianou A, Merlini L, Poletti PA, Platon A, Delattre BM, Rager O, Burkhardt K, Becker M. Orbital tumours and tumour-like lesions: exploring the armamentarium of multiparametric imaging. Insights Imaging. 2016;7(1):43–68. https://doi.org/10.1007/s13244-015-0443-8. Epub 2015 Oct 31. PMID: 26518678; PMCID: PMC4729705.
2. Abussuud Z, Ahmed S, Paluzzi A. Surgical approaches to the orbit: a neurosurgical perspective. J Neurol Surg B Skull Base. 2020;81(4):385–408. https://doi.org/10.1055/s-0040-1713941. Epub 2020 Sep 9. PMID: 33209566; PMCID: PMC7661317.
3. Martins C, Costa e Silva IE, Campero A, Yasuda A, Aguiar LR, Tatagiba M, Rhoton A. Microsurgical anatomy of the orbit: the rule of seven. Anat Res Int. 2011;2011:468727. https://doi.org/10.1155/2011/468727.
4. Rootman J. Diseases of the orbit. 2nd ed. Lippincott, Williams and Wilkins; 2002.
5. Rootman J. Orbital surgery: a conceptual approach. 2nd ed. Lippincott, Williams and Wilkins; 2013.

12 Intraconal Tumors

Chiman Jeon

Anatomy

The orbit is divided into intraconal and extraconal spaces that are separated by the extraocular muscles and connected at the orbital apex [1]. The intraconal space is located within the musculofascial cone of the extraocular muscles and their surrounding fascia. The extraconal space refers to the intraorbital space that lies outside of the extraocular muscles within the bony walls. Posteriorly at the orbital apex, all extraocular muscles except the inferior oblique muscle originate from the annulus of Zinn [2].

The intraconal space contains critical anatomical structures including the ophthalmic artery (OA), the optic nerve (ON), the oculomotor nerve (superior and inferior divisions), the nasociliary branch of the ophthalmic division of the trigeminal nerve, and the abducens nerve, which are surrounded by the intraconal fat [1, 3]. The lateral boundary of the intraconal space comprises the ON and its associated neurovascular structures, including the OA, nasociliary nerve, long ciliary artery, and long ciliary nerve [3]. The superior and inferior limits are bounded by the anterior ethmoidal and posterior ethmoidal neurovascular bundles and the inferior rectus muscle, respectively. The anterior and posterior boundaries consist of the globe and annulus of Zinn, respectively. The medial rectus muscle forms the medial boundary of the pyramid-shaped medial intraconal space [3].

Innervation of the superior rectus and levator muscles comes from the superior division of the oculomotor nerve, while the inferior rectus, medial rectus, and inferior oblique muscles are innervated by the inferior division of the oculomotor nerve. The lateral rectus muscle is solely innervated by the abducens nerve, which runs in the lateral intraconal space after entering the orbit through the superior orbital fissure and annulus of Zinn [2].

The extraconal space harbors the anterior portion of the superior ophthalmic vein, the lacrimal and frontal branches of CN V1, the lacrimal apparatus, and extraconal orbital fat.

A thorough knowledge of the orbital vascular supply is crucial for intraconal dissection in achieving satisfactory clinical outcomes. It is accepted that there is great variability in the neurovascular supply. The area lateral to the ON, within the intraconal space, is rich in small arteries and arterioles [4]. The OA gives rise to the central retinal, long and short ciliary, supraorbital, medial and lateral palpebral, lacrimal, recurrent meningeal, ethmoidal, supratrochlear, and dorsal nasal arteries [5, 6]. It exits the optic canal and the annular tendon at their most lateral aspect, inferior to the intraorbital ON [6]. The

C. Jeon (✉)
Department of Neurosurgery, Korea Universtiy Ansan Hospital, Korea University College of Medicine, Ansan, Republic of Korea

T. H. Schwartz et al. (eds.), *Endoscopic Transorbital Surgery of the Orbit, Skull Base and Brain*,
https://doi.org/10.1007/978-3-031-59504-2_12

OA continues anteromedially and gives off the posterior and anterior ethmoidal arteries, which course inferior to the superior oblique muscle to exit the orbit via their respective ethmoidal foramina [5]. The branches of the OA that supply the contents of the orbit and the ON are the central retinal artery (CRA) and the ciliary arteries. The CRA is usually the first branch of the OA and arises in proximity to the ciliary ganglion before the OA ascends steeply to cross over the ON. It pierces through the ON's dural sheath approximately 1 cm behind the globe to course anteriorly adjacent to and more distally within the ON. Posterior ciliary arteries branch off the OA in two forms. Two long posterior ciliary arteries travel within the sclera to supply the ciliary muscle and iris, while short posterior ciliary arteries supply the anterior ON and peripapillary choroid [7]. Anterior ciliary arteries arise from the branches of the OA that supply the rectus muscles [7].

Pathologies

A variety of benign and malignant tumors of different origins and histologic types can arise in the orbit. Orbital tumors can be classified as primary tumors (meaning they originated from orbital structures), secondary tumors (meaning they extend into the orbit from surrounding structures outside the orbit such as eyelids, paranasal sinus, nasopharynx, or brain), and orbital metastases [8–10]. Anatomically, they are also divided into intraconal, extraconal, and intracanalicular, based on the tumor's relationship with the musculofascial cone, with the intracanalicular group of tumors being those lesions that are at least partially within the optic canal [9]. Primary tumors of the orbit are less common than those arising from adjacent structures. About two thirds of the primary orbital tumors are benign, with higher incidences of malignant tumors in elderly patients [11–13]. Ohtsuka et al. have reported that in the intraconal area, the most common tumors in adults are cavernous hemangioma, optic nerve sheath meningioma (ONSM), and orbital schwannoma, while the most common tumors in children are optic nerve glioma, hemorrhagic lymphangioma, and rhabdomyosarcoma [14].

Cavernous hemangioma constitutes the most common benign tumor of the intraconal region in adults, representing 5–15% of all orbital masses [1, 15, 16]. It tends to involve predominantly the middle third of the orbit, especially lateral to the ON in the intraconal compartment of the left orbit [4]. It is the second most frequent cause of unilateral proptosis after thyroid-associated orbitopathy [15]. ONSM occurs more often in adults, representing approximately 2% of all orbital tumors [17, 18]. Primary ONSM arises from either the intraorbital or intracanalicular portion of the arachnoid sheath surrounding the ON; secondary ONSM typically originates intracranially and invades the orbit and optic canal secondarily [18]. Isolated optic nerve glioma is usually seen in pediatric patients and traditionally associated with neurofibromatosis type 1 [16, 19]. This intraconal tumor, which is restricted to the ON, without extension to the chiasm or posteriorly, is traditionally lumped together with chiasmatic tumors or another optic pathway involvement [19]. Its pathology is mostly low-grade pilocytic astrocytoma. Other benign neoplasms also include orbital schwannomas and neurofibromas [1, 20]. Orbital schwannoma commonly arises from sensory nerves, most frequently the supraorbital and supratrochlear nerves, especially in the superior orbit [20].

On the other hand, common malignant lesions in adults include non-Hodgkin's lymphoma, orbital metastases, and sinonasal malignancies penetrating into the orbit [1, 21]. For pediatric patients, infantile hemangiomas and rhabdomyosarcomas are the most common benign and malignant primary pathologies, respectively [1].

Clinical Presentation

Patients with primary or secondary orbital tumors usually present with exophthalmos, diplopia, swelling, pain, tearing, and blurred vision [9]. Although exophthalmos is a common sign in orbital tumors, this sign can be seen in other conditions, such as thyroid disease, orbital varices, collagen vascular disease, prolapse of intracranial contents into the orbit, and congenital defect of the orbital wall [9]. Specifically, intraconal tumors tend to present with early vision loss, extraocular muscle paresis, diplopia, and axial proptosis [15]. In contrast, extraconal tumors tend to manifest early as proptosis, displacement of the globe, diplopia, and late vision loss. Intracanalicular tumors (within the optic canal) tend to cause early vision loss, ON head edema, and appearance of optociliary shunt vessels on the surface of the optic discs, with minimal or no proptosis [15].

Approach Selection

Although the incidence of orbital tumors is relatively low, the surgical strategy with respect to choosing the most appropriate approach is crucial to achieve the best clinical outcome [22]. As a rule, cosmetics and accessibility are both considered in the management of orbital tumors [23, 24]. With the evolution of endoscopic skull base techniques, there are two main types of minimally invasive approaches to intraorbital tumors: endoscopic endonasal and transorbital approaches. The endoscopic transorbital approach (ETOA) is a novel technique that has overcome the limited endonasal surgical corridor, thereby providing straightforward access to the contents of the orbit as well as the intracranial compartments, including the anterior and middle fossa and lateral cavernous sinus [23, 25–30]. It has the advantage of providing a shorter, unencumbered access to the target lesion that minimizes the extent of tissue dissection and eases its dissection. Notwithstanding, orbital surgery has been traditionally considered challenging because it requires scrupulous dissection of the delicate intraorbital structures. The lack of definite anatomical reference points also makes it risky, thus potentially leading to loss of the surgeon's orientation [31]. In this regard, appropriate approach selection is of utmost importance in managing the intraorbital lesions to minimize the risk of surgery-related complications.

The location of the orbital tumor with respect to the ON is paramount in dictating the most appropriate surgical approach. Paluzzi et al. proposed a clock model as a simple algorithm that guides the selection of the most appropriate approach for intraorbital pathologies in relation to the ON [15]. The group recommended either transcranial approaches, such as a frontotemporal craniotomy with orbitozygomatic osteotomy, a lateral orbitotomy, an anterior medial orbitotomy, or an endoscopic endonasal approach (EEA) according to its corresponding clock position relative to the ON [15]. Such extraorbital approaches may accompany the risk of brain retraction and temporalis muscle atrophy as well as injury to the frontal branches of the facial nerve [29]. On the other hand, Moe et al. first introduced a pure ETOA along with the concept of four quadrants of the orbit for anterior skull base pathology [23]. They recommended that the selection of surgical approach is dependent on which quadrant of the orbit is most closely involved with or is the most direct route to the lesion of interest. The four quadrants are accessed as follows: precaruncular for the medial quadrant, superior eyelid crease for the superior quadrant, lateral retrocanthal for the lateral quadrant, and the preseptal lower eyelid for the inferior quadrant [23]. Likewise, we have recently developed a neuro-topographic four-zone model (zones I–IV) of the orbit for approaching both intraconal and extraconal lesions, with the epicenter around the ON on the coronal plane for the selection of optimal endoscopic approaches (Fig. 12.1) [22]. We demonstrated that ETOA achieved successful resection of the orbital tumors with acceptable morbidity via the superolateral trajectory along the orbit (zones I and II). No patient treated with ETOA in our series underwent an orbitozygomatic osteotomy or a lateral orbitotomy. EEA provided excellent exposure of the orbital lesions inferomedial to the ON for orbital decompression (zones III and IV), demonstrating favorable resection outcomes [22].

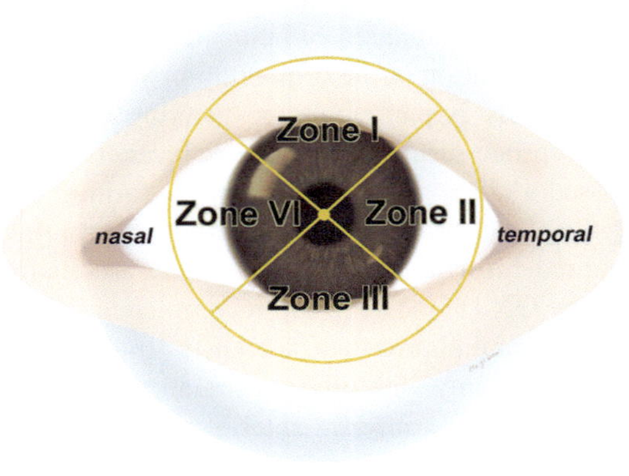

Fig. 12.1 Artist rendition of the four-zone model with its epicenter around the optic nerve (yellow dot) on the coronal plane, consisting of zones I and II (temporal side) and zones III and IV (nasal side)

Surgical Technique

Approaches to Zones I and II

A skin marking is made at the lateral half of the superior eyelid crease line for patients with an eyelid crease and at the same length along supraciliary line for those without an eyelid crease [32]. The line is extended approximately 1 cm laterally over the lateral orbital rim. A lubricated corneal protector is placed over the ipsilateral eye to avoid corneal abrasion. A skin incision is made after infiltration of a local anesthetic with a mixture of 2% lidocaine with 1:100,000 epinephrine and 0.5% bupivacaine [32]. The skin and orbicularis muscle flap are elevated and extended superolaterally until the lateral orbital rim is reached. Utmost care must be taken to avoid trauma to the levator muscle and aponeurosis. A periosteal incision is made on the lateral orbital rim after blunt dissection to the periosteum. The periosteum is elevated with the Freer periosteal elevator. Although the lateral orbital rim is not usually removed for orbital tumors during ETOA, a lateral orbitotomy can be performed as needed according to the size and location of the tumor. A rigid 0° endoscope is introduced into the surgical corridor, while the periorbita is gently retracted medially with a Silastic sheet to avoid excessive orbit soft tissue compression. The subperiosteal dissection then proceeds to the superior and inferior orbital fissures with care not to violate the periorbita as prolapsing orbital fat will make the subsequent dissection more difficult.

The lateral orbital wall (composed of the greater wing of the sphenoid bone) is carefully drilled using a high-speed 3-mm coarse diamond burr from lateral to medial. The extent of bone removal can be tailored to the surgical plan. Great care should be taken while drilling the lateral orbital wall to prevent the orbital fat from being caught in the high-speed drill, which could result in damage to the rectus muscles.

Approaches to Zones III and IV

Both EEA and ETOA can provide access to the inferomedial aspect of the intraconal region in the orbit. According to the neuro-topographic four-zone model, EEA can provide excellent exposure of the orbital tumors inferomedial to the ON, especially those located in the mid and posterior medial orbit and orbital apex [20, 22, 33]. On the other hand, as Moe et al. reported in their series, ETOA can also permit surgical resection of the intraconal tumors located inferiorly and medially, which predominantly involve either zone III or zone IV according to the four-zone model, via the dissection corridor between the medial and inferior rectus muscles [22, 23]. For the intraconal tumors predominantly involving the zone III, ETOA with a transconjunctival incision can be employed to access the orbital floor; for those predominantly occupying the medial intraconal space, which corresponds to the zone IV, ETOA with a transconjunctival precaruncular incision can be used [22, 23, 34]. However, both transorbital routes can be more challenging when the intraconal tumors are located in the medial orbital apex due to the narrow working space between the medial orbital wall and the globe. Depending on the size and location of the tumor, ETOA can be combined with EEA in a multiportal technique in order to expose the lateral or posterior part of the orbit as well as the inferomedial part of the ON [22, 35]. Such a combined endoscopic multiportal approach allows for adequate exposure of the surgical field.

Intraconal Tumor Resection

Under the guidance of neuronavigation, the periorbita overlying the lesion of interest is appropriately opened parallel to the medial/lateral rectus muscles. A working space between the extraocular muscles is created after the extraconal fat is removed. Preserving the extraconal fat not only helps to preserve orbital volume but also minimizes the risk of medial/lateral rectus scarring and entrapment. The intraconal fat is entered above or below the medial/lateral rectus muscles. With blunt dissection, the intraorbital structures and the tumor are progressively identified through the space between the extraocular muscles, taking care not to manipulate the ventral side of the muscles to avoid damage to neural motor fibers. Once the capsule of the tumor is identified, it is then carefully followed, and a 270° dissection from the surrounding fat and other orbital tissue may be performed using blunt dissectors, gentle traction, dynamic retraction, low bipolar cauterization, and sharp dissection, taking care not to damage the rectus muscles, the ON, and the ciliary ganglion. It should be kept in mind that direct dissection between the tumor and the ON should be avoided when the intraconal tumor is abutting the ON [1]. This is crucial as even minor manipulation could end up in damage to the ON or in OA vasospasm, which both could threaten the patient's vision [1]. It is widely accepted that the use of monopolar cautery should be avoided within the orbit as it can result in an increased risk of thermal conduction to adjacent critical neural structures [36]. Also, sharp cutting instruments should be used cautiously; otherwise, they can increase the risk of bleeding from inadvertent arterial injury. Given that clear dissection may not always be possible, it becomes very difficult to make a decision in balancing functional preservation and radicality of resection [33]. Total resection must be balanced against the risk of iatrogenic morbidity, and it is thus recommended to discuss with the patient before surgery to clarify the priorities of the surgical procedure. Excessive fixed retraction should also be avoided to prevent compromising the surrounding critical neurovascular structures.

Complications

It is imperative that extreme care is taken to minimize the retraction-induced pressure on the globe, which may induce the oculo-cardiac reflex, while dissecting the periorbita or drilling the greater sphenoid wing [22, 29]. Furthermore, an elevated intraocular pressure due to excessive globe retraction during ETOA might lower the ocular perfusion pressure, potentially leading to perioperative visual loss [37]. Both the endoscope and instruments should therefore be withdrawn intermittently from the operative corridor while checking for a change in the pupil size or shape [22, 29, 38, 39].

Vascular injuries can occur, especially when dealing with intraconal lesions. Injury to intraorbital vessels can lead to catastrophic sequelae, including orbital hematomas and complete blindness. Injury to the OA, which is located inferolateral to the ON, is rare owing to its anatomic location. Damage to the ciliary arteries from the OA may lead to severe visual impairment [40]. In addition, injury to the CRA, one of the first branches of the OA, can cause sudden painless loss of vision. Arterial branches to the medial rectus muscle are known to be most commonly injured. On the other hand, injuries to muscular branches are rare.

Orbital hematoma may occur in case of blood vessel injuries [41]. Meticulous hemostasis should be achieved at the end of the procedure in order to avoid increasing the intraorbital pressure. Transient diplopia may also occur if extraocular muscles are manipulated or impaired, whereas permanent diplopia is a relatively rare event. Enophthalmos may occur when there is a decrease in orbital volume, due to either excessive removal of orbital fat or intraorbital fat herniation [40].

Case Example

A 46-year-old man presented with progressive proptosis in the left eye. Preoperative MRI scans demonstrated a hyperintense, rounded mass occupying the intraconal space in the left orbit (Fig. 12.2). The intraconal mass was shown to compress the ON in a superomedial direction in zones II and III. An ETOA was performed, and a GTR was achieved (Fig. 12.3). He underwent an ETOA with gross total removal of the lesion. The pathologic diagnosis revealed a schwannoma. Proptosis immediately improved after surgery. Transient diplopia was observed after resection, but it recovered by the 3-month follow-up.

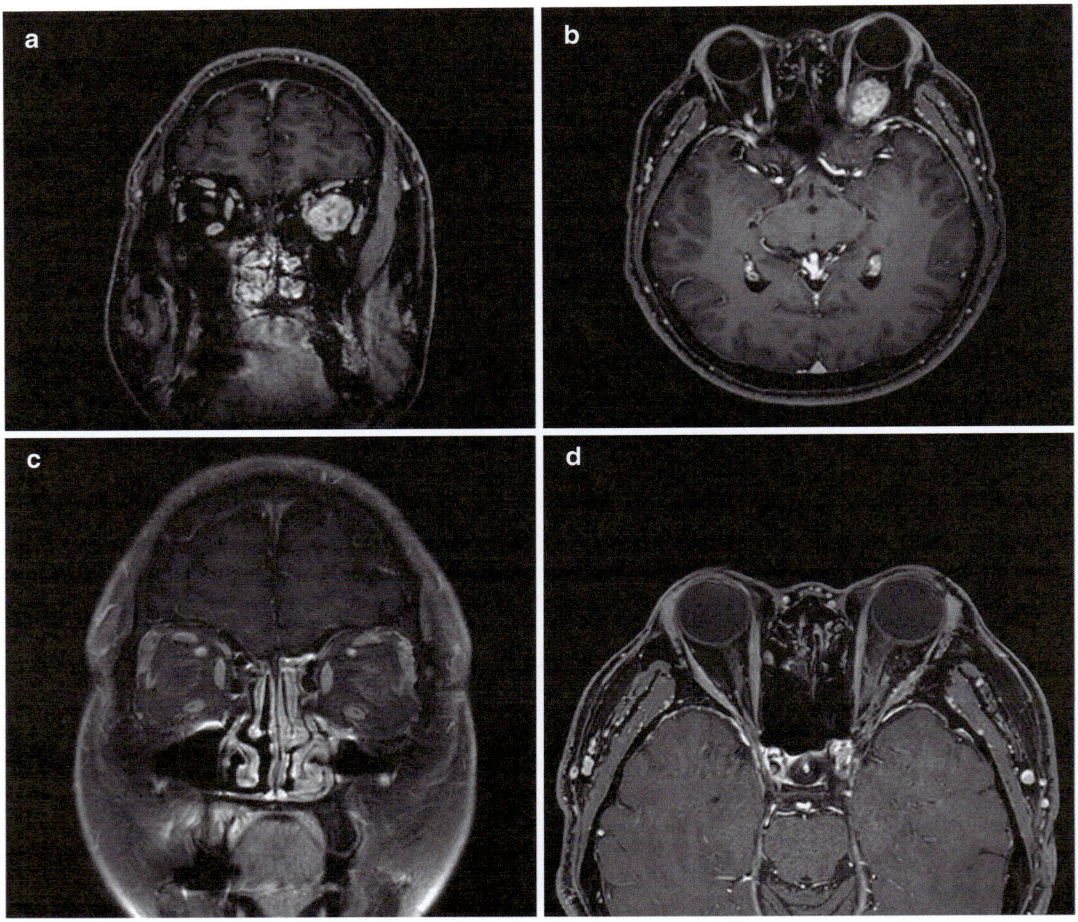

Fig. 12.2 Preoperative contrast-enhanced MRI scans in coronal (**a**) and axial (**b**) views of an intraconal schwannoma in the left orbit. Postoperative MRI (**c** and **d**) showed gross total resection of the lesion after endoscopic transorbital superior eyelid approach

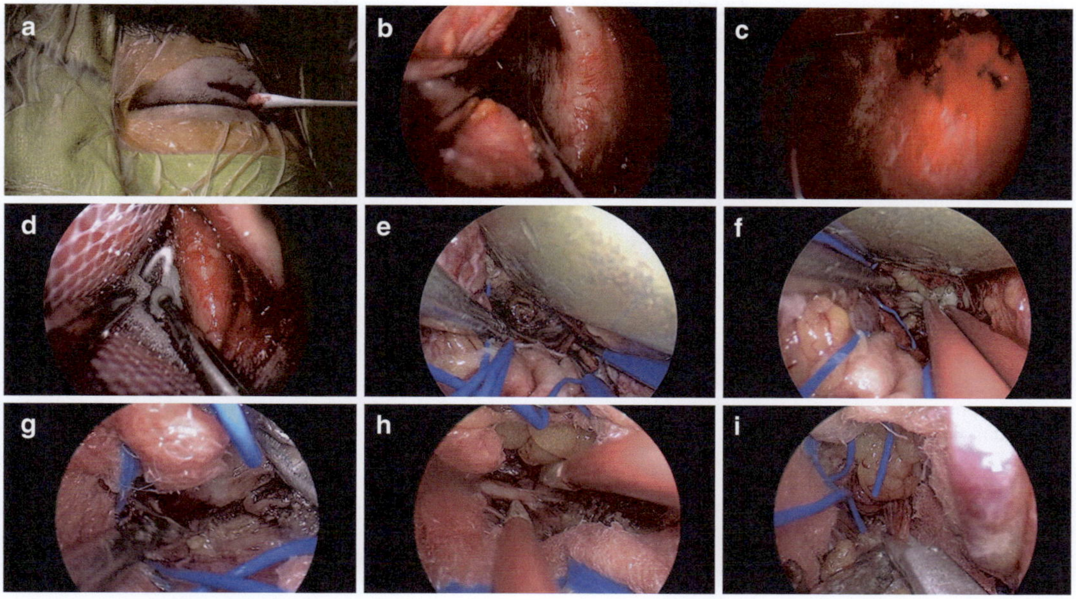

Fig. 12.3 Intraoperative endoscopic transorbital images (case example). A skin incision along the lateral half of the left superior eyelid crease (**a**). Intraoperative endoscopic transorbital views of a subperiosteal dissection (**b**), exposure of superior orbital fissure (**c**), drilling of the lateral orbital wall with a high-speed drill (**d**), exposure of an intraconal tumor through a working corridor between rectus muscles after opening of the periorbita (**e**), low power bipolar coagulation of the tumor (**f**), circumferential dissection off the surrounding structures (**g**) and oculomotor nerve (**h**), and final cut freeing the tumor from the intraconal space (**i**)

Conclusion

Intraorbital surgery can be challenging due to its anatomical complexity and the presence of important structures in a narrow working space. Careful preoperative planning with a multidisciplinary team approach is invaluable and can facilitate the maximal safe resection of orbital tumors with minimal morbidity and good cosmetic and functional outcomes. It can be achieved by choosing the most anatomically favorable surgical approach for the lesion of interest to minimize or avoid manipulation of the intraorbital vascular supply and the ON. Without open transcranial approaches, minimally invasive ETOA can provide 360° circumferential access to the entire orbit with acceptable morbidity based on a neurotopographic four-zone model with the epicenter around the ON on the coronal plane. Depending on the size and location of the tumor, a combined endoscopic multiportal technique, such as ETOA combined with EEA, can be considered, focusing on the advantages and limiting the restrictions of each approach.

References

1. Mueller SK, Bleier BS. Endoscopic surgery for intraconal orbital tumors. HNO. 2022;70(5):345–51. https://doi.org/10.1007/s00106-022-01156-y.
2. Rene C. Update on orbital anatomy. Eye (Lond). 2006;20(10):1119–29. https://doi.org/10.1038/sj.eye.6702376.
3. Bleier BS, Healy DY Jr, Chhabra N, Freitag S. Compartmental endoscopic surgical anatomy of the medial intraconal orbital space. Int Forum Allergy Rhinol. 2014;4(7):587–91. https://doi.org/10.1002/alr.21320.
4. McNab AA, Selva D, Hardy TG, O'Donnell B. The anatomical location and laterality of orbital cavernous haemangiomas. Orbit. 2014;33(5):359–62. https://doi.org/10.3109/01676830.2014.915329.

5. Lieber S, Fernandez-Miranda JC. Anatomy of the orbit. J Neurol Surg B Skull Base. 2020;81(4):319–32. https://doi.org/10.1055/s-0040-1715096.
6. Hayreh SS, Dass R. The ophthalmic artery: II. Intra-orbital course. Br J Ophthalmol. 1962;46(3):165–85. https://doi.org/10.1136/bjo.46.3.165.
7. Hayreh SS. The ophthalmic artery: III. Branches. Br J Ophthalmol. 1962;46(4):212–47. https://doi.org/10.1136/bjo.46.4.212.
8. Shinder R, Al-Zubidi N, Esmaeli B. Survey of orbital tumors at a comprehensive cancer center in the United States. Head Neck. 2011;33(5):610–4. https://doi.org/10.1002/hed.21498.
9. Margalit N, Ezer H, Fliss DM, Naftaliev E, Nossek E, Kesler A. Orbital tumors treated using transcranial approaches: surgical technique and neuroophthalmogical results in 41 patients. Neurosurg Focus. 2007;23(5):E11. https://doi.org/10.3171/FOC-07/11/E11.
10. Darsaut TE, Lanzino G, Lopes MB, Newman S. An introductory overview of orbital tumors. Neurosurg Focus. 2001;10(5):E1. https://doi.org/10.3171/foc.2001.10.5.2.
11. Goto H, Yamakawa N, Komatsu H, Asakage M, Tsubota K, Ueda SI, et al. Clinico-epidemiological analysis of 1000 cases of orbital tumors. Jpn J Ophthalmol. 2021;65(5):704–23. https://doi.org/10.1007/s10384-021-00857-1.
12. Maroon JC, Kennerdell JS. Microsurgical approach to orbital tumors. Clin Neurosurg. 1979;26:479–89. https://doi.org/10.1093/neurosurgery/26.cn_suppl_1.479.
13. Aftahy AK, Krauss P, Barz M, Wagner A, Meyer B, Negwer C, et al. Surgical treatment of intraorbital lesions. World Neurosurg. 2021;155:e805–e13. https://doi.org/10.1016/j.wneu.2021.09.011.
14. Ohtsuka K, Hashimoto M, Suzuki Y. A review of 244 orbital tumors in Japanese patients during a 21-year period: origins and locations. Jpn J Ophthalmol. 2005;49(1):49–55. https://doi.org/10.1007/s10384-004-0147-y.
15. Paluzzi A, Gardner PA, Fernandez-Miranda JC, Tormenti MJ, Stefko ST, Snyderman CH, et al. "Round-the-clock" surgical access to the orbit. J Neurol Surg B Skull Base. 2015;76(1):12–24. https://doi.org/10.1055/s-0033-1360580.
16. Caballero-Garcia J, Aparicio-Garcia C, Linares-Benavides YJ, Lopez-Sanchez M, Abreu-Perdomo FA, Huanca-Amaru J. Minimally invasive 360-degree approach to intraconal orbital tumors. Am J Ophthalmol. 2021;224:301–9. https://doi.org/10.1016/j.ajo.2020.07.035.
17. Eddleman CS, Liu JK. Optic nerve sheath meningioma: current diagnosis and treatment. Neurosurg Focus. 2007;23(5):E4. https://doi.org/10.3171/FOC-07/11/E4.
18. Solli E, Turbin RE. Primary and secondary optic nerve sheath meningioma. J Neurol Surg B Skull Base. 2021;82(1):27–71. https://doi.org/10.1055/s-0041-1723801.
19. Shofty B, Ben-Sira L, Kesler A, Jallo G, Groves ML, Iyer RR, et al. Isolated optic nerve gliomas: a multicenter historical cohort study. J Neurosurg Pediatr. 2017;20(6):549–55. https://doi.org/10.3171/2017.6.PEDS17107.
20. Chaskes MB, Rabinowitz MR. Orbital schwannoma. J Neurol Surg B Skull Base. 2020;81(4):376–80. https://doi.org/10.1055/s-0040-1713935.
21. Palmisciano P, Ferini G, Ogasawara C, Wahood W, Bin Alamer O, Gupta AD, et al. Orbital metastases: a systematic review of clinical characteristics, management strategies, and treatment outcomes. Cancers (Basel). 2021;14(1):94. https://doi.org/10.3390/cancers14010094.
22. Jeon C, Hong SD, Woo KI, Seol HJ, Nam DH, Lee JI, et al. Use of endoscopic transorbital and endonasal approaches for 360 degrees circumferential access to orbital tumors. J Neurosurg. 2020;135:103. https://doi.org/10.3171/2020.6.JNS20890.
23. Moe KS, Bergeron CM, Ellenbogen RG. Transorbital neuroendoscopic surgery. Neurosurgery. 2010;67(3 Suppl Operative):ons16–28. https://doi.org/10.1227/01.NEU.0000373431.08464.43.
24. Bejjani GK, Cockerham KP, Kennerdel JS, Maroon JC. A reappraisal of surgery for orbital tumors. Part I: Extraorbital approaches. Neurosurg Focus. 2001;10(5):E2. https://doi.org/10.3171/foc.2001.10.5.3.
25. Dallan I, Castelnuovo P, Locatelli D, Turri-Zanoni M, AlQahtani A, Battaglia P, et al. Multiportal combined transorbital transnasal endoscopic approach for the management of selected skull base lesions: preliminary experience. World Neurosurg. 2015;84(1):97–107. https://doi.org/10.1016/j.wneu.2015.02.034.
26. Di Somma A, Andaluz N, Cavallo LM, de Notaris M, Dallan I, Solari D, et al. Endoscopic transorbital superior eyelid approach: anatomical study from a neurosurgical perspective. J Neurosurg. 2018;129(5):1203–16. https://doi.org/10.3171/2017.4.JNS162749.
27. Locatelli D, Pozzi F, Turri-Zanoni M, Battaglia P, Santi L, Dallan I, et al. Transorbital endoscopic approaches to the skull base: current concepts and future perspectives. J Neurosurg Sci. 2016;60(4):514–25.
28. Jeon C, Hong CK, Woo KI, Hong SD, Nam DH, Lee JI, et al. Endoscopic transorbital surgery for Meckel's cave and middle cranial fossa tumors: surgical technique and early results. J Neurosurg. 2018;131:1126–35. https://doi.org/10.3171/2018.6.JNS181099.
29. Kong DS, Young SM, Hong CK, Kim YD, Hong SD, Choi JW, et al. Clinical and ophthalmological outcome of endoscopic transorbital surgery for cranioorbital tumors. J Neurosurg. 2018;131(3):667–75. https://doi.org/10.3171/2018.3.JNS173233.
30. Ramakrishna R, Kim LJ, Bly RA, Moe K, Ferreira M Jr. Transorbital neuroendoscopic surgery for the treatment of skull base lesions. J Clin Neurosci. 2016;24:99–104. https://doi.org/10.1016/j.jocn.2015.07.021.

31. Zoli M, Sollini G, Milanese L, La Corte E, Rustici A, Guaraldi F, et al. Endoscopic approaches to orbital lesions: case series and systematic literature review. J Neurosurg. 2020;134:608. https://doi.org/10.3171/2019.10.JNS192138.
32. In Woo K, Kong DS, Park JW, Kim M, Kim YD. Orbital decompressive effect of endoscopic transorbital surgery for sphenoorbital meningioma. Graefes Arch Clin Exp Ophthalmol. 2021;259(4):1015–24. https://doi.org/10.1007/s00417-020-05008-9.
33. Shin M, Kondo K, Hanakita S, Suzukawa K, Kin T, Shojima M, et al. Endoscopic transnasal approach for resection of locally aggressive tumors in the orbit. J Neurosurg. 2015;123(3):748–59. https://doi.org/10.3171/2014.11.JNS141921.
34. Moe KS. The precaruncular approach to the medial orbit. Arch Facial Plast Surg. 2003;5(6):483–7. https://doi.org/10.1001/archfaci.5.6.483.
35. Ciporen JN, Moe KS, Ramanathan D, Lopez S, Ledesma E, Rostomily R, et al. Multiportal endoscopic approaches to the central skull base: a cadaveric study. World Neurosurg. 2010;73(6):705–12. https://doi.org/10.1016/j.wneu.2010.03.033.
36. Bleier BS, Castelnuovo P, Battaglia P, Turri-Zanoni M, Dallan I, Metson R, et al. Endoscopic endonasal orbital cavernous hemangioma resection: global experience in techniques and outcomes. Int Forum Allergy Rhinol. 2016;6(2):156–61. https://doi.org/10.1002/alr.21645.
37. Kim W, Moon JH, Kim EH, Hong CK, Han J, Hong JB. Optimization of orbital retraction during endoscopic transorbital approach via quantitative measurement of the intraocular pressure—[SevEN 006]. BMC Ophthalmol. 2021;21(1):76. https://doi.org/10.1186/s12886-021-01834-5.
38. Kong DS, Kim YH, Hong CK. Optimal indications and limitations of endoscopic transorbital superior eyelid surgery for spheno-orbital meningiomas. J Neurosurg. 2020;134(5):1472–9. https://doi.org/10.3171/2020.3.JNS20297.
39. Park HH, Hong SD, Kim YH, Hong CK, Woo KI, Yun IS, et al. Endoscopic transorbital and endonasal approach for trigeminal schwannomas: a retrospective multicenter analysis (KOSEN-005). J Neurosurg. 2020;133(2):467–76. https://doi.org/10.3171/2019.3.JNS19492.
40. Castelnuovo P, Turri-Zanoni M, Battaglia P, Locatelli D, Dallan I. Endoscopic endonasal management of orbital pathologies. Neurosurg Clin N Am. 2015;26(3):463–72. https://doi.org/10.1016/j.nec.2015.03.001.
41. Sellari-Franceschini S, Dallan I, Bajraktari A, Fiacchini G, Nardi M, Rocchi R, et al. Surgical complications in orbital decompression for Graves' orbitopathy. Acta Otorhinolaryngol Ital. 2016;36(4):265–74. https://doi.org/10.14639/0392-100X-1082.

Part V

Skull Base Pathology: Middle Fossa

13 Endoscopic Transorbital Skull Base Approach to the Meckel's Cave

Doo-Sik Kong

Meckel's cave (MC) is a natural aperture that lies between the petrous apex's meningeal dura propria and periosteal layers in the medial portion of the middle cranial fossa. MC acts as a conduit for the trigeminal nerve as it passes from the prepontine cistern toward the cavernous sinus [1, 2]. It contains the Gasserian ganglion and proximal rootlets of the trigeminal nerve [3]. Surgical access to the MC remains challenging due to its deep-seated location and surrounding critical neurovascular structures (Fig. 13.1).

Historically, surgical approaches to Meckel's cave have included anterolateral, lateral, and posterolateral approaches (Fig. 13.2). However, these conventional approaches require brain retraction that risks venous sacrifice and traumatic injury to normal tissue. Excessive retraction of the temporalis muscle may lead to atrophy and a cosmetic defect. Occasionally, injury to the vein of Labbe may result in a postoperative venous infarction. To decrease brain retraction and gain a more favorable angle of attack, traditional skull base approaches often require quite extensive osteotomies, resulting in a long operative time to reach the lesion and to reconstruct the skull defect. In recent years, with the introduction of minimally invasive techniques and with the use of the endoscope, minimally invasive surgical corridors to the deep skull base compartments have been developed. Nevertheless, endoscopic endonasal (EE) approaches still require dissection near the internal carotid artery (ICA) and/or mobilization with trauma and possible destruction of the normal pterygopalatine neurovascular contents.

D.-S. Kong (✉)
Department of Neurosurgery, Samsung Medical Center, Sungkyunkwan University, Seoul, Republic of Korea

T. H. Schwartz et al. (eds.), *Endoscopic Transorbital Surgery of the Orbit, Skull Base and Brain*,
https://doi.org/10.1007/978-3-031-59504-2_13

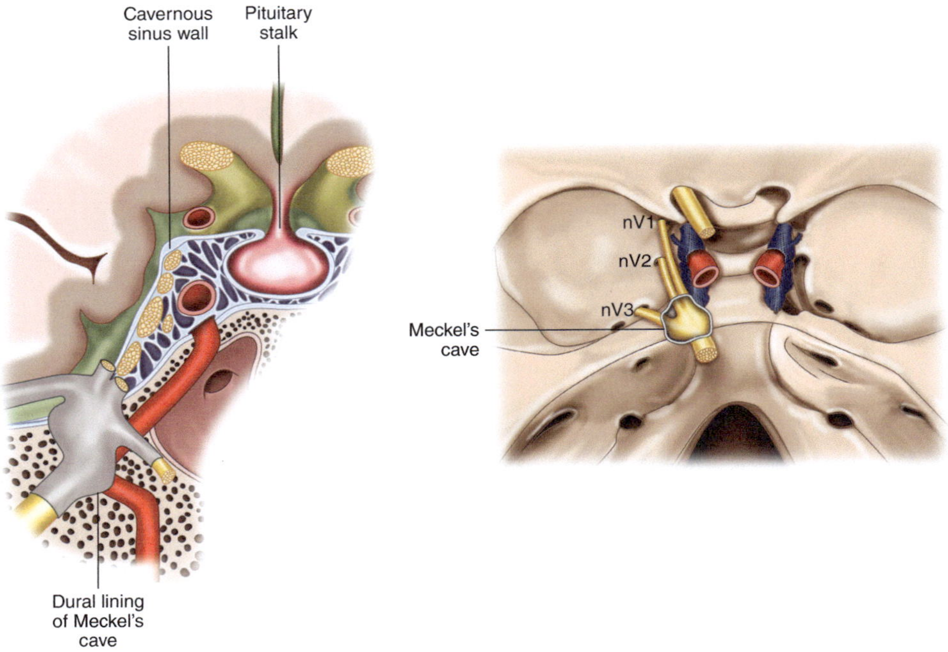

Fig. 13.1 Illustration of the Meckel's cave

Advantages of the Transorbital Corridor

Significant advances have been made in the field of endoscopy with the design of new dedicated instruments. These tools have not only transformed and invigorated the endonasal approach, but their application to transorbital surgery has improved the working angles, shortened the working distances, and optimized visualization of deep anatomy by bringing the target closer to the operative field [4–6], thereby improving cosmetic results and potentially decreasing surgical morbidity [7, 8].

The endonasal revolution introduced the front-door concept [5], an anteromedial corridor using the endoscopic endonasal route, which also requires a transpterygoid approach to sufficiently access MC. This approach includes an uncinectomy, posterior ethmoidectomy, wide sphenoidotomy, and wide maxillary antrostomy with lateral exposure of the infraorbital fissure with its neurovascular structures to increase the working space to provide a panoramic view [7]. Whether destroying these normal structures to gain access to the target lesion is justifiable remains controversial. In addition, the endoscopic endonasal approach sometimes has to cross the plane of the internal carotid artery, vidian canal, and the trigeminal branches, which requires a long working distance where only limited manipulation of the instruments is possible due to its far-lateral location in the lateral recess of the sphenoid sinus. Sometimes, if the lateral recess of the sphenoid sinus is not well developed, extensive drilling of thick pterygoid bone and lateral sphenoid bone is required to create an adequate working space.

The transorbital route provides an alternative anterolateral corridor to reach the MC. It has some advantages over the endonasal route in that it does not require crossing of the internal carotid artery and trigeminal branches and provides a shorter working distance, resulting in easier surgical manipulation. It also has advantages over the cranio-orbito-zygomatic approaches in that it does not leave a skull base defect, has a small skin eyelid incision, and avoids atrophy of the temporalis muscle postoperatively. Compared to

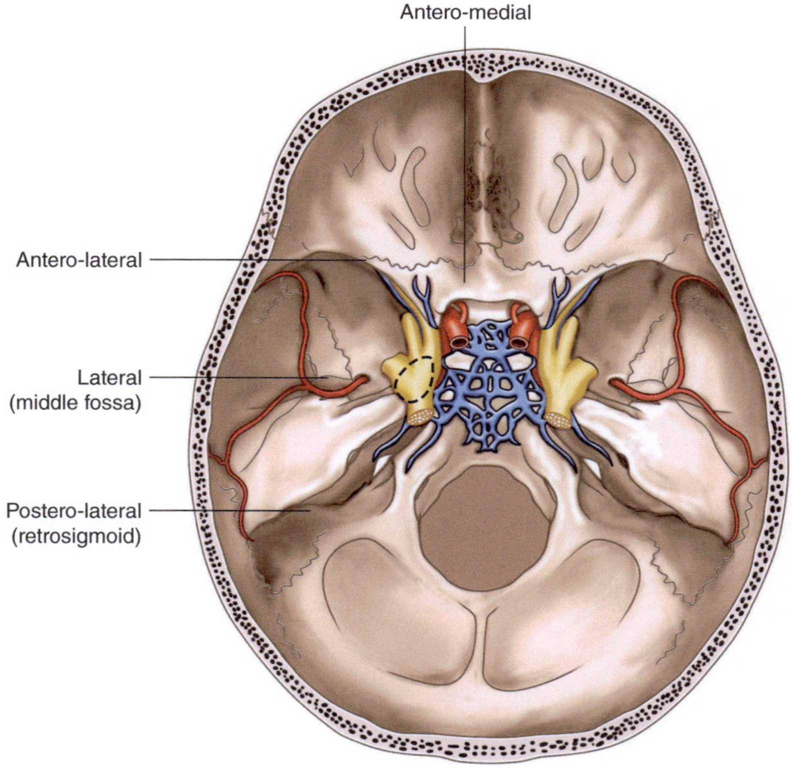

Fig. 13.2 Surgical approaches to the Meckel's cave lesions

the lateral approach using the subtemporal extra- or intradural route, the transorbital route avoids retraction of the temporal lobe, thereby reducing the risk of injury to the vein of Labbe.

Classification of Meckel's Cave Schwannoma (Trigeminal Schwannoma)

The most common type of tumor that occurs in MC is the trigeminal schwannoma. Therefore, the incidence and classification of this tumor should be studied before applying transorbital surgery to trigeminal schwannoma. Although trigeminal schwannomas are the most common nonvestibular schwannomas, they are a rare disease entity, comprising only 0.8–8% of all intracranial schwannomas and 0.07–0.36% of all intracranial tumors [9]. Trigeminal schwannomas can occur anywhere along the path of the nerve and are capable of extending intradurally into the middle and posterior fossa and extracranially into the orbit, pterygopalatine, and infratemporal fossa [9]. Trigeminal schwannomas have been classified according to their geographical complexities and anatomic varieties by several outstanding neurosurgeons [10, 11]. Commonly used classification includes middle fossa type (type A); posterior fossa root type (type B); dumbbell type, with both middle and posterior fossa components (type C); and tumors extending into the extracranial compartment (type D). Depending on the division of CN V involved, type D tumors are further classified into ophthalmic division (D1), maxillary division (D2), and mandibular division (D3) subtypes [10]. Based on this classification, we analyzed the clinical outcomes of endoscopic transorbital surgery for trigeminal schwannomas and reported that endoscopic transorbital surgery had an excellent outcome after surgery for middle fossa or dumbbell-type schwannomas, with over 90% gross- or near-total resection (unpublished).

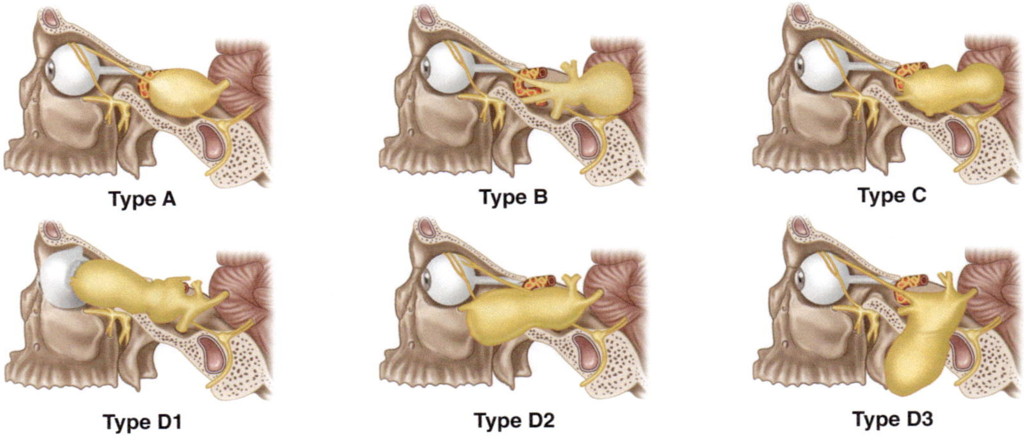

Fig. 13.3 Classification of trigeminal schwannoma (modified Samii classification). Trigeminal schwannomas are classified into middle cranial fossa tumors (type A), posterior fossa tumors (type B), dumbbell-shaped tumors (type C), and extracranial extension (type D). Type D tumors are subclassified as ophthalmic division (D1), maxillary division (D2), and mandibular division (D3) [12]

According to our study, appropriate indicators for endoscopic transorbital surgery include schwannomas centered in the middle fossa such as middle or middle and posterior fossa tumors, as well as the so-called "dumbbell"-type tumors and V1-based schwannomas involving the orbit. However, V2- or V3-based schwannomas are more easily removed with the endoscopic endonasal approach (Fig. 13.3).

Surgical Step

The transorbital surgical procedure is developed from modified Krönlein operation [13]. The major difference from the previous procedure is the introduction of endoscopy. With the help of endoscopy, the main target lesions can be extended to intracranial lesions as well as orbital lesions.

Patient Position

The patient is usually placed in the supine position on a horseshoe head plate. Excessive extension or flexion of the head should be avoided. I generally recommend a neutral head position with a slight turn to the other side; however, I favor a neutral position for schwannomas. Surgeons usually stand on the side ipsilateral to the tumor (Fig. 13.4).

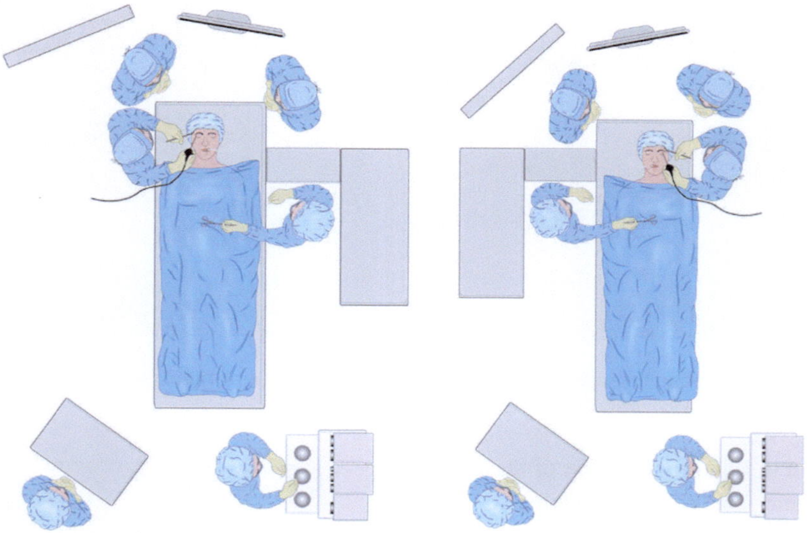

Fig. 13.4 Patient position. For both right-side and left-side lesions, the surgeon usually stands on the side ipsilateral to the tumor

Orbital Phase (Skin Incision to the Exposure of Orbital Wall)

The orbital phase includes a superior eyelid incision followed by suborbicular dissection to reach the lateral orbital rim and periosteum. Usually, skin incision along the superior eyelid can be extended laterally 1 or 2 cm lateral to the lateral canthus to avoid inadvertent injury to the frontal branch of the facial nerve (Fig. 13.5). Alternatively, a sub-eyebrow incision can be done as per the surgeon's preference. However, in such cases, more care should be taken to reach the lateral orbital rim because the superior orbital rim might be exposed first. After skin incision, dissection under the orbicularis muscle should be performed without injuring the orbital septum. In most cases, division of the orbicularis is carried out at the same time as the skin incision, because the orbicularis muscle is very thin. Thus, additional incision in the orbicularis muscle is not required. The anterior lamella consists of the skin and orbicularis oculi muscle, while the posterior lamella extends from the levator aponeurosis, Muller's muscle, and palpebral conjunctiva [4]. The orbital septum arises from the periosteum at the arcus marginalis and fuses with the levator aponeurosis near the tarsus. The orbital septum is often covered by preseptal fat tissue. Care should be taken to maintain the layer of preseptal fat tissue layer. Once the lateral orbital rim is palpated with a freer elevator or finger, a periosteal incision with a monopolar cautery is made along the superolateral orbital rim. The periosteum is fused with the periorbita at the level of the orbit, and periosteal elevation is the same analogous to periorbital elevation, in which the orbital structures can be separated from the lateral orbital wall without cutting the lateral canthal ligament. It is one of the surgical tips where a silastic sheet is used to keep the periorbita intact. Protection of the periorbita prevents the disrupted periorbital fat from obstructing the surgical view. It also evenly distributes retraction pressure to the orbital globe. Until this step, all surgical procedures can be performed with the naked eye or in an exoscopic view. Thereafter, a 4-mm straight rigid endoscope with a high-definition camera (Karl Storz, Tuttlingen, Germany) held by an assistant or a pneumatic holder (UniArm; Mitaka Kohki, Tokyo, Japan) is introduced into the surgical field. Under the endoscopic view, the periorbital membrane is carefully elevated from the lateral orbital wall. Several bridging vessels are

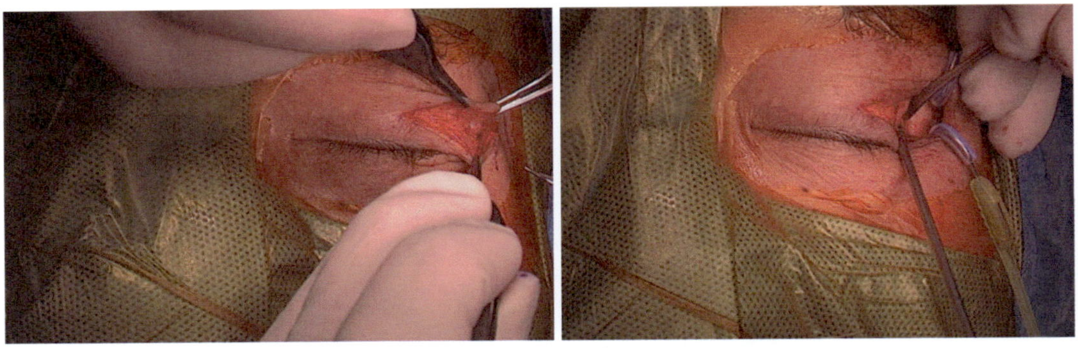

Fig. 13.5 Skin incision along the superior eyelid crease. The orbicularis oris muscle is incised, while preserving the orbital septum. Then the lateral orbital rim is exposed and incised

found and cut during the elevation of the periorbital membrane. The recurrent meningeal artery or meningolacrimal branch may pass through the cranio-orbital foramen near the front of the superior orbital fissure, while the temporozygomatic branches pass through the nameless foramen near the inferior orbital fissure in most cases. The superior and inferior orbital fissures are important landmarks of the boundary of the transorbital approach.

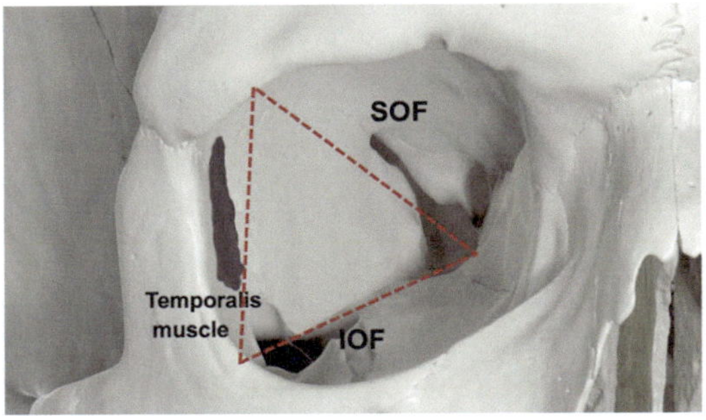

Fig. 13.6 The imaginary line of the transorbital triangle. Transorbital triangle is bordered by superior orbital fissure (SOF), inferior orbital fissure (IOF), and temporalis muscle. Drilling of this boundary exposes the middle cranial fossa

Bony Phase

Initial drilling of the bone can be performed with a 4-mm coarse diamond burr or cutting burr. First, the zygomatic process within the lateral orbital wall should be drilled vertically, resulting in the exposure of the temporalis muscle. From the perspective of orbital bony anatomy, the superior orbital fissure, inferior orbital fissure, and temporalis muscle form a triangle, the so-called the transorbital triangle, a gateway to the middle fossa, cavernous sinus, and MC (Fig. 13.6).

Once the temporalis muscle is exposed, it should be oriented vertically in the endoscopic view to avoid disorientation. The lateral orbital wall is composed mostly of the greater sphenoid bone, and the shape of the cross-sectional image on the lateral part of the greater sphenoidal wing represents an inverted triangle. Within this inverted triangular line, drilling of the bone should be performed safely until the temporal dura is exposed. Drilling should be directed from the lateral to medial. After full exposure of the temporal dura, the lesser sphenoidal bone can then be drilled out to slightly expose the frontal dura and the sphenoidal ridge. Thereafter, it is critical to flatten the temporal floor bone. Preoperative lumbar drainage of the cerebrospinal fluid for at least 6 h is useful to reduce temporal lobe retraction. After bone work is completed, the meningo-orbital band, which is a tight adhesive tissue between the periorbital membrane and temporal lobe, is easily found and should be detached, as would be done in the traditional transcranial approach. Dural coagulation with bipolar cautery can induce shrinkage of the temporal dura, which makes separation of the temporal lobe from the outer membrane of the cavernous sinus easier. Then, interdural dissection is performed along the cleavage between the dura propria of the temporal lobe and the lateral membrane of the cavernous sinus. In most cases of schwan-

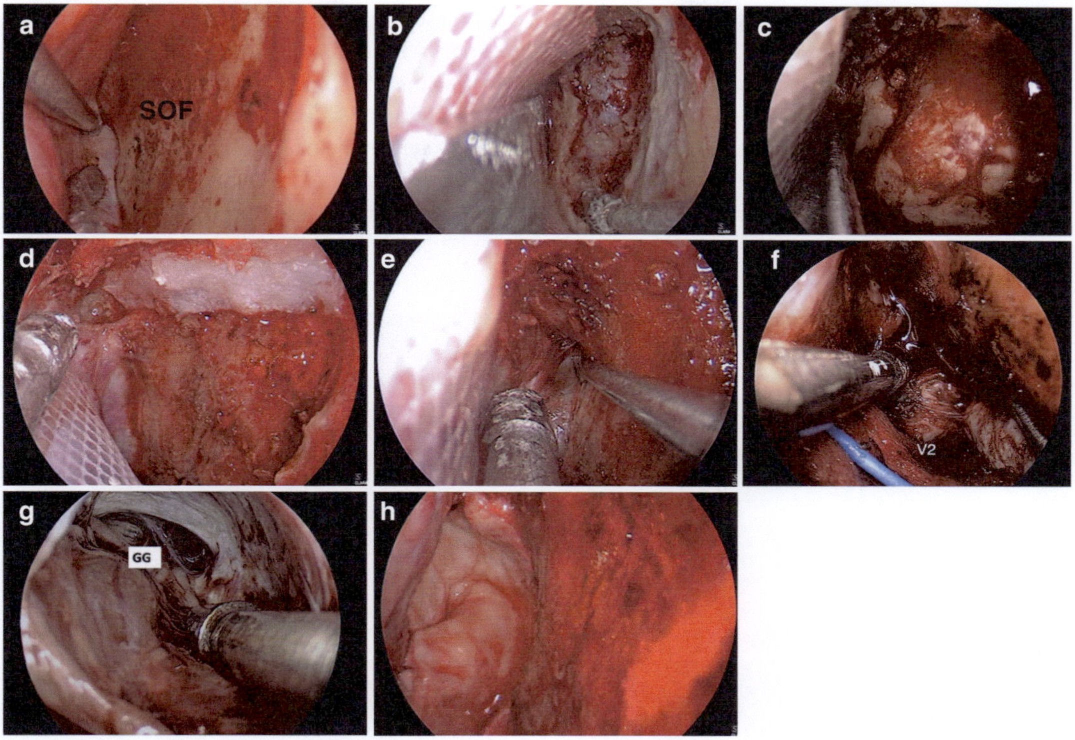

Fig. 13.7 Intraoperative endoscopic transorbital views. (**a**) When the periorbita is elevated from the lateral orbital wall, the superior orbital fissure (SOF) is a landmark of the middle cranial fossa. (**b**) After exposure of the temporalis muscle by drilling of the zygomatic bone, the direction of the temporalis muscle should be oriented vertically. Then, drilling of the greater sphenoid bone exposes the temporal dura. Then, drilling of the greater sphenoidal bone is performed in a lateral to medial direction. (**c**) To expose the lateral surface of the superior orbital fissure, the sagittal crest must be taken out. (**d**) When anterior temporal dura is fully exposed, the meningo-orbital band (MOB) attachment between the temporal dura and the periorbita should be identified and cut to facilitate entry into the cavernous sinus (white material is bone wax to control bone bleeding). (**e**) Interdural dissection between the dura propria of the temporal lobe and the lateral wall of the cavernous sinus will expose the tumor capsule. (**f**) In some cases, the distal V2 nerve sometimes can be found during internal debulking of the tumor. (**g**) Finally, the Gasserian ganglion of the trigeminal nerve is identified coming from the porus trigeminus. (**h**) To reconstruct the cavernous sinus defect, DuraGen or allodermal graft is applied

noma involving the MC, the anteromedial triangle, composed of space between V1 and V2, is the preferred corridor to access the MC and the cavernous sinus (Fig. 13.7).

Cavernous and MC Phase

As a dura propria of the temporal lobe is taken off little by little from the lateral membrane of the cavernous sinus, the protruding portion of the cavernous sinus is exposed. The space between the V1 and V2 nerve (anteromedial triangle) is the most favored corridor. Based on the origin and location of the schwannoma, the anterolateral triangle (the space between the V2 and V3 nerves) or the Kawase triangle (lateral border to the V3 nerve) can also be selected as the surgical corridor. It is recommended that the direction of the incision be parallel to the direction of the V1 or V2 nerve pathway. After exposing the tumor capsule, internal debulking of the lesion is initiated, followed by dissection of the external capsule of the lesion from the surrounding brain tissue. The consistency of schwannomas varies from case to case. Therefore, a ring curettage or an ultrasonic aspirator can be helpful in debulking the tumor. In some cases, the inferolateral trunk of the internal carotid artery supplies to the medial portion of the tumor. In such cases, excessive bleeding may occur inadvertently if the tumor is removed blindly. Therefore, blind dissection should be avoided to prevent inadvertent neurovascular injury. After removal of the tumor, the porus trigeminus (an inlet of the trigeminal nerve to the MC from the posterior cranial fossa) can be identified and the surrounding cranial nerves such as the oculomotor or trochlear nerve may be observed. The abducens nerve is often shifted medially by the tumor mass (Fig. 13.8).

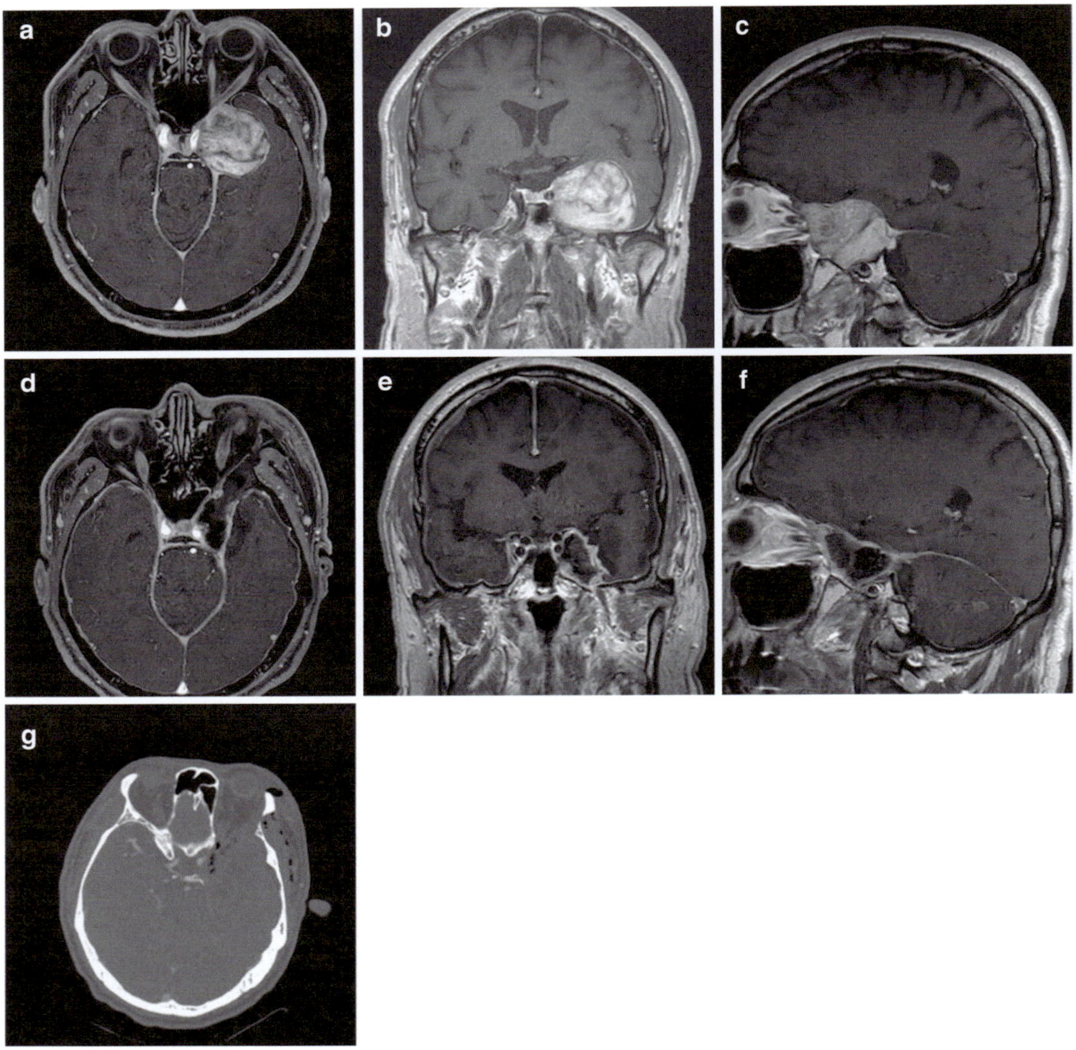

Fig. 13.8 Case illustration. A 62-year-old man with a trigeminal schwannoma was treated with endoscopic transorbital surgery. Preoperative symptoms included a slight tingling sensation on the face. Preoperative axial (**a**) T1-weighted MR image showing tumor and internal carotid artery shifted medially by the tumor mass. Preoperative coronal (**b**) and sagittal (**c**) contrast-enhanced T1-weighted MR images show a huge schwannoma mass involving the Meckel's cave and middle cranial fossa. Postoperative axial (**d**), coronal (**e**), and sagittal (**f**) contrast-enhanced T1-weighted MR images demonstrate a gross total resection of the tumor. (**g**) A postoperative bony CT scan reveals the defect of the greater sphenoid bone on the left side

Reconstruction Phase

In theory, the transorbital approach to MC is entirely extradural or interdural work. Therefore, the incidence of a cerebrospinal fluid leak should be very low, as was shown in our retrospective multicenter study (unpublished). This means that postoperative lumbar drainage is not necessary after schwannoma removal. To reconstruct the skull base defect, the opening of the porus trigeminus can be obstructed by a collagen matrix (DuraGen, Integra Neurosciences, Plainsboro, NJ), and the defect on the cavernous sinus between V1 and V2 can be closed with allodermal graft material such as the AlloDerm or fascia lata followed by the placement of an absorbable fibril sealant patch (TachoSil, Takeda, Japan). Fat tissue graft is not required in every case. To prevent postoperative enophthalmos, posterior displacement of the eyeball within the orbit and the placement of an alloplastic resorbable polydioxanone sheet (PDS sheet) may be used depending on the surgeon's preference. The periosteum is sutured with a 5.0 vicryl suture, and the subcutaneous tissue is sutured with 5.0 absorbable vicryl suture. Finally, a 6.0 rapid absorbable monofilament suture is done for eyelid closure.

Complications

Postoperative complications include approach-related complications and surgical resection-related morbidities. One of the key parameters of minimally invasive endoscopic skull base surgery is the reduction in approach-related morbidity. During the resection of the schwannoma arising from MC, common neurosurgical morbidities include injury to the internal carotid artery or vein of Labbe and neurological deficits associated with facial sensation such as corneal keratopathy and adjacent cranial nerve (oculomotor, trochlear, and abducens nerves) injury. In our data (unpublished) from 50 patients who underwent endoscopic transorbital surgery, we encountered 7 cases of transient diplopia, 1 case of permanent diplopia, 4 cases of transient ptosis, 1 case of permanent ptosis, 7 cases of corneal keratopathies, 5 cases of mastication difficulties, and 14 cases of neuralgic pain requiring medication. However, all these complications were related to the tumor location involving the orbit, previous history of surgery or radiation therapy, or the presence of recurrence. Despite the application of this novel technique, these neurovascular injuries are unavoidable, with transcranial microscopic surgery. However, with special attention to approach-related complications, we encountered only 2 cases of wound infection in 50 patients. In addition, there were no postoperative cerebrospinal fluid leaks, visual dysfunction, or vascular injury of the vein of Labbe due to excessive retraction of the temporal lobe.

Conclusions

Endoscopic transorbital surgery is an ideal technique for the treatment of well-selected schwannomas involving the MC. Some tumors extending to the distal branches or involving the posterior fossa can be treated using an endoscopic endonasal or posterior approach. The transorbital approach results in minimal neurovascular deficits and a very low rate of cerebrospinal fluid leaks. However, as with any new approach, there is an anatomical and technical learning curve that must be overcome to apply this technique safely in our patients.

References

1. Malhotra A, Tu L, Kalra VB, et al. Neuroimaging of Meckel's cave in normal and disease conditions. Insights Imaging. 2018;9(4):499–510.
2. Janjua RM, Al-Mefty O, Densler DW, Shields CB. Dural relationships of Meckel cave and lateral wall of the cavernous sinus. Neurosurg Focus. 2008;25(6):E2.
3. Kawase T, Toya S, Shiobara R, Mine T. Transpetrosal approach for aneurysms of the lower basilar artery. J Neurosurg. 1985;63(6):857–61.
4. Laleva L, Spiriev T, Dallan I, et al. Pure endoscopic lateral orbitotomy approach to the cavernous sinus, posterior, and infratemporal fossae: anatomic study. J Neurol Surg B Skull Base. 2019;80(3):295–305.
5. Kassam AB, Prevedello DM, Carrau RL, et al. The front door to Meckel's cave: an anteromedial corridor

via expanded endoscopic endonasal approach—technical considerations and clinical series. Neurosurgery. 2009;64(3 Suppl):ons71–82; discussion ons82–73.
6. Truong HQ, Sun X, Celtikci E, et al. Endoscopic anterior transmaxillary "transalisphenoid" approach to Meckel's cave and the middle cranial fossa: an anatomical study and clinical application. J Neurosurg. 2018;130(1):227–37.
7. Suero Molina E, Revuelta Barbero JM, Ewelt C, Stummer W, Carrau RL, Prevedello DM. Access to Meckel's cave for biopsies of indeterminate lesions: a systematic review. Neurosurg Rev. 2021;44(1):249–59.
8. Fortes FS, Sennes LU, Carrau RL, et al. Endoscopic anatomy of the pterygopalatine fossa and the transpterygoid approach: development of a surgical instruction model. Laryngoscope. 2008;118(1):44–9.
9. Park HH, Hong SD, Kim YH, et al. Endoscopic transorbital and endonasal approach for trigeminal schwannomas: a retrospective multicenter analysis (KOSEN-005). J Neurosurg. 2020;133(2):467–76.
10. Samii M, Migliori MM, Tatagiba M, Babu R. Surgical treatment of trigeminal schwannomas. J Neurosurg. 1995;82(5):711–8.
11. Fukaya R, Yoshida K, Ohira T, Kawase T. Trigeminal schwannomas: experience with 57 cases and a review of the literature. Neurosurg Rev. 2010;34(2):159–71.
12. Kong DS, Kim YH, Lee WJ, Kim YH, Hong CK. Indications and outcomes of endoscopic transorbital surgery for trigeminal schwannoma based on tumor classification: a multicenter study with 50 cases. J Neurosurg. 2022;138(6):1653–61. https://doi.org/10.3171/2022.9.JNS22779.
13. Berke RN. A modified Kronlein operation. Trans Am Ophthalmol Soc. 1953;51:193–231.

14 Cavernous Sinus

Alberto Di Somma, Alejandra Mosteiro, Isam Alobid, and Joaquim Enseñat

Abbreviations

III	Oculomotor nerve
IV	Trochlear nerve
V_1	Ophthalmic division of the trigeminal nerve
V_2	Maxillary division of the trigeminal nerve
V_3	Mandibular division of the trigeminal nerve
VI	Abducens nerve
VII	Facial nerve
VIII	Vestibulocochlear nerve
CS	Cavernous sinus
cICA	Cavernous segment of the internal carotid artery
GSPN	Great superficial petrosal nerve
ICA	Internal carotid artery
IOF	Inferior orbital fissure
LSW	Lesser sphenoid wing
MOB	Meningo-orbital band
pICA	Petrous segment of the internal carotid artery

The cavernous sinus (CS) is a beautiful, delicate, and complex venous entity within the sphenoidal and temporal skull base, comprising multiple neurovascular relations. As coined by Parkinson [1], this "anatomic jewel box" has attracted the attention of pioneer neurosurgeons who have provided detailed descriptions through cadaveric and intraoperative studies. Indeed, the composite anatomy of the CS and the proximity to crucial neural and vascular structures have generated great controversy regarding the optimal surgical approach to this area, with many lesions considered unresectable and prone to nonsurgical management [2–4]. Even when conventional transcranial approaches are, thus far, the gold standard [5–9], the direct pathway afforded by ventral routes like the transorbital (TO) avenue and the minimally disruptive manipulation granted by the endoscopic techniques have rekindled the surgical intention to this area [10–16]. Still, it is only through extensive anatomic expertise that this region becomes a scrutable surgical site.

This chapter starts with a concise review of the anatomic fundamentals to understand the CS area. Then, a step-by-step explanation on how to approach the CS through the superior eyelid TO approach is provided. Emphasis is made on key anatomical references and how to perform interdural and extradural peeling of the CS. Potential applications of this approach will be discussed and clarified with illustrative surgical cases. The

A. Di Somma (✉) · A. Mosteiro · J. Enseñat
Department of Neurological Surgery, Hospital Clínic de Barcelona, Barcelona, Spain

I. Alobid
Rhinology Unit and Smell Clinic, ENT Department, Hospital Clínic de Barcelona, Barcelona, Spain
e-mail: ialobid@clinic.cat

T. H. Schwartz et al. (eds.), *Endoscopic Transorbital Surgery of the Orbit, Skull Base and Brain*,
https://doi.org/10.1007/978-3-031-59504-2_14

major advantages and limitations of this ventral endoscopic pathway will be compared to other endoscopic and transcranial alternatives. Finally, some advice on how to avoid complications will be given.

Concise Surgical Anatomy of the Cavernous Sinus

Since the earliest descriptions from Taptas [17], Dolenc [18], Umanksy [19], Bowder [20], and Parkinson [21], the CS has been well outlined from the transcranial [22–30] and the endoscopic endonasal [31–34] perspectives. Here, we will unveil the CS from an endoscopic TO view, emphasizing the key landmarks to navigate this structure from this relatively novel standing point [35].

The Cavernous Sinus

The CS is a paired boat-shaped structure with a prow directed anteriorly towards the superior orbital fissure (SOF), which will become a valuable reference for surgical orientation during TO approach and a wide stern facing posteriorly at the junction of the basilar and the superior and inferior petrosal sinuses [36]. The CS is delimited by five walls conformed by dura folds over an osseous scaffold and divided into four venous spaces according to the course of the intracavernous internal carotid artery (cICA) [37]. The sinus also serves as a passage area for the third (III), fourth (IV), and sixth (VI) cranial nerves, the first (V_1) and second (V_2) division of the fifth nerve, and the sympathetic plexus towards the orbit. Of note, the III, IV, V_1, and V_2 travel in the lateral surface of the CS and will be in intimate relation to the surgical corridor. Meanwhile, medially, the CS is in contact with the sella turcica and the pituitary gland. Moreover, the CS establishes a network of anastomosis with the surrounding sinuses and veins, which increases the difficulty of the endoscopic procedure due to potential bleeding; the main connections to be aware of are the intercavernous, basilar, and petrosal sinuses; the ophthalmic veins; the veins of the foramen rotundum, ovale, and spinosum; and the deep and superficial middle cerebral veins.

The Lateral Wall of the Cavernous Sinus

The lateral wall of the CS is of utmost importance in the TO approach, becoming the main surgical reference. It is composed of a two-layer dura fold, as an extension of the dura lining the middle cranial fossa. At the inferolateral edge of the sinus, right above the V_2 branch, the inner (endosteal) and the outer (meningeal) layers separate; the former extends medially to form the medial sinus wall, which then bends at the roof of the CS to encircle the pituitary gland; and the outer layer extends upwards and forms the lateral wall of the CS as the dura propria [38].

As first described by Umansky et at. [19], the two-layer frame enables to perform an interdural dissection of the CS, where the semitransparent inner layer allows an exploration of the nerves coursing the lateral wall (III, IV, V_1, V_2) without penetrating the intracavernous space [18]. The foramen rotundum and indeed V_2 will become key structures during the interdural peeling of the CS. For some authors, the lateral wall of the CS ends at the superior edge of V_2 [18, 19, 27, 30, 38].

From the SOF, the lateral wall [38] can be followed along the middle cranial fossa extending posterior up to the petrous apex and petroclival fissure, inferiorly, and to the petroclinoid ligament and the trigeminal porus, superiorly.

Here, the oculomotor nerve is seen coursing lateral to the optic strut, at the lower margin of the anterior clinoid, as the most superior of all neural structures of the lateral wall of the CS. In the posterior part of the roof of the CS, the oculomotor nerve is seen entering the oculomotor triangle. This same triangle serves as an entrance point for the trochlear nerve, in a rather posterolateral position compared to the oculomotor. The trochlear nerve is also seen coursing the lateral wall of the CS, right below the III nerve, until it reaches the anterior clinoid process, where it bends medially and over the III to enter the SOF. The trochlear nerve is a landmark delimitating two anatomical triangles (the supratrochlear and infratrochlear) that serve as key landmarks to identify the ICA from a TO perspective.

Also within the lateral wall, the ophthalmic division of the trigeminal nerve courses under the IV nerve. Posteriorly, the ophthalmic branch joins the Gasserian ganglion, located just lateral to the CS within the Meckel's cave. In turn, the maxillary division courses in the inferior margin of the CS lateral wall; at the inferomedial region of the middle cranial fossa, V_2 is seen traversing the foramen rotundum towards the pterygopalatine fossa. It is in this point of transition, over the V_2 nerve, where the dura of the lateral wall unfolds into the two layers, separated by a trabecula of fibrous adhesions, which can be sharply divided to start the interdural dissection from a TO route [38].

Rather posteriorly and laterally within the middle fossa, the mandibular division of the trigeminal nerve is seen entering the foramen ovale into the infratemporal fossa. Of note, the V_3 branch does not properly pertain to the lateral wall of the CS; therefore, exposing V_3 requires an extradural peeling of the middle cranial fossa floor or, alternatively, cutting off the dura fibers that separate V_3 from the lateral wall of the sinus during an interdural peeling.

The Anterior Wall of the Cavernous Sinus

From the lateral orbital corridor, the anterior wall of the CS is the first one coming into view after adequate bone work [13]. This wall extends from the SOF to the anterior clinoid process, the optic strut, and the carotid sulcus inferiorly. From a TO perspective, in the medial aspect, this wall is limited by the meningo-orbital band (MOB), superiorly, and by the foramen rotundum, inferiorly, while in the lateral aspect, it is limited by the dura of the temporal pole.

The Roof of the Cavernous Sinus

The roof of the CS extends between the anterior and posterior clinoid processes; from the anterior petroclinoid ligament laterally, to the *diaphragma sellae* medially, covering the lateral margin of the sella. The dura covering the anterior clinoid process and the optic strut extends medially to form the upper and lower dural rings, delineating the clinoid segment of the ICA. From a TO perspective, the roof of the CS can be reached after an anterior clinoidectomy or after the peeling of the lateral wall of the CS.

The Medial Wall of the Cavernous Sinus

The medial wall of the CS [32] is the only one conformed by a single dura layer. The sellar part of the medial wall is in continuation with the *diaphragma sellae* folding inferiorly and wrapping the pituitary gland. Meanwhile, the sphenoidal part of the medial wall is formed by the endosteal layer covering the sphenoid bone in continuation with the sellar floor. As previously advanced, this medial wall is somewhat hidden from the lateral TO perspective; it can only be reached after intracavernous dissection in a lateral to medial fashion.

The Posterior Wall of the Cavernous Sinus

From the petrous apex and petroclival fissure, the posterior wall of the CS extends towards the posterior clinoid process. At the inferior margin of the posterior wall, Dorello's canal, enclosed by Grüber's petrosphenoid ligament, serves as the entry point for the VI nerve. The posterior wall of the CS can be explored after peeling the lateral wall or after intracavernous dissection.

Anatomical Triangles Within the Cavernous Sinus

Several dura folds serve as anatomic triangles for surgical orientation. Of particular interest, in the lateral wall of the CS, the supratrochlear (Dolenc's) [39] and infratrochlear (Parkinson's) [21] triangles are delimited by the III and IV and the IV and V_1 nerves, respectively, and provide safe access points into the CS. Also, a wider triangle is encountered between V_1 and V_2, Mullan's anteromedial triangle [40], which can also give access to the most anterolateral area of the CS. A thorough description of these triangles is beyond the scope of this chapter.

Endoscopic Superior Eyelid Transorbital Approach to the Cavernous Sinus

The TO approach offers a straight route to the CS, particularly directed to its lateral wall. This is achieved by either an interdural or an extradural dissection of the two layers that integrate the lateral wall of the sinus [13, 14, 38]. Commonly, both dissecting techniques are used in combination to increase the exposure of the parasellar area. Moreover, the peeling of the CS is also intended to mobilize the temporal lobe laterally to gain an extradural access to Meckel's cave [41, 42], the tentorial area [43, 44], and the posterior cranial fossa [45]. From the TO perspective, the intracavernous component per se, though rarely targeted during surgery, can be accessed and anatomically explored through triangular zones lying between the neurovascular structures of the lateral wall.

Among the described skin incisions for the TO approach [46], in our institution we opt for the superior eyelid crease incision. A stepwise description of the surgical technique will be provided in the following lines.

Intraoperative Neurophysiologic Monitoring of Oculomotor Nerves

Given the proximity to the oculomotor and trigeminal cranial nerves, intraoperative neurophysiologic monitoring is considered mandatory in our center. Nonetheless, monitoring the extraocular muscle function is controversial and may pose technical difficulties during orbital manipulation due to the surgical approach. The oculoplastic surgeon introduces the hookwire needles into the superior oblique (IV) and external rectus (VI) muscles via transconjunctival. The needle to the inferior rectus (III) is introduced transcutaneous. Continuous spontaneous electromyographic (sEMG) activity is registered, while triggered EMG (tEMG) is performed for ad hoc identification of a cranial nerve if necessary [47]. Corticobulbar motor-evoked potentials (CoMEPs) are also obtained periodically throughout the surgery [48].

Skin Incision and Working Space

The skin incision is made in the superior eyelid crease to minimize cosmetic defects (surgical wound hidden with opened eyes). It is advisable to mark the incision in the awake patient, before undergoing the induction of anesthesia, as this may distort the wrinkle patter in the eyelid. Alternatively, in the asleep patient, elevating the eyelid in a physiological manner can reveal the natural wrinkles, and the same effect can be sought laterally to stress the lateral canthal lines. The cut is made with a cold steel scalpel or electrocautery, extending from the level of the supraorbital notch to the level of the lateral orbital canthus; at this point, the incision is curved laterally, to prevent it from coursing over the lateral canthal tendon. Below the skin, the fibers of the orbicularis oculi muscle are identified and divided to reveal the pretarsal fascia, a white plane connecting the septum and the *levator palpebrae* muscle. This avascular plane must be preserved and followed superiorly until the superior orbital rim and the frontal process of the zygoma are recognized. Traction stitches are placed to keep the superior eyelid incision open (Fig. 14.1).

The periosteum overlying the superolateral orbital rim is sharply divided and dissected towards the orbit while preserving the periorbital fascia for close-up reconstruction at the end of the surgery. Dynamic retraction is applied to displace the orbit medially so the endoscope can be inserted at the superolateral corner of the surgical corridor. At this point, identification of the infe-

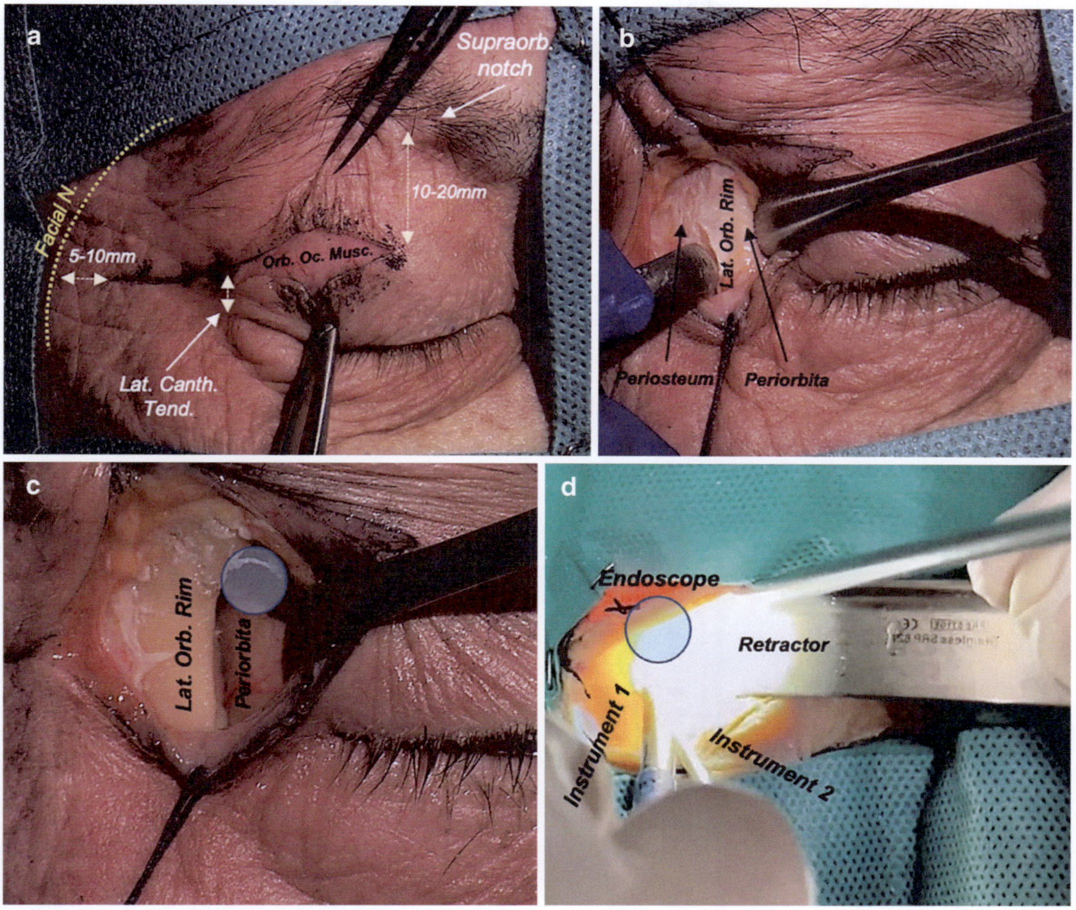

Fig. 14.1 Skin incision for a superior eyelid transorbital approach. (**a**) The incision is made on the superior eyelid crease, from the level of the supraorbital notch to the lateral canthus; here, the incision is curved laterally to prevent injury to the lateral canthal tendon. Care must be taken not to extend it too laterally as to transgress the frontalis branch of the facial nerve. The orbicularis orbital muscle is exposed and its fibers dissected. (**b**) The white plane of the pretarsal fascia is preserved and followed towards the lateral orbital rim. The periosteum is cut. (**c**) A plane is created between the lateral orbital wall laterally and the periorbita medially, and the endoscope can be inserted (blue circle). (**d**) For a four-hand technique, the retractor will keep the periorbita medially and away from the corridor, the endoscope is kept at the superolateral quadrant, and two instruments are manipulated in the inferior quadrants

rior (IOF) and superior (SOF) orbital fissures serves for anatomical orientation before proceeding with the removal of the lateral orbital wall. The spatula should always be kept to follow the direction of the IOF. Systematic check of the pupil size, every 20 min, is advisable throughout the duration of the surgery; in case a dilated pupil is noticed, it is advisable to wait until spontaneous reversal [46].

Bone Work

The lateral wall of the orbit extends between the IOF and SOF and is comprised of the greater sphenoid wing (GSW) and part of the body of the zygoma (orbital surface of the zygomatic body). As this bony concavity is gently drilled, the deep temporalis fascia is exposed, and, deeper into the corridor, the dura protecting the temporal pole is uncovered. The floor of the middle cranial fossa should be flattened [49, 50]; this is particularly intricate at the most medial part, where the sagittal crest [51] penetrates between the SOF and the temporal lobe. The floor of the middle fossa should be drilled out until the foramen rotundum is opened and V_2 exposed; optionally, further removal of the floor can be done to facilitate the access towards deep-seated structures, like the petrous apex and petroclival region [50]. Adequate identification of V_2 is paramount, as it harbors the natural limit of the two dura layers constituting the lateral wall of the CS. Ultimately, V_2 will be the starting point of the interdural peeling. The drilling is then turned to the lesser sphenoid wing (LSW), which separates the dura over the temporal and the frontal lobes, and it can be extended further superiorly and anteriorly to expose the dura overlying the frontobasal lobe but also medially to remove the lateral attachment of the anterior clinoid (thus exposing the base of the anterior clinoid). The aim of the superomedial bone removal is to expose the MOB (Fig. 14.2).

In brief, after proper skin incision and intraorbital endoscopic bone exposure and drilling, the following structures need to be identified and exposed before moving forward: superiorly, the

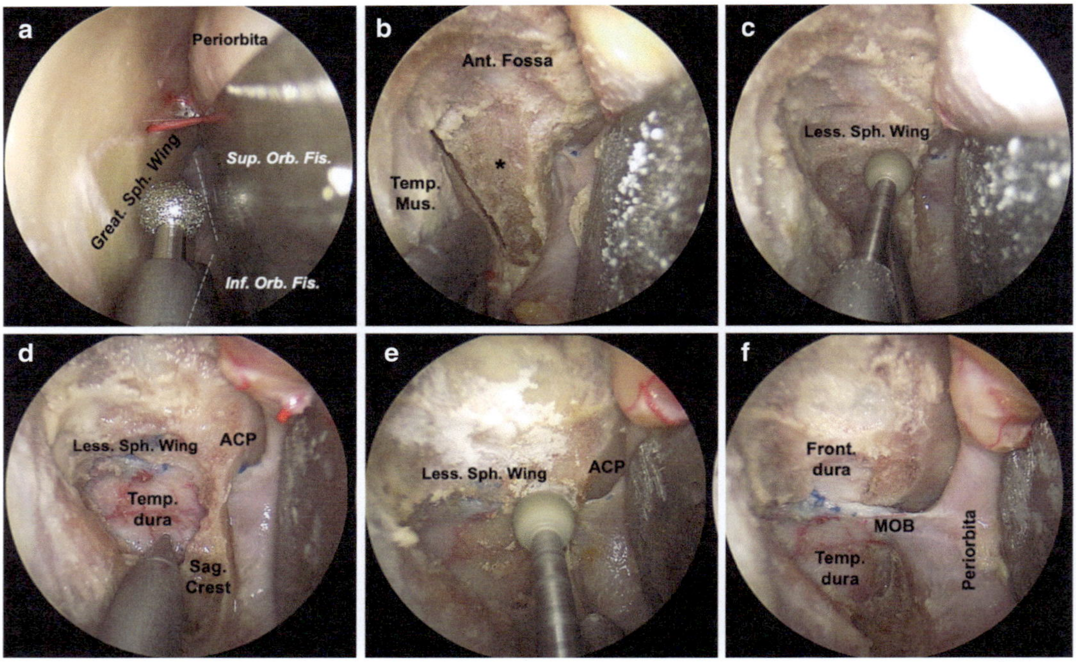

Fig. 14.2 Bone work during the lateral transorbital approach to the middle fossa and cavernous sinus. (**a**) The superior (SOF) and inferior (IOF) orbital fissures are key anatomic landmarks (dotted white lines). The spatula is maintained parallel to the IOF, in a vertical plane. The lateral wall of the orbit extending from the SOF and IOF and comprising the greater sphenoid wing is drilled. (**b**) The deep fascia of the temporalis muscle is uncovered. The last piece of greater sphenoid wing lying in a vertical portion adopts a "V" shape (*) that serves as an orientation for drilling and uncovering the dura overlying the temporal pole. (**c**) A qualitative change in the bone composition is noticed once the drilling passes from the greater sphenoid wing of the lateral orbit wall to the same structure that covers the anterior temporal pole dura ("V" structure). (**d**) The dura covering the temporal pole is exposed. The sagittal crest is the triangle-shaped bone lying between the SOF and the temporal lobe. Drilling continues towards the lesser sphenoid wing and the anterior cranial fossa. (**e**) The lesser sphenoid wing should be removed up to its most medial part, the lateral insertion of the anterior clinoid process (ACP). (**f**) Once the SOF is completely opened, the meningo-orbital band (MOB) is seen

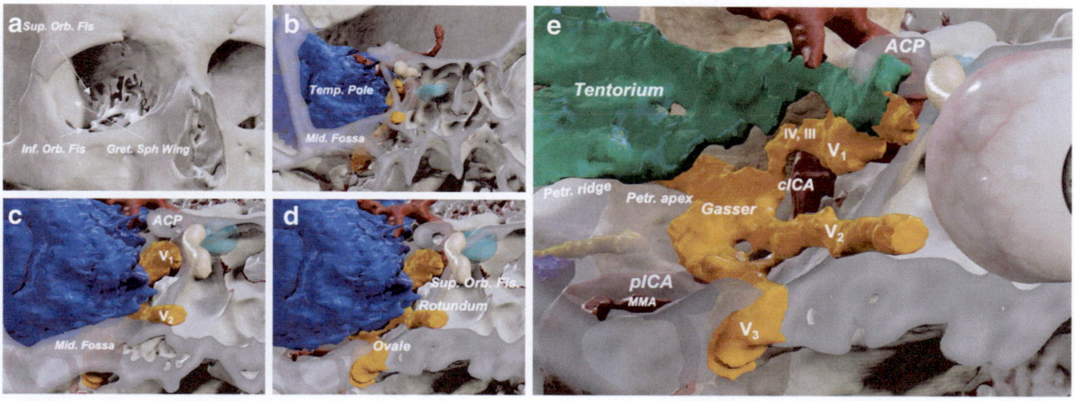

Fig. 14.3 Three-dimensional reconstruction of the bone work phase (Brainlab workstation). (**a**) View of the osseous components of the right orbit. (**b–d**) Details of the anatomic relation between the neural and osseous structures related with the transorbital approach to the cavernous sinus. (**b**) The V_1 nerve is seen exiting the middle cranial fossa through the superior orbital fissure, while the V_2 nerve is seen entering the foramen rotundum towards the pterygopalatine fossa. (**c**) V_1 is encountered right below the anterior clinoid process (ACP). (**d**) Both V_1 and V_2 course in intimate contact with the temporal lobe (blue). (**e**) A detail of the neurovascular structures traversing the medial aspect of the middle fossa is shown. *pICA and cICA* petrous and cavernous segments of the internal carotid artery, *MMA* middle meningeal artery, *ACP* anterior clinoid process, *III* oculomotor nerve, *IV* trochlear nerve, V_1 ophthalmic division of the trigeminal nerve, V_2 maxillary branch of the trigeminal nerve, V_3 mandibular branch of the trigeminal nerve

lesser sphenoid wing (flattened) and the frontobasal dura (or the bone corresponding to the frontobasal area/orbital roof that needs to be flattened); inferiorly, the middle cranial fossa floor (flattened down at least up to expose the crista ovale [52]); supero-medially, the MOB, in close relation with the base of the anterior clinoid; and inferomedially, the foramen rotundum, in close relation with the base of the sagittal crest (Fig. 14.3).

Peeling of the Lateral Wall of the Cavernous Sinus

Once the bone work is accomplished, the interdural and extradural planes need to be identified. Afterwards, the peeling should start at the level of the foramen rotundum/V_2. The MOB [13] can be cut to obtain further mobilization of the temporal dura laterally, yet it is not indispensable. Neurophysiologic stimulation of the intended site of cut can help avoid injuring one of the cranial nerves (Fig. 14.4). Hence, the exposure of the lateral wall of the CS can be obtained through an interdural or an extradural peeling, or a combination of the two. Via the TO pathway, it is generally achieved starting from an interdural dissection.

Interdural Dissection

At the foramen rotundum, V_2 marks the point where the junction of the two dura layers is naturally distinguished [38, 52], and a sharp division with a dissector directed upwards will separate the two layers aside [13]. The temporal lobe, protected by the meningeal layer, is freed from the dura attachments and laterally displaced as the interdural dissection moves superiorly and posteriorly, revealing the lateral wall of the cavernous sinus protected by the endosteal dura layer [18] (Fig. 14.5). The cranial nerves III, IV, V_1, and V_2 become apparent in the lateral sinus wall; meanwhile, in the floor of the middle fossa, the V_3

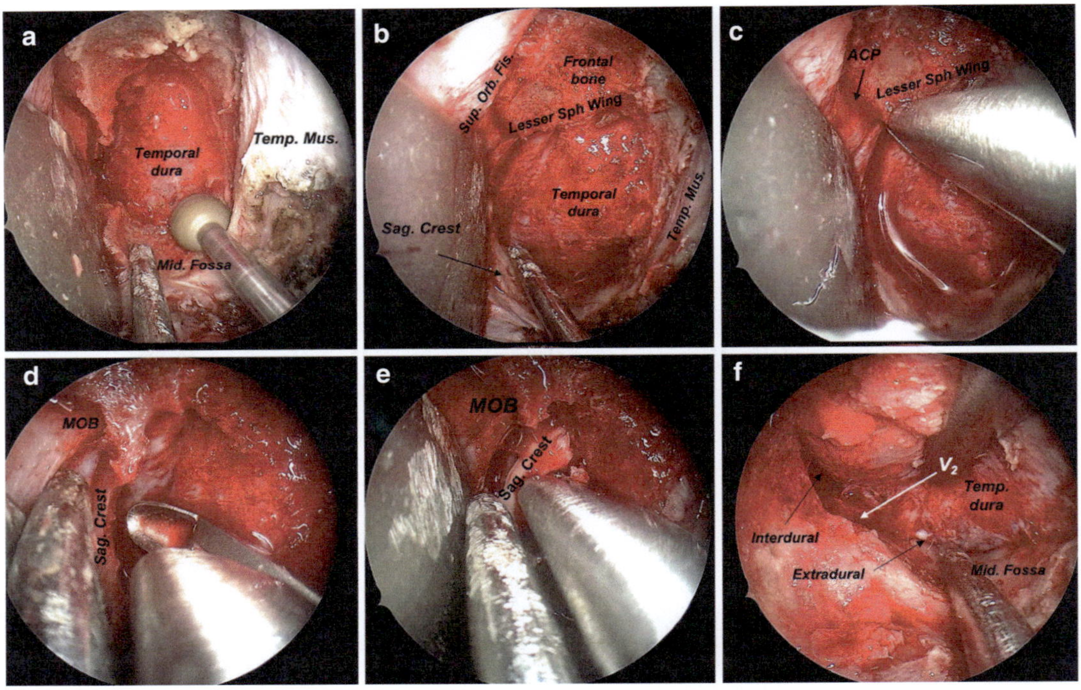

Fig. 14.4 Illustrative surgical case of peeling of the lateral wall of the cavernous sinus via a left superior eyelid transorbital approach. (**a**) Drilling the greater sphenoid wing at the lateral wall of the orbit exposes the deep fascia of the temporalis muscle, the dura overlying the temporal pole, and the floor of the middle cranial fossa. (**b**) The spatula that follows the direction of the IOF and is placed in the vertical plane retracting the periorbita medially is advanced to reveal the superior orbital fissure (SOF). (**c**) Drilling the lesser sphenoid wing up to its most medial extension (i.e., the lateral insertion of the anterior clinoid process, ACP) is needed. (**d**) The sagittal crest is a constant anatomic landmark in the lateral transorbital approach. This is a triangular-shaped bone ridge extending between the SOF and the temporal dura in the vertical plane. (**e**) The sagittal crest should be completely removed to free the way into the interdural plane of dissection. However, once the crest is removed, the spatula retracting the periorbita may lose a point of stability, so this maneuver should be done as last step before interdural peeling starts. (**f**) Finally, the floor of the middle fossa floor is flattened, and an extradural exploration is performed by spearing the dura over the basal temporal lobe. The V_2 nerve entering the foramen rotundum is another major landmark in this approach

nerve is seen coming from the infratemporal fossa though the foramen ovale and joining at the Gasserian ganglion. This branch is not part of the sinus wall (Fig. 14.6).

Extradural Dissection

The extradural peeling involves the separation of the dura proper of the temporal lobe away from the lateral wall of the CS. The dissection is, in this case, initiated at the inferomedial surface of the temporal lobe (see Fig. 14.5), at the level of the floor of the middle fossa. The floor of the middle fossa is exposed epidurally, until the foramen spinosum with the middle meningeal artery is encountered laterally, the foramen rotundum with V_2 is encountered medially, and the foramen ovale with V_3 is seen posteriorly. The epidural plane can be followed further posterior until the petrous ridge and apex are reached. Cutting off the dura extending between V_2 and V_3 will communicate the interdural and extradural spaces, thus increasing the exposure and maneuverability in the lateral cavernous region.

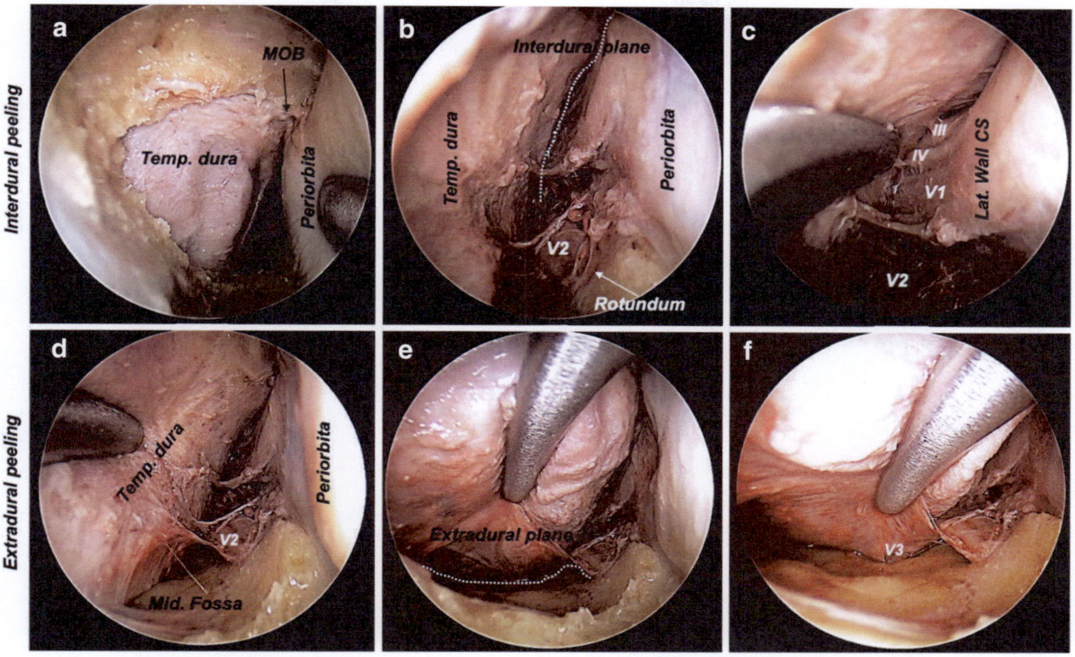

Fig. 14.5 Interdural and extradural peeling of the lateral wall of the cavernous sinus (right orbit). (Cadaveric dissections). (**a**) The meningo-orbital band (MOB) extending between the periorbita and the dura covering the temporal and frontal lobes, seen after opening the superior orbital fissure. The MOB can be cut to facilitate the interdural peeling, though it is not mandatory. (**b**) The interdural plane is the virtual space between the inner and outer dural layers that conform the lateral wall of the cavernous sinus. The interdural peeling starts at the level of the foramen rotundum, where gentle traction of the dura covering the V_2 nerve naturally opens this plane of dissection. (**c**) As the dissection proceeds further up and deep, the cranial nerves running on the lateral wall of the cavernous sinus become visible, protected by the thin layer of inner dura. Some fibrous adhesions joining the inner and outer layers of dura may need to be sharply cut to proceed with the peeling. (**d**) The extradural plane is the virtual space between the dura propria of the temporal lobe (an extension of the outer dura layer of the lateral wall of the cavernous sinus) and the bony floor of the middle cranial fossa. (**e**) The interdural peeling starts laterally to the V_2 branch, and it continues further lateral and deeper, until the middle meningeal artery and the V_3 branch (foramen ovale) are encountered, respectively. (**f**) Cutting the dura layer separating V_2 and V_3 will communicate the interdural and extradural planes and increase the exposure and maneuverability in the cavernous area

Intracavernous Dissection

For anatomic purposes, an exploration of the contents of the inner cavernous sinus will be provided. Opening the interdural plane reveals the lateral wall of the cavernous sinus protected by the thin inner dura layer. The cranial nerves that run in this lateral wall are seen from superior to inferior: the oculomotor (III) and trochlear (IV) and the ophthalmic (V_1) and maxillary (V_2) divisions of the trigeminal nerve. V_3 does not pertain to the lateral wall of the cavernous sinus, but it rather runs in the middle fossa floor until it enters the foramen ovale towards the infratemporal fossa. Parkinson's infratrochlear triangle is delimited by the IV and V_1 nerves. Mullan's anteromedial triangle is limited by V_1 and V_2. Opening Parkinson's triangle affords direct access to the cavernous segment of the internal carotid artery (ICA). Opening Mullan's triangle by gentle retraction of V_1 exposes the abducens (VI) nerve and more deeply, also the ICA accompanied by the sympathetic plexus (Fig. 14.7).

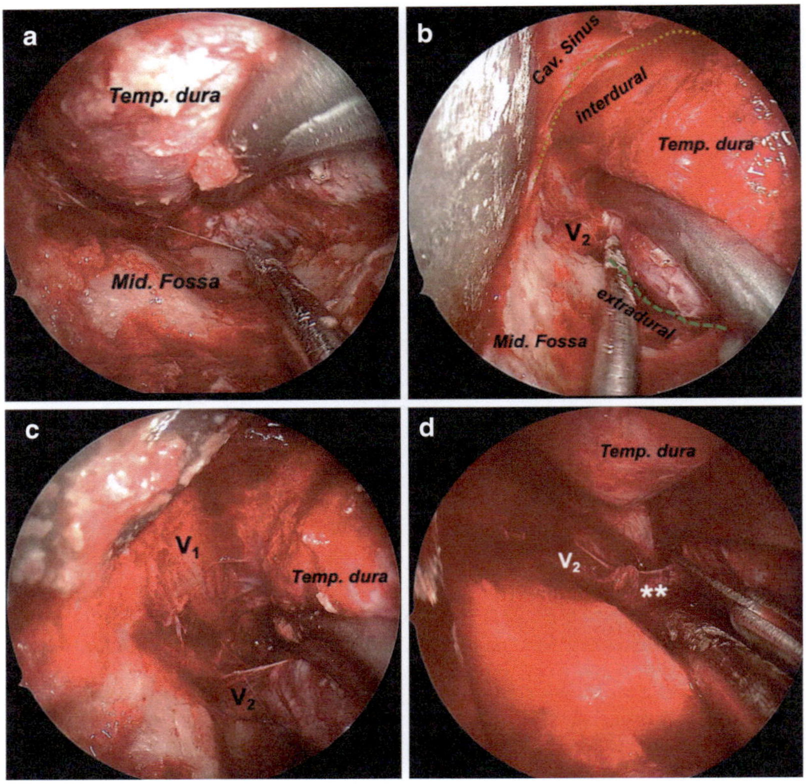

Fig. 14.6 Interdural peeling of the lateral wall of the cavernous sinus (in continuation with Fig. 14.4). (Intraoperative images following Fig. 14.4). (**a**) The interdural dissection begins at the level of the foramen rotundum, where the dura covering V_2 is distracted upwards to reveal the plane of dissection between the inner and outer dura layers. (**b**) The temporal lobe, protected by the meningeal layer, is freed from the arachnoid attachments and laterally displaced as the interdural dissection moves superiorly and posteriorly, revealing the lateral wall of the cavernous sinus protected by the endosteal dura layer. (**c**) The cranial nerves III, IV, V_1, and V_2 become apparent in the lateral wall of the cavernous sinus. (**d**) Meanwhile, in the floor of the middle fossa, the V_3 nerve is seen coming from the foramen ovale and joining at the Gasserian ganglion

Cranial Nerves Course from a Transorbital Perspective

From the TO perspective, the cavernous course of the related cranial nerves can be inspected (Figs. 14.8 and 14.9). V_1 is seen traversing from the superior orbital fissure towards the Gasserian ganglion (GG). V_2 is seen coming out from the pterygopalatine fossa through the foramen rotundum and coursing posteriorly towards the GG. Meanwhile, V_3 can only be seen if an extradural peeling of the middle cranial fossa is performed, or if the dura bands extending between V_2 and V_3 are cut. V_3 runs within the middle fossa floor as it emerges from the infratemporal fossa through the foramen ovale to join the GG. The dura propria of the GG can be opened to enter the virtual arachnoid space of the Meckel's cave, containing the trigeminal root fibers (see dotted lines in Fig. 14.8b). The trigeminal root can be followed further posteriorly, traversing the trigeminal porus towards the posterior fossa. Here, the trigeminal nerve crosses in intimate relation to the tentorial inci-

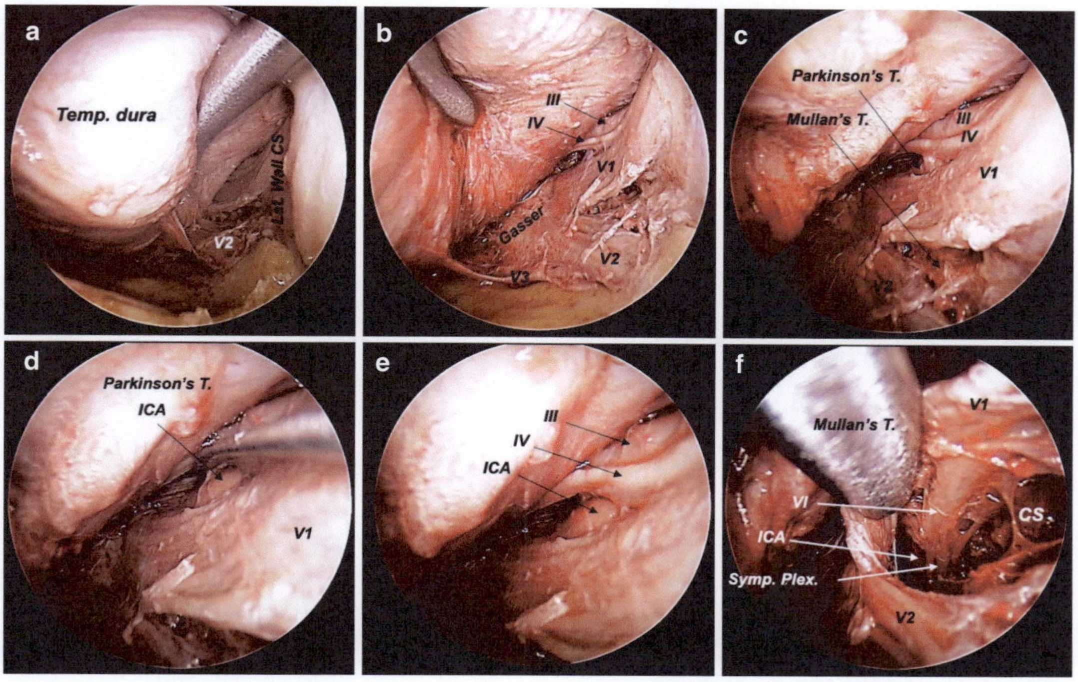

Fig. 14.7 Triangles in the lateral wall of the cavernous sinus and their contents. (Cadaveric dissections). (**a**) The temporal dura has been retracted laterally and superiorly, to reveal the epidural and interdural planes, separated by a band of dura propria at the level of V_2. The lateral wall of the cavernous sinus protected by the thin inner dura layer comes into view. (**b**) As the interdural peeling extends posteriorly, the cranial nerves running within the lateral wall of the cavernous sinus are encountered, namely, the oculomotor (III) and trochlear (IV), coming from the oculomotor triangle at the roof of the cavernous sinus and reaching the anterior clinoid process to enter the orbit. Then, V_1 and V_2 are seen extending from the Gasserian ganglion towards the superior orbital fissure and foramen rotundum, respectively. Meanwhile, V_3, also coming from the Gasserian ganglion, does not pertain to the lateral wall of the cavernous sinus; it rather runs in the middle fossa floor until entering the foramen ovale towards the infratemporal fossa. (**c**) Parkinson's infratrochlear triangle is delimited by the IV and V_1 nerves. Mullan's anteromedial triangle is limited by V_1 and V_2. (**d, e**) Opening Parkinson's triangle affords direct access to the cavernous segment of the internal carotid artery (ICA). (**f**) Opening Mullan's triangle by gentle retraction of V_1 exposes the abducens (VI) nerve and more deeply, also the ICA accompanied by the sympathetic plexus

sura and enters the anterior surface of the pons (see Fig. 14.8a–c).

The *III* and *IV* cranial nerves share a similar trajectory within the lateral wall of the CS (its superior aspect). They run from the anterior clinoid process towards Hakuba's oculomotor triangle, located at the posterior part of the roof of the CS. Hakuba's triangle, delimited by the petroclinoid and interclinoid ligaments, can be opened to unveil the course of these nerves within the basal cisterns. The *III* nerve is seen coursing between the posterior cerebral artery (PCA) and the superior cerebellar artery (SCA) before entering the midbrain at the interpeduncular fossa (see Fig. 14.8d–f). Meanwhile, the *IV* nerve courses above the SCA, within the pontomesencephalic sulcus, to reach its apparent origin in the posterior surface of the midbrain (see Fig. 14.8c).

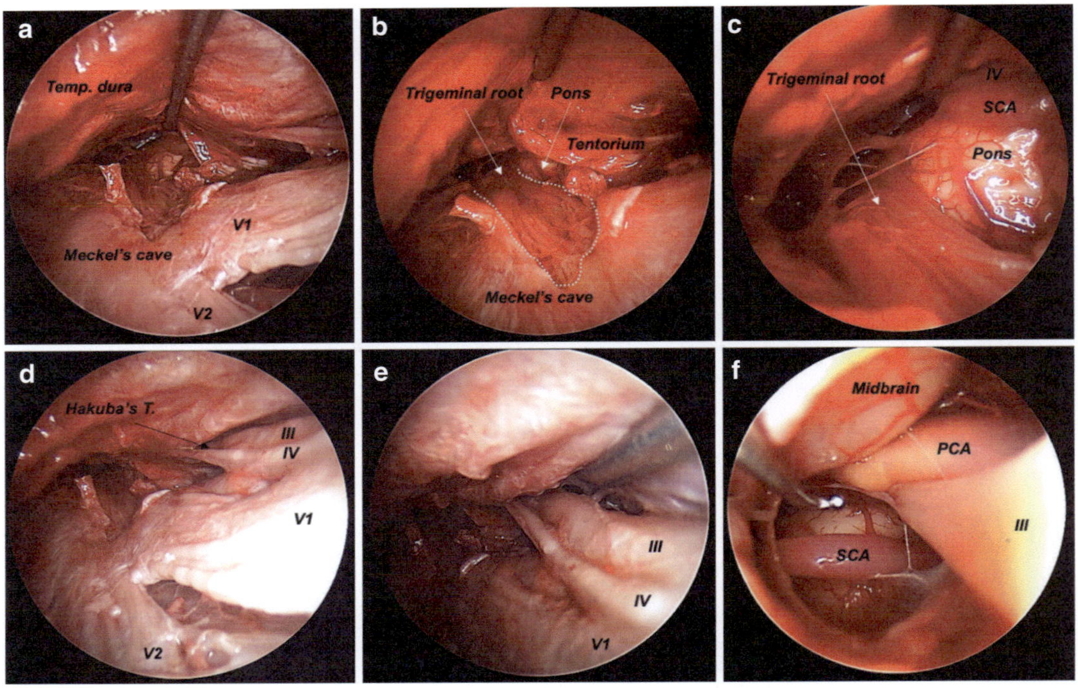

Fig. 14.8 Intracavernous course of the oculomotor, trochlear and trigeminal nerves. (Cadaveric dissections). (**a**) Opening of the dura propria of the Gasserian ganglion opens the arachnoid cage known as Meckel's cave and reveals the fibers of the trigeminal root. (**b**) The trigeminal root can be followed posteriorly by opening the trigeminal porus, in intimate relation to the tentorial incisura. (**c**) The trigeminal root is ultimately seen at its apparent origin in the surface of the pons. The trochlear nerve is seen here coursing posteriorly along the ponto-mesencephalic sulcus, above the superior cerebellar artery (SCA), towards its point of emergence at the posterior midbrain. (**d**, **e**) In the roof of the cavernous sinus, Hakuba's oculomotor triangle is encountered. This triangle, delimited by the petroclinoid ligaments, serves as the point of entrance for both the III and IV cranial nerves. (**f**) Opening if Hakuba's triangle reveals the apparent origin of the III nerve, at the interpeduncular cistern of the midbrain. The III nerve is seen coursing between the posterior cerebral artery (PCA) and the SCA

Finally, the *IV* nerve has a purely intracavernous trajectory and can be seen if the Mullan's triangle is opening (between V_1 and V_2). Within the CS, the *VI* nerve courses in intimate contact to the ICA, in a rather inferior position. However, as the trajectory is followed deeper, the VI nerve adopts a rather lateral position towards the posterior wall of the CS. The VI nerve pierces the posterior wall of the CS towards the posterior cranial fossa. Concretely, the VI nerve passes under Grüber petrosphenoidal ligament, delimiting the so-called Dorello's canal (see Fig. 14.9).

Closure and Reconstruction

The reconstruction obeys the same principles mentioned elsewhere in this book. Recapitulating, autologous fat, fixed with fibrin glue, is used to obliterate the surgical cavity. Then, fascia lata is used to sustain the material in place. Importantly, the periosteum overlying the lateral orbital rim must be consciously closed with running sutures. Finally, the orbicularis oculi muscle and the eyelid skin are closed with simple or continuous sutures [47].

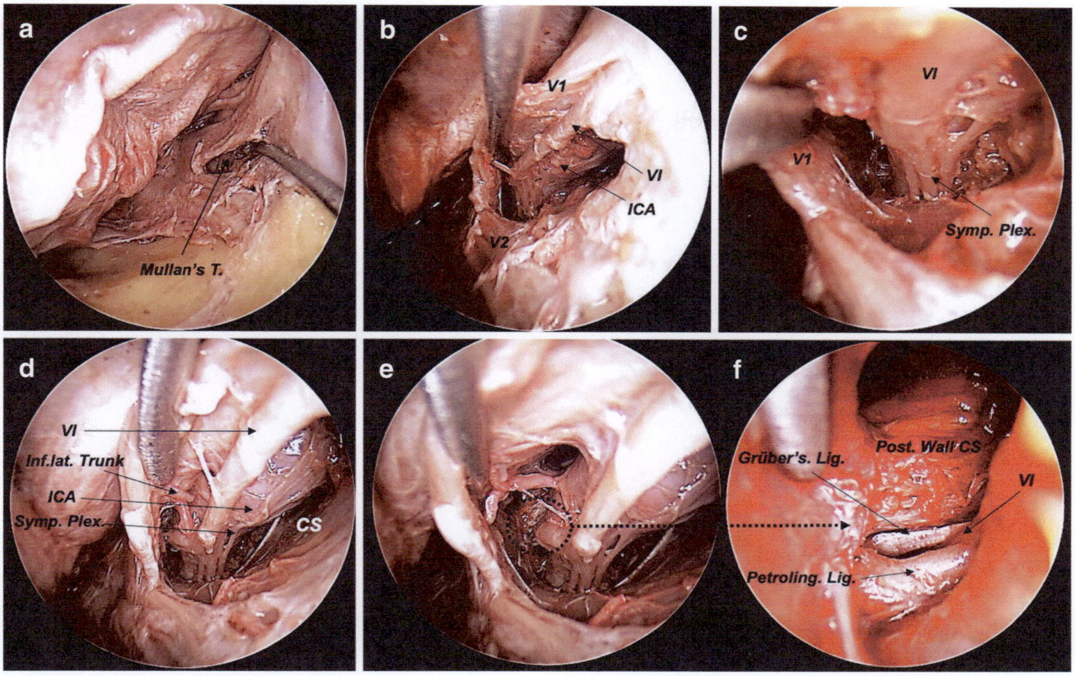

Fig. 14.9 Intracavernous course of the abducens nerve. (Cadaveric dissections). (**a**) Mullan's anteromedial triangle is delimited by the first and second trigeminal branches. (**b**) Opening Mullan's triangle reveals the VI cranial nerve, running in close contact to the internal carotid artery (ICA). (**c**) At the surface of the ICA, the fibers of the sympathetic plexus are seen. (**d**) The inferolateral trunk is the intracavernous branch coming from the lateral surface of the horizontal segment of ICA. (**e**) The VI nerve courses inferior to the ICA, and as the trajectory becomes deeper, it adopts a rather lateral position towards the posterior wall of the cavernous sinus. (**f**) At the posterior wall of the cavernous sinus, the VI nerve passes under Grüber's petrosphenoidal ligament towards the posterior fossa. Grüber's ligament thus delimits the so-called Dorello's canal. Inferiorly, the ICA is seen passing under the petrolingual ligament, to become extracavernous; this is the transition to the lacerum segment

Surgical Applications of the Transorbital Route to the Cavernous Sinus

Following the established levels of difficulty for the TO surgery, an example is provided for the level 4, biopsy of an intracavernous lesion, and level 5, resection of an intracavernous and posterior fossa lesion.

Illustrative Case 1: Biopsy of an Intracavernous Sinus Lesion

A 49-year-old male presented with diplopia and a right VI nerve palsy. The MRI revealed an extra-axial hyper-enhancing lesion within the cavernous sinus (a–d). The lesion engulfed the cavernous internal carotid artery (cICA) and seems to be completely intracavernous. The differential diagnosis comprised meningioma, schwannoma, hemangioma, hemangiopericytoma or an inflammatory/lymphomatous lesion (Fig. 14.10a–d). A biopsy was deemed necessary for diagnostic purposes, and the lateral transorbital approach was chosen as a direct route to the lesion.

A superior eyelid crease incision was chosen, and a lateral orbital wall craniectomy was performed. Special attention was directed to remove the sagittal crest completely (Fig. 14.10e) to gain appropriate access to the tumoral area within the

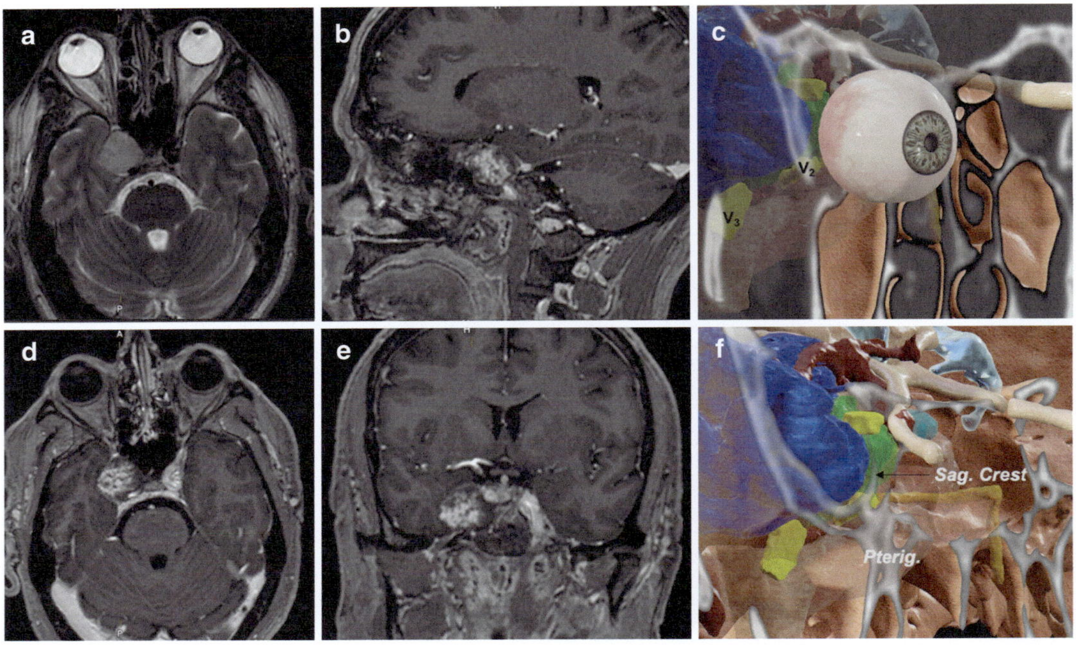

Fig. 14.10 Transorbital endoscopic approach to biopsy a cavernous hemangioma (case presentation and preoperative planning). (**a**) T2-weighed and (**b–d**) T1 contrast-enhanced magnetic resonance image showing an extra-axial lesion (25 mm) within the lateral wall of the right cavernous sinus. The lesion is surrounding the internal carotid artery. It shows and heterogeneous enhancing pattern. (**e**) Preoperative planning 3D reconstructions obtained with Brainlab workstation. The lesion (green) is seen medial to the lateral wall of the CS, delimited by the first and second divisions of the trigeminal nerve (V_1, V_2). (**f**) Complete drilling of the sagittal crest is essential to enter the plane between the temporal lobe (blue) and the CS. Note that the working area is located within the middle cranial fossa, just above the pterygoid

lateral wall of the CS. After interdural peeling of the lateral wall of the cavernous sinus, the lesion was accessed through the infratrochlear triangle, between the IV and V_1 cranial nerves. A biopsy of the intracavernous lesion was obtained, by entering the most superficial and anterior part of the tumor emerging at the surface of the lateral CS wall. Intraoperative pathological inspection informed of a hemangioma, amenable to radiotherapy; therefore, further resection was deemed unnecessary. Hemostasis was later achieved by means of thrombin agents and mechanical compression. After radiotherapy, partial remission of the ophthalmoparesis was gained as well as a reduced diameter of the lesion at the last follow-up (Fig. 14.11a–d). Postoperatively, no new deficits were seen. The palpebral edema resolved within 10 days, and the eyelid scar is barely noticed (Fig. 14.11e).

Illustrative Case 2: Combined Transorbital and Endonasal Approach for a Tumor Within the Cavernous Sinus and Clival Region

The TO route is one of the strategies to consider when resecting a tumor extending from the clival region and invading the CS. Of help in this scenario is the combined TO-endonasal approach, where the TO corridor will expose the cavernous component of the tumor lateral to the ICA, while the endonasal transclival venue will reach the clival component and the cavernous portion medial to the ICA.

A 33-year-old woman complaining of paresthesia in the territory of the left V_3 nerve underwent a brain MRI. The findings were compatible with a petroclival tumor with invasion of the CS, right Meckel's cave, anterior and middle fossa, and orbital apex (Fig. 14.12). After careful dis-

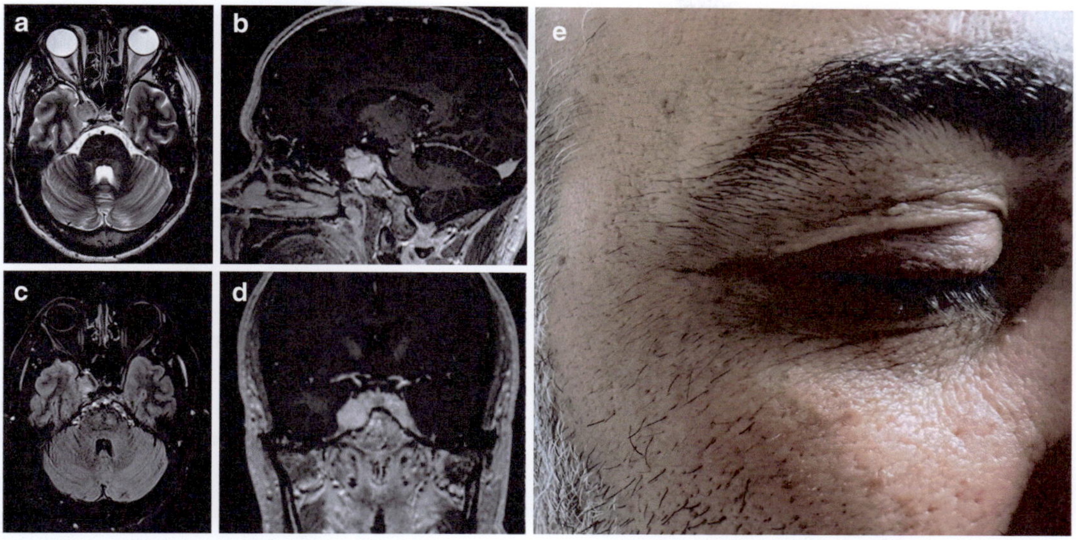

Fig. 14.11 Transorbital endoscopic approach to biopsy a cavernous hemangioma (surgical outcome). (**a–d**) Follow-up MRI after radiotherapy treatment showing a diminished diameter of the intracavernous lesion. (**e**) Cosmetic outcome after the superior eyelid incision and lateral orbital craniectomy

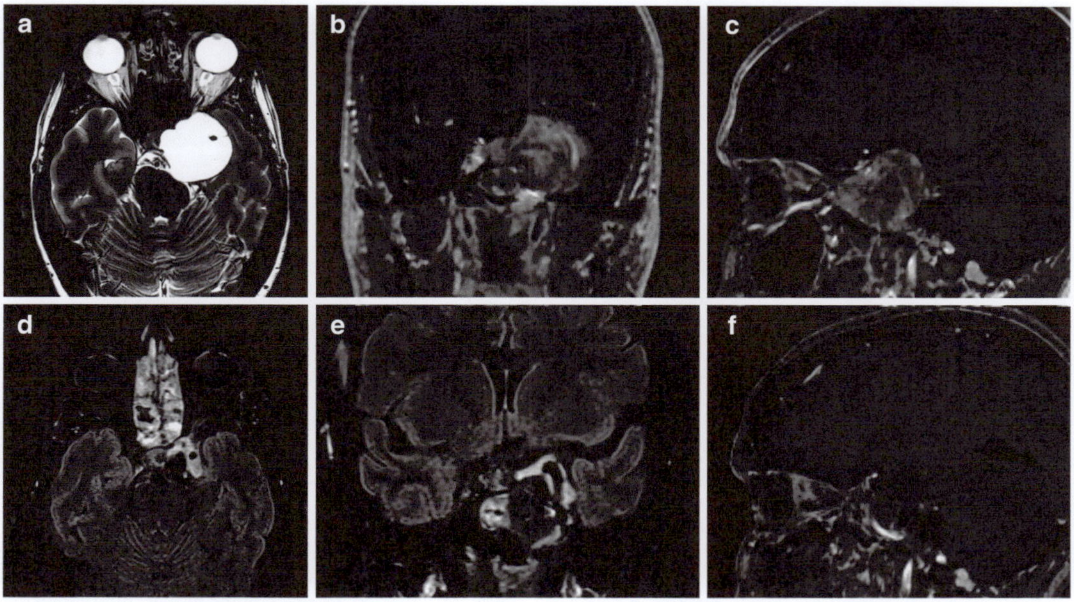

Fig. 14.12 Combined transorbital-endonasal resection of a clival chondrosarcoma invading the left cavernous sinus (case presentation and outcomes). (**a–c**) Preoperative MRI study showing a left extra-axial lesion comprising the cavernous sinus and orbital apex and extending to the anterior and middle cranial fossa, the petrous apex, and petroclival areas. The lesion completely engulfed the internal carotid artery. Differential diagnosis included a chordoma, chondrosarcoma, and meningioma. (**d**, **e**) Postoperative MRI showing a small remanent of tumor capsule, adherent to the internal carotid artery and lateral cavernous sinus wall (cranial nerves). (**f**) The extent of resection was 92%. No postoperative complications were seen on the MRI study

cussion within the skull-base unit, a combined transorbital-endonasal approach was planned.

In collaboration with the oculoplastic surgeon, a superior eyelid incision and a conventional lateral orbital wall craniectomy were performed. Simultaneously, the ENT team obtained a nasoseptal flap and performed a middle turbinectomy and sphenoidotomy, followed by the neurosurgical team fulfilling a middle transclival approach. From the TO perspective (Fig. 14.13), after the bone work phase with removal of the sagittal crest and lesser sphenoid wing, the MOB was exposed and cut. The anterior surface of the tumor was seen emerging in the interdural space. The tumor capsule was opened, and tumor debulking was started by simple aspiration, given the friable consistency of the lesion. The Doppler ultrasound was used when in doubt for internal carotid artery preservation; similarly, tEMG was used to identify the presence of cranial nerves embedded within the tumor mass. Debulking was continued until the posterior wall of the cavernous sinus was encountered medially and inferiorly (see Fig. 14.13e) and until the internal carotid was identified laterally and posteriorly (see Fig. 14.13f). A near total resection of the tumor was achieved (EOR 92%), with a small remanent of tumor capsule (yellow) enclosing the internal

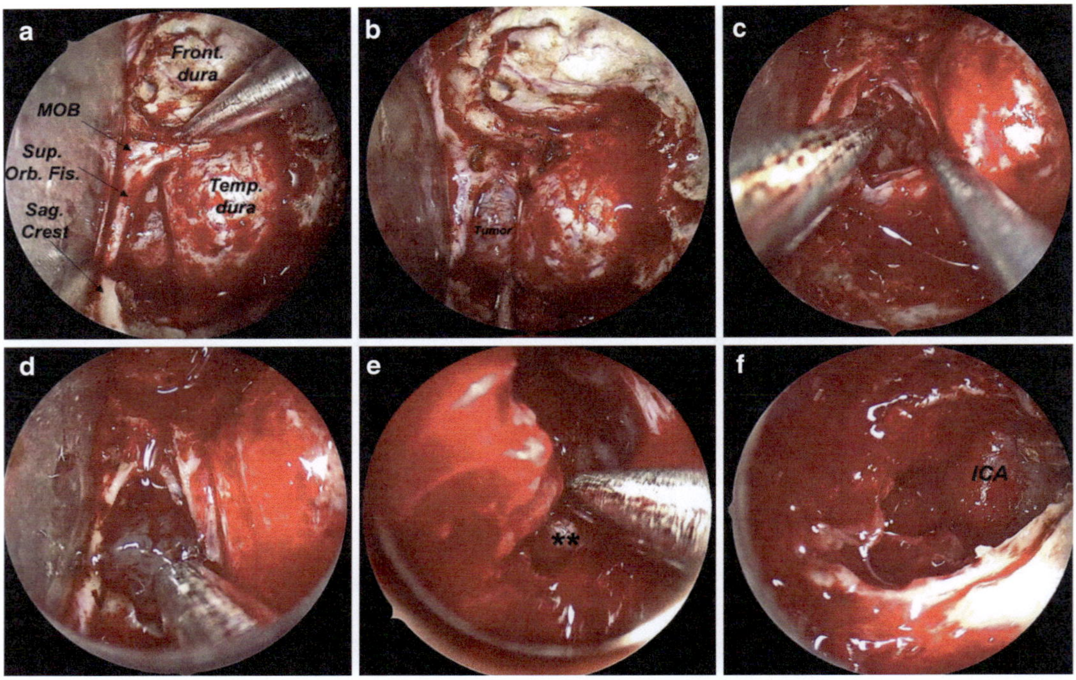

Fig. 14.13 Combined transorbital-endonasal resection of a clival chondrosarcoma (intraoperative view from the transorbital route). (**a**) Once the bone work is accomplished, the periorbita and the superior orbital fissure are retracted medially (with a spatula placed in the perpendicular plane), and the dura over the temporal pole and basal frontal lobes is exposed. The meningo-orbital (MOB) band is seen extending from the superior orbital fissure to the temporal and frontal dura. (**b**) Attention should be paid to the complete removal of the sagittal crest before starting the interdural peeling of the lateral wall of the cavernous sinus (CS). Sectioning the MOB exposes the interdural plane in the lateral wall of the CS; in this case, the plane has already been divided by the tumor. (**c**, **d**) The tumor capsule is opened and an extracavernous debulking of the tumor is performed. (**e**) Medially, the tumor capsule is left intact, because of the intimate adhesion to the cranial nerves running in the inner layer of the lateral wall of the CS. (**f**) The carotid artery (ICA) was identified within the tumor mass and preserved during the resection. The point of encounter with the endonasal route was located at the inferomedial margin of the transorbital working area (double asterisk). Once the corresponding resection was completed from the transorbital corridor, this surgical standing point served for checking the carotid integrity during the most upper and lateral part of the endonasal resection

carotid and lateral wall of the cavernous sinus (see Fig. 14.12d–f). The lesion was categorized as a WHO grade 2 chondrosarcoma, and adjuvant radiotherapy was indicated. No postoperative deficits were encountered, and moderate palpebral edema resolved within 1 week. No late ocular deformities were developed. The patient is now completely asymptomatic and follow-up imaging shows no signs of lesion regrowth.

Comparison with the Alternative Transcranial and Endonasal Approaches

After the pioneer work of Parkinson [21] and Browder [20], the first surgical series accessing the CS came from Yasargil [53], who used a pterional intradural transsylvian approach to the parasellar area. Entry to the CS through a subtemporal approach was introduced by Hakuba et al. [22], who performed a peeling of the lateral wall of the sinus from a lateral to medial extradural dissection of the middle cranial fossa. It was Dolenc who combined the pterional and subtemporal intra- and extradural approaches to the CS [5, 6, 18], providing access to the lateral wall, the infratrochlear, anteromedial, and paramedial triangles, by means of a medial to lateral middle fossa dissection. More recently, Al-Mefty popularized the zygomatic and orbitozygomatic approach to the CS [7, 8]. Conventional transcranial approaches rely on extensive bone removal and a certain extent of brain retraction to provide a comfortable working exposure of the CS. In these approaches, control of the proximal and distal internal carotid artery is also sought.

In the orbitozygomatic approach [8, 54], a cranio-orbital flap including the sphenoid bone, the lateral orbit, and the zygomatic arch provides simultaneous access to the cranium and orbit [55]. Drilling of the Glasscock triangle is necessary to gain proximal control of the ICA, and removal of the orbital roof, SOF, and anterior clinoid provides control of the supraclinoid carotid. Conversely, gaining control of the ICA through the endoscopic TO approach has its limitations, as bone removal and temporary clip application are not straightforward through this surgical corridor. When this vascular control is considered essential, relying on endovascular balloon placement in a hybrid operating room could become a convenient solution [56, 57].

By means of interdural peeling, the orbitozygomatic approach exposes the lateral wall of the cavernous sinus, the Meckel's cave, and the petrous apex, in a similar extent to the TO route, but with greater retraction of the temporal lobe. Entry to the CS is also through Parkinson's triangle, although this is somewhat eased from the orbitozygomatic lateral perspective, as the vector of the surgical approach falls perpendicular to the lateral wall of the sinus. In the TO route, removal of the lateral orbital rim permits further lateral angulation of the vector of approach and a more favorable working angle towards the CS [14, 41, 58]. On the contrary, the natural course of the TO corridor directly leading towards the petrous apex and Meckel's cave is more convenient than the lateral exposure provided by the orbitozygomatic approach. This is especially relevant in cases of trigeminal schwannomas, where the longitudinal axis of the tumor follows the same vector of the surgical corridor, making these lesions particularly amenable from the TO perspective [59].

Reconstruction after an orbitozygomatic craniotomy is laborious, and special care should be given to potential opening of the frontal sinus. This transgression of the paranasal cavities is virtually inexistent in the TO approach, thus minimizing the risk of postoperative CSF fistula. In addition to the long skin scar, temporalis muscle disinsertion and drilling of the pterion contribute to cosmetic disfiguration in the orbitozygomatic approach. These all can be avoided by the TO route; yet enophthalmos and palpebral retractions could become an issue in this case.

A significant evolution of the transcranial approaches towards less invasive procedures was the keyhole concept. Concretely, the microscopic-based lateral TO [9, 14, 60, 61] and the subtemporal [62, 63] keyhole approaches provided more conservative anterolateral and lateral routes to the CS and Meckel's cave. However, the main limitation with these keyhole strategies is the narrow surgical corridor, transforming the surgical field into a dark and uncomfortable area. The ultimate advance in the minimally invasive trend was the combination of these small ports with the endoscopic armamentarium [64].

The extended endonasal endoscopic approach can provide access to the anterior and middle walls of the CS, by means of an ethmoido-pterygo-sphenoidal removal [10, 12]. If drilling is extended laterally to the parasellar ICA, the lateral wall of the CS can also be exposed [34] by retracting the ICA and the VI cranial nerve medially. From the endonasal perspective [11], an anteromedial corridor can be opened to reach the lateral CS and Meckel's cave [65]. Arguably, exposure of these lateral components of the CS is more feasible through the TO route, as it avoids an extensive exposure and manipulation of the ICA.

Conversely, to access the medial CS the endonasal corridor is superior to the TO. After opening the floor and lateral aspects of the sella, an arachnoid plane can be opened between the pituitary gland and the anterior bend of the internal carotid; the gland is retracted medially, and the medial wall of the CS comes into view [34]. This anteromedial approach to the CS has some advantages as assured by Cavallo et al. [11]: the medial wall of the CS is thin and conformed by a single dura layer; moreover, it has some weak points around the SOF plexus and cranial nerves through which access to intracavernous tumors is eased; in addition, the anteroinferior venous space is predominant in most of the cases [36, 66]. Still, these potential advantages mostly apply to pituitary adenomas extending to the CS [67] and not to other tumoral or vascular lesions. Plus, a major drawback of the anterior corridor is dealing with hypothetical injury to the ICA, which is the main boundary in the lateral extension of the surgical corridor.

Complementing the limitations of the endonasal approach, the endoscopic lateral TO access is a direct route to the lateral wall of the CS [9, 13–15]. Compared to the subtemporal and orbitozygomatic approaches, the need for temporal lobe retraction is remarkably reduced but at the expense of less surgical freedom in the posterior region of the cavernous sinus, particularly in the vertical plane [41].

An endoscopic alternative to the endonasal and TO corridors is the transoral transmaxillary approach described by Couldwell et al. [68], through which the CS can be exposed from the pterygopalatine fossa by enlarging the foramen rotundum. Each of these endoscopic approaches provides a certain degree of surgical exposure and a specific working angle; therefore judiciously combining two or more of these ports can enhance surgical maneuverability and increase the success rates, and it also facilitates cooperation between participating surgeons and reduces the tendency to instrument crowding seen in endoscopic procedures.

Potential Complications and Final Remarks

The most frequent complication after a TO approach to the CS area is ophthalmoparesis, most frequently an exotropia due to a III nerve palsy, in contrast with the ventral endonasal approach which tends to affect predominantly the VI nerve. Injury or manipulation of the trigeminal ganglion or its branches may result in facial numbness or neuralgia. To minimize the risk of nerve damage, intraoperative electrophysiological monitoring is advised; however, maintaining the extraocular muscles recording needles in place while orbital retraction is applied for surgical purposes is challenging.

Entering the CS could result in the potentially fatal laceration of the ICA, but an otherwise inadvertent injury to a hypophyseal branch could result in pituitary dysfunction. The use of endovascular procedures to gain proximal and even distal control of the carotid artery could help perform the intracavernous maneuvers more safely; this requires a hybrid operating room and the collaboration of a vascular neurosurgeon. Alternatively, proximal control of the carotid can be obtained at the cervical level if considered imperative. Besides, identifying the small intracavernous branches of the internal carotid can be difficult, particularly due to the continuous venous bleeding within the sinus. The use of fluorescent dyes, such as the indocyanine green, could facilitate the process of arterial identification. Still, a full pituitary hormone analysis is recommended perioperatively.

Conclusions

In this chapter a brief anatomic review of the cavernous sinus anatomy as seen via the TO pathway has been provided. As well, some clinical illustrative cases have been shown.

Anatomic studies and preliminary surgical case series have given proof that the endoscopic lateral TO approach is a feasible alternative to access and treat lesions within the lateral wall of the cavernous sinus, the petrous apex, Meckel's cave, and the tentorial area. Moreover, intracavernous access can be exploited with biopsy or respective aims. Still, surgical expertise and comprehensive anatomical knowledge are required, positioning these surgical targets in the culminating learning process of the TO surgery [69]. Individual assessment of each case will determine if the well-established transcranial approaches can be substituted by the TO route.

References

1. Parkinson D. The cavernous sinus. In: Dolenc VV, editor. The cavernous sinus. New York: Springer; 1987. p. 3–29.
2. Fariselli L, Biroli A, Signorelli A, Broggi M, Marchetti M, Biroli F. The cavernous sinus meningiomas' dilemma: surgery or stereotactic radiosurgery? Rep Pract Oncol Radiother. 2016;21(4):379–85.
3. Raheja A, Couldwell WT. Cavernous sinus meningioma with orbital involvement: algorithmic decision-making and treatment strategy. J Neurol Surg B Skull Base. 2020;81(4):348–56.
4. Corniola MV, Roche PH, Bruneau M, Cavallo LM, Daniel RT, Messerer M, et al. Management of cavernous sinus meningiomas: consensus statement on behalf of the EANS skull base section. Brain Spine. 2022;2:100864.
5. Dolenc VV. A combined epi- and subdural direct approach to carotid-ophthalmic artery aneurysms. J Neurosurg. 1985;62(5):667–72.
6. Dolenc VV. Transcranial epidural approach to pituitary tumors extending beyond the sella. Neurosurgery. 1997;41(3):542–50; discussion 51–2.
7. al-Mefty O, Anand VK. Zygomatic approach to skull-base lesions. J Neurosurg. 1990;73(5):668–73.
8. Heth JA, Al-Mefty O. Cavernous sinus meningiomas. Neurosurg Focus. 2003;14(6):e3.
9. Matsuo S, Komune N, Iihara K, Rhoton AL. Translateral orbital wall approach to the orbit and cavernous sinus: anatomic study. Oper Neurosurg (Hagerstown). 2016;12(4):360–73.
10. Cappabianca P, Alfieri A, de Divitiis E. Endoscopic endonasal transsphenoidal approach to the sella: towards functional endoscopic pituitary surgery (FEPS). Minim Invasive Neurosurg. 1998;41(2):66–73.
11. Cavallo LM, Cappabianca P, Galzio R, Iaconetta G, de Divitiis E, Tschabitscher M. Endoscopic transnasal approach to the cavernous sinus versus transcranial route: anatomic study. Neurosurgery. 2005;56(2 Suppl):379–89; discussion 379–89.
12. Cappabianca P, de Divitiis E. Endoscopic endonasal transsphenoidal surgery. New York: Springer; 2003.
13. Dallan I, Di Somma A, Prats-Galino A, Solari D, Alobid I, Turri-Zanoni M, et al. Endoscopic transorbital route to the cavernous sinus through the meningo-orbital band: a descriptive anatomical study. J Neurosurg. 2017;127(3):622–9.
14. Altay T, Patel BC, Couldwell WT. Lateral orbital wall approach to the cavernous sinus. J Neurosurg. 2012;116(4):755–63.
15. Bly RA, Ramakrishna R, Ferreira M, Moe KS. Lateral transorbital neuroendoscopic approach to the lateral cavernous sinus. J Neurol Surg B Skull Base. 2014;75(1):11–7.
16. Di Somma A, Andaluz N, Cavallo LM, Topczewski TE, Frio F, Gerardi RM, et al. Endoscopic transorbital route to the petrous apex: a feasibility anatomic study. Acta Neurochir. 2018;160(4):707–20.
17. Taptas JN. The so-called cavernous sinus: a review of the controversy and its implications for neurosurgeons. Neurosurgery. 1982;11(5):712–7.
18. Dolenc V. Direct microsurgical repair of intracavernous vascular lesions. J Neurosurg. 1983;58(6):824–31.
19. Umansky F, Valarezo A, Elidan J. The superior wall of the cavernous sinus: a microanatomical study. J Neurosurg. 1994;81(6):914–20.
20. Browder J. Treatment of carotid artery cavernous sinus fistula: report of a case. Arch Ophthalmol. 1937;18:95–102.
21. Parkinson D. A surgical approach to the cavernous portion of the carotid artery: anatomical studies and case report. J Neurosurg. 1965;23:474–83.
22. Hakuba A, Tanaka K, Suzuki T, Nishimura S. A combined orbitozygomatic infratemporal epidural and subdural approach for lesions involving the entire cavernous sinus. J Neurosurg. 1989;71(5 Pt 1):699–704.
23. Harris FS, Rhoton AL. Anatomy of the cavernous sinus. A microsurgical study. J Neurosurg. 1976;45(2):169–80.
24. Kawase T, van Loveren H, Keller JT, Tew JM. Meningeal architecture of the cavernous sinus: clinical and surgical implications. Neurosurgery. 1996;39(3):527–34; discussion 34–6.
25. Krisht A, Barnett DW, Barrow DL, Bonner G. The blood supply of the intracavernous cranial nerves: an anatomic study. Neurosurgery. 1994;34(2):275–9.
26. Sekhar LN, Burgess J, Akin O. Anatomical study of the cavernous sinus emphasizing operative approaches and related vascular and neural reconstruction. Neurosurgery. 1987;21(6):806–16.

27. Seoane E, Rhoton AL, de Oliveira E. Microsurgical anatomy of the dural collar (carotid collar) and rings around the clinoid segment of the internal carotid artery. Neurosurgery. 1998;42(4):869–84.
28. Seoane E, Tedeschi H, de Oliveira E, Wen HT, Rhoton AL. The pretemporal transcavernous approach to the interpeduncular and prepontine cisterns: microsurgical anatomy and technique application. Neurosurgery. 2000;46(4):891–8.
29. Yasuda A, Campero A, Martins C, Rhoton AL, Ribas GC. The medial wall of the cavernous sinus: microsurgical anatomy. Neurosurgery. 2004;55(1):179–89; discussion 89–90.
30. Yasuda A, Campero A, Martins C, Rhoton AL, de Oliveira E, Ribas GC. Microsurgical anatomy and approaches to the cavernous sinus. Neurosurgery. 2005;56(1 Suppl):4–27.
31. Knosp E, Kitz K, Steiner E, Matula C. Pituitary adenomas with parasellar invasion. Acta Neurochir Suppl (Wien). 1991;53:65–71.
32. Fernandez-Miranda JC, Zwagerman NT, Abhinav K, Lieber S, Wang EW, Snyderman CH, et al. Cavernous sinus compartments from the endoscopic endonasal approach: anatomical considerations and surgical relevance to adenoma surgery. J Neurosurg. 2018;129(2):430–41.
33. Erdogan U, Turhal G, Kaya I, Biceroglu H, Midilli R, Gode S, et al. Cavernous sinus and parasellar region: an endoscopic endonasal anatomic cadaver dissection. J Craniofac Surg. 2018;29(7):e667–e70.
34. Abuzayed B, Tanriover N, Gazioglu N, Ozlen F, Cetin G, Akar Z. Endoscopic anatomy and approaches of the cavernous sinus: cadaver study. Surg Radiol Anat. 2010;32(5):499–508.
35. Di Somma A, Andaluz N, Cavallo LM, de Notaris M, Dallan I, Solari D, et al. Endoscopic transorbital superior eyelid approach: anatomical study from a neurosurgical perspective. J Neurosurg. 2018;129(5):1203–16.
36. Rhoton AL, Hardy DG, Chambers SM. Microsurgical anatomy and dissection of the sphenoid bone, cavernous sinus and sellar region. Surg Neurol. 1979;12(1):63–104.
37. Bouthillier A, van Loveren HR, Keller JT. Segments of the internal carotid artery: a new classification. Neurosurgery. 1996;38(3):425–32.
38. Perneczky A, Knosp E, Matula C. Cavernous sinus surgery. Approach through the lateral wall. Acta Neurochir. 1988;92(1–4):76–82.
39. Dolenc VV. Anatomy and surgery of the cavernous sinus. Vienna: Springer, Springer; 1989.
40. Mullan S. Treatment of carotid-cavernous fistulas by cavernous sinus occlusion. J Neurosurg. 1979;50:131–44.
41. Lima LR, Beer-Furlan A, Prevedello DM, Carrau RL, Servián-Duarte DA, Galarce MG, et al. Minimally invasive approaches to the lateral cavernous sinus and Meckel's cave: comparison of transorbital and subtemporal endoscopic techniques. World Neurosurg. 2020;141:e86–96.
42. Di Somma A, Langdon C, de Notaris M, Reyes L, Ortiz-Perez S, Alobid I, et al. Combined and simultaneous endoscopic endonasal and transorbital surgery for a Meckel's cave schwannoma: technical nuances of a mini-invasive, multiportal approach. J Neurosurg. 2020;134(6):1836–45.
43. De Rosa A, Di Somma A, Mosteiro A, Ferrés A, Reyes LA, Roldan P, et al. Superior eyelid endoscopic transorbital approach to the tentorial area: a qualitative and quantitative anatomic study. Front Surg. 2022;9:1007447.
44. Lin BJ, Hong KT, Chung TT, Liu WH, Hueng DY, Chen YH, et al. Endoscopic transorbital transtentorial approach to middle incisural space: preclinical cadaveric study. Acta Neurochir. 2019;161(4):831–9.
45. García-Pérez D, Abarca J, González-López P, Nieto J, Lagares A, Paredes I. A frontal route to middle and posterior cranial fossa: quantitative study for the lateral transorbital endoscopic approach and comparison with the subtemporal approach, vol. 167. World Neurosurg; 2022. p. e236.
46. Moe KS, Bergeron CM, Ellenbogen RG. Transorbital neuroendoscopic surgery. Neurosurgery. 2010;67(3 Suppl Operative):ons16–28.
47. López JR, Legatt AD. Monitoring surgery around the cranial nerves. Handb Clin Neurol. 2022;186:319–51.
48. Kodama K, Kothbauer KF, Deletis V. Mapping and monitoring of brainstem surgery. Handb Clin Neurol. 2022;186:151–61.
49. Di Somma A, Sanchez España JC, Alobid I, Enseñat J. Endoscopic superior eyelid transorbital approach: how I do it. Acta Neurochir. 2022;164(7):1953–9.
50. Guizzardi G, Mosteiro A, Hoyos J, Ferres A, Topczewski T, Reyes L, et al. Endoscopic transorbital approach to the middle fossa: qualitative and quantitative anatomic study. Oper Neurosurg (Hagerstown). 2022;23(4):e267–e75.
51. Corrivetti F, de Notaris M, Di Somma A, Dallan I, Enseñat J, Topczewski T, et al. "Sagittal crest": definition, stepwise dissection, and clinical implications from a transorbital perspective. Oper Neurosurg (Hagerstown). 2022;22(5):e206–e12.
52. Yanez-Siller JC, Noiphithak R, Martinez-Perez R, Dallan I, Moe KS, Revuelta Barbero JM, et al. The "Crista Ovale": a reliable anatomical landmark in transorbital endoscopic approaches to the middle cranial fossa. Oper Neurosurg (Hagerstown). 2022;24:e172.
53. Otani N, Wada K, Toyooka T, Fujii K, Kobayashi Y, Mori K. Operative surgical nuances of modified extradural temporopolar approach with mini-peeling of dura propria based on cadaveric anatomical study of lateral cavernous structures. Surg Neurol Int. 2016;7(Suppl 16):S454–8.
54. Goel A, Shenoy A, Shah A, Goel N, Vutha R, Hawaldar A. Cavernous hemangioma of cavernous sinus: an outcome report of 45 surgically treated patients. World Neurosurg. 2022;159:381–9.

55. Shimizu S, Tanriover N, Rhoton AL, Yoshioka N, Fujii K. MacCarty keyhole and inferior orbital fissure in orbitozygomatic craniotomy. Neurosurgery. 2005;57(1 Suppl):152–9; discussion 152–9.
56. Zhang Y, Tian Z, Li C, Liu J, Yang X. A modified endovascular treatment protocol for iatrogenic internal carotid artery injuries following endoscopic endonasal surgery. J Neurosurg. 2019;132(2):343–50.
57. Zhang N, Xin WQ. Application of hybrid operating rooms for clipping large or giant intracranial carotid-ophthalmic aneurysms. World J Clin Cases. 2020;8(21):5149–58.
58. Noiphithak R, Yanez-Siller JC, Revuelta Barbero JM, Otto BA, Carrau RL, Prevedello DM. Comparative analysis between lateral orbital rim preservation and osteotomy for transorbital endoscopic approaches to the cavernous sinus: an anatomic study. Oper Neurosurg (Hagerstown). 2019;16(1):86–93.
59. Kong DS, Kim YH, Lee WJ, Hong CK. Indications and outcomes of endoscopic transorbital surgery for trigeminal schwannoma based on tumor classification: a multicenter study with 50 cases. J Neurosurg. 2022;138(6):1653–61.
60. Chabot JD, Gardner PA, Stefko ST, Zwagerman NT, Fernandez-Miranda JC. Lateral orbitotomy approach for lesions involving the middle fossa: a retrospective review of thirteen patients. Neurosurgery. 2017;80(2):309–22.
61. Priddy BH, Nunes CF, Beer-Furlan A, Carrau R, Dallan I, Prevedello DM. A side door to Meckel's cave: anatomic feasibility study for the lateral transorbital approach. Oper Neurosurg (Hagerstown). 2017;13(5):614–21.
62. Taniguchi M, Perneczky A. Subtemporal keyhole approach to the suprasellar and petroclival region: microanatomic considerations and clinical application. Neurosurgery. 1997;41(3):592–601.
63. Pichierri A, D'Avella E, Ruggeri A, Tschabitscher M, Delfini R. Endoscopic assistance in the epidural subtemporal approach and Kawase approach: anatomic study. Neurosurgery. 2010;67(3 Suppl Operative):ons29–37.
64. Perneczky A, Fries G. Endoscope-assisted brain surgery: Part 1—Evolution, basic concept, and current technique. Neurosurgery. 1998;42(2):219–24; discussion 24–5.
65. Kassam AB, Prevedello DM, Carrau RL, Snyderman CH, Gardner P, Osawa S, et al. The front door to Meckel's cave: an anteromedial corridor via expanded endoscopic endonasal approach—technical considerations and clinical series. Neurosurgery. 2009;64(3 Suppl):ons71–82; discussion ons82–3.
66. Inoue T, Rhoton AL, Theele D, Barry ME. Surgical approaches to the cavernous sinus: a microsurgical study. Neurosurgery. 1990;26(6):903–32.
67. Yokoyama S, Hirano H, Moroki K, Goto M, Imamura S, Kuratsu JI. Are nonfunctioning pituitary adenomas extending into the cavernous sinus aggressive and/or invasive? Neurosurgery. 2001;49(4):857–62.
68. Couldwell WT, Sabit I, Weiss MH, Giannotta SL, Rice D. Transmaxillary approach to the anterior cavernous sinus: a microanatomic study. Neurosurgery. 1997;40(6):1307–11.
69. Di Somma A, Kong DS, de Notaris M, Moe KS, Sánchez España JC, Schwartz TH, et al. Endoscopic transorbital surgery levels of difficulty. J Neurosurg. 2022;137:1187.

15 Spheno-Orbital Meningiomas: Indications and Limitations

Iacopo Dallan, Giacomo Fiacchini, Miriana Picariello, Lodovica Cristofani Mencacci, and Paolo Castelnuovo

Introduction

Spheno-orbital meningiomas (SOMs) are a unique type of intracranial meningioma that arise from the dura mater overlying the greater or the lesser wing of the sphenoid. From an epidemiological point of view, SOMs comprise between 4% and 9% of all meningiomas [1]. So, they should be considered a rare disease. Habitually SOMs have been managed via traditional transcranial approaches, namely pterional, frontotemporal, frontotemporal orbito-zygomatic approach (FTOZ) that can be associated with some degree of cosmetic and functional impairment [2]. As with all other meningiomas, the decision-making process for SOMs must be tailored to each patient's needs. Mass effect of the tumor, age, general conditions, comorbidities, team expertise, QoL, and patients' wishes should be taken into account. From a biological and pathological point of view, these tumors not infrequently show, at least partially, an en plaque growing pattern associated with hyperostotic bone [3, 4]. Due to their area of origin, SOMs present distinct surgical challenges because they can involve important structures, such as periorbita, extraconal muscles, orbital contents, superior orbital fissure (SOF) and cavernous sinus (CS), temporal and infratemporal fossa, optic canal, and even brain and intracranial vessels. In this sense, one of the key points in SOMs management is the multi-compartmental involvement often seen with these tumors, which usually requires adequate exposure and extensive bone work.

Review of Literature and Personal Considerations on SOM Management

Even with conventional, very extensive, transcranial surgeries, these lesions can usually not be radically extirpated because of their innate characteristics, such as a highly infiltrative nature and high degree of anatomic complexity [1, 5, 6]. The infiltrative growth and pattern of spread make total resection simply impossible [7]. In this respect, due to the expected biological toll of traditional approaches and radical resection, minimally invasive alternatives and a function-sparing philosophy make sense. That said, one of the major questions, related to SOM management, is to find a good balance between resection and QoL after surgery. Should the primary goal of

I. Dallan (✉) · G. Fiacchini · M. Picariello
L. Cristofani Mencacci
ENT Unit, Azienda Ospedaliero-Universitaria Pisana, Pisa, Italy

P. Castelnuovo
ENT Department, University of Insubria, Varese, Italy

T. H. Schwartz et al. (eds.), *Endoscopic Transorbital Surgery of the Orbit, Skull Base and Brain*, https://doi.org/10.1007/978-3-031-59504-2_15

surgery in SOMs always be a complete and radical resection? It is our personal viewpoint that achieving the highest Simpson resection grade should not always be the goal of surgery. As a matter of fact, in the last decade, we have observed a clear shift toward function-sparing surgery [2, 3, 7–12]. A "wise" resection, regardless the approach, followed by radiotherapy or radiosurgery could be considered a valid alternative to traditional, transcranial-based management. This is even more so the case for recurrent or residual disease. In this respect, the natural history of SOMs reveals that not infrequently, during long-term follow-up, recurrences appear [13]. And so, the search for a more conservative, QoL-oriented strategy has become mainstream in SOM management. Among minimally invasive procedures, the superior eyelid, endoscopically assisted, transorbital approach (SEA) represents an interesting option, to be considered in selected cases. The periorbital corridor provides a potential route to reach the anterior and middle cranial fossa in a minimally invasive fashion [14]. In this respect SEA provides adequate working space and freedom of movement to deal with such complex regions and lesions. Furthermore, SEA can be integrated into a combined approach, giving rise to what is also known as a multiport paradigm. Schematically speaking, SEA offers several advantages: short distance to the target, reduced temporalis muscle disruption, limited craniectomy, small skin incision, adequate freedom of movement, and reduced length of stay.

Surgical Considerations and Possible Candidates: The Good, the Bad, and the Ugly

At the time of this writing, due to the low incidence of these tumors and the relatively recent introduction of transorbital endoscopically assisted approach, we affirm that there's no clear and sound agreement on the indications and contraindications. Kong and colleagues have proposed some insights on this topic [7], but clear indications for surgery are lacking. NCCN guidelines recommend intervention for lesions >3 cm, but observation for smaller lesions is predicated on the tumor's anatomical proximity to neurovascular structures. So, the closer the lesion is to critical structures, the less is the size of the tumor factors into the decision-making process. In other words, smaller lesions, close to the optic nerve and other critical structures should be seriously evaluated as possible surgical candidates. According to Kong et al. [7] in the presence of neurological or orbital symptoms, or in the case of a tumor larger than 2 cm, regardless of the presence of symptoms, surgery should be strongly considered. Based on our experience and on available data, some conclusions can be drawn.

More than 10 years of experience [15] has convinced us that endoscopic SEA is a safe and effective alternative to transcranial approaches in selected cases of SOMs, where the planned primary objective is to obtain a maximally safe resection, aimed at symptom relief, rather than a gross total resection at any cost [2, 3]. We agree with Chotai and Schwartz when they state that exclusive use of the Simpson grading score (SGS) as an outcome parameter might lead to misinterpretation of the postoperative data [16]. Hence, evaluating the postoperative residual tumor volume by MRI will likely be more important than the Simpson grade. However, as previously said, it remains which meningiomas will be optimally treated via this novel route.

Another critical factor in selecting patient for the SEA is the experience of the surgical team. While large lesions (>6 cm) are not ideal candidate for SEA, perhaps more important than the dimension itself is the multi-compartmental behavior of the tumor. In 2021 Kong et al. proposed, as exclusion criteria for SEA, the involvement of the anterior clinoid process (ACP) or the middle cerebral arteries. We partially agree with this statement since ACP involvement is not a true contraindication to SEA, especially when the intracranial part of the lesion is small and the need of vascular dissection of the ICA is limited. It should be emphasized that the addition of a lateral orbital rim osteotomy greatly increases the working space in both the lateral and medial directions, thus allowing a safe and adequate resection in the ACP and surrounding areas.

According to Kong [7], the decision regarding whether or not to perform a lateral orbital rim osteotomy is made according to the lateral extent of the tumor. This author states that lateral orbital rim osteotomy significantly increases surgical access to the lateral extent of the tumor. In our opinion the real advantage of lateral orbital rim osteotomy is much more evident when working medially, in the ACP and surrounding areas. The efficacy of SEA appears to be diminished when dealing with large lesions extending laterally and posteriorly (toward the squamous part of the temporal bone) and inferiorly (toward the temporal or infratemporal fossa). In the case of lesions extending inferiorly to the floor of the middle fossa and even the infratemporal fossa, positioning, namely, increasing the forward inclination of the head, can be very helpful [7]. Despite this, tumors extending inferiorly are challenging to manage via the transorbital route. It appears clear that for such lesions, a traditional frontotemporal or even FTOZ is by far more effective. Lastly, extensive intracranial pathology could be considered a relative contraindication to pure SEA, and it represents another factor to be kept in mind when choosing the surgical approach.

While SEA is a valuable option for tumors with minimal involvement of orbital structures, there is no effective approach for pathology with extensive orbital invasion.

In Fig. 15.1 we have tried to give a general and schematic overview of our philosophy.

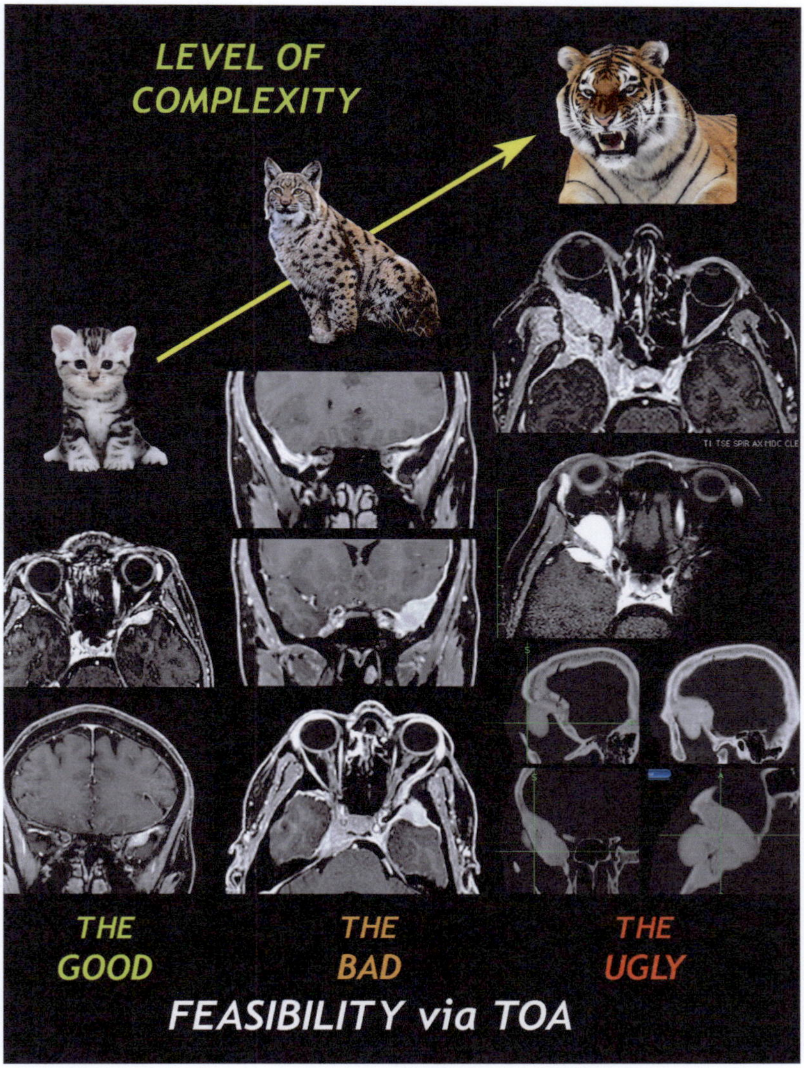

Fig. 15.1 General and schematic overview of philosophy

Factors Affecting Outcome and Recurrence

The subtype and anatomic extent of the SOM are a strong factor determining the ability to obtain a gross total resection (GTR) [7]. It is not surprising that the en plaque type is associated with a lower rate of GTR, clearly because of the diffuse involvement of several skull base compartments. Cavernous sinus invasion is another critical factor that limits resection. With CS or SOF involvement, the goal of surgery is to resect all tumors except the part involving the CS or SOF itself. Lateral orbital rim orbitotomy seems to increase the ability to obtain GTR, clearly enhancing the ability to safely dissect in critical areas. Furthermore, orbital, orbital apex invasion, SOF, infratemporal fossa, or paranasal sinuses involvement should be considered an independent factor for recurrence [17].

Conclusions

Transorbital approaches are a valid option to accomplish function-sparing strategies, possibly integrated in a truly multidisciplinary policy that eventually includes postoperative radiotherapy. Performance status indexes are very important parameters to be considered in the postoperative period, probably more important than a mere analysis of Simpson grade [2]. Subtotal resection followed by stereotactic radiosurgery presents a similar recurrence-free survival as GTR. In conclusion, we consider small- to medium-sized SOMs with limited lateral and inferior extension and minimal invasion of the orbital structures to be ideal candidates for SEA, even in the recurrent setting.

References

1. Shrivastava RK, Sen C, Costantino PD, Della Rocca R. Sphenoorbital meningiomas: surgical limitations and lessons learned in their long-term management. J Neurosurg. 2005;103(03):491–7.
2. Locatelli D, Restelli F, Alfiero T, Campione A, Pozzi F, Balbi S, Arosio A, Castelnuovo P. The role of the transorbital superior eyelid approach in the management of selected spheno-orbital meningiomas: in-depth analysis of indications, technique, and outcomes from the study of a cohort of 35 patients. J Neurol Surg B Skull Base. 2020;83(2):145–58. https://doi.org/10.1055/s-0040-1718914.
3. Dallan I, Sellari-Franceschini S, Turri-Zanoni M, de Notaris M, Fiacchini G, Fiorini FR, Battaglia P, Locatelli D, Castelnuovo P. Endoscopic transorbital superior eyelid approach for the management of selected spheno-orbital meningiomas: preliminary experience. Oper Neurosurg (Hagerstown). 2018;14(3):243–51. https://doi.org/10.1093/ons/opx100.
4. Park HH, Yoo J, Yun IS, Hong CK. Comparative analysis of endoscopic transorbital approach and extended minipterional approach for sphenoid wing meningiomas with osseous involvement: preliminary surgical results. World Neurosurg. 2020;139:e1–e12. https://doi.org/10.1016/j.wneu.2020.01.115.
5. Pompili A, Derome PJ, Visot A, Guiot G. Hyperostosing meningiomas of the sphenoid ridge—clinical features, surgical therapy, and long-term observations: review of 49 cases. Surg Neurol. 1982;17(06):411–6.
6. Ringel F, Cedzich C, Schramm J. Microsurgical technique and results of a series of 63 spheno-orbital meningiomas. Neurosurgery. 2007;60(04 Suppl 2):214–21.
7. Kong DS, Kim YH, Hong CK. Optimal indications and limitations of endoscopic transorbital superior eyelid surgery for spheno-orbital meningiomas. J Neurosurg. 2020;134(5):1472–9.
8. Almeida JP, Omay SB, Shetty SR, Chen YN, Ruiz-Treviño AS, Liang B, Anand VK, Levine B, Schwartz TH. Transorbital endoscopic eyelid approach for resection of sphenoorbital meningiomas with predominant hyperostosis: report of 2 cases. J Neurosurg. 2018;128(6):1885–95. https://doi.org/10.3171/2017.3.JNS163110.
9. Corvino S, Sacco M, Somma T, Berardinelli J, Ugga L, Colamaria A, Corrivetti F, Iaconetta G, Kong DS, de Notaris M. Functional and clinical outcomes after superior eyelid transorbital endoscopic approach for spheno-orbital meningiomas: illustrative case and literature review. Neurosurg Rev. 2022;46(1):17. https://doi.org/10.1007/s10143-022-01926-w.
10. Dallan I, Castelnuovo P, Locatelli D, Turri-Zanoni M, AlQahtani A, Battaglia P, Hirt B, Sellari-Franceschini S. Multiportal combined transorbital transnasal endoscopic approach for the management of selected skull base lesions: preliminary experience. World Neurosurg. 2015;84(1):97–107. https://doi.org/10.1016/j.wneu.2015.02.034.
11. Di Somma A, Guizzardi G, Valls Cusiné C, Hoyos J, Ferres A, Topczewski TE, Mosteiro A, De Rosa A, Solari D, Cavallo LM, Reyes L, Enseñat J. Combined endoscopic endonasal and transorbital approach to skull base tumors: a systematic literature review.

J Neurosurg Sci. 2022;66(5):406–12. https://doi.org/10.23736/S0390-5616.21.05401-1.
12. Goncalves N, Lubbe DE. Transorbital endoscopic surgery for sphenoid wing meningioma: long-term outcomes and surgical technique. J Neurol Surg B Skull Base. 2020;81(4):357–68. https://doi.org/10.1055/s-0040-1713854.
13. Saeed P, van Furth WR, Tanck M, Kooremans F, Freling N, Streekstra GI, Regensburg NI, van der Sprenkel JW, Peerdeman SM, van Overbeeke JJ, Mourits MP. Natural history of spheno-orbital meningiomas. Acta Neurochir. 2011;153(2):395–402. https://doi.org/10.1007/s00701-010-0878-0.
14. Alqahtani A, Padoan G, Segnini G, Lepera D, Fortunato S, Dallan I, Pistochini A, Abdulrahman S, Abbate V, Hirt B, Castelnuovo P. Transorbital transnasal endoscopic combined approach to the anterior and middle skull base: a laboratory investigation. Acta Otorhinolaryngol Ital. 2015;35(3):173–9.
15. Dallan I, Cristofani-Mencacci L, Fiacchini G, Turri-Zanoni M, van Furth W, de Notaris M, Picariello M, Alexandre E, Georgalas C, Bruschini L. Endoscopic-assisted transorbital surgery: where do we stand on the Scott's parabola? Personal considerations after a 10-year experience. Front Oncol. 2022;12:937818. https://doi.org/10.3389/fonc.2022.937818.
16. Chotai S, Schwartz TH. The Simpson grading: is it still valid? Cancers (Basel). 2022;14(8):2007. https://doi.org/10.3390/cancers14082007.
17. Mariniello G, de Divitiis O, Corvino S, Strianese D, Iuliano A, Bonavolontà G, Maiuri F. Recurrences of spheno-orbital meningiomas: risk factors and management. World Neurosurg. 2022;161:e514–22. https://doi.org/10.1016/j.wneu.2022.02.048.

Spheno-Orbital Meningiomas: Results

16

Alberto Daniele Arosio, Giorgio Sileo, Pierlorenzo Veiceschi, Davide Locatelli, and Paolo Castelnuovo

Abbreviations

ACF Anterior cranial fossa
CAD Computer-aided design
CAM Computer-aided manufacturing
EI Exophthalmos index
EOR Extent of resection
eTOAs Endoscopic transorbital approaches
FTOZ Frontotemporal-orbitozygomatic
GSW Greater sphenoidal wing
GTR Gross total resection
ILTEA Infero-lateral transorbital endoscopic approach
IOF Inferior orbital fissure
LSW Lesser sphenoidal wing
MCA Middle cerebral artery
MCF Middle cranial fossa
MRI Magnetic resonance imaging
OEM Ocular extrinsic muscle
PA Pterional approach
PET-CT Positron emission tomography–computed tomography
PFS Progression-free survival

Alberto Daniele Arosio, Giorgio Sileo, and Pierlorenzo Veiceschi equally contributed to the manuscript and share the first authorship.

Davide Locatelli and Paolo Castelnuovo equally share the last authorship.

A. D. Arosio (✉) · G. Sileo
Division of Otorhynolaryngology, Department of Biotechnology and Life Sciences, "Ospedale di Circolo e Fondazione Macchi", University of Insubria, Varese, Italy

P. Veiceschi
Division of Neurosurgery, Department of Biotechnology and Life Sciences, "Ospedale di Circolo e Fondazione Macchi", University of Insubria, Varese, Italy

D. Locatelli
Division of Neurosurgery, Department of Biotechnology and Life Sciences, "Ospedale di Circolo e Fondazione Macchi", University of Insubria, Varese, Italy

Head and Neck & Forensic Dissection Research Center (HNS&FDRc), Department of Biotechnology and Life Sciences, University of Insubria, Varese, Italy

Research Center for Pituitary Adenomas and Sellar Pathology, University of Insubria, Varese, Italy
e-mail: davide1.locatelli@uninsubria.it

P. Castelnuovo
Division of Otorhynolaryngology, Department of Biotechnology and Life Sciences, "Ospedale di Circolo e Fondazione Macchi", University of Insubria, Varese, Italy

Head and Neck & Forensic Dissection Research Center (HNS&FDRc), Department of Biotechnology and Life Sciences, University of Insubria, Varese, Italy

Research Center for Pituitary Adenomas and Sellar Pathology, University of Insubria, Varese, Italy

T. H. Schwartz et al. (eds.), *Endoscopic Transorbital Surgery of the Orbit, Skull Base and Brain*,
https://doi.org/10.1007/978-3-031-59504-2_16

RT Radiotherapy
SEA Superior eyelid approach
SOM Spheno-orbital meningiomas

Introduction

SOMs are extra-axial neoplasms with epicenter of growth based on the sphenoid ridge. In large surgical series, SOMs account approximately for 2–9% of overall intracranial meningiomas [1–3]. They are also referred as "en plaque meningiomas" for the peculiarly "carpet-like" infiltrative diffusion across the fronto-temporo-sphenoidal dura, and for the wide hyperostotic spreading along the sphenoid crest [4], characteristics believed to be responsible of their high recurrence rate after surgery [5].

Due to those features, in about 70% of the cases, SOMs exhibit a multicompartmental involvement [6]. In fact, they may extend forward into the orbit, medially toward the cavernous sinus, posteriorly into the anterior (ACF) and middle cranial fossa (MCF), and inferolaterally in the infratemporal and temporal fossa [7–9].

The most common presenting symptoms include unilateral proptosis (84%), visual impairment (46%), visual field deficits (31%), and diplopia (22%) [1]. Proptosis is considered the most common sign, with incidence varying between 33% [10] and 95% [4].

A recent meta-analysis on SOM management, analyzing a total of 1486 patients, has demonstrated that external anterolateral transcranial approaches represent a safe and effective treatment for patients presenting with visual or neurological deficits [1]. Nonetheless, due to the nature of tumor spread, the tendency of a multicompartmental extension and the close relationship with critical neurovascular structures (e.g., optic nerve and cerebral vessels), SOMs represent a true surgical challenge: complete Simpson I resection is not easy to achieve, often requiring skull base craniotomies or additional craniofacial osteotomies, burdened by considerable invasiveness and sometimes resulting in large gaps in the skull base or esthetic defects (e.g., bone depressions, temporal muscle atrophy, and surgical scars) [7].

No surgical consensus on the best treatment strategy for SOMs has been reached in the past 40 years. Indeed, a multitude of opinions exist regarding the ideal surgical approach, the optimal degree of tumor resection or decompression of the hyperostotic bone to obtain, how to manage periorbital invasion, and how best to reconstruct the dura and orbital walls [1].

For this reason, especially in the last decade, much research has been directed toward less invasive approaches, capable of reducing the surgical morbidity and the esthetic damage, without compromising functional outcome. In the wake of the need for interdisciplinary collaboration, technological advances, and greater expertise, pioneering techniques have been developed for the treatment of pathologies extended to the orbit [11]. Therefore, more conservative endoscopic transorbital approaches have been proposed for selected cases [12].

In the previously mentioned systematic review performed in 2020, only 3 out of 38 studies (8%) reported on eTOAs for SOM resection; however, in recent years these surgical procedures are growing in popularity, and, in the last 2 years, a total of five studies on eTOAs have been published. Augmented by improvements in radiosurgery and conformal radiotherapeutic modalities, eTOAs have contributed to a progressive evolution in management of SOMs: the primary endpoint now being to pursue maximal safe resection, as opposed to the unconditioned goal of radical resection pursued by the classical approaches. Tables 16.1 and 16.2 disclose some of the most relevant case series reporting on surgical management of SOMs with external transcranial approaches and endoscopic transorbital approaches, respectively. This panorama, rich in surgical options, demands more complex planning for each case, where the analysis of multiple variables is needed to choose the most appropriate approach for each patient.

The present chapter will provide technical notes for endoscopic surgical approaches for SOM management, as well a critical analysis of the surgical and functional results compared to traditional external approaches. The aim is to provide information and tips that should guide surgeons in their clinical practice. We will also propose a new treatment allocation algorithm for the management of SOMs.

Table 16.1 Review of the literature reporting some of the most relevant studies on surgical management of SOMs with external craniotomy approaches

Author, year	Pts	Sex (%)	Mean age (years)	Location (%)	Presenting symptoms (%)	Procedure (%)	Histology (%)	Postoperative complications (%)	Tumor resection (%)	Outcome (%)	Mean F.U. (months)
Boari et al., 2013	40	• F 35 (87.5) • M 5 (12.5)	52.5	• SOF 18 (45) • CS 10 (25)	• Proptosis 40 (100) • Visual impairment 18 (45) • TF swelling 9 (22.5) • Visual field deficit 7 (17.5) • Diplopia 6 (15) • CN V impairment 2 (5) • Pain 4 (10)	Frontotemporal approach	Meningioma I 40 (100)	• Amaurosis 1 (2.5) • Diplopia 2 (5) • CSFL 2 (5) • Wound complication 2 (5)	• GTR 23 (56.1) • STR 18 (43.9)	• Visual improvement 11 (27.5) • Visual field improvement 7 (17.5) • Proptosis improvement 37 (92.5)	72.6
Talacchi et al., 2014	47	• F 26 (55.4) • M 21 (44.6)	57	• GSW 47 (100) • ITO extraconal 40 (85.1) • ITO intraconal 14 (29.7) • Temporobasal region 22 (46.8) • Frontobasal region 9 (19.1) • CS 22 (46.8)	• Proptosis 45 (95.7) • Visual impairment 24 (51) • OEM deficit 18 (38.2) • Temporal swelling 21 (44.6)	Frontotemporal approach	• Meningioma I 46 (97.9) • Meningioma II 1 (2.1)	• Diplopia 5 (10.6) • Extradural hematoma 2 (4.2) • CSFL 1 (2.1) • Wound complication 1 (2.1) • Endocarditis 1 (2.1)	• GTR 24 (51) • STR 23 (49)	• Visual deterioration 2 (4.2) • OEM deterioration 1 (2.1)	52

(continued)

Table 16.1 (continued)

Author, year	Pts	Sex (%)	Mean age (years)	Location (%)	Presenting symptoms (%)	Procedure (%)	Histology (%)	Postoperative complications (%)	Tumor resection (%)	Outcome (%)	Mean F.U. (months)
Terrier et al., 2017	130	• F 119 (91.5) • M 11 (8.5)	51.2	• GSW 119 (91.5) • TF 73 (56.1) • ITF 25 (19.2) • Temporal lobe 58 (44.6) • ITF 25 (19.2) • ITO intra-/extraconal 73 (56.1) • CS 11 (8.5)	• Proptosis 123 (94.6) • Visual impairment 49 (37.7) • Retro-orbital pain 17 (13) • OEM deficit 13 (10)	Frontotemporal approach + superolateral orbitotomy	Meningioma I 130 (100)	• Enophthalmos 3 (2.3) • OEM palsy 21 (16.1) • CN V dysfunction 6 (4.6)	• GTR 10 (7.7) • NTR 87 (66.9) • STR 43 (33.1)	• Proptosis improvement 72 (55.4) • Visual improvement 22 (16.9) • Visual deterioration 33 (25.4)	72
Najafabadi et al., 2021	19	• F 18 (94.7) • M 1 (5.3)	47	n.a.	• Proptosis 16 (84.2) • Visual impairment 10 (52.6) • VF deficit 8 (42.1)	Pterional approach + OWD	Meningioma I 19 (100)	• CN V dysfunction 6 (31.6) • CN VII dysfunction 3 (15.8) • Wound complication 1 (5.3) • Orbital cellulitis 1 (5.3)	• GTR 14 (73.7) • STR 5 (26.3)	• Proptosis improvement 16 (84.2) • Visual improvement 8 (42.1) • Visual stabilization 2 (10.5) • VF improvement 8 (42.1)	24
Dalle Ore et al., 2021	54	• F 45 (83.3) • M 9 (16.7)	52.1	• ITO 46 (85.2)	• Proptosis 40 (74.1) • Visual impairment 28 (51.8) • Headache 22 (40.7) • OEM deficit 11 (20.4)	Frontotemporal approach ± orbital reconstruction	• Meningioma I 46 (85.2) • Meningioma II 8 (14.8)	• Seizure 2 (3.7) • OEM deficit 8 (14.8) • Wound complication 4 (7.4) • Pneumocephalus 1 (1.8)	• GTR 9 (16.6) • STR 36 (66.6)	• Proptosis improvement 29 (53.7) • Visual improvement 12 (22.2) • Visual stabilization 41 (75.9) • EOM improvement 6 (11.1)	30

Dos Santos et al., 2022	40	• F 35 (87.5) • M 5 (12.5)	49.5	n.a.	• Proptosis 36 (90) • Visual impairment 26 (65) • Motility deficit 8 (20) • Pain 8 (20)	Pretemporal craniotomy + superolateral orbitotomy	• Meningioma I 39 (97.5) • Meningioma II 1 (2.5)	• Surgical site infection 3 (7.5) • Seizures 3 (7.5) • Strokes 2 (5) • Pulmonary thromboembolism 1 (2.5) • Diabetes insipidus 1 (2.5) • CSFL 1 (2.5) • Enophthalmos 1 (2.5)	• GTR 26 (65)	• Visual improvement 13 (32.5) • Motility improvement 2 (5) • Pain improvement 5 (12.5)	39

ACF anterior cranial fossa, *CN* cranial nerve, *CR* complete remission, *CS* cavernous sinus, *Fb* frontal bone, *GSW* greater sphenoidal wing, *ILTEA* inferolateral transorbital endoscopic approach, *ITF* infratemporal fossa, *ITO* *intraorbital*, *LCEA* lateral canthal endoscopic approach, *MCF* middle cranial fossa, *OD* optic nerve decompression, *OWD* orbital wall decompression, *Pb* parietal bone, *SETOA* *superior eyelid transorbital endoscopic approach*, *TEPS* *trans*-ethmoid-pterygoid-sphenoidotomy, *TF* temporal fossa, *UPS* upper parapharyngeal space, *VF* visual field, *Zb* zygomatic bone

Table 16.2 Review of the literature reporting case series of endoscopic transorbital management for SOMs

Author, year	Pts	Sex (%)	Mean age (years)	Location (%)	Presenting symptoms (%)	Procedure (%)	Histology (%)	Postoperative complications (%)	Tumor resection (%)	Outcome (%)	Mean F.U. (months)
Dallan et al., 2017	14	• F 12 (85.7) • M 2 (14.3)	51 (mean)	• ITO extraconal 5 (35.7) • ITO intra-/extraconal 1 (7.1) • GSW, LSW 6 (42.8) • GSW 3 (21.4) • MCF 11 (78.6) • Fb 5 (35.7) • Zb, Pb 2 (14.3) • ACF 2 (14.3) • Sphenoid, pterygoid 2 (14.3) • ITF, UPS 1 (7.1) • Temporal lobe 1 (7.1)	• Proptosis 14 (100) • Visual impairment 6 (42.8) • Diplopia 7 (50) • Palpebral ptosis 1 (7.1) • OEM impairment 1 (7.1)	• SETOA 9 (64.3) • SETOA + TEPS 3 (21.4) • SETOA + transnasal OWD 1 (7.1) • SETOA + transnasal OD 1 (7.1)	• Meningioma I 11 (78.6) • Recurrent meningioma I 3 (21.4)	• Diplopia 3 (21.4) • Palpebral edema 4 (28.6) • V1/2 hypoesthesia 4 (28.6) • Upper eyelid necrosis 1 (7.1) • Keratitis 1 (7.1) • Abduction impairment 1 (7.1)	• STR 9 (64.3) • GTR 3 (21.4) • NTR 2 (14.3)	• Proptosis improvement 14 (100) • Diplopia resolution 4 (28.6)	25
Almeida et al., 2017	2	• F 2 (100)	59 (mean)	• ITO extraconal, GSW 1 (50) • ITO extraconal, GSW, MCF 1 (50)	• Proptosis 2 (100) • Visual impairment 2 (100)	SETOA + transnasal OD 2 (100)	• Meningioma I 1 (50) • Recurrent meningioma I 1 (50)	• Palpebral edema and ptosis 1 (50)	STR 2 (100)	• Proptosis improvement 2 (100) • Visual improvement 2 (100)	2

Lubbe et al., 2020	21	• F 20 (95.2) • M 1 (4.8)	48.8 (mean)	GSW 21 (100)	• NLP 5 (23.8) • Proptosis 20 (95.2) • Visual impairment 16 (76.2) • Pain 16 (76.2) • Diplopia 3 (14.3)	LCEA + transnasal OD 21 (100)	• Meningioma I 20 (95.2) • Meningioma II 1 (4.8)	• SOF syndrome 1 (4.8)	STR 21 (100)	• NLP 5 (23.8) • Proptosis improvement 19 (90.5) • Visual improvement 9 (42.8)	12
Jeon et al., 2021	1	F 1 (100)	52	ITO extraconal, GSW 1 (100)	Proptosis 1 (100)	SETOA 1 (100)	Meningioma I 1 (100)	–	GTR 1 (100)	Proptosis improvement 1 (100)	6
Kong et al., 2021	41	• F 36 (87.8) • M 5 (12.2)	52 (mean)	• ITO intra-/extraconal 28 (68.2) • CS 15 (36.6) • TF 18 (43.9) • ITF 9 (21.9)	• Proptosis 20 (4.9) • Visual impairment 3 (7.3)	• SETOA 19 (46.3) • SETOA + lateral orbitotomy 22 (4.9)	• Primary 34 (82.9) • Recurrent 7 (17) • Meningioma (I) 39 (95.1) • Meningioma (II) 2 (4.9)	• CFSL 2 (4.9) • Wound complication 2 (4.9)	• GTR 21 (51.2) • STR 20 (48.8)	• Proptosis improvement 20 (48.8) • Visual improvement 2 (4.9)	n.a.
Colombo et al., 2022	3	F 3 (100)	59 (mean)	• ITO extraconal 3 (100) • GSW, LSW 2 (66.6) • MCF, ACF 1 (33.3)	• Proptosis 3 (100) • Visual impairment 2 (66.6) • Eye pain 1 (33.3)	ILTEA 3 (100)	• Meningioma I 2 (66.6) • Meningioma II 1 (33.3)	–	• STR 2 (66.6) • GTR 1 (33.3)	• Proptosis improvement 2 (66.6) • Visual improvement 1 (33.3) • Visual impairment 1 (33.3)	12
Henderson et al., 2022	1	F 1 (100)	60	GSW, temporal lobe 1 (100)	Headache, temporal lobe dysfunction 1 (100)	SETOA 1 (100)	Meningioma I 1 (100)	–	GTR 1 (100)	–	n.a.

(continued)

Table 16.2 (continued)

Author, year	Pts	Sex (%)	Mean age (years)	Location (%)	Presenting symptoms (%)	Procedure (%)	Histology (%)	Postoperative complications (%)	Tumor resection (%)	Outcome (%)	Mean F.U. (months)
Corvino et al., 2022	1	F 1 (100)	53	GSW, LSW, CS, temporal lobe, ITO extraconal 1 (100)	Proptosis 1 (100)	SETOA 1 (100)	Meningioma I 1 (100)	Transient diplopia 1 (100)	STR 1 (100)	Proptosis improvement 1 (100)	n.a.

ACF anterior cranial fossa, *CR* complete remission, *CS* cavernous sinus, *Fb* frontal bone, *GSW* greater sphenoidal wing, *ILTEA* inferolateral transorbital endoscopic approach, *ITF* infratemporal fossa, *ITO* *in*tra*o*rbital, *LCEA* lateral canthal endoscopic approach, *MCF* middle cranial fossa, *OD* optic nerve decompression, *OEM* ocular extrinsic muscles, *OWD* orbital wall decompression, *Pb* parietal bone, *SETOA* *s*uperior *e*yelid *t*rans*o*rbital endoscopic *a*pproach, *TEPS* *trans*-ethmoid-pterygoid-sphenoidotomy, *TF* temporal fossa, *UPS* upper parapharyngeal space, *Zb* zygomatic bone

Surgical Approaches: Techniques and Historical Evolution

The Wait-and-See Policy

SOMs are characterized by a slow growth rate, comparable with asymptomatic meningiomas. Saeed et al. retrospectively reviewed 90 patients diagnosed with SOMs, performing a volumetric magnetic resonance imaging (MRI)-based analysis in a subset of 32 of them [9]. A median annual growth rate of 0.3 cm^3/year was observed, with a 60-fold difference between the fastest- and the slowest-growing SOMs found. The factors significantly associated with higher growth rates were large initial tumor volume and proportionally greater soft tissue component. A nonsignificant trend for increased growth rate was found for younger age ($p = 0.346$). In light of these considerations, the authors suggested an annual follow-up encompassing MRI and ophthalmological evaluation for asymptomatic patients, whereas they proposed a 6-month follow-up in case of SOMs with large volume, proportionally greater soft tissue component, fast growth rate (>1 cm^3/year), or optic canal involvement.

Indeed, a significant proportion of patients in this series experienced worsening of the proptosis (20/90, 22%) or visual deterioration over the years, with 59/90 patients (65%) developing optic neuropathy. Therefore, the wait-and-see policy should be carefully counterbalanced by the opportunity for surgical intervention, with either transcranial or endoscopic approaches, which according to the most recent evidence are effective in improving visual acuity, visual field deficits, and symptomatic proptosis [1, 7, 13, 14].

Cranial Open Approaches

Surgical resection is the cornerstone of SOM treatment, which can relieve the mass effect and related symptoms. Among the "classical" neurosurgical anterolateral approaches, the pterional approach (PA) has been considered, for a long time, the gold-standard procedure [15]. It allows early exposure of the meningioma through a direct corridor to the dura along the sphenoid ridge. A standard pterional craniotomy is usually sufficient to manage most lateral sphenoid wing meningiomas [16]. A case illustration is provided in Fig. 16.1.

However, many variations of the PA exist, and the craniotomy may be extended on the temporal or frontal side as needed, according to the location of the tumor and its dural attachment. A recent systematic review enrolling 1486 patients affected by SOMs confirms that the extended pterional approach is the most widely used approach, applied in 97% of studies [1].

In cases of hyperostosis of the greater sphenoid wing, with involvement of the orbit and the floor of the MCF, an additional skull base osteotomy may be adopted [17]. The most common skull base extension of the pterional approach is represented by the front-temporal-orbito-zygomatic (FTOZ) approach. In the case of SOMs, it facilitates the removal of the involved bone of the posterolateral orbit, both superiorly and inferiorly to the superior orbital fissure (SOF). Moreover, the broad exposure of the MCF floor also facilitates the access to the posterior portion of the tumor, medially to the foramen rotundum and foramen ovale, via an extradural corridor [18, 19].

Among other skull base extensions, the lateral orbital osteotomy (orbitocranial or cranio-orbital approach) can be performed in selected cases, especially in case of involvement of the greater sphenoid wing or the external orbital wall with minimal dural invasion. However, even in the case of large lateral sphenoid wing tumors, a cranio-orbital or orbito-zygomatic osteotomy is not necessary, since it provides an additional invasiveness without real benefit [20, 21].

Classical neurosurgical approaches, although widely used, are burdened by high morbidity, high mortality (up to 6%) [9] and recurrences, with subtotal resection rates being higher than for meningiomas in other locations [12, 22]. Even if craniotomies guarantee a wide surgical exposure, resections are subtotal in anywhere from 10% to 80% of the cases, with reported recurrent rates varying from 8% to as high as 56% [23, 24]. These disappointing results are related to the

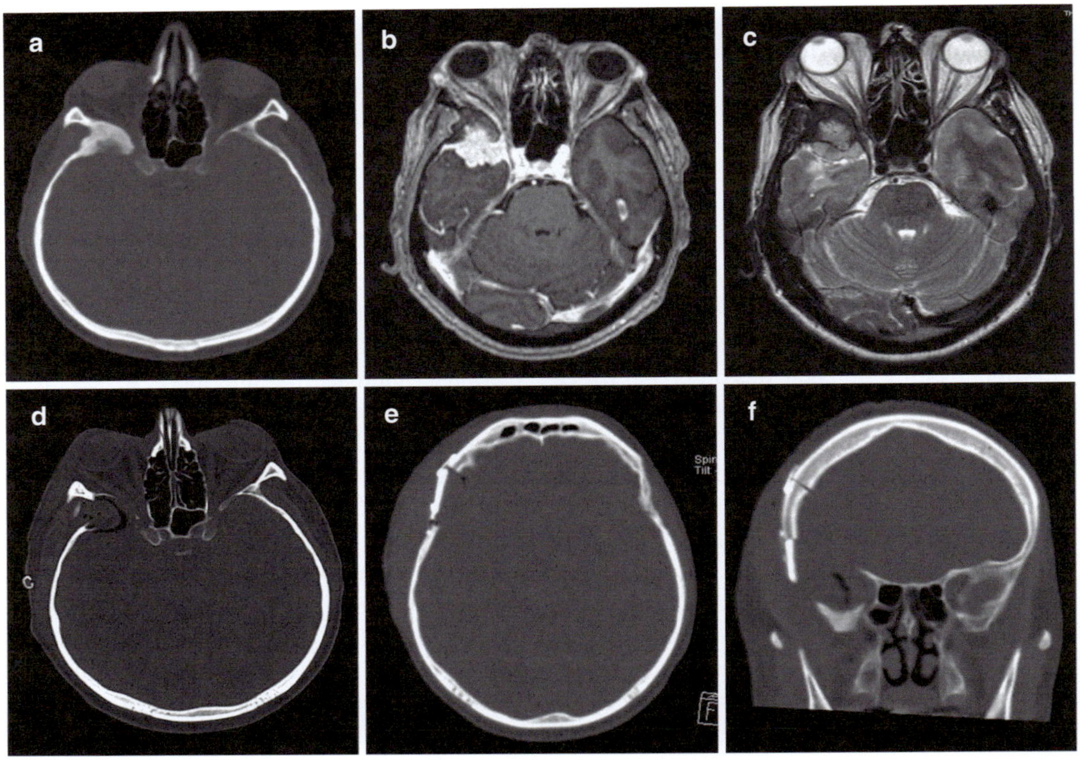

Fig. 16.1 Microsurgical removal of a right SOM with pterional craniotomy. Case illustration of a 54-year-old male complaining of visual impairment in the right superior and inferior temporal hemifield. At clinical examination, a right cranial nerve VI deficit and diplopia in the extreme degrees of lateral gaze were pointed out. An axial CT scan with bone window (**a**) highlighted a right sphenoid wing meningioma; on axial T1 weighted-image MRI with contrast enhancement (**b**), an extensive dural infiltration was observed; moreover, on axial T2-weighted image MRI (**c**), the right optic nerve appeared to be tortuous and compressed at the level of the orbital apex. Patient underwent microsurgical pterional craniotomy with total removal of the lesion. Postoperative axial (**d**, **e**) and coronal (**f**) CT scans demonstrated the extensive drilling of the right lesser sphenoid wing, with unroofing of the optic canal. To achieve a Simpson 1 grade, the infiltrated dura mater was removed. The greater sphenoid wing was also drilled out for oncological purposes and reconstructed by an acrylic resin cranioplasty

intricate and subtle location of the disease, as well as to its widespread involvement of the bone and dura. Given these facts, a progressive shift has occurred toward a "symptoms-oriented surgery," mainly aimed at optic nerve decompression (in case of optic neuropathy) and proptosis reduction, which is now possible with the use of eTOAs. A growing body of literature is progressively establishing the efficacy and safety of less invasive approaches to achieve reduced morbidity [12]. Those approaches will be reviewed in the following sections.

Endoscopic and Combined Approaches

Superior Eyelid Approach (SEA)

A brief description of the SEA is here provided, as performed by the senior authors and already depicted in previous papers [6, 25–27]. A case illustration is provided in Fig. 16.2.

Under general anesthesia, the patient is placed supine with the head in the neutral position. A skin incision is made on a superior eyelid crease and a

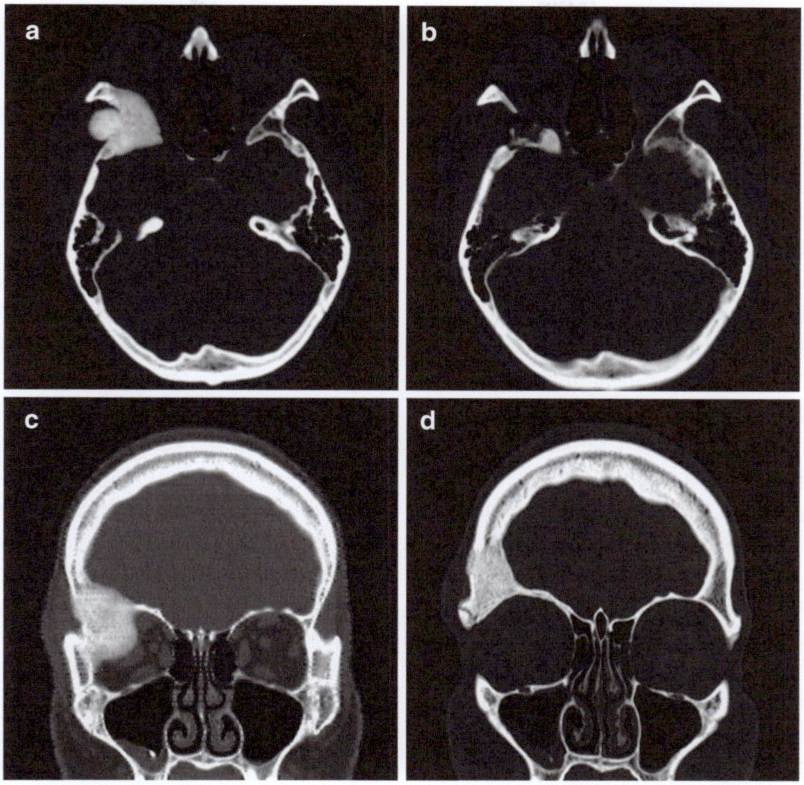

Fig. 16.2 Subtotal removal of a SOM via superior eyelid approach. Case illustration of a 53-year-old lady who had been reporting right fronto-parietal headache and ipsilateral epiphora for the previous 2 years. At clinical evaluation exophthalmos and reduction of visual acuity in the right eye were observed. A brain MRI revealed a right SOM. At the axial (**a**) and coronal (**c**) CT scan, an extensive hyperostosis of the greater and lesser sphenoid wing was observed, with marked orbital and temporal bone involvement. The patient underwent subtotal removal of the neoformation via transorbital route and contextual debulking of the hyperostotic bone tissue (Simpson IV), as demonstrated by postoperative axial (**b**) and coronal (**d**) CT scan

skin-orbicularis muscular flap is raised. In this phase, stitches and small silastic tubes help in creating adequately wide access and reducing the risk of iatrogenic damage to the skin. Suborbicularis dissection is performed in a supero-lateral direction until exposure of the orbital rim, paying attention not to damage the underlying orbital septum and the levator palpebrae muscle. Once the lateral orbital rim is exposed, a careful subperiosteal dissection of the periorbit from the orbital bones is performed until the superior and inferior orbital fissures, as well as the optic canal, are clearly identified. During this phase, the lacrimal gland is detached in a subperiosteal plane, and the underlying bony area can be drilled away to provide wider access, the so-called "lacrimal keyhole" area, which represents a good space to rest the endoscope during surgery [13].

Care must be taken to avoid opening of the periorbita in order to prevent the orbital fat from protruding into the surgical field. Bridging vessels can be seen and sacrificed without risk during this phase. In 50–60% of the patients, Hyrtl's foramen or meningo-orbital foramen is seen close to the SOF. The foramen typically accommodates the connecting vessel between the orbital branch of the anterior division of the middle meningeal artery and the lacrimal branch of the ophthalmic artery, which should be cauterized and cut [28].

Once the intraorbital landmarks are identified, endoscopic holding systems can be used, if available. The greater sphenoidal wing (GSW) is drilled gradually to expose the temporalis muscle, which is an important anatomical landmark. To approach the MCF, the GSW should be drilled out as far as the dura mater, in a lateral to medial direction. In this phase, venous bleeding is controlled with hemostatic agents and bony wax or by avoiding irrigation during diamond burr work. The superomedial boundary of the approach is defined by the SOF, the inferomedial border is defined by the inferior orbital fissure (IOF), and the lateral boundary is delineated by the temporalis muscle. The approach may be partially prolonged superiorly to the lesser sphenoidal wing (LSW) toward the anterior clinoid process. If required, the frontal bone can be partially resected and the spheno-orbital sinus coagulated. This approach enables direct access to the cavernous sinus (lateral wall) and the Gasserian ganglion, as well as adequate exposure of the MCF floor. When the pathology involves the intracranial compartment, the dura may be safely opened, usually under neuronavigation guidance. The intracranial component is debulked with the help of an ultrasonic aspirator or by simple suction alone. In tumors involving the ocular structures, the periorbital layer is identified and opened. In some cases, the periorbit and extraocular muscles, such as the lateral rectus muscle, are infiltrated by the tumor. In these cases, attention must be paid to preserve the extraocular muscles as well as the neurovascular structures in order to avoid permanent diplopia. More research is needed with the use of ultrasound and nerve monitoring to assist more complete resection of the orbital component [13].

For tumors extending to the temporal floor or infratemporal fossa, a lateral orbital rim osteotomy may be helpful, as well as increased forward inclination of the head and a wider skin incision.

Surgical exposure and maneuverability might still be a concern and demand for more extended or multiportal approaches.

For an ACF approach, the craniotomy removes the orbital part of the frontal bone, along with part of the LSW, while GSW is left untouched. The dura is exposed and the extent of the dural incision is adjusted according to the extent of tumor involvement.

During closure, when the dura is partially or completely removed, it is reconstructed in a standard multilayer fashion with dural substitutes and the help of fibrin glue. Free fat tissue from the abdomen can be harvested and grafted to fill the empty space intradurally. Orbital reconstruction is debated in the literature. Some authors advocated the use of artificial bone plates to prevent postoperative pulsatile enophthalmos, which in the authors' opinion is hardly ever observed, so that usually no bony reconstruction is necessary. Filling the orbital empty space with autologous fat graft is usually sufficient to prevent postoperative enophthalmos and to support eventual skull base reconstruction. Small periorbital openings may be safely repaired. Finally, subcutaneous tissue and skin are sutured layer by layer.

Inferolateral Transorbital Endoscopic Approach (ILTEA)

This approach has been proposed to efficiently manage the intraorbital component of the lesions in cases of limited intracranial extension and without involvement of the optic canal, which would demand other ancillary procedures to obtain decompression at this level [8, 29]. A subciliary incision is carried out 2 mm below the ciliary margin from the inferior punctum to the lateral canthus, extending laterally and superiorly in a laugh line. After incision of the orbicularis oculi muscle, the orbital septum is followed inferiorly toward its insertion on the orbital floor and laterally toward the lateral canthal ligament. The periosteum is incised from the midpoint of the inferior orbital rim to the lateral canthal ligament, which allows to gain the correct dissection plane. The intraorbital phase of the surgery proceeds as described for SEA under 0° endoscopic guidance.

Combined Multiportal Approaches

Multiportal transorbital and transnasal approaches have been proposed and described in order to overcome some limits of the pure transorbital or lateral approaches. A case illustration is provided in Fig. 16.3.

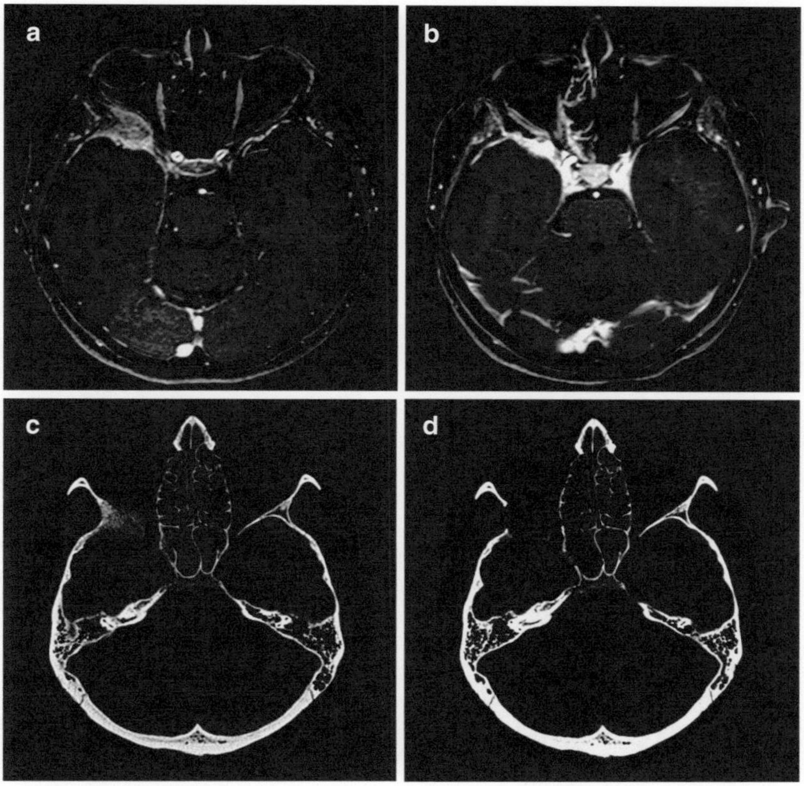

Fig. 16.3 Removal of a SOM by means multiportal approach (endoscopic endonasal + transorbital transpalpebral). A 44-year-old woman, due to the onset of right eyelid diplopia and ptosis, underwent brain MRI (**a**) and CT scan (**c**) with evidence of a right spheno-orbital extra-axial lesion compatible with meningioma. The patient was operated on by a combined approach targeting total removal of the lesion (Simpson 3). By means of a super eyelid approach, the intra-orbital component was removed until the dura of the middle cranial fossa was exposed and coagulated. With the endonasal approach, a medial maxillectomy with right spheno-ethmoidectomy was carried on; after removal of the posterior wall of the maxilla, the hyperostotic component involving the pterygoid and basisphenoid up to the region of the foramen lacerum (not accessible by transorbital approach) was drilled out. The patient experienced complete resolution of the symptoms. Good surgical results are demonstrated on follow-up images (**b–d**)

Goncalves et al. proposed a multistep combined endoscopic transorbital approach for the management of SOMs, with the major advantage of stabilizing and improving the vision by performing a medial optic canal decompression prior to accessing the main intracranial and orbital components of the tumor [13]. This reduces the risk of compressive damage to the optic nerve, which may occur during traditional approaches and may worsen visual outcomes. The first phase of the surgery is a medial optic canal decompression which can be performed via endonasal or multiportal precaruncular and endonasal approaches. The advantage of using a precaruncular approach in combination with the endonasal route in the authors' opinion is to overcome the herniation of orbital fat and periorbit into the ethmoid cavity after removal of the posterior portion of the lamina papyracea. This is achieved with the use of a ribbon (dural) retractor inserted through the precaruncular window to protect the orbit, improving the visualization of the optic canal. The following phases of the surgery are performed as already described for SEA. The transorbital phase might be performed with a lateral canthal incision combined with a 6 mm burr hole, drilled just behind the lateral orbital rim, leaving at least 5 mm of orbital rim intact. The added hole allows for extra instrument manipulation in a more narrow surgical field, as compared to the SEA [30].

Dallan et al. reported a preliminary experience on five cadaveric specimens and four patients with the combined multiportal transnasal transorbital endoscopic approach for the management of selected complex skull base pathologies [31]. Among the four clinical cases presented, three were affected by SOMs and were managed with SEA combined with a transnasal-transpterygoid approach. The details of the transnasal procedure are beyond the scope of this chapter; however, this corridor allows the surgical window to be expanded to include the sphenoid sinus region, pterygoid plates, and parapharyngeal region, as well as the infratemporal and pterygopalatine fossa.

Radiation Therapy

Radiotherapy (RT), both conventional and stereotactic, is an important addition to modern treatment of extra-axial lesions. It is beyond the scope of this chapter to cover this topic; however, some basic indications will be herein provided. The literature advises the use of postoperative RT for atypical grade II meningiomas, while for grade I lesions, indications for postoperative RT are controversial due to limited expected effects [32]. Radiation therapy is increasingly being used to control tumor remnants after meningioma surgery and to treat progressive unresectable disease. There is no evidence that early radiation therapy is better than delaying RT until tumor progression [18]. Surgical resection is encouraged for symptomatic SOMs [33], but in case of extension beyond accessible anatomical regions, a subtotal resection may also be appropriate. Cavernous sinus disease is a good indication for radiosurgery or stereotactic radiotherapy [34, 35], and much data exist suggesting that radiotherapy may help to control residual intraorbital meningioma [10]. In our clinic, patients are followed up with serial MRIs, and, in case of volumetric enlargement of the tumor remnant, radiation treatment is started.

Critical Analysis of Results

Published studies on surgical intervention for SOMs in the literature reported a considerable improvement of vision in around 30–90% of patients, visual fields in 20–85%, and proptosis in 60–100%. All this at the expense of a non-negligible rate of permanent complications, ranging from 20% to 45% [14].

In the last decades, a variety of different approaches have been described, and changes in indications for primary intervention and re-intervention were observed, along with differences in postoperative follow-up policy and functional outcomes surveillance. This composite panorama has become even more complex with the recent introduction and increasing diffusion of eTOAs for the treatment of SOMs, which demands a careful and critical analysis of the results in terms of resection rate, incidence of complications, and functional outcomes.

Surgical Resection

In his pioneering work, Simpson described five different grades of meningioma surgical resection, from the lowest (grade I), which is the complete removal of the tumor with the underlying bone and associated dura, to the highest (grade V), a simple decompression eventually associated with a biopsy [36]. However, for SOMs the definition of the extent of resection (EOR) is not uniform among studies, in part due to the difficulties to adapt the Simpson grade, originally applied for convexity meningiomas: some authors consider only Simpson grade I as a gross total resection (GTR) [37], while others define GTR as Simpson I, II, and III [5]. Thereby, the lack of consensus about basic concepts hinders direct comparisons.

Considering that subtotal resection of the affected bone is associated with an increased risk of recurrence and the potential need for revision surgery or radiotherapy, with their accompanying risks, the extent of surgical resection is an important goal for surgical planning [1]. Regarding traditional craniotomies for SOMs, resection rates ranging from 60% to 100% have been reported in the literature [38–40]. Mariniello et al. reported on 60 patients treated with lateral orbitotomy (15/60, 25%), supraorbital-pterional approach (42/60, 70%), and a FOTZ approach (3/60, 5%) reporting complete tumor removal (Simpson grades I and II) in 40/60 cases (66.6%) and a recurrence rate of 42.3% (52/60), with 84.6% (44/60 patients) achieving tumor control after two or more surgeries [41]. In their experience, the recurrence rate was correlated with Simpson grade of resection and intraorbital tumor location: significantly higher rates of recurrence were recorded for the orbital apex type (50%) and diffuse forms (60%). Amirjamshidi et al. described a series of 88 SOMs treated with fronto-temporal approach or lateral orbitotomy, reporting Simpson grade I to II in all cases, 12/88 cases (13.6%) of tumor recurrence, with only 2 cases requiring reoperation [42]. More recently, Terrier et al. [20] retrospectively analyzed 130 consecutive patients undergoing surgery for SOMs via frontotemporal craniotomy, reporting Simpson grades I and II in 97/130 patients (74.6%).

Data regarding results of eTOAS in terms of extent of resection are more scant in the literature, and GTR rates are either equivalent or lower than craniotomy approaches. Locatelli et al. compared SEA and craniotomy approaches in terms of EOR and found that the former were significantly associated with higher rates of subtotal resections ($p = 0.005$, OR of STR = 12.07) [7]. These data are not surprising since eTOAs are mainly performed with the intent of obtaining clinical improvement rather than for pursuing GTR. Residual tumors are often located in areas that are more difficult to manage with such minimally invasive approaches. Kong et al. [6] reported a mean degree of resection of 83.9% in a series of 41 patients treated with eTOAs, with 68.3% (28/41 patients) of them showing extracranial compartments involvement such as the orbit, cavernous sinus, and infratemporal fossa. GTR was achieved in 21/41 patients (51.2%), while subtotal resection was achieved in the remaining 20/41 patients (48.8%). Statistical analysis of the factors associated with incomplete resection alone showed that the "en plaque" type of meningioma ($p < 0.01$) and cavernous invasion ($p < 0.01$) were significant factors both in univariate and multivariate analysis. According to the new concept of GTR (complete resection or intended subtotal resection, thus excluding the presence of cavernous sinus invasion from the independent variables due to preoperative planning of leaving intentional residual tumor in this site), univariate regression analysis showed that factors associated with lower GTR rates were the "en plaque" meningioma pattern (11.5% vs. 93.3%, $p < 0.01$), the absence of lateral orbital rim osteotomy (26.3% vs. 54.5%, $p < 0.01$), and the involvement of critical areas ($p < 0.01$) such as the temporal floor or infratemporal fossa (16.7% vs. 60.9%), the orbit (19% vs. 65%), and the medial one-third of the greater sphenoid wing (18.5% vs. 85.7%). Of all these factors, only the "en plaque" type and the absence of orbital rim osteotomy maintained statistical significance in multivariate analysis ($p < 0.01$).

With regard to tumor location, Masalha et al. [5] reported that intraconal and cavernous sinus infiltrations, observed in 23 out of 65 patients, were associated with significantly worse progression-free survival (PFS) compared to other locations ($p = 0.017$). Moreover, in the authors' experience, patients with WHO grade I SOMs showed improved PFS than patients with WHO grade II tumors in both univariate and multivariate analysis ($p = 0.00076$ and $p = 0.0029$, respectively).

It is interesting to note that tumor recurrence has been shown to be unlikely in cases where subtotal resection has been performed despite the presence of an aggressive histological tumor grade and in the absence of additional therapy. This has led to the hypothesis that it is possible that tumor remnants may remain dormant and cease to grow [13]. On the other hand, positron emission tomography/computed tomography (PET-CT) studies reported the presence of pathological hyperostotic cells in areas not identified by surgeons, supporting the need for a maximum resection [43]. In the authors' opinion, a careful balance between the risk of recurrence and the invasiveness of the surgical approach is the key that should guide the surgical planning, with the aim to obtain the safest maximal resection and seek symptom improvement.

Postoperative Complications

A direct comparison of complications occurring after external craniotomy approaches and eTOAs for SOM management is not easy to perform due to inevitable bias related to surgical technique, extent of resection and the aim of surgery. With regard to craniotomy approaches, systemic complications occur infrequently but need to be taken into account, especially in cases of fragile and/or older patients. Santos et al. analyzed a series of 40 patients treated with pretemporal craniotomy, associated with superolateral orbitotomy, and reported surgical site infections in 3/40 cases (7.5%), postoperative seizures in 3/40 cases (7.5%), strokes in 2/40 cases (5%), pulmonary thromboembolism and insipidus diabetes in 1 case each (2.5%). Moreover, one patient presented a cerebrospinal fluid fistula, requiring revision surgery [23]. With regard to local complications after external approaches, they might occur in up to one in five patients. In the literature the most common postoperative complications are oculomotor palsy and trigeminal dysfunction [1]. The former ranges between 0% and 16% [20] although rates as high as 31% have been reported [40], especially when radical resection is performed in patients with cavernous sinus and/or SOF involvement. This wide range could be explained by the fact that extrinsic muscle disturbances are considered to be multifactorial, both neurological and muscular, due to the dissection of the periorbita. In the work by Najafabadi et al. [14], the most common postoperative complications were hyperesthesia of the maxillary nerve (31%) and eyebrow asymmetry due to deficit of the frontal branch of the facial nerve (15.7%).

In the subgroup analysis including studies using the (extended) pterional approach, Fisher et al. [1] reported unspecified cranial nerves deficits in 23% of patients, followed by ophthalmoplegia (20%), diplopia (17%), ptosis (17%), and trigeminal hypesthesia (15%). Complications regarding visual acuity and visual field in this group occurred in respectively 5% and 4% of the cases.

A correlation with EOR and extension of SOMs to critical anatomical areas can be noticed according to some authors. Masalha et al. observed that GTR, defined as Simpson grades I–III, significantly increased ($p = 0.0107$) neurological deficits of the trigeminal nerve [5]. Trigeminal dysfunction, which could be avoided by reducing the drilling around the SOF, foramen rotundum, and foramen ovale, is reported to occur between 3.0% and 23% of cases [40, 44]. Hyperpathic trigeminal syndrome involves mostly the V1 and V2 divisions and can be treated with adjusted doses of gabapentin or carbamazepine; in all the patients treated by Terrier et al., the initial doses could be tapered within 9 months after surgery [20]. Visual deterioration is another severe postoperative complication that must be considered, as it may occur in 11–31% of cases [45]. In this regard, Terrier et al. reported blindness in 5.6% of patients treated [20].

Functional and Esthetic Outcomes

A postoperative follow-up at least of 2 years is required for SOMs. This also applies to the evaluation of functional outcomes, as deterioration in visual outcomes and recrudescence of proptosis tend to develop even years after surgery. Therefore, a thorough analysis of such outcomes is not immediate, since the majority of SOM studies are represented by small case series with short postoperative surveillance. A brief overview of functional and esthetic outcomes will be provided for both external and endoscopic approaches.

Visual Outcomes

Visual loss in patients affected by SOMs occurs as a result of compressive optic neuropathy. A systematic review and meta-analysis of visual outcomes following optic nerve decompression for chronic compressive optic neuropathy showed that at least 60% of patients show improvement in vision [46]. The factors that were statistically significant in predicting improvement were the absence of optic disc atrophy, small tumor size, primary resection, soft tumor consistency, clear dissection plane, absence of cavernous sinus involvement, and a complete tumor excision. Moreover, the duration of symptoms and preoperative vision status were noted to be significant prognosticators for visual outcomes, even if little chance of improvement is expected in cases with poor preoperative visual acuity.

With regard to SOMs, according to the meta-analysis performed by Fisher et al., surgery is effective in improving visual acuity and visual field deficits, respectively, in 91% and 87% of the cases [1]. Moreover, almost all patients with ophthalmoplegia as a presenting symptom showed improvement after surgery. For patients treated with craniotomy approaches, improvements in visual outcomes are variable in the literature, with reported rates ranging from 28% to 70% [10, 13, 39, 44]. While performing optic nerve decompression for sphenoid wing meningioma using an open surgical approach in 25 patients, Shrivastava et al. observed that only 28% of patients experienced an improvement in visual acuity and 72% of patients experienced no change in vision [47]. Dos Santos et al. analyzed the surgical outcomes of 40 patients treated with pretemporal craniotomy and lateral orbitotomy, mainly focusing on proptosis evaluation: 78% of patients' long-term visual acuity was maintained or improved [23].

Less data has been published regarding visual outcomes after eTOAs for SOM management. Almeida et al. reported two cases treated with endoscopic SEA for sphenoid wing meningioma and showed an improvement in visual acuity and proptosis at 1 month postoperatively [48]. In a preliminary analysis of seven cases treated using the combined endoscopic transnasal and lateral orbitotomy approach, Lubbe et al. reported stabilization and improvement over time in optic nerve function in all patients, apart from the patient presenting with no light perception vision. Five of seven patients had dramatic visual improvement, with an average 2.7-line increase in Snellen acuity within 6 weeks after surgery. On the contrary, if compared to visual acuity, brightness, chromatic appreciation, relative afferent pupillary deficits, and visual fields showed slower recovery time, with deficits still noted at the sixth postoperative week [30]. Interestingly, in the authors' opinion, the key to improve or stabilize visual outcomes is early decompression of the canal: performing this as the first step of the surgery ensures that the optic nerve does not get compressed during resection of the sphenoid wing meningioma through the lateral approach. In the large series described by Kong et al., the authors reported restoring of the visual function in two of three patients presenting with preoperative visual impairment [6].

In a previous experience, our group [12] reported on results of a series of 14 cases of SOMs treated via transorbital endoscopic and superior eyelid approach. No cases of visual deficit or impairment were observed postoperatively, as well as no new onset or worsening of diplopia. Moreover, in four cases the preoperative diplopia disappeared at the last follow-up. More recently, our group reported on 35 patients treated for SOMs with eTOA, combined or purely craniotomy approaches with a mean follow-up of 31.5 months: after 1 year, only one case of postoperative stable new-onset visual deficit after a combined procedure was observed, without new deficit regarding ocular extrinsic muscle (OEM) motility and visual field, independently from the procedure performed. Looking more specifically at the endoscopic procedures, of the 13 patients who underwent an endoscopic SEA affected preoperatively by visual (6 patients), OEM (4 patients), and visual field deficits (3 patients), after surgery we observed a visual improvement in 4 patients ($p = 0.043$), an OEM improvement in 3 patients ($p = 0.007$), and visual-field improvement in 1 patient ($p = 0.001$), whereas the remaining 5 patients preoperatively impaired remained stable. No worsening of the preoperative deficits was observed at long-term follow-up [7].

To sum up, the evidence shows that surgery is effective in improving visual acuity and visual field deficits, regardless of the surgical approach. Of course, surgeons should assess predictors for postoperative visual outcomes in order to foresee results and to correctly perform preoperative counseling. According to the literature, optic canal involvement is a negative predictor for postoperative proptosis, visual acuity, and visual field deficits; periorbital involvement is a negative predictor for postoperative visual acuity, whereas intracranial involvement is a negative predictor for postoperative visual field deficits [1, 20, 49]. In their regression analysis, Najafabadi et al. found that preoperative visual function and extension of hyperostosis were strong predictors of poorer postoperative visual outcomes. This suggests that surgery might be beneficial, even with minimal visual impairment or hyperostosis, to prevent further worsening [14]. Moreover, if patients are operated earlier, the risk for new complications decreases, as cranial nerves are less at risk if compression is lower.

Proptosis

As described previously, proptosis is the most common clinical sign of SOMs. It is cosmetically deforming, and in the long term, it might affect vision due to corneal exposure or stretching of the optic nerve [30]. Several factors may be involved in its pathophysiological mechanism: it may be caused by the hyperostotic reaction of the bone caused by tumor infiltration, by the intraorbital tumor growth or by the venous drainage blockage due to infiltration of the SOF [20, 37].

Proptosis is therefore one of the main outcomes of interest for SOM surgical resection. Generally speaking, surgery is effective at alleviating proptosis. In the literature review performed by Terrier et al., a mean rate of improvement was reported in 84.7% of the 787 patients treated with traditional craniotomy approaches [20]. The meta-analysis performed by Fisher et al. reported a 96% rate of improvement, with 846/965 patients over 29 studies experiencing proptosis reduction [1].

One issue when evaluating results in terms of proptosis improvement is that the criteria used for assessing its severity may vary from series to series, being measured with Hertel's exophthalmometer [30] or calculated with radiological measurements [20]. Scarone et al. [37] defined the exophthalmos index (EI) and quantified proptosis reduction by comparison of preoperative and postoperative MRI and/or computed tomography (CT) scans. The distance in millimeters from the most anterior aspect of the globe on a section including the lens to a line between the anterior tips of the frontal processes of the zygomas was measured: the ratio between this measure in the affected eye and the same measure in the contralateral eye was defined as the EI. In their series of 30 patients treated with standard frontotemporal approach without orbital reconstruction, Scarone et al. reported EI improvement at the first radiological follow-up (median 12 months) in 27 patients (90%) and at the last radiological follow-up (median 61 months) in 28 patients (93%).

Less has been published on the reduction in proptosis using the transorbital approach if compared to traditional craniotomy approaches, but these minimally invasive approaches appear to be effective. In their initial experience, Lubbe et al. reported promising results in the initial postoperative period, with an average statistically significant reduction of 2 mm ($p = 0.0054$). However, proptosis recurrence was reported by 1 year [13]. More recently, three patients treated with ILTEA reported by Colombo et al. experience postoperative improvement after surgery [8]. With regard to SEA, the literature review performed by Corvino et al. [50] disclosed five studies reporting a total of 66 patients, with a 100% rate of proptosis improvement [6, 7, 51, 52].

Excision of the periorbita seems to have a positive effect on proptosis reduction, while radiological involvement of the optic canal is a predictor for residual postoperative proptosis [20, 49]. Other factors might explain persistence and/or worsening of the proptosis during the follow-up, such as subtotal tumor resection, growth of residual tumor, intraconal tumor involving the periorbita, and fibrous scar tissue replacing hyperostotic bone. Interestingly, in the work by Scarone et al. [37] in the interval between the first and final imaging follow-up, the EI improved in only 8 patients (20%), worsened in 15 patients (50%), and showed no variation in 7 patients (30%). The role of subtotal resection and the possibility for residual tumor growth in worsening the proptosis is debatable. Lubbe et al. suggested that residual tumor might be the cause for a trend in proptosis worsening in the follow-up after subtotal resection with endoscopic approaches [30]. However, Santos et al. suggested that even an incomplete removal of the tumor could provide good late outcomes [23]. Indeed, in their series of 40 patients treated with pretemporal craniotomy, associated with supero-lateral orbitotomy with a median follow-up of 39 months, the authors reported lower quantifiable proptosis in the STR group than the GTR group (2.5 ± 2.1 mm vs. 3.8 ± 3.2 mm).

Therefore, as for visual outcomes, proptosis evaluation in the postoperative follow-up should be assessed in the long term, as both further improvement and worsening might occur.

Orbital Reconstruction

While reconstruction of the orbital rim is always necessary, the need for orbital wall reconstruction is debated in the literature. Proponents of bony reconstruction deem it a necessity to reduce the risk of CSF leakage, infection, pulsatile enophthalmos, and diplopia [53]. Moreover, reconstructed orbits might provide better fronto-temporal scalp cosmesis [23]. Indeed, when orbital reconstruction is performed, Terrier et al. reported a statistically significant association with better esthetic results ($p = 0.0001$) and less temporal muscular atrophy ($p = 0.01$) and found that only 10.0% of patients (13/117) were unsatisfied with the esthetic outcome [20]. Differently, according to Talacchi et al., there are no functional reasons to advocate reconstruction after two-wall resection, and, if necessary, corrective surgery might also be a staged procedure [54]. Moreover, reconstructive osteoplasty of the orbital cavity can be challenging, because of the presence of different planes of curvature and thickness, and must achieve perfect symmetry to the contralateral eye in order to obtain excellent outcomes. In this regard Goertz et al. reported their experience with the use of computer-aided design (CAD) and computer-aided manufacturing (CAM) customized implants in a single-step procedure for orbital reconstruction. According to the authors, there is no need to reconstruct the orbital walls completely as supero-lateral orbital rim reconstruction is sufficient to provide good cosmetic outcomes [55]. Dalle Ore et al. stressed the importance of performing forced duction eye testing before closure to rule out extraocular muscle entrapment [56].

The occurrence of pulsatile enophthalmos is variable in the literature, and this event has been described also in the cases in which bony orbital reconstruction is performed, with percentages ranging from 2.3% to 30% of the cases [1, 20, 48, 54]. Hence, for many authors orbital reconstruction is not mandatory in most cases: Dos Santos et al. reported only one case of enophthalmos in the late follow-up [23]; whereas Maroon et al. [57] and Mariniello et al. [58] did not observe any of these complications. This also applies for endoscopic approaches for SOM management. In these cases, the lateral orbital wall is usually not reconstructed, thus granting proper proptosis correction and pleasant esthetic results, considering that the orbital rim is left intact [13]. With regard to the periorbita, some authors advocate preserving it to prevent enophthalmos [54, 59]; however, its resection is critical to maximally reduce proptosis and should be done if tumor infiltration is appreciated. Small periorbital openings can be managed with simple bipolar coagulation or fibrin glue if more extensive, and they are generally not causative of clinical sequelae [7, 12].

Indications and Limits of Endoscopic Approaches for SOM Management

From a purely anatomical point of view, endoscopic SEA is an optimal option when patients complain of ocular-related symptoms and pathology has spread to the intraorbital area, lateral to the optic nerve. Even in the case of extensive pathologies with locations in the ACF, MCF, LSW, and GSW, such minimally invasive approach may help in relieving symptoms. However, the management of the intradural portion should be limited within 1 cm from the dural opening, in order to avoid complications that are difficult to handle without resorting to an open procedure. Moreover, this approach allows early assessment of periorbital invasion and can be indicated to avoid extensive surgical scars in patients already operated with transcranial approaches or treated with RT/radiosurgery [7].

Indications are constantly increasing thanks to several advantages, such as the minimally invasive nature, direct access to the target with reduced bone destruction and minimal brain manipulation, early tumor devascularization, shorter hospital stay, and rapid patient recovery [50].

However, different concerns have been raised regarding endoscopic transorbital approaches. The main concern is the risk of orbital injury and bradycardia, due to activation of the oculocardiac reflex during the manipulation of the orbital globe. In this regard, intermittent globe relaxation is important to minimize the risk of increased intraorbital pressure [60]. Surgical maneuverability may also represent an issue, due to the narrow surgical corridor, although combining a lateral orbital rim osteotomy might increase the working space and the chance to obtain GTR. According to Kong et al., the endoscopic transorbital approach is not indicated in case of tumor diameter more than 6 cm or involvement of the anterior clinoid process or middle cerebral arteries [6]. While the superolateral part of the orbit and the middle cranial fossa can be easily addressed with such approaches, inferior extension toward the infratemporal and temporal fossa might be challenging and require multiportal approaches in most of the cases [27].

Management Proposal

SOMs are a cluster of meningiomas originating from the sphenoid ridge that invade the neighboring compartments. Like for many other intracranial meningiomas, surgery should aim for complete tumor removal, with excision of both the dura of origin and the hyperostosis, including an extra safety margin. According to the dictates of Simpson I, this logic would be conceptually curative. However, SOMs often extend to "do-not touch areas" such as the superior orbital fissure and cavernous sinus, precluding a true radical surgery. Furthermore, hyperostosis is often so prominent that it is not always possible to drill out all the pathological bone.

Therefore the primary objectives of surgery may conflict, one being gross total resection of the lesion (including its bony part and the dural implant) and the other being improvement in the patient's quality of life. In light of this, alternative surgical strategies aimed at obtaining the so-called maximal safe subtotal resection has become the goal for SOM management in recent years [7].

As previously described, historically these tumors were treated only by the traditional anterolateral craniotomy approaches (e.g., PA, FTOZ), but nowadays the endoscope-assisted transorbital approaches have entered the skull base armamentarium offering new treatment strategies.

The study by Locatelli et al. published in 2022 [7] has demonstrated that craniotomy approaches for SOMs can obtain higher tumor removal rates compared with transorbital ones. However, both surgical strategies offer an improvement for preoperative visual deficits (intended as visual field defects, diplopia, and proptosis); moreover, in this case series, there was a unique improvement in extrinsic ocular muscle function in patients undergoing transorbital surgery. This led the authors to conclude that, given the infiltrative characteristics of SOMs, it may not always be appropriate to proceed with a radical intent. An alternative strategy aimed at symptom improvement that considers patients' comorbidities in the surgical planning might be appropriate as well, rather than seeking a gross total resection at all costs. In this setting, transorbital approaches configure themselves alongside, and sometimes as an alternative to traditional open craniotomies.

But When to Choose One Approach Over the Other?

To answer this question, several considerations must be made. Anatomically speaking, anterolateral craniotomies (possibly accompanied by skull base extensions) ensure an excellent exposure of the lateral wall and the roof of the orbit, as well as reaching the intradural compartments. Endoscopic transorbital approaches, instead, allow resection of the lateral orbital wall, to examine any infiltration of the periorbita and to drill the hyperostotic bone with optimal decompression of the SOF [12, 48, 61]. Obviously, absent any orbital involvement or visual symptoms, transorbital approaches lose their value [7]. In the case of extensive intradural diffusion, the classic craniotomy approaches should be preferred, although in promising anatomical transorbital studies, it appears that deep regions such as Meckel's cavity and the mesial part of the temporal lobe can be reached (see other chapters in this textbook) [62, 63].

Whether neurovascular encasement by tumor is a contraindication to transorbital surgery is debatable. This same debate occurred in the early years of endonasal surgery, and as surgeons gained experience, vascular involvement became more manageable. Ultimately, the surgeon must know their limitations and abilities, and if they are technically unable to perform vascular dissections transorbitally, this will be a contraindication in their hands.

In patients carrying intraorbital symptomatic relapses who have already undergone craniotomies or radiation therapy, transorbital approaches represent naive route, in which the anatomy is not distorted by scar tissue.

Likewise, in patients with a low Karnofsky performance status, advanced age (>75 years), and/or with comorbidities, the use of an endoscopic approach may be appropriate as opposed to extensive and long surgeries, with their inherently higher risk of systemic complications. In this sense, the patients' preference shouldn't be neglected: after adequate counseling, the choice of the patient to proceed with a less invasive approach mainly intended to relieve symptoms should be considered in the surgical planning.

To summarize, several factors should be analyzed in conjunction with the anatomical location and extension of the pathology, in order to carefully select the most appropriate approach for each patient. In such a composite panorama, with several options and strategies available, the focus should be the aim of the surgery combined with the characteristics of each unique patient. Figure 16.4 attempts to visually summarize all the critical factors to consider according to the authors' opinion for the management of spheno-orbital meningiomas.

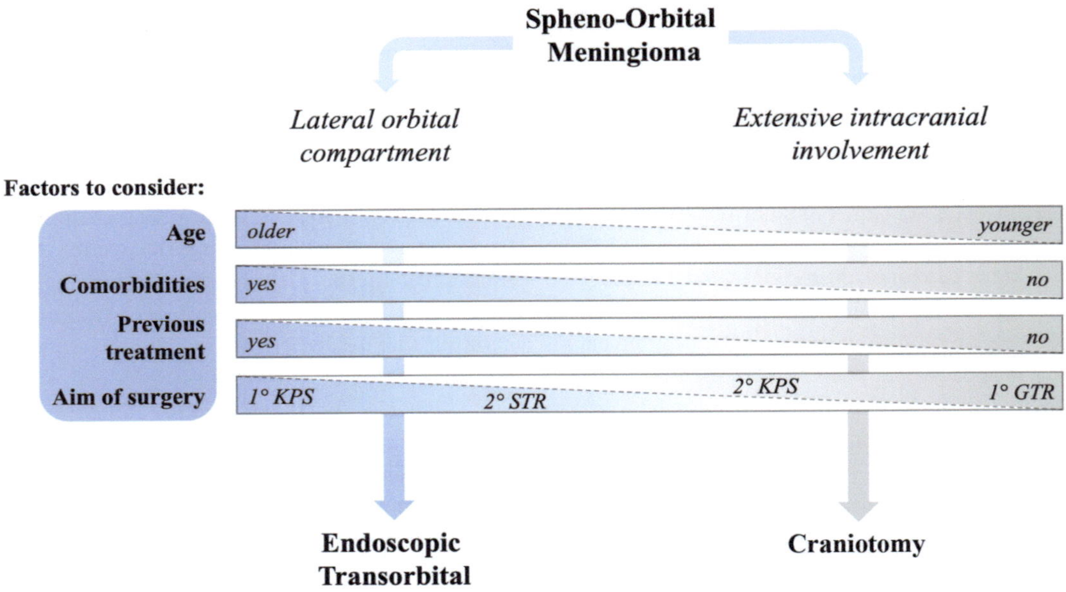

Fig. 16.4 Proposal of a treatment allocation algorithm for the management of spheno-orbital meningiomas (SOMs). Invasion of the lateral orbital compartment is the prerequisite for the indication to perform an endoscopic superior eyelid approach. When both craniotomic and transorbital approaches may be indicated from an anatomical point of view, a series of factors may help in determining surgical aim and choose the most appropriate surgical corridor. When a planned subtotal resection is the objective, the analysis of performance indexes such as KPS and mRS should be the outcome that deserves to be primarily considered; in cases where a GTR is considered safely achievable, Simpson grades 0/I should be the objective. *GTR* gross total resection, *KPS* Karnofsky Performance Status, *STR* subtotal resection. (With permissions from Locatelli D et al., The Role of the Transorbital Superior Eyelid Approach in the Management of Selected Spheno-orbital Meningiomas: In-Depth Analysis of Indications, Technique, and Outcomes from the Study of a Cohort of 35 Patients. J Neurol Surg B Skull Base. 2022;83:145–58)

Conclusion

Surgical management of SOMs still provides a challenge to the surgeons. Different surgical approaches can be employed in their management, with the extended pterional one being the most commonly used to date. The aim of surgery should be to obtain the maximum safe resection that can improve or, at least, to prevent further deterioration of the patient's quality of life. The extent of resection should always be counterbalanced between the risk of complications, the likelihood of recurrence, and the possible need for second operation or radiotherapy following subtotal resection. In this regard, transorbital and combined multiportal approaches might be indicated in selected cases in order to obtain symptomatic relief, with reduced risk of complications. With new opportunities in mind, the surgeon should train to perform an accurate preoperative evaluation of both goals and hazards, in order to properly select the patient who might benefit from surgery.

In conclusion, to manage SOMs in a modern and effective way, well-trained multidisciplinary teams are needed, wielding dedicated technological equipment and confident with both endoscopic and traditional craniotomy surgical techniques.

Acknowledgments ADA is a PhD student of the "Biotechnologies and Life Sciences" course at University of Insubria, Varese, Italy.

References

1. Fisher FL, Zamanipoor Najafabadi AH, Schoones JW, Genders SW, Furth WR. Surgery as a safe and effective treatment option for spheno-orbital meningioma: a systematic review and meta-analysis of surgical techniques and outcomes. Acta Ophthalmol. 2021;99:26–36.
2. Jääskeläinen J. Seemingly complete removal of histologically benign intracranial meningioma: late recurrence rate and factors predicting recurrence in 657 patients. A multivariate analysis. Surg Neurol. 1986;26:461–9.
3. Stafford SL, Perry A, Suman VJ, Meyer FB, Scheithauer BW, Lohse CM, et al. Primarily resected meningiomas: outcome and prognostic factors in 581 Mayo Clinic patients, 1978 through 1988. Mayo Clin Proc. 1998;73:936–42.
4. Pieper DR, Hanada Y. Hyperostosis associated with meningioma of the cranial base: secondary changes or tumor invasion. Neurosurgery. 1999;44(4):742–6; discussion 746–7.
5. Masalha W, Heiland DH, Steiert C, Krüger MT, Schnell D, Scheiwe C, et al. Progression-free survival, prognostic factors, and surgical outcome of spheno-orbital meningiomas. Front Oncol. 2021;11:672228.
6. Kong D-S, Kim YH, Hong C-K. Optimal indications and limitations of endoscopic transorbital superior eyelid surgery for spheno-orbital meningiomas. J Neurosurg. 2021;134:1472–9.
7. Locatelli D, Restelli F, Alfiero T, Campione A, Pozzi F, Balbi S, et al. The role of the transorbital superior eyelid approach in the management of selected spheno-orbital meningiomas: in-depth analysis of indications, technique, and outcomes from the study of a cohort of 35 patients. J Neurol Surg B Skull Base. 2022;83:145–58.
8. Colombo G, Ferreli F, Baram A, Mercante G, Riva M, Di Maria A, et al. Inferolateral transorbital endoscopic approach for spheno-orbital meningiomas. J Craniofac Surg. 2022;33:e260–5.
9. Saeed P, van Furth WR, Tanck M, Kooremans F, Freling N, Streekstra GI, et al. Natural history of spheno-orbital meningiomas. Acta Neurochir. 2011;153:395–402.
10. Schick U, Hassler W. Management of meningiomas en plaque of the sphenoid wing. J Neurosurg. 2006;104:208.
11. Moe KS, Bergeron CM, Ellenbogen RG. Transorbital neuroendoscopic surgery. Oper Neurosurg. 2010;67:ons16–28.
12. Dallan I, Sellari-Franceschini S, Turri-Zanoni M, de Notaris M, Fiacchini G, Fiorini FR, et al. Endoscopic transorbital superior eyelid approach for the management of selected spheno-orbital meningiomas: preliminary experience. Oper Surg. 2018;14:243–51.
13. Goncalves N, Lubbe DE. Transorbital endoscopic surgery for sphenoid wing meningioma: long-term outcomes and surgical technique. J Neurol Surg B Skull Base. 2020;81:357–68.
14. Zamanipoor Najafabadi AH, Genders SW, van Furth WR. Visual outcomes endorse surgery of patients with spheno-orbital meningioma with minimal visual impairment or hyperostosis. Acta Neurochir. 2021;163:73–82.
15. Adegbite AB, Khan MI, Paine KWE, Tan LK. The recurrence of intracranial meningiomas after surgical treatment. J Neurosurg. 1983;58:51.
16. Cappabianca P, Solari D. Meningiomas of the skull base. New York: Thieme; 2011.
17. Al-Mefty O. Clinoidal meningiomas. J Neurosurg. 1990;73:840–9.
18. Bikmaz K, Mrak R, Al-Mefty O. Management of bone-invasive, hyperostotic sphenoid wing meningiomas. J Neurosurg. 2007;107:905–12.
19. Leake D, Gunnlaugsson C, Urban J, Marentette L. Reconstruction after resection of sphenoid wing meningiomas. Arch Facial Plast Surg. 2005;7:99–103.
20. Terrier L-M, Bernard F, Fournier H-D, Morandi X, Velut S, Hénaux P-L, et al. Spheno-orbital meningiomas surgery: multicenter management study for complex extensive tumors. World Neurosurg. 2018;112:e145–56.
21. Hendricks BK, Cohen-Gadol AA. The extended pterional craniotomy: a contemporary and balanced approach. Oper Surg. 2020;18:225–31.
22. De Jesús O, Toledo MM. Surgical management of meningioma en plaque of the sphenoid ridge. Surg Neurol. 2001;55:265–9.
23. dos Santos AG, Paiva WS, da Roz LM, Santo MPE, Teixeira MJ, Figueiredo EG, et al. Spheno-orbital meningiomas: is orbit reconstruction mandatory? Long-term outcomes and exophthalmos improvement. Surg Neurol Int. 2022;13:318.
24. Boari N, Gagliardi F, Spina A, Bailo M, Franzin A, Mortini P. Management of spheno-orbital en plaque meningiomas: clinical outcome in a consecutive series of 40 patients. Br J Neurosurg. 2013;27:84–90.
25. Locatelli D, Dallan I, Castelnuovo P. Surgery around the orbit: how to select an approach. J Neurol Surg B Skull Base. 2020;81:409–21.
26. Dallan I, Castelnuovo P, Turri-Zanoni M, Fiacchini G, Locatelli D, Battaglia P, et al. Transorbital endoscopic assisted management of intraorbital lesions: lessons learned from our first 9 cases. Rhinology. 2016;54:247–53.
27. Di Somma A, Andaluz N, Cavallo LM, de Notaris M, Dallan I, Solari D, et al. Endoscopic transorbital superior eyelid approach: anatomical study from a neurosurgical perspective. J Neurosurg. 2018;129:1203–16.
28. Erdogmus S, Govsa F. Importance of the anatomic features of the lacrimal artery for orbital approaches. J Craniofac Surg. 2005;16:957–64.
29. Ferrari M, Schreiber A, Mattavelli D, Belotti F, Rampinelli V, Lancini D, et al. The inferolateral transorbital endoscopic approach: a preclinical anatomic study. World Neurosurg. 2016;90:403–13.

30. Lubbe D, Mustak H, Taylor A, Fagan J. Minimally invasive endo-orbital approach to sphenoid wing meningiomas improves visual outcomes—our experience with the first seven cases. Clin Otolaryngol. 2017;42:876–80.
31. Dallan I, Castelnuovo P, Locatelli D, Turri-Zanoni M, AlQahtani A, Battaglia P, et al. Multiportal combined transorbital transnasal endoscopic approach for the management of selected skull base lesions: preliminary experience. World Neurosurg. 2015;84:97–107.
32. Combs SE, Ganswindt U, Foote RL, Kondziolka D, Tonn J-C. State-of-the-art treatment alternatives for base of skull meningiomas: complementing and controversial indications for neurosurgery, stereotactic and robotic based radiosurgery or modern fractionated radiation techniques. Radiat Oncol. 2012;7:226.
33. Honig S, Trantakis C, Frerich B, Sterker I, Schober R, Meixensberger J. Spheno-orbital meningiomas: outcome after microsurgical treatment: a clinical review of 30 cases. Neurol Res. 2010;32:314–25.
34. Lee JYK, Niranjan A, McInerney J, Kondziolka D, Flickinger JC, Lunsford LD. Stereotactic radiosurgery providing long-term tumor control of cavernous sinus meningiomas. J Neurosurg. 2002;97:65–72.
35. Minniti G, Clarke E, Cavallo L, Osti MF, Esposito V, Cantore G, et al. Fractionated stereotactic conformal radiotherapy for large benign skull base meningiomas. Radiat Oncol. 2011;6:36.
36. Simpson D. The recurrence of intracranlal meningiomas after surgical treatment. J Neurol Neurosurg Psychiatry. 1957;20(1):22–39.
37. Scarone P, Leclerq D, Héran F, Robert G. Long-term results with exophthalmos in a surgical series of 30 sphenoorbital meningiomas: clinical article. J Neurosurg. 2009;111:1069–77.
38. Nakamura M, Roser F, Jacobs C, Vorkapic P, Samii M. Medial sphenoid wing meningiomas: clinical outcome and recurrence rate. Neurosurgery. 2006;58:626–39.
39. Ringel F, Cedzich C, Schramm J. Microsurgical technique and results of a series of 63 spheno-orbital meningiomas. Oper Neurosurg. 2007;60:214–22.
40. Mirone G, Chibbaro S, Schiabello L, Tola S, George B. En plaque sphenoid wing meningiomas: recurrence factors and surgical strategy in a series of 71 patients. Oper Neurosurg. 2009;65:ons100–9.
41. Mariniello G, de Divitiis O, Corvino S, Strianese D, Iuliano A, Bonavolontà G, et al. Recurrences of spheno-orbital meningiomas: risk factors and management. World Neurosurg. 2022;161:e514–22.
42. Amirjamshidi A, Abbasioun K, Amiri R, Ardalan A, Hashemi SR. Lateral orbitotomy approach for removing hyperostosing en plaque sphenoid wing meningiomas. Description of surgical strategy and analysis of findings in a series of 88 patients with long-term follow up. Surg Neurol Int. 2015;6:79.
43. Kunz WG, Jungblut LM, Kazmierczak PM, Vettermann FJ, Bollenbacher A, Tonn JC, et al. Improved detection of transosseous meningiomas using ^{68}Ga-DOTATATE PET/CT compared with contrast-enhanced MRI. J Nucl Med. 2017;58:1580–7.
44. Sandalcioglu IE, Gasser T, Mohr C, Stolke D, Wiedemayer H. Spheno-orbital meningiomas: interdisciplinary surgical approach, resectability and long-term results. J Craniofac Surg. 2005;33:260–6.
45. Heufelder MJ, Sterker I, Trantakis C, Schneider J-P, Meixensberger J, Hemprich A, et al. Reconstructive and ophthalmologic outcomes following resection of spheno-orbital meningiomas. Ophthalmic Plast Reconstr Surg. 2009;25:223–6.
46. Carlson A, Stippler M, Myers O. Predictive factors for vision recovery after optic nerve decompression for chronic compressive neuropathy: systematic review and meta-analysis. J Neurol Surg B. 2012;74:020–38.
47. Shrivastava RK, Sen C, Costantino PD, Della Rocca R. Sphenoorbital meningiomas: surgical limitations and lessons learned in their long-term management. J Neurosurg. 2005;103:491–7.
48. Almeida JP, Omay SB, Shetty SR, Chen Y-N, Ruiz-Treviño AS, Liang B, et al. Transorbital endoscopic eyelid approach for resection of sphenoorbital meningiomas with predominant hyperostosis: report of 2 cases. J Neurosurg. 2018;128:1885–95.
49. Yannick N, Patrick F, Samuel M, Erwan F, Pierre-Jean P, Michel J, et al. Predictive factors for visual outcome after resection of spheno-orbital meningiomas: a long-term review. Acta Ophthalmol. 2012;90:e663–5.
50. Corvino S, Sacco M, Somma T, Berardinelli J, Ugga L, Colamaria A, et al. Functional and clinical outcomes after superior eyelid transorbital endoscopic approach for spheno-orbital meningiomas: illustrative case and literature review. Neurosurg Rev. 2022;46:17.
51. Dallan I, Cristofani-Mencacci L, Fiacchini G, Caniglia M, Sellari-Franceschini S, Berrettini S. When multidisciplinary surgical trans-orbital approaches should be considered to reach the skull base. Acta Otorhinolaryngol Ital. 2021;41:S59–66.
52. De Rosa A, Pineda J, Cavallo LM, Di Somma A, Romano A, Topczewski TE, et al. Endoscopic endo- and extra-orbital corridors for spheno-orbital region: anatomic study with illustrative case. Acta Neurochir. 2019;161:1633–46.
53. Kim W, Ghodrati F, Mozaffari K, Samarage HM, Zhang AB, Pradhan A, et al. Endoscopic endonasal approach for resection of a recurrent spheno-orbital meningioma resulting in complete resolution of visual symptoms: a case report and review of literature. J Neurooncol. 2022;160:545–53.
54. Talacchi A, De Carlo A, D'Agostino A, Nocini P. Surgical management of ocular symptoms in spheno-orbital meningiomas. Is orbital reconstruction really necessary? Neurosurg Rev. 2014;37:301–10.
55. Goertz L, Stavrinou P, Stranjalis G, Timmer M, Goldbrunner R, Krischek B. Single-step resection of sphenoorbital meningiomas and orbital reconstruction using customized CAD/CAM implants. J Neurol Surg B. 2020;81:142–8.
56. Dalle Ore CL, Magill ST, Rodriguez Rubio R, Shahin MN, Aghi MK, Theodosopoulos PV, et al.

Hyperostosing sphenoid wing meningiomas: surgical outcomes and strategy for bone resection and multidisciplinary orbital reconstruction. J Neurosurg. 2021;134:711–20.

57. Maroon JC, Kennerdell JS, Vidovich DV, Abla A, Sternau L. Recurrent spheno-orbital meningioma. J Neurosurg. 1994;80:202–8.
58. Mariniello G, Maiuri F, Strianese D, Donzelli R, Iuliano A, Tranfa F, et al. Spheno-orbital meningiomas: surgical approaches and outcome according to the intraorbital tumor extent. Zentralbl Neurochir. 2008;69:175–81.
59. Demonte F, Tabrizi P, Culpepper SA, Suki D, Soparkar CNS, Patrinely JR. Ophthalmological outcome after orbital entry during anterior and anterolateral skull base surgery. J Neurosurg. 2002;97:851–6.
60. Stonnington HO, Turcotte EL, Di Nome MA, Lettieri SC, Mrugala MM, Porter AB, et al. Commentary: Transorbital endoscopic eyelid approach for resection of spheno-orbital meningioma: 2-dimensional operative video. Oper Neurosurg. 2022;23:e195–6.
61. Locatelli D, Pozzi F, Turri-Zanoni M, Battaglia P, Santi L, Dallan I, Castelnuovo P. Transorbital endoscopic approaches to the skull base: current concepts and future perspectives. J Neurosurg Sci. 2016;60(4):514–25.
62. Jeon C, Hong C-K, Woo KI, Hong SD, Nam D-H, Lee J-I, et al. Endoscopic transorbital surgery for Meckel's cave and middle cranial fossa tumors: surgical technique and early results. J Neurosurg. 2019;131:1126–35.
63. Priddy BH, Nunes CF, Beer-Furlan A, Carrau R, Dallan I, Prevedello DM-S. A side door to Meckel's cave: anatomic feasibility study for the lateral transorbital approach. Oper Surg. 2017;13:614–21.

17 The Lateral Transorbital Approach for Removal of Select Sphenoid Wing and Middle Fossa Meningiomas

Kate U. Rosen, John K. Chae, Joseph A. Carnevale, Evan D. Bander, Kyle J. Godfrey, and Theodore H. Schwartz

Abbreviations

EEA	Endoscopic endonasal approach
EOR	Extent of resection
GTR	Gross-total resection
ICA	Internal carotid artery
NTR	Near-total resection
OGM	Olfactory groove meningioma
PS	Planum sphenoidale
SSM	Suprasellar meningioma
STR	Subtotal resection
TCA	Transcranial approach
PSM	Planum sphenoidale meningioma
TOA	Lateral transorbital approach
TS	Tuberculum sellae
TSM	Tuberculum sella meningioma

Kate U. Rosen and John K. Chae share primary authorship.

K. U. Rosen · J. K. Chae · J. A. Carnevale (✉)
E. D. Bander
Department of Neurological Surgery, Weill Cornell Medicine/New York Presbyterian Hospital, New York, NY, USA
e-mail: qiz9012@nyp.org; nhc9003@nyp.org; joc3003@nyp.org; evb2005@nyp.org

K. J. Godfrey
Division of Oculoplastic Surgery, Department of Ophthalmology, Weill Cornell Medicine/New York Presbyterian Hospital, New York, NY, USA
e-mail: kyg9004@med.cornell.edu

Introduction

The lateral transorbital approach (LTOA) is a relatively new approach to the skull base that has only recently been applied in vivo in the management of complex skull base pathology [1–3]. The LTOA derives its philosophical and technical roots from the endoscopic endonasal approach (EEA). Compared to the EEA, the lateral limits of which are classically the paraclival and parasellar internal carotid artery (ICA), the exposure provided by LTOA begins, in a general sense, where EEA leaves off, namely, lateral to the ICA. The LTOA utilizes natural planes superolateral to the orbit as a corridor to access the cavernous sinus, Meckel's cave, middle cranial fossa, and portions of the anterior fossa, posterior fossa, infratemporal fossa, and the parapharyngeal space [1, 4].

T. H. Schwartz
Department of Neurosurgery, Weill Cornell Medicine, NewYork–Presbyterian Hospital, New York, NY, USA
e-mail: schwarh@med.cornell.edu

T. H. Schwartz et al. (eds.), *Endoscopic Transorbital Surgery of the Orbit, Skull Base and Brain*,
https://doi.org/10.1007/978-3-031-59504-2_17

The conventional transcranial and transfacial approaches for lesions situated in the anatomical areas exposed by the LTOA can be challenging in the presence of important neurovascular structures, requiring greater degrees of dissection and brain retraction to achieve optimal surgical windows [5, 6]. TOA, in comparison, allows the potential for lower morbidity, better cosmetic outcomes, and faster postoperative recovery period [2, 5, 7]. Moreover, unlike the EEA and its inherent risk of postoperative CSF leak, TOA carries a lower risk of CSF leak because the intraocular contents act as a natural tamponade [8]. However, since TOA involves retraction of the orbit, it introduces a new set of potential complications including diplopia, ptosis, proptosis, and vision changes, but these ophthalmologic changes are often temporary and transient [7].

Meningiomas are the most common benign intracranial tumor. Unless small and asymptomatic, surgery remains the first-line therapy for most meningiomas that require treatment. Meningiomas are classified based on their dural attachments, which are not equally distributed along the meninges [9, 10]. One area of predisposition is the sphenoid wing. These include meningiomas of the lateral, mid-, and medial sphenoid wing (with and without cavernous sinus invasion), middle fossa, and spheno-orbital subtypes. The transorbital approach (TOA) is a novel minimally invasive alternative to open craniotomy suitable for removal of select spheno-orbital, sphenoid wing, and middle fossa meningiomas. Since other chapters in this book focus on spheno-orbital meningiomas, this particular chapter will describe the TOA specifically for sphenoid wing and middle fossa meningiomas, which represent 8–10% and 1–2% of all intracranial meningiomas respectively [9, 10].

Case Selection

Sphenoid wing meningiomas have been divided into several subtypes, which will be quickly reviewed here. Cushing and Eisenhardt [9] were the first to classify sphenoid ridge meningiomas [11]. They distinguished between globoid tumors with nodular shape and en plaque tumors, which are flat and spread along the entire ridge. The globoid meningiomas were divided into three groups: (1) inner or medial, (2) middle, and (3) lateral/pterional. A more modern classification was proposed by Roser et al. In their schema, there are seven categories [12]. Group I, medial sphenoid wing, no cavernous sinus infiltration; Group II, medial sphenoid wing with cavernous sinus infiltration; Group III, middle sphenoid wing; Group IV, lateral sphenoid wing; Group V, en plaque, no cavernous sinus infiltration; Group VI, en plaque with cavernous sinus infiltration; Group VII, pure intraosseous.

Middle fossa meningiomas can also be subdivided into subtypes based on location. In one classification, they have been divided into three separate groups: those that arise medially from the lateral wall of the cavernous sinus, those that arise from the floor of the middle fossa, and those that arise laterally from the convexity [13]. If >50% of the tumor's dural attachment arises from any of these locations, they are classified as such.

Since the TOA provides a limited corridor and since the goal of meningioma surgery is maximal safe cytoreduction, it is important to carefully select cases in the right location to achieve the surgical goals [14]. In general, we aim to remove all the soft tissue mass compressing the brain, as much bone hyperostosis as safely possible, with the goal of correcting any exophthalmos. Tumor invading the orbit or cavernous sinus is approached less aggressively, particularly if there aren't symptoms related to mass effect, since radiosurgery can be effectively employed as a surgical adjunct.

In our experience, the sphenoid wing tumors that are most suitable for TOA are Group I, medial sphenoid wing, no cavernous sinus infiltration; Group II, medial sphenoid wing with cavernous sinus infiltration (goal of surgery is removal of extra-cavernous tumor only); Group III, middle sphenoid wing; Group V, en plaque, no cavernous sinus infiltration; Group VI, en plaque with cavernous sinus infiltration (goal of surgery is removal of extra-cavernous tumor only); Group VII, pure intraosseous (goal is decompression of bone if there is proptosis, cosmetic issues, or mass effect on brain). The middle fossa tumors are suitable for TOA, those arising from the lateral wall of the cavernous sinus and the floor. Those arising from the convexity are generally too lateral for TOA and likely more suitable for a lateral approach.

The Lateral Transorbital Approach

After general anesthesia, the patient is positioned supine with the head placed in Mayfield pin fixation and registered to the frameless stereotactic equipment. Topical proparacaine is applied to each eye, which is protected with a sterile corneal shield intraoperatively. The patient is subsequently prepped and draped in the usual fashion. For optimal cosmetic outcomes, the incision is made along the superior eyelid crease (Fig. 17.1a). The orbicularis oculi muscle is divided with a monopolar, and the arcus marginalis is cut at the orbital rim. A subperiosteal plane is created with a periosteal elevator and carried into the orbit (Fig. 17.1b). For larger meningiomas we sometimes remove the lateral orbital rim to create more room. This can be helpful to expose more laterally for middle fossa floor meningioma or Types II, V, and VI meningiomas with lateral extension. The superior orbital fissure (SOF) is a key landmark in the posterolateral aspect of the dissection. The orbital contents are retracted medially with care, and in order to prevent complications stemming from prolonged retraction and high intraorbital pressure, intermittent relaxation is done (approximately every 20 min) with diligent monitoring of the pupil. The triangular wedge of greater sphenoid wing between the superior and inferior orbital fissure is drilled until the temporal dura is in contact with the temporalis muscle and the sagittal crest is removed (Fig. 17.1c). All hyperostotic bone is removed. The meningo-orbital band is transected taking care to avoid entering the superior orbital fissure. This also facilitates anterior clinoidectomy, which is performed if needed by drilling the bone

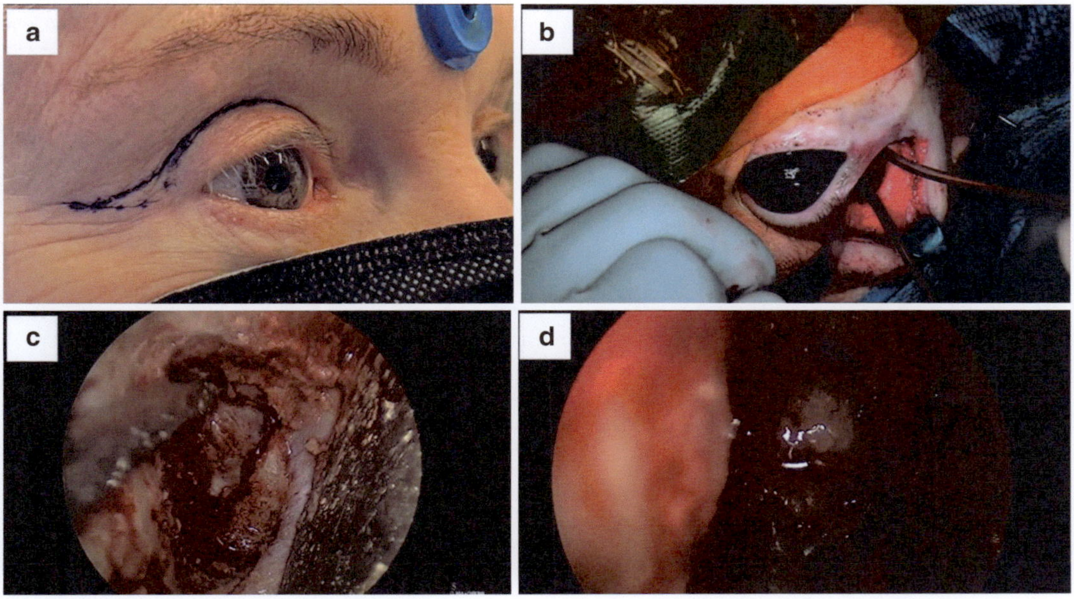

Fig. 17.1 (**a**) Preoperative image of transorbital approach incision made along the superior eyelid crease. (**b**) Intraoperative image of open eyelid incision with the orbicularis oculi muscle divided and the arcus marginalis cut at the orbital rim showing the subperiosteal plane carried into the orbit. (**c**) Endoscopic intraoperative view of the triangular wedge of greater sphenoid wing between the superior and inferior orbital fissure drilled showing the temporal dura. (**d**) Endoscopic intraoperative view of tumor being removed

up over the superior orbital fissure. If needed, the middle fossa dura is dissected off the lateral wall of the cavernous sinus and Meckel's cave to increase exposure.

Tumor resection proceeds with internal debulking followed by extra-capsular dissection. Endonasal instruments are helpful and well-suited for the LTOA. A 0° endoscope is used for most of the operation, which makes surgery more straightforward. The scope can be held by a third individual or placed on a scope holder. Frequent irrigation through an external sheath keeps the scope clean.

After tumor resection (Fig. 17.1d), the dura is closed with an inlay-onlay button closure with AlloMax. This is overlaid with autologous fat, both to prevent CSF leak and to prevent enophthalmos, which is then covered by Tisseel (Baxter) fibrin glue. PDS can be used to reconstruct the lateral orbit if needed. The periosteum, orbicularis oculi, and skin are closed with 5-0 BioSyn, 7-0 Vicryl, and 6-0 plain gut sutures, respectively. The corneal shields are removed, and erythromycin ointment is prophylactically applied to the eye, which is then covered with a pressure patch.

Case Examples

Sphenoid Wing Meningiomas

A 60-year-old woman presented with transient memory loss and aphasia. MRI revealed a Group III 1.5 × 1.6 cm left middle sphenoid wing meningioma with hyperostosis of the sphenoid wing and edema in the temporal lobe (Fig. 17.2). She underwent a LTOA for GTR of the soft tissue and hyperostosis (Fig. 17.3). Pathology revealed a WHO Grade I meningioma. Postoperatively she noted a visual decline in the left eye and was found to have a subretinal hemorrhage (Terson's syndrome). She underwent an open vitrectomy repair. At 18 months her vision is OD 20/40 and OS 20/150 but correctable. Her tumor has not recurred.

A 55-year-old woman presented with an enlarging right 2.8 × 2.5 cm Group I medial sphenoid wing meningioma without cavernous sinus infiltration and adjacent hyperostosis (Fig. 17.4). She underwent LTAO for GTR of the tumor and hyperostotic bone (Fig. 17.5). Pathology was WHO Grade II. Postoperatively she developed transient diplopia and numbness around the eye

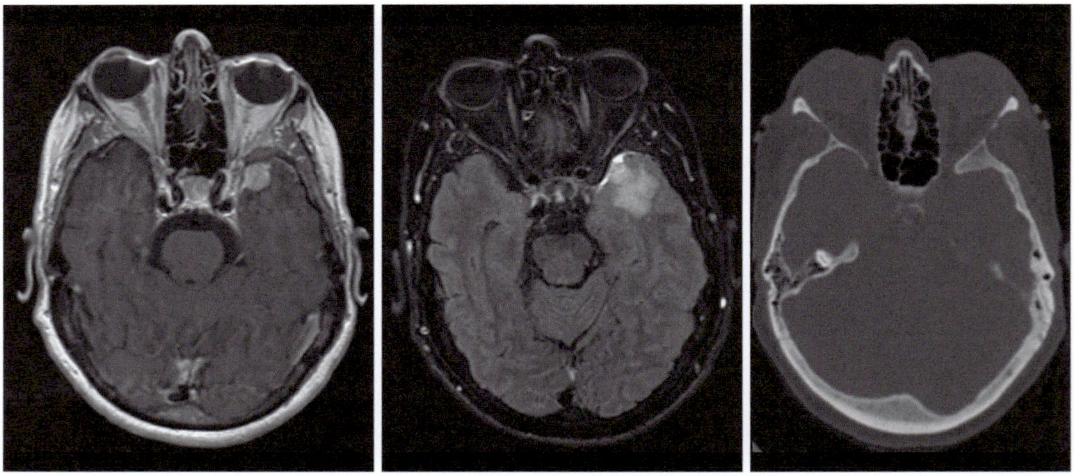

Fig. 17.2 Preoperative axial imaging (left, T1 post-contrast; middle, FLAIR; right, CT bone window) showing a Group III 1.5 × 1.6 cm left middle sphenoid wing meningioma with hyperostosis (right) of the sphenoid wing and edema (middle) in the temporal lobe

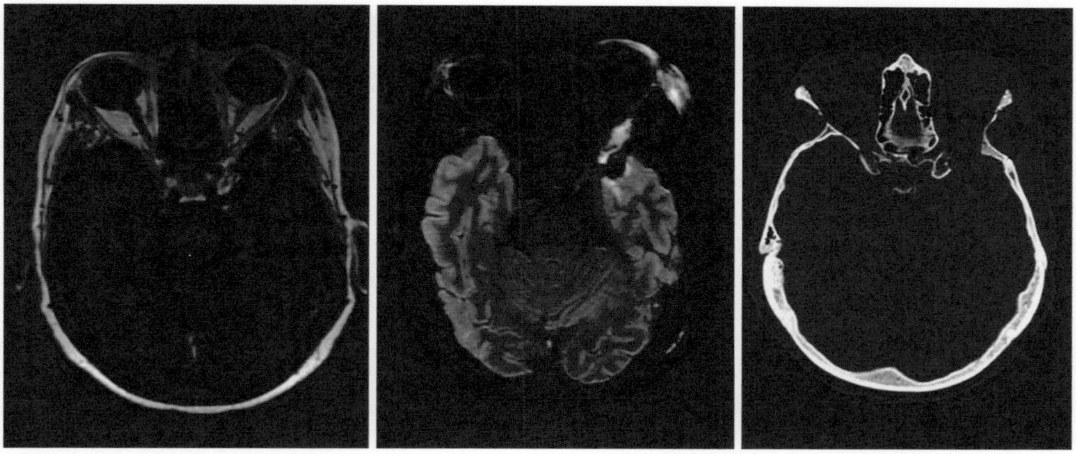

Fig. 17.3 Postoperative axial imaging (left, T1 post-contrast; middle, FLAIR; right, CT bone window) following LTOA for GTR of the soft tissue mass and hyperostosis

Fig. 17.4 Preoperative axial (left) and coronal (right) MRI showing a right 2.8 × 2.5 cm Group I medial sphenoid wing meningioma without cavernous sinus infiltration and adjacent hyperostosis

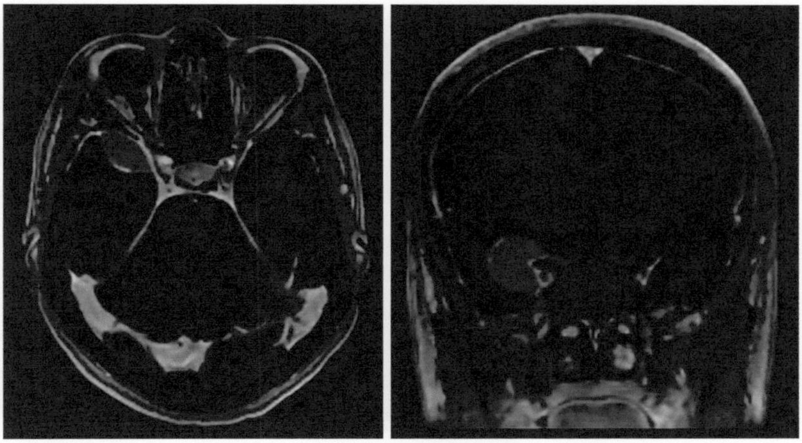

Fig. 17.5 Postoperative axial (left) and coronal (right) MRI following LTAO for GTR of the tumor and hyperostotic bone

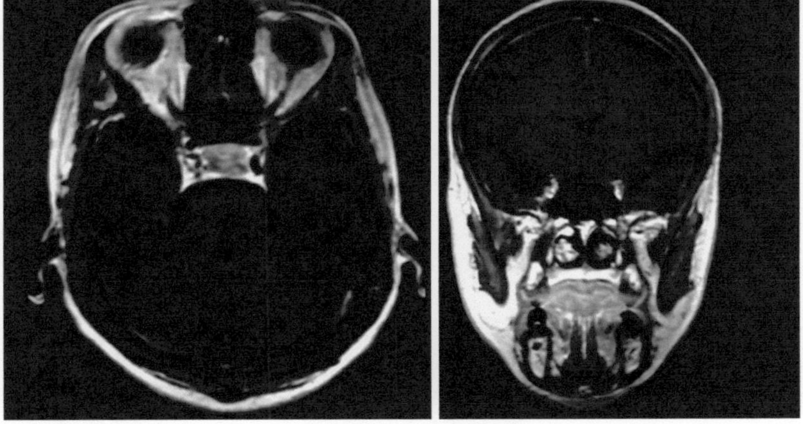

which gradually improved. She developed a pseudomeningocele which was resolved with lumbar drainage (of note, autologous fat was not placed over the closure). At 15 months, the tumor has not recurred.

A 71-year-old man presented with a 3.3 × 3.1 cm right-sided meningioma with significant FLAIR signal abnormality in the temporal lobe that could be classified either as a Group 1 medial sphenoid wing meningioma without cavernous invasion or a middle fossa meningioma arising from the lateral wall of the cavernous sinus (Fig. 17.6). He underwent a LTOA for GTR of tumor (Fig. 17.7). Pathology revealed a WHO Grade I meningioma. Postoperatively he complained of diplopia and gaze paresis which returned to baseline over time.

Middle Fossa Meningiomas

A 39-year-old woman presented with intractable seizures and a 2.7 × 2.1 cm left middle fossa meningioma arising from the lateral wall of the cavernous sinus with significant surrounding edema (Fig. 17.8). She underwent a LTAO for GTR (Fig. 17.9). Pathology revealed a meningioma with central necrosis and markedly elevated Ki-67 and prominent neutrophilic infiltrate without brain invasion. One year after surgery, she is seizure-free on one medication with no evidence of tumor recurrence.

A 71-year-old woman presented with a 1.5 × 1.5 cm middle fossa floor meningioma with extensive surrounding vasogenic edema (Fig. 17.10). She underwent LTAO for GTR

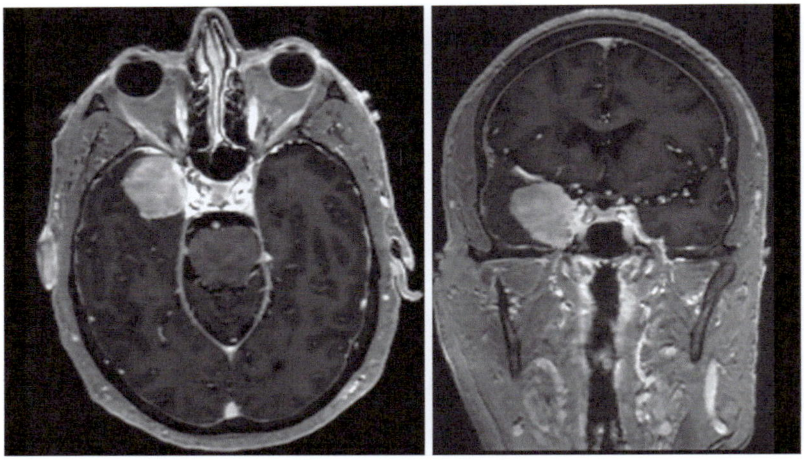

Fig. 17.6 Preoperative axial (left) and coronal (right) MRI showing a 3.3 × 3.1 cm right-sided meningioma that could be classified either as a Group 1 medial sphenoid wing meningioma without cavernous invasion or a middle fossa meningioma arising from the lateral wall of the cavernous sinus

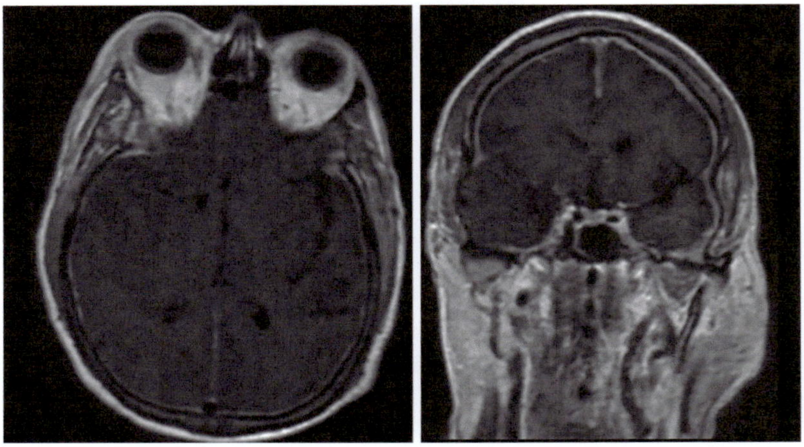

Fig. 17.7 Postoperative axial (left) and coronal (right) MRI following LTOA for GTR of tumor

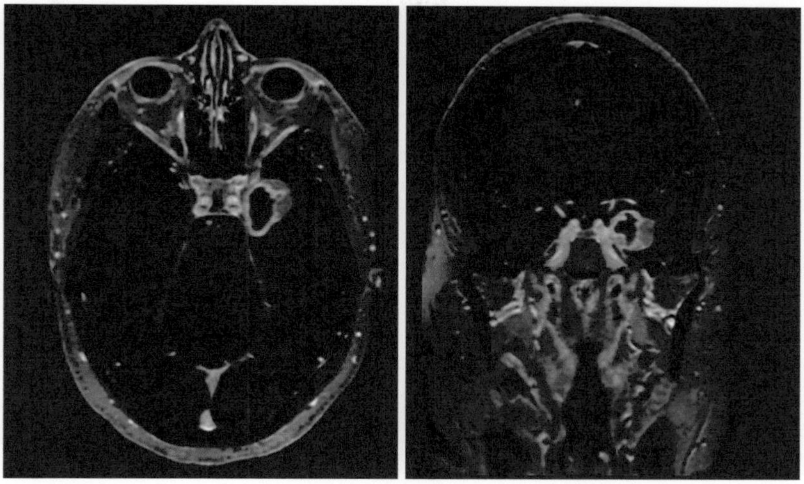

Fig. 17.8 Preoperative axial (left) and coronal (right) MRI showing a 2.7 × 2.1 cm left middle fossa meningioma arising from the lateral wall of the cavernous sinus with significant surrounding edema

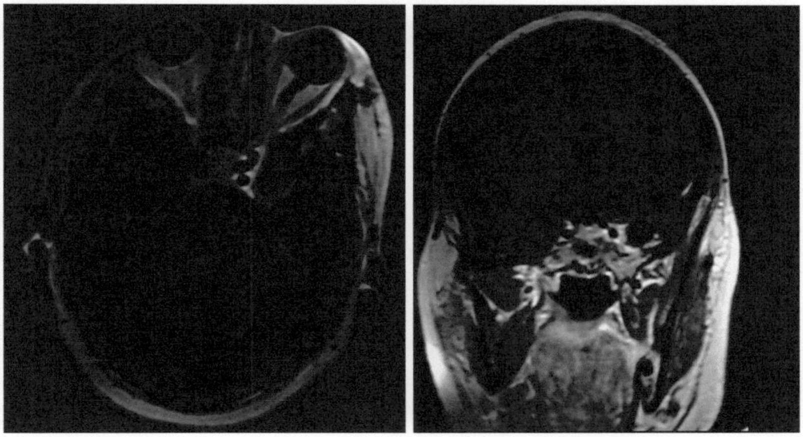

Fig. 17.9 Postoperative axial (left) and coronal (right) MRI following a LTAO for GTR

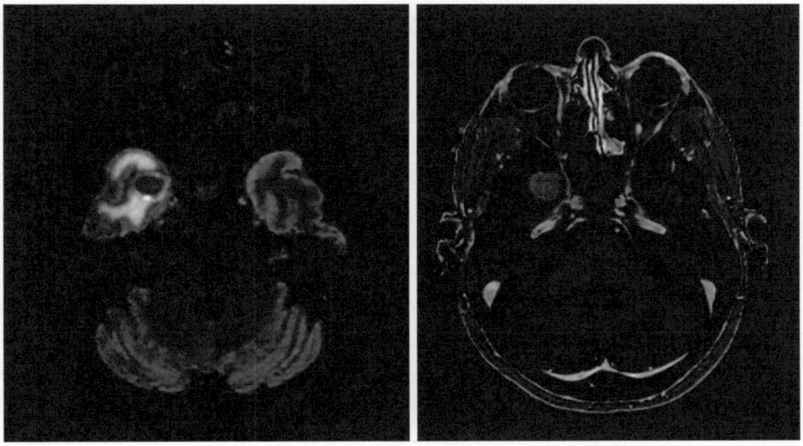

Fig. 17.10 Preoperative axial FLAIR (left) and axial post-contrast (right) MRI showing a 1.5 × 1.5 cm middle fossa floor meningioma with extensive surrounding vasogenic edema (Fig. 17.10). She underwent LTAO for GTR

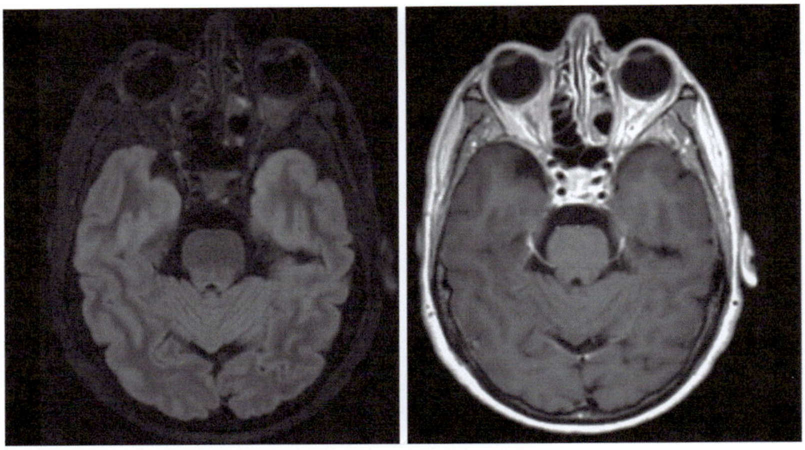

Fig. 17.11 Postoperative axial FLAIR (left) and axial post-contrast (right) MRI following LTAO showing resolution of FLAIR signal and GTR of tumor

(Fig. 17.11). Pathology revealed WHO Grade II meningioma. At 9 months follow-up, she is doing well with no complaints and no tumor recurrence.

Discussion

The purpose of meningioma care is to minimize disease progression and symptoms for the remainder of a patient's lifetime. To this end, the goal of surgery is generally maximal safe removal of the tumor, its dural attachment, and all infiltrated bone [14]. Given the efficacy of stereotactic radiosurgery (SRS) for controlling growth of small residual bits of tumor, achieving a Simpson Grade I resection at the cost of a new neurological deficit is difficult to justify. That said, maximal resection remains a priority. The LTOA provides excellent exposure to specific areas of the skull base, which makes it a suitable minimally invasive alternative to craniotomy.

In this chapter we have outlined a variety of sphenoid wing and middle fossa meningioma locations suitable for LTOA and provided case examples. A few points are worth discussing. First, our GTR rate, which included removal of the dural attachment and all infiltrated bone, was achieved in all patients. It is important to highlight that since the trajectory of the TOA is ventral, the tumor is approached at its base, like a convexity meningioma through a craniotomy or a tuberculum meningioma through EEA. This vector necessitates removal of the infiltrated bone for adequate tumor exposure, which may provide more durable tumor control than a more lateral approach, where the hyperostosis is not always drilled out as completely. On the other hand, the narrow corridor may limit the field of view and thwart removal of an extensive dural tail or laterally situated hyperostosis. An open approach would be better suited for such a situation, which is why case selection and careful review of preoperative films are so important for achieving a successful result.

The second important point is that the morbidity of our cases was somewhat higher than expected. Our case of retinal hemorrhage was concerning. Although repairable with surgery, if the incidence of Terson's is high in this approach, the risk would not justify its use. However, to date, our case is the only one reported in the literature following TOA, so we feel that this outcome was an exception, rather than common [15]. Our second complication was a pseudomeningocele, which resolved with lumbar drainage. In this case, we had a large dural opening, and we failed to place abdominal fat in the cavity. For meningiomas, it is now our convention to place a lumbar drain at the start of the operation and close with fat for these high-flow leaks. This protocol is not *required* in all LTOA cases that extend intradurally but may be helpful for those that leave a very large dural opening. This will depend on the size of the tumor and its attachment. As with EEA, LD placement may be useful for high-risk leaks to prevent postoperative pseudomeningoceles [16, 17]. This might include patients not only with large dural openings but also with prior radiation, diabetes, and/or high BMI.

Skull base meningiomas are more likely to be WHO Grade I, associated with memory deficits and at risk for subtotal resection and recurrence due to the limited working angles offered by most conventional open craniotomy approaches [9, 18–22]. In terms of cell markers, middle fossa meningiomas in particular are associated with higher CD34 levels and negative EMA and are less likely to be p53- or Ki67-positive, altogether suggesting a cellular profile that is more differentiated with less malignant/oncogenic potential [9]. Surprisingly, of our five cases, there were two Grade II meningiomas and one with an unusual pathology that might forebode a more rapid growth rate. It's unclear why our cases were not representative of typical histology in this location. Further experience will be required to explore this phenomenon.

Meningioma remains the most common indication for TOA [7]. However, the most common location approach has been spheno-orbital meningiomas. Few prior reports of sphenoid wing meningioma and even fewer middle fossa meningiomas have been described. Park et al. reported 11 cases of sphenoid wing meningiomas removed through LTOA, and GTR was achieved in 9/11 cases [23]. Unlike our series, theirs included three Grade IV cases of the lateral sphenoid wing, and they were able to achieve GTR in all of these. The two STRs were in cases with cavernous sinus invasion. There was one CSF leak. They compared these results to those achieved with a mini-pterional and found they were similar, although the LTOA cases had less blood loss and shorter operative time and shorter length of stay.

In a systematic review of 193 TOA cases, 60 complications were reported, the most common of which were diplopia (38.3%) and ptosis (20%) [7]. However, all but one of these were transient and/or managed conservatively, not requiring any additional procedural intervention. Ptosis and diplopia are common transient symptoms after TOA that result from orbital swelling and, as such, should not be considered complications any more than redness, swelling, and numbness around a scalp incision [1]. In another series of 45 consecutive TOA cases from 2006 to 2013 (pathologies not limited to meningioma), there were only three complications—namely, ptosis, epiphora, and enophthalmos [2], suggesting that TOA, despite its inherent ophthalmologic risks, has low morbidity.

At our institution, we compared the supraorbital approach (SOA), EEA, and TOA for skull base meningioma in a variety of locations—mostly olfactory groove and anterior clinoid for the SOA, planum sphenoidale and tuberculum for the EEA, and spheno-orbital, sphenoid wing, and middle fossa for TOA [24]. Vision improvement was similar among the three approaches (67–69%). The rates of GTR were overall higher in the SOA (92%) and EEA (84%) than that in TOA (50%), but when the spheno-orbital cases were removed from the TOA group, in GTR was not the goal of surgery, the GTR rate was 100%.

Conclusions

LTOA provides a direct minimal access corridor to certain well-selected sphenoid wing and middle fossa meningiomas. LTOA minimizes brain retraction, maximizes bone removal at the start of the operation, and provides a high rate of GTR. Transient ptosis and diplopia are common but resolve over time. CSF leaks and pseudomeningoceles may occur, and placement of lumbar drains and closure with onlay fat graft may be helpful for prevention.

References

1. Di Somma A, Kong D-S, de Notaris M, Moe KS, Sánchez España JC, Schwartz TH, et al. Endoscopic transorbital surgery levels of difficulty. J Neurosurg. 2022;137(4):1187–90.
2. Ramakrishna R, Kim LJ, Bly RA, Moe K, Ferreira M. Transorbital neuroendoscopic surgery for the treatment of skull base lesions. J Clin Neurosci. 2016;24:99–104.

3. Moe KS, Bergeron CM, Ellenbogen RG. Transorbital neuroendoscopic surgery. Neurosurgery. 2010;67(3 Suppl Operative):ons16–28.
4. Gerges MM, Godil SS, Younus I, Rezk M, Schwartz TH. Endoscopic transorbital approach to the infratemporal fossa and parapharyngeal space: a cadaveric study. J Neurosurg. 2019;133(6):1948–59.
5. Yoo J, Park HH, Yun I-S, Hong C-K. Clinical applications of the endoscopic transorbital approach for various lesions. Acta Neurochir (Wien). 2021;163(8):2269–77.
6. Jeon C, Hong C-K, Woo KI, Hong SD, Nam D-H, Lee J-I, et al. Endoscopic transorbital surgery for Meckel's cave and middle cranial fossa tumors: surgical technique and early results. J Neurosurg. 2018; https://doi.org/10.3171/2018.6.JNS181099.
7. Vural A, Carobbio ALC, Ferrari M, Rampinelli V, Schreiber A, Mattavelli D, et al. Transorbital endoscopic approaches to the skull base: a systematic literature review and anatomical description. Neurosurg Rev. 2021;44(5):2857–78.
8. Schwartz TH, Henderson F, Di Somma A, Kong D-S, de Notaris M, Enseñat J, et al. Endoscopic transorbital surgery: another leap of faith? World Neurosurg. 2022;159:54–5.
9. Sun C, Dou Z, Wu J, Jiang B, Iranmanesh Y, Yu X, et al. The preferred locations of meningioma according to different biological characteristics based on voxel-wise analysis. Front Oncol. 2020;10:1412.
10. Hosainey SAM, Bouget D, Reinertsen I, Sagberg LM, Torp SH, Jakola AS, et al. Are there predilection sites for intracranial meningioma? A population-based atlas. Neurosurg Rev. 2022;45(2):1543–52.
11. Cushing H. Meningiomas: their classification, regional behavior, life history, and surgical end result. Springfield: Charles C Thomas; 1938.
12. Roser F, Nakamura M, Jacobs C, Vorkapic P, Samii M. Sphenoid wing meningiomas with osseous involvement. Surg Neurol. 2005;64(1):37–43; discussion 43.
13. Magill ST, Sughrue ME, Rodriguez LR, McDermott MW. Middle fossa meningiomas. In: Meningiomas, Part II. Elsevier; 2020. p. 65–7.
14. Schwartz TH, McDermott MW. The Simpson grade: abandon the scale but preserve the message. J Neurosurg. 2020; https://doi.org/10.3171/2020.6.JNS201904.
15. Foulsham W, North VS, Botsford BW, Dinkin MJ, Henderson F, Godfrey KJ, et al. Multilayered macular hemorrhages as an unusual complication of transorbital neuroendoscopic surgery. Am J Ophthalmol Case Rep. 2022;26:101556.
16. Cohen S, Jones SH, Dhandapani S, Negm HM, Anand VK, Schwartz TH. Lumbar drains decrease the risk of postoperative cerebrospinal fluid leak following endonasal endoscopic surgery for suprasellar meningiomas in patients with high body mass index. Oper Neurosurg (Hagerstown). 2018;14(1):66–71.
17. Zwagerman NT, Wang EW, Shin SS, Chang Y-F, Fernandez-Miranda JC, Snyderman CH, et al. Does lumbar drainage reduce postoperative cerebrospinal fluid leak after endoscopic endonasal skull base surgery? A prospective, randomized controlled trial. J Neurosurg. 2018; https://doi.org/10.3171/2018.4.JNS172447.
18. Sade B, Chahlavi A, Krishnaney A, Nagel S, Choi E, Lee JH. World Health Organization Grades II and III meningiomas are rare in the cranial base and spine. Neurosurgery. 2007;61(6):1194–8; discussion 1198.
19. Kane AJ, Sughrue ME, Rutkowski MJ, Shangari G, Fang S, McDermott MW, et al. Anatomic location is a risk factor for atypical and malignant meningiomas. Cancer. 2011;117(6):1272–8.
20. Cornelius JF, Slotty PJ, Steiger HJ, Hänggi D, Polivka M, George B. Malignant potential of skull base versus non-skull base meningiomas: clinical series of 1,663 cases. Acta Neurochir (Wien). 2013;155(3):407–13.
21. Lemée J-M, Corniola MV, Da Broi M, Joswig H, Scheie D, Schaller K, et al. Extent of resection in meningioma: predictive factors and clinical implications. Sci Rep. 2019;9(1):5944.
22. Liouta E, Koutsarnakis C, Liakos F, Stranjalis G. Effects of intracranial meningioma location, size, and surgery on neurocognitive functions: a 3-year prospective study. J Neurosurg. 2016;124(6):1578–84.
23. Park HH, Yoo J, Yun I-S, Hong C-K. Comparative analysis of endoscopic transorbital approach and extended mini-pterional approach for sphenoid wing meningiomas with osseous involvement: preliminary surgical results. World Neurosurg. 2020;139:e1–12.
24. Carnevale JA, Schwartz TH. Minimal access endonasal, supraorbital and transorbital surgery for skull base meningiomas in the anterior and middle fossa. J Neurosurg. (Submitted for publication).

Transorbital Endoscopic Skull Base Surgery for Intra-axial Mesial Temporal Lobe Tumors

18

Hun Ho Park and In-Sik Yun

Introduction

The mesial temporal lobe (MTL) is the most medial part of the temporal lobe where various skull base and vascular pathologies can arise exclusively. Traditional transcranial approaches have been used successfully to manage lesions within MTL, but the laterally oriented entry point inevitably involved temporal lobe retraction and breach of the lateral neocortex to arrive at the targets. The entire length of MTL could not be exposed without some degree of temporal lobe retraction or resection that put the bridging veins and optic radiation at risk. Concurrent advances in neuroendoscopy and its instruments have enabled to overcome these limitations of traditional open craniotomies. The basic principles of traditional approaches involved removal of more bone to avoid brain retraction, whereas minimally invasive surgery entailed using endoscopes through "well-placed" small openings to avoid brain retraction. The benefits of endoscopic endonasal approach (EEA) over open craniotomies, in selected cases of median and paramedian skull base lesions, have been well documented for over a decade [1–3]. Unfortunately, the endoscopic passage through the nasopharynx had anatomical boundaries and drawbacks to access the lateral portion of the skull base including MTL [4, 5]. Since the advent of endoscopic transorbital approach (ETOA), it has gained increasing popularity as a feasible surgical corridor for selected cases of various extra-axial lesions around MTL [6–8]. The feasibility and application of ETOA have recently expanded to intra-axial lesions in MTL. In this chapter, the endoscopic anatomical view of MTL is demonstrated, and the clinical aspects are assessed for patients undergoing ETOA for intra-axial temporal lobe tumors.

H. H. Park (✉)
Department of Neurosurgery, Gangnam Severance Hospital, Yonsei University, Seoul, South Korea

I.-S. Yun
Department of Oculoplastic Surgery, Gangnam Severance Hospital, Yonsei University, Seoul, South Korea

Indications

- Cavernous malformation
- Mesial temporal lobe low-grade glioma
- Temporal lobe high-grade glioma
- Dysembryoplastic neuroepithelial tumor

Surgical Steps

Surgical Trajectory

ETOA followed the long axis of the hippocampus, sparing the lateral neocortex including the Meyer's loop (green arrow, Fig. 18.1). The lateral-to-medial direction of ETOA pointed

T. H. Schwartz et al. (eds.), *Endoscopic Transorbital Surgery of the Orbit, Skull Base and Brain*,
https://doi.org/10.1007/978-3-031-59504-2_18

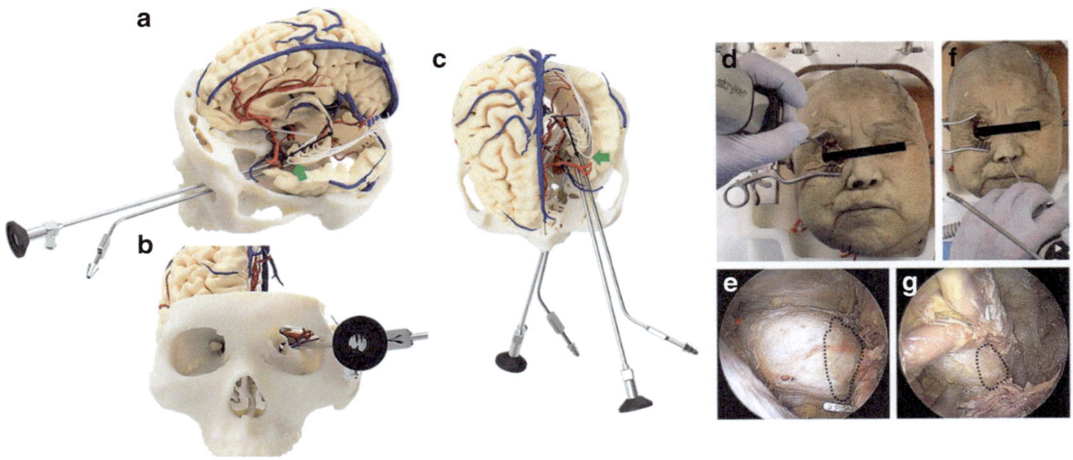

Fig. 18.1 Schematic illustrations of the surgical trajectory of ETOA to MTL. (**a–c**) Oblique (**a**) and surgeon's (**b**) view demonstrating that the long axis of MTL (black arrow) including the uncus is in line with the natural surgical trajectory of ETOA compared to EEA (**c**). The lateral neocortex and the optic tract including the Meyer's loop (green arrow) can be spared with both approaches. Cadaveric views of the surgical trajectory of EEA and ETOA. (**f**, **g**) The medial-to-lateral trajectory of EEA, allowing access to MTL (black dotted circle) with some difficulties, especially at the most mesial segment as demonstrated through the external (**f**) and internal (**g**) views of the cadaver. (**d**, **e**) The lateral-to-medial trajectory of ETOA, pointing toward MTL (black dotted circle) with ease is shown through the external (**d**) and internal (**e**) views of the cadave

toward MTL with ease compared to the medial-to-lateral direction of the endoscopic endonasal approach (EEA).

First Step: Extra-dural Stage

A superior eyelid incision, extending toward the lateral canthus, is made (Fig. 18.2a). Then, the orbicularis muscle is raised subperiosteally from the superolateral border of the orbital rim to avoid lacrimal gland injury. The orbit is detached in the same manner from superolateral to inferomedial direction until the optic canal (OC), SOF, and inferior orbital fissure (IOF) can be identified (Fig. 18.2b, c). For bone drilling, a self-retaining and malleable retractor is placed over the orbit for orbital protection and retraction. The greater wing of the sphenoid bone (GWS) underneath the temporalis muscle is drilled until the muscle fascia is exposed (Fig. 18.2d). The exposure creates more room to get to the deeper segments of GWS without added orbital retraction. The drilling of GWS continues until SOF, IOF, and the temporal base are reached to expose the frontal and temporal dura and the temporalis muscle fascia completely (Fig. 18.2e). The meningo-orbital band (MOB) holding the temporal dura to the temporal base is cut for the lateral mobilization of MTL and minimization of orbital retraction during the intradural stage to MTL (Fig. 18.2f–h).

Second Step: Intradural Stage

The temporal dura is incised in a rectangular fashion for the complete exposure of the temporal lobe including the inferior temporal gyrus (ITG), occipitotemporal gyrus (OTG), and the parahippocampal gyrus (PHG). A cortisectomy is made along the rhinal sulcus (RS) between OTG and PHG (Fig. 18.3a). Then, PHG is aspirated with a suction until the temporal horn is opened to expose the head of the hippocampus (Fig. 18.3b). Once inside the temporal horn, the head, body, and tail of the hippocampus are resected until the collateral trigone (CT) is identified (Fig. 18.3c). Care is taken not to injure the collateral eminence (CE) on the lateral side and the lateral geniculate body (LGB) on the medial

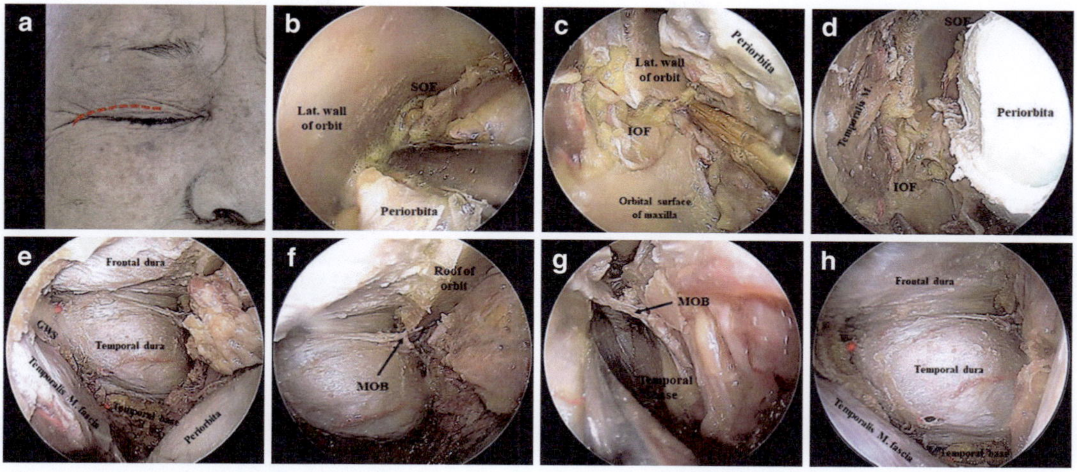

Fig. 18.2 Cadaver dissection, extra-dural stage of a right ETOA for MTL with a 0° endoscope. (**a**) A skin incision is made along the crease of the superior eyelid (red dotted line), extending toward the lateral canthus. (**b**, **c**) After subperiosteal elevation of the orbicularis muscle, the periorbita is detached from the lateral wall of the orbit until the superior orbital fissure (SOF) and inferior orbital fissure (IOF) are identified. (**d**) The bone beneath the temporalis muscle is first drilled until the fascia of the muscle is exposed. The drilling increases the surgical corridor while reducing the retraction of the orbit. (**e**) The drilling continues until SOF and IOF are opened, which are the superomedial and inferolateral borders of craniectomy, respectively. (**f**, **g**) The meningo-orbital band (MOB) is identified upon opening of SOF, which is cut for the lateral mobilization of MTL. (**h**) The final exposure of the extradural stage showing the frontal and temporal dura, temporalis muscle fascia, greater wing of the sphenoid bone (GWS), and the temporal base

side (Fig. 18.3d). The remaining structures of MTL including the uncus are aspirated in a subpial manner, so as not to breach the ambient and Sylvian cisterns (Fig. 18.3e). The neurovascular structures within the ambient and Sylvian cisterns including the crus cerebri, optic tract, oculomotor nerve, anterior choroidal artery (AChoA), posterior cerebral artery (PCA), and middle cerebral artery (MCA) are identified and preserved (Fig. 18.3f). MTL can be resected selectively and exclusively without injury to irrelevant structures (Fig. 18.3g, h).

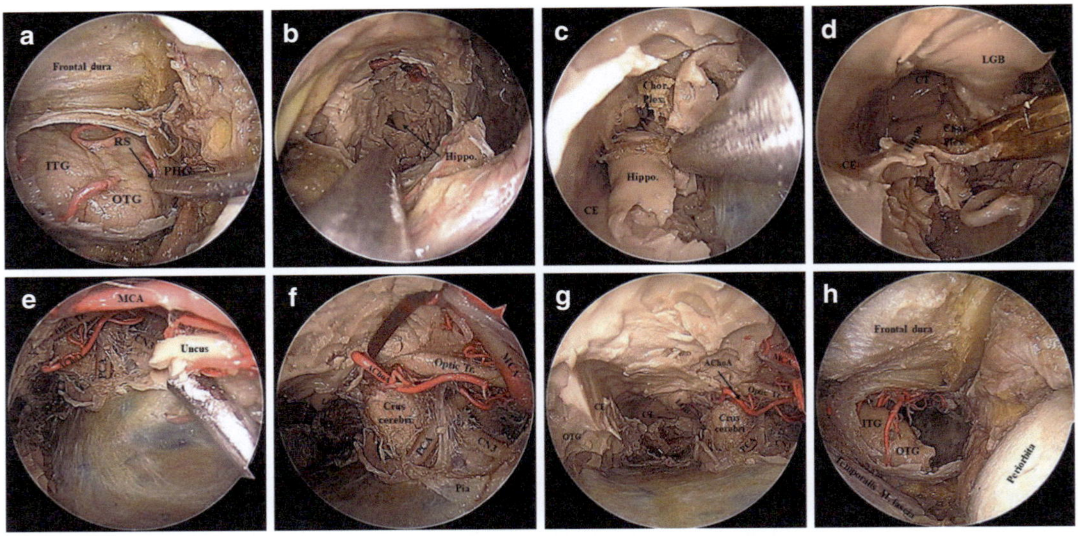

Fig. 18.3 Cadaver dissection, intradural stage of a right ETOA for MTL with a 0° endoscope. (**a**) The dura is removed, exposing the anterior surface of the temporal lobe including the inferior temporal gyrus (ITG), occipitotemporal gyrus (OTG), and the parahippocampal gyrus (PHG). A cortisectomy is made where the suction tip is, medial to OTG and along the rhinal sulcus (RS). (**b**) PHG is aspirated until the temporal horn of the lateral ventricle is opened, exposing the hippocampus. (**c**) Upon entry of the temporal horn, the head, body, and tail of the hippocampus next to the collateral eminence (CE) are identified and aspirated. (**d**) The hippocampus and PHG are resected until the collateral trigone (CT) is reached. Care is taken not to damage the lateral geniculate body (LGB) and CE. (**e**) After the resection depth has been reached, the structures of MTL including the uncus are removed in a subpial manner. (**f**–**h**) The views of MTL with a 0° endoscope after complete resection of MTL. The medial and close up (**f**), the lateral and superficial (**g**), and the extradural views of MTL (**h**). The optic tract, crus cerebri, oculomotor nerve, middle cerebral artery (MCA), posterior cerebral artery (PCA), and anterior choroidal artery (AChoA) are observed over the pia. The lateral neocortex of the temporal lobe is preserved after complete resection of MTL

Case Example

A 16-year-old male patient presented with a history of generalized seizures at the clinic. T2-weighted magnetic resonance imaging (MRI) showed a well-circumscribed and non-enhancing mass in the left MTL (Fig. 18.4a–d). Histological diagnosis was positive for an isocitrate dehydrogenase (IDH)-mutant World Health Organization (WHO) grade II astrocytoma, and a gross-total resection was performed by ETOA without any manipulation or injury to the lateral neocortex including the Meyer's loop. The postoperative course was unremarkable for any visual field deficits or hemiparesis (Fig. 18.4e–h).

The key steps of the surgery were as follows:

During the extra-dural stage of the surgery, GWS underneath the temporalis muscle was drilled until the muscle fascia was exposed. The drilling continued until the SOF, IOF, and the temporal bases were reached to expose the frontal and temporal dura completely (Fig. 18.5a–c). The MOB holding the temporal dura to the temporal base was cut for the lateral mobilization of MTL and minimization of orbital retraction (Fig. 18.5b). The natural line of sight pointed directly to MTL after the dural opening (Fig. 18.5d). For the intradural stage of the surgery, the white matter of PHG was aspirated after identifying OTG and PHG (Fig. 18.5e). A subpial resection of PHG was per-

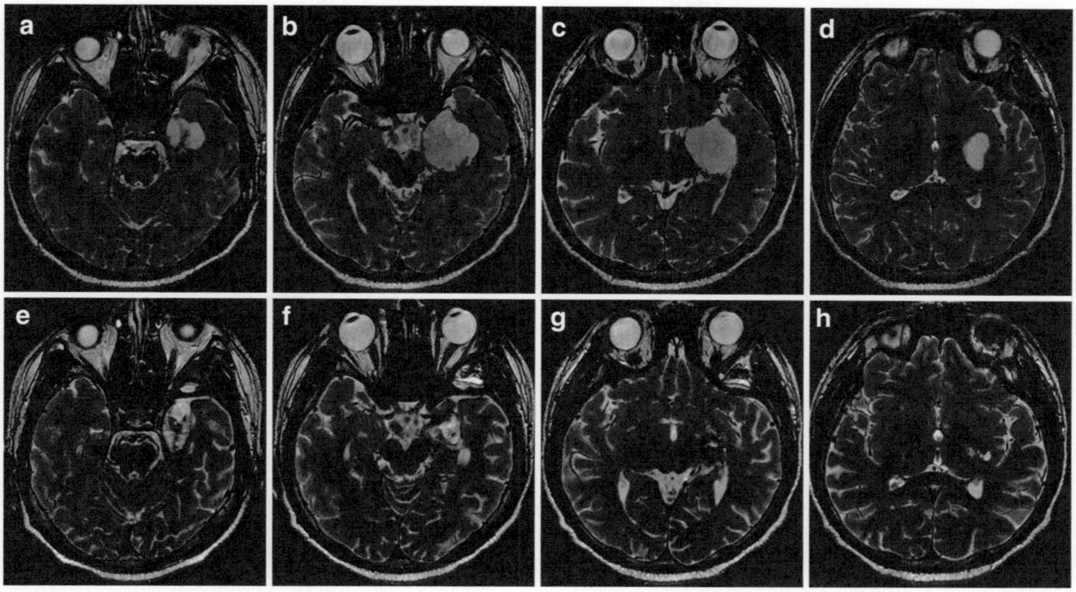

Fig. 18.4 Pre- (**a**–**d**) and postoperative (**e**–**h**) T2-weighed axial MR images of ETOA for an isocitrate dehydrogenase (IDH)-mutant World Health Organization (WHO) grade II astrocytoma, exclusively located in MTL

formed until the Sylvian and ambient cisterns were reached (Fig. 18.5f–h). The temporal horn of the lateral ventricle was exposed after resecting PHG, the head, and the body of the hippocampus (Fig. 18.5i, j). Subpial resection of MTL including the amygdala (Fig. 18.5k) could preserve the neurovascular structures within the ambient cistern (Fig. 18.5l). Bleeding control was performed with surgicel and fibrin glue (Fig. 18.5m). For closure, the dura was approximated with nonabsorbable suture after inlay artificial dura (Fig. 18.5n). The dural defect was reinforced with onlay artificial dura (Fig. 18.5o) and fleece-coated fibrin glue patch (Fig. 18.5p).

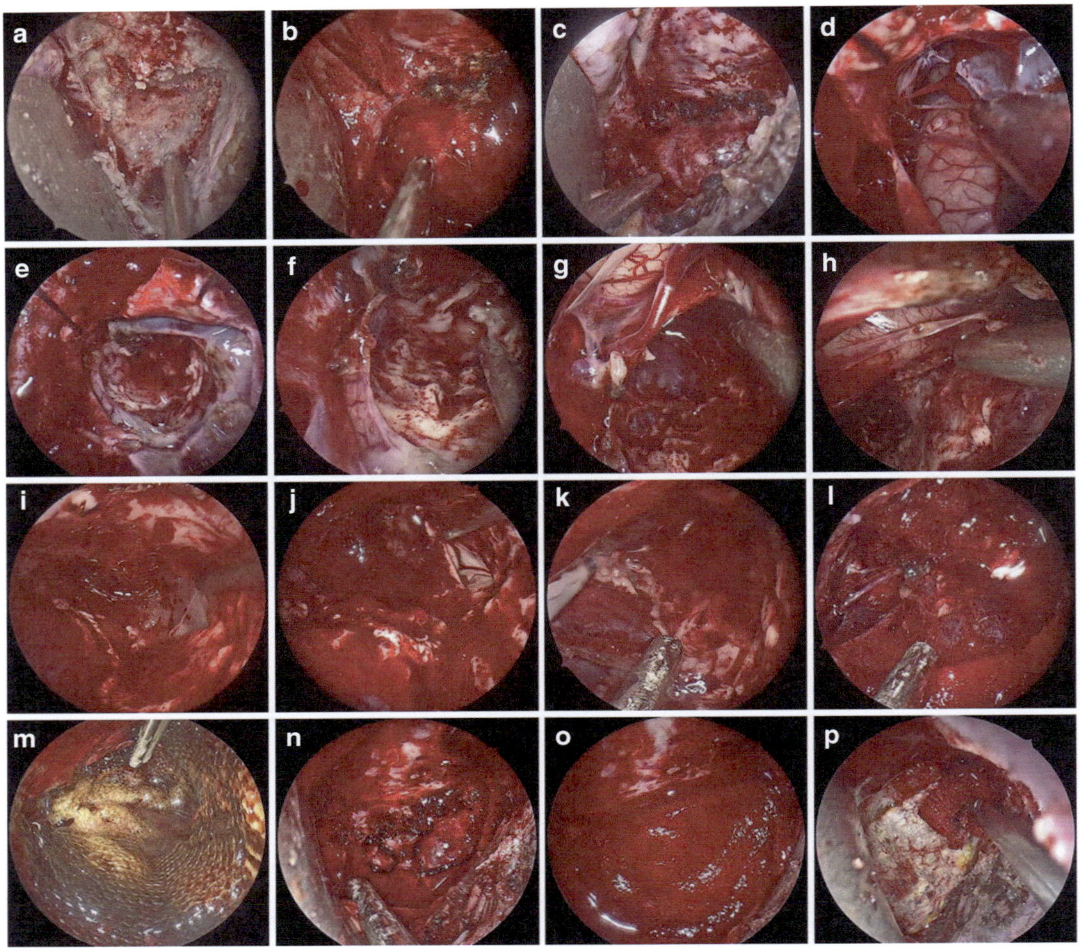

Fig. 18.5 Intraoperative photographs of the surgical steps to MTL. (**a**–**c**) Drilling of GWS until exposure of the frontal and temporal dura. (**b**) MOB cut to mobilize MTL and reduce orbital retraction. (**d**) Natural line-of-sight pointing at MTL after dural opening. (**e**–**h**) Subpial resection of MTL over the Sylvian and ambient cisterns. (**i**, **j**) Opening of the temporal horn after resection of PHG and hippocampus. (**k**, **l**) Resection of the amygdala and MTL, preserving the neurovascular structures within the ambient cistern. (**m**–**p**) For closure, bleeding control with surgicel and fibrin glue (**m**), dural approximation with suture and inlay artificial dura (**n**), and dural reinforcement with onlay artificial dura (**o**) and fleece-coated fibrin glue patch (**p**)

Tips and Tricks to Avoid Complications

Maneuver

There is a lack of surgical freedom for ETOA, even compared to the most minimally invasive transcranial approach under the cadaveric setting [9]. The reduced instrument maneuverability of ETOA requires the surgeon to be more precautious than in a transcranial approach when performing a subpial resection of MTL near the ambient and Sylvian cisterns. PCA injury during subpial dissection of the tumor can occur and vascular injury in an endoscopic surgery with a limited surgical window is not easy to control.

Bleeding Control

There is difficulty in determining the surgical depth and handling of the bipolar electrocautery for any endoscopic surgery. Therefore, an adequate surgical corridor for temporary clipping and direct compression should always be obtained, and dissection should be performed following standard microsurgical principles, on top of classic endoscopic endonasal maneuvers. Hemostasis should be achieved with readily available hemostatic matrix and absorbable oxidized regenerated cellulose, but not heavily relied upon. ETOA for intra-axial lesions should be performed by those who have previous experience in both microsurgical and endoscopic endonasal techniques and ample training with cadaveric specimens.

Cerebrospinal Fluid (CSF) Leaks

A CSF leak is not a major concern for ETOA, unlike EEA [6–8]. Despite the unavailability of a nasoseptal flap in ETOA, dural approximation with in- and onlay artificial dura substitute and reinforcement with fleece-coated fibrin glue patch is effective enough to prevent a CSF leak [6–8]. However, CSF leaks do occur, so care should be taken with the reconstruction. A CSF leak after ETOA could be easier to solve than EEA with continuous lumbar drainage and/or additional abdominal fat graft reinforcement since pressure from the orbit itself serves as a buttress that facilitates dural healing.

Orbital Injury

Visual loss as a consequence of orbital injury after ETOA has not been reported to date. Extensive drilling of GWS and lateral mobilization of MTL by cutting the MOB minimizes the need for orbital retraction. Quantitative measurement of intraocular pressure is essential, and studies are underway for the optimization of orbital retraction during ETOA [10].

Enophthalmos

A wedge-shaped piece of polymerized absorbable buttress can be placed over the orbital wall defect to prevent postoperative enophthalmos.

References

1. Cappabianca P, Cavallo LM, Esposito F, De Divitiis O, Messina A, De Divitiis E. Extended endoscopic endonasal approach to the midline skull base: the evolving role of transsphenoidal surgery. Adv Tech Stand Neurosurg. 2008;33:151–99. https://doi.org/10.1007/978-3-211-72283-1_4.
2. Castelnuovo P, Dallan I, Battaglia P, Bignami M. Endoscopic endonasal skull base surgery: past, present and future. Eur Arch Otorrinolaringol. 2010;267:649–63. https://doi.org/10.1007/s00405-009-1196-0.
3. Kasemsiri P, Carrau RL, Ditzel Filho LF, Prevedello DM, Otto BA, Old M, et al. Advantages and limitations of endoscopic endonasal approaches to the skull base. World Neurosurg. 2014;82:S12–21. https://doi.org/10.1016/j.wneu.2014.07.022.
4. Kalinin P, Sharipov O, Kutin M, Fomichev D, Gavrjushin A, Polev G, et al. Amygdalohippocampectomy via the lateral extended transsphenoidal endoscopic approach through the pterygopalatine fossa: an anatomic study. World Neurosurg. 2017;103:457–64. https://doi.org/10.1016/j.wneu.2017.04.052.
5. Park HH, Ronconi D, Hanakita S, Watanabe K, Labidi M, Bernat AL, et al. Endoscopic endonasal approach to the mesial temporal lobe: anatomical study and clinical considerations for a selective amygdalohippocampectomy. Acta Neurochir. 2020;162:881–91. https://doi.org/10.1007/s00701-019-04163-1.
6. Park HH, Hong SD, Kim YH, Hong CK, Woo KI, Yun IS, et al. Endoscopic transorbital and endonasal approach for trigeminal schwannomas: a retrospective multicenter analysis (KOSEN-005). J Neurosurg. 2020;133:467–76. https://doi.org/10.3171/2019.3.JNS19492.
7. Park HH, Yoo J, Yun IS, Hong CK. Comparative analysis of endoscopic transorbital approach and extended mini-pterional approach for sphenoid wing meningiomas with osseous involvement: preliminary surgical results. World Neurosurg. 2020;139:e1–12. https://doi.org/10.1016/j.wneu.2020.01.115.
8. Yoo J, Park HH, Yun IS, Hong CK. Clinical applications of the endoscopic transorbital approach for various lesions. Acta Neurochir. 2021; https://doi.org/10.1007/s00701-020-04694-y.
9. Noiphithak R, Yanez-Siller JC, Revuelta Barbero JM, Cho RI, Otto BA, Carrau RL, et al. Comparative analysis of the exposure and surgical freedom of the endoscopic extended minipterional craniotomy and the transorbital endoscopic approach to the anterior and middle cranial fossae. Oper Neurosurg (Hagerstown). 2019;17:174–81. https://doi.org/10.1093/ons/opy309.
10. Kim W, Moon JH, Kim EH, Hong CK, Han J, Hong JB. Optimization of orbital retraction during endoscopic transorbital approach via quantitative measurement of the intraocular pressure—[SevEN 006]. BMC Ophthalmol. 2021;21:76. https://doi.org/10.1186/s12886-021-01834-5.

19 Endoscopic Transorbital Approach for the Insular Tumors

Eui Hyun Kim

Insular Gliomas

The insula is an anatomical structure seated deep inside the Sylvian fissure. Although it has been associated with sensorimotor processing, socio-emotional processing, and cognitive functions, the insula is one of the least understood regions of the brain [1]. Insular gliomas are one of the most common pathologies found in this region [2]. Maximal resection is essential for better survival outcomes in both low- and high-grade gliomas [3]. Increased anatomical knowledge, advances in microsurgical technique, and functional mapping have contributed to the improvement of surgical outcomes for insular gliomas. However, surgical removal of insular gliomas still remains a major challenge [4–7].

Insular gliomas can be approached through the Sylvian fissure (trans-Sylvian approach) or through the frontal and temporal operculum (transcortical approach). While the surgical approach is selected based on the dominance of the brain, the extent of the tumor, and the surgeon's preference, these lateral approaches and their combinations can result in significant postoperative morbidity. The most vulnerable structure encountered during surgical resection is the middle cerebral artery (MCA) and its branches. Injury of the long insular perforating arteries is frequently associated with infarction in the corona radiata, which results in serious contralateral motor dysfunction [8].

E. H. Kim (✉)
Department of Neurosurgery, Yonsei University College of Medicine, Seoul, South Korea

Brain Tumor Center, Endoscopic Skull Base Center, Severance Hospital, Seoul, South Korea
e-mail: euihyunkim@yuhs.ac

Anatomical Considerations

The classical transcranial approach for resection of insular gliomas requires a large opening with wide exposure of the frontal and temporal lobes. On the other hand, insular tumor can be approached in a less invasive manner using ETOA. The long axis of the insula is in the anterior-to-posterior direction. ETOA is more advantageous considering its approach trajectory is in alignment with the long axis of the insula (Fig. 19.1).

Another important advantage of ETOA is that the MCA and its branches are less likely to be violated compared with in conventional lateral approach through a standard craniotomy. M2 and its branches cover the lateral surface of the insula tumor, and the risk of vasospasm in the MCA and its branches can be one of the most devastating complications during surgical resection of the insular tumors using transcranial lateral approaches [9, 10]. In ETOA, the tumor removal starts at the most anterior side, where a safe window can be found between M2 and its branches

T. H. Schwartz et al. (eds.), *Endoscopic Transorbital Surgery of the Orbit, Skull Base and Brain*,
https://doi.org/10.1007/978-3-031-59504-2_19

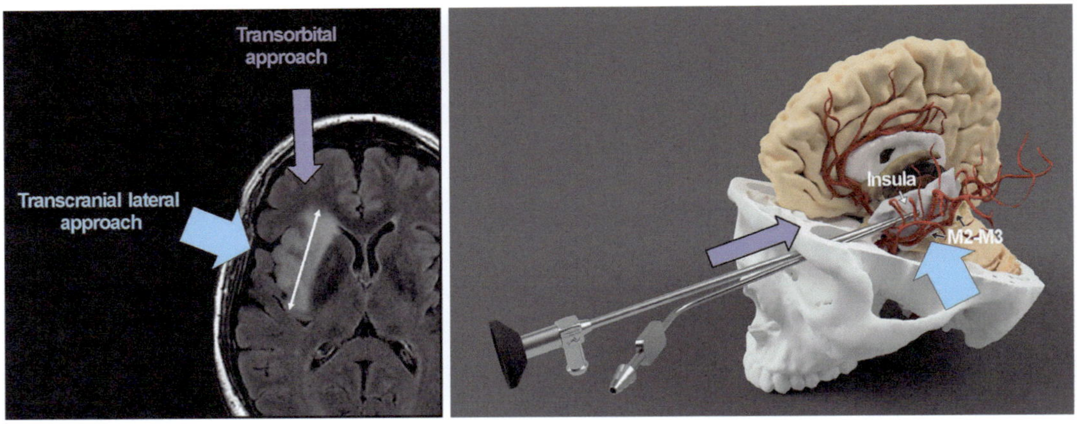

Fig. 19.1 Schematic illustration of the endoscopic transorbital approach (ETOA, purple arrow) in contrast to transcranial lateral approaches (blue arrow) in an axial view of FLAIR magnetic resonance and in a three-dimensional model

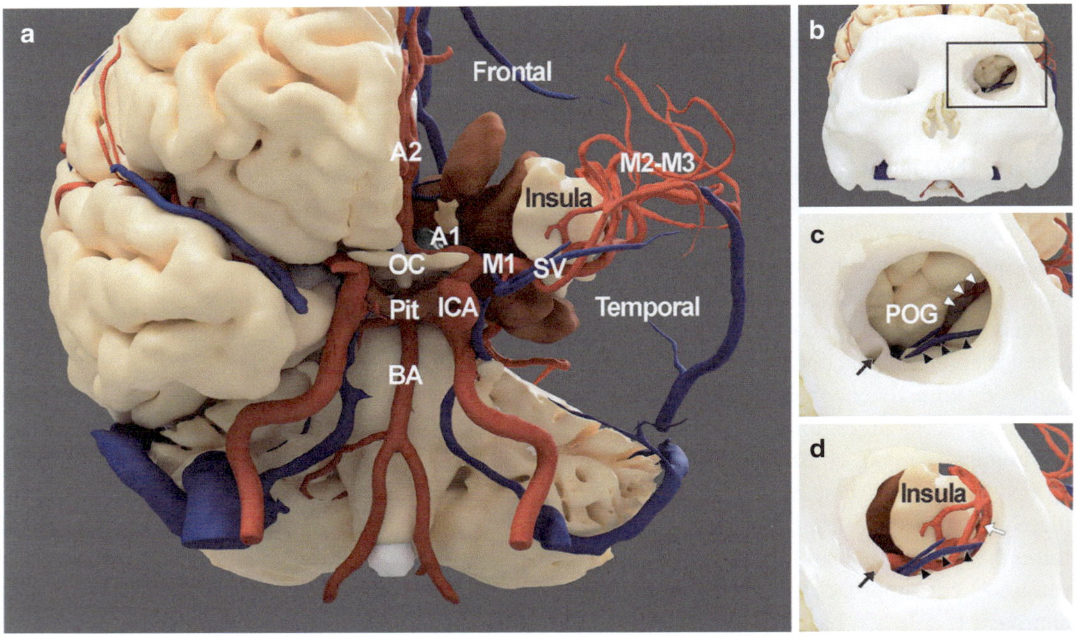

Fig. 19.2 Endoscopic transorbital approach (ETOA) and its relevant neurovascular anatomical structures in a three-dimensional model. (**a**) The front view of a brain shows the three-dimensional anatomical relationship between insular and middle cerebral artery (MCA) and its branches. Most of MCA and its branches run along the inferior and lateral surface of the insula. (**b**) After superior and lateral orbital wall are removed, frontal and temporal lobes are exposed. At the medial margin, a medial end of superior orbital fissure (black arrow) is identified. (**c** and **d**) Posterior orbital gyrus is located above the Sylvian vein (black arrow heads) in the Sylvian fissure (white arrow heads) hindering the accessibility to the insula under EOTA. After posterior orbital gyrus is removed, anterior surface of insular is exposed, where a small window can be made without violation of MCA and its branches. *BA* basilar artery, *ICA* internal carotid artery, *OC* optic chiasm, *Pit* pituitary gland, *POG* posterior orbital gyrus, *SV* Sylvian vein

laterally and the lenticulostriate arteries arising medially from proximal M1 [11]. After tumor removal commences, the lateral margin of the tumor can then be removed in a subpial dissection with minimal chance of violating M2 and its branches (Fig. 19.2).

Advantages of ETOA in the Resection of Insular Gliomas

- The insula is a structure with an elongated shape along the anteroposterior axis, which is similarly aligned with the axis of the ETOA.
- The lateral part of an insular glioma can be removed in a subpial manner, which minimizes violation of MCA and its branches.

Surgical Technique

The ETOA was performed as described in the previous literature [12]. Heads were placed in a supine position with more extension than usually required for conventional ETOA in order to enhance accessibility to the frontal region. A skin incision was made along the lateral part of the eyelid and extended to the lateral orbital rim. The orbicularis oculi muscle was incised parallel to its fibers and retracted. The undersurface of the muscle was dissected until the orbital rim and the fronto-zygomatic sutures were identified. After lateral orbitotomy, subperiosteal dissection was performed circumferentially along the orbital wall and deep into the orbital apex. The periorbita was gently retracted medially and inferiorly together with its intraorbital contents using a malleable retractor system. During dissection, the meningolacrimal artery was identified and cut. The sphenoid bone was drilled out with a high-speed electrical drill, which was extended down to the inferior orbital fissure and above the superior orbital fissure. Excision of the meningo-orbital band greatly facilitated orbital retraction and generated a much more spacious working area. Extensive drilling was continued until the lateral sphenoid ridge was completely drilled out with wide exposure of the frontal and temporal dura.

A vertical dural incision was made crossing the dural fold at the level of the sphenoid ridge, and then dural cuff was retracted with several sutures. The Sylvian fissure covered by thick arachnoid membrane was exposed. The overlying arachnoid membrane was opened preserving the Sylvian vein. After opening the anterior ramus of the Sylvian fissure, the M2 segment of the MCA was first identified. As Sylvian dissection was extended medially along the M2 segment of the MCA, the bifurcation and lateral lenticulostriate arteries were identified. Then, the M2 segment was traced along the surface of the insula posterolaterally with dissection of the Sylvian fissure. Between the lateral lenticulostriate artery and the vertical part of the M2 segment of the MCA, a small window was made on the posterior orbital gyrus. The safe entry point into the insula was not covered by the M2 segment of the MCA, unlike its lateral surface that was crowded with M2 and its major branches. Subpial resection of the insula was performed using an ultrasonic aspirator. Without violation of the M2 and its branches, the insula was removed effectively and safely.

Case Illustration

A 59-year-old male patient was referred for a glioma pathologically proven by stereotactic biopsy. Magnetic resonance imaging (MRI) confirmed a non-enhanced tumor mass in the right insula in continuity with the medial temporal lobe via temporal stem (Fig. 19.3). The patient was right-handed and did not show any neurological signs. The possibility of surgical resection under ETOA was tested by preoperative three-dimensional simulation and found to be feasible. A 3-cm long skin incision was made along the right upper eyelid crease with lateral extension. After incision of the orbicularis oculi muscle, the periosteal layer was exposed and separated from the lateral orbital rim and wall. The outer surface of the frontal branch of the zygoma was also separated from the temporalis muscle. After a large piece of lateral orbit was removed, the periorbital layer was further dissected deep into the orbit and lifted from the superior and lateral orbital wall. Then, the greater wing of the sphenoid bone was extensively drilled out with exposure of the frontal and temporal dura. The lesser wing of the

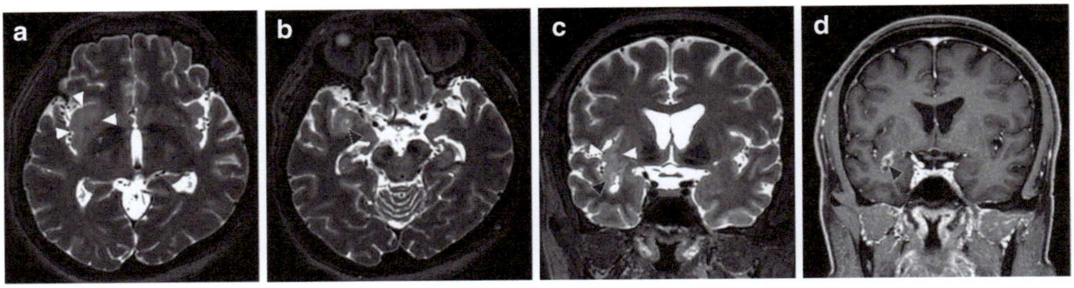

Fig. 19.3 Preoperative magnetic resonance imaging. (**a**–**c**) T2-weighted axial and coronal images show diffuse infiltrative glioma (white arrow heads) in the right insula and medial temporal lobe. (**d**) T1-weighted coronal image revealed that temporal part of the tumor is enhanced with contrast media (black arrow heads)

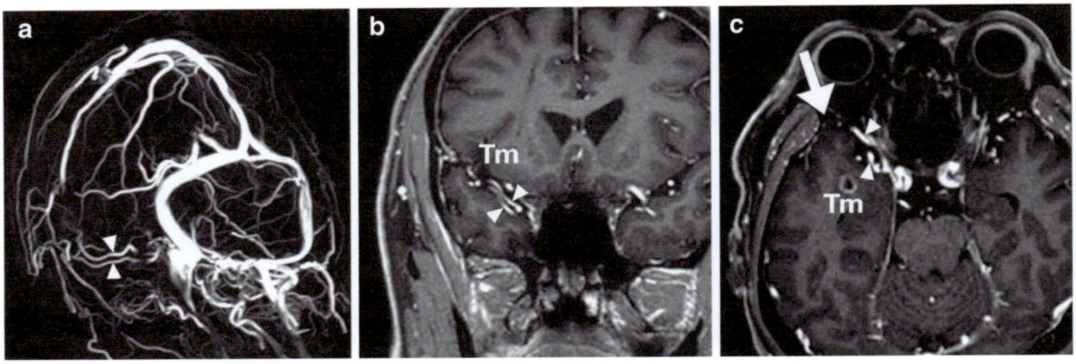

Fig. 19.4 The presence of sphenoparietal sinus is evaluated by magnetic resonance imaging. (**a**) Magnetic resonance venography shows two major Sylvian veins (white arrow heads) running medially. (**b**) These two Sylvian veins run far medially without merging to dural sinus at the level of sphenoid ridge. (**c**) Owing to the absence of prominent sphenoparietal sinus, surgical corridor to the insula is safely secured under endoscopic transorbital approach (white arrow). *Tm* tumor

sphenoid (sphenoid ridge) was also carefully drilled out completing wide dural exposure. Meningo-orbital band was coagulated and cut to more retract the periorbita from the orbital wall generating more sufficient surgical working space. As the sphenoparietal sinus was not developed in this patient as confirmed by preoperative MRI venogram, the dural layer was safely incised from the frontal to the temporal vertically crossing sphenoid ridge dura, and its leaflets were retracted with several sutures (Fig. 19.4). After identifying the Sylvian veins, the arachnoid membrane was opened just above not to injure Sylvian veins. The MCA bifurcation was identified at the medial margin.

The posterior orbital gyrus was localized with the aid of neuro-navigation system, which was partially removed until the anterior surface of the insula tumor was exposed (Fig. 19.5). After identification of a safe window at the anterior tumor surface, several tiny vessels were coagulated, and small cortisectomy was done to make an entry point. After checking tumor consistency, tumor removal was continued by using an ultrasonic aspirator. We first identified the medial margin of the tumor with exposure of the grey matter, which was extended posteriorly. Motor-evoked potential with subcortical mapping [13] was frequently performed to estimate the distance from the internal capsule. After we reached the posterior margin of the tumor along the medial border, then the main tumor mass was removed safely. The most lateral part of the tumor was removed with subpial dissection and the M2, and its branches were not violated during tumor removal (Fig. 19.6).

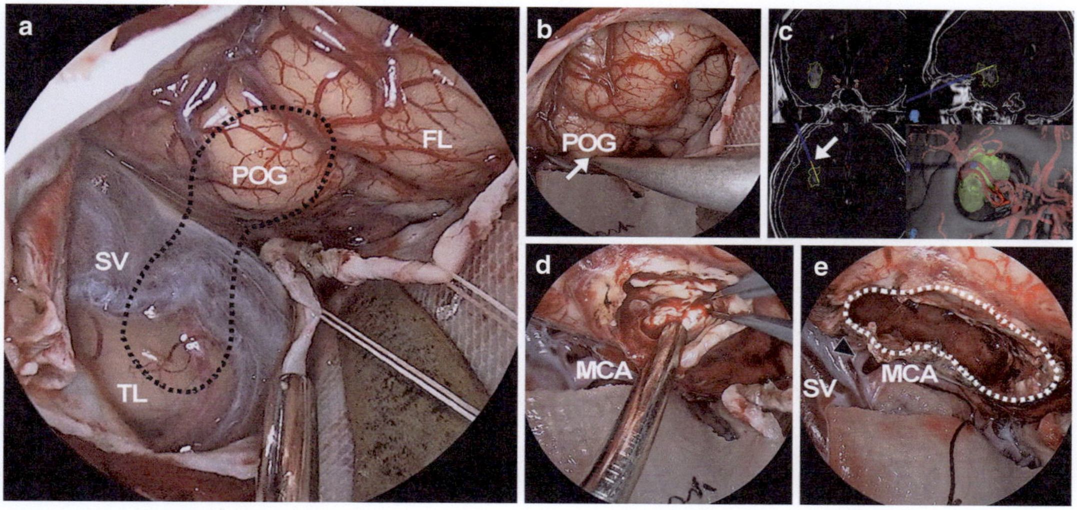

Fig. 19.5 Intradural procedure during endoscopic transorbital approach (ETOA) for right insular glioma. (**a**) After dural opening, frontal and temporal lobe are exposed. Imaginary boundary of tumor in the insula and medial temporal lobe is marked (black dotted line). Posterior orbital gyrus is located above the Sylvian vein and middle cerebral artery in the Sylvian fissure and occupies the surgical route to the insula under ETOA. (**b** and **c**) Posterior orbital gyrus is localized in the aid of neuro-navigation system. The neuro-navigation system demonstrates that the navigation probe (white arrow) is aiming at the insula. (**d** and **e**) Posterior orbital gyrus is removed (white dotted line) until anterior surface of insula is fully exposed. *FL* frontal lobe, *MCA* middle cerebral artery, *POG* posterior orbital gyrus, *SV* Sylvian vein, *TL* temporal lobe

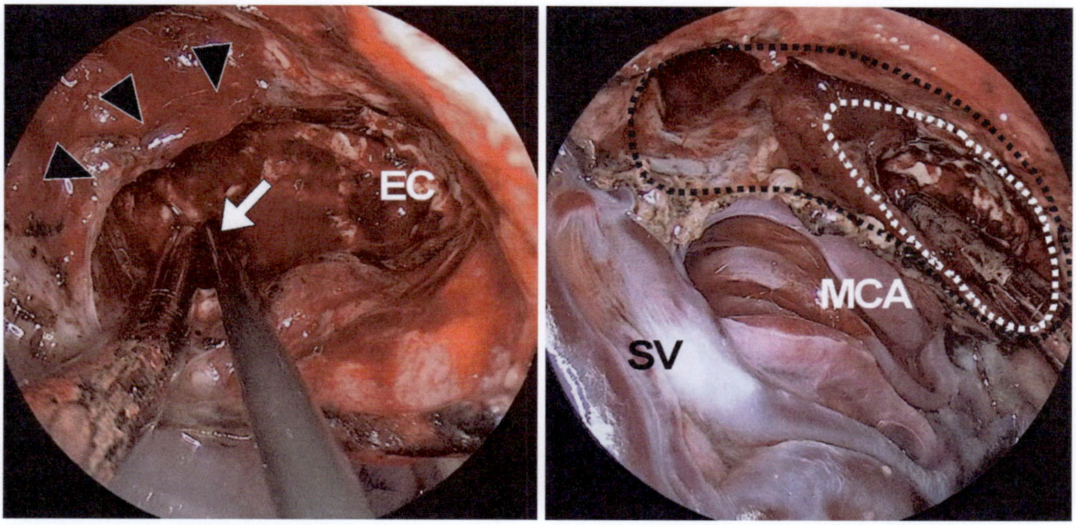

Fig. 19.6 Removal of insular tumor under endoscopic transorbital approach. (Left) After removal of the majority of the tumor, cortical spinal tract is localized under monopolar stimulation for subcortical mapping (white arrow). Most of overlying pial layer at the lateral surface of insular tumor is well preserved after tumor removal in a subpial manner (black arrow heads). (Right) After tumor removal, resection margin of insular tumor is marked (white dotted line), while the resection margin of posterior orbital gyrus is more anteriorly located (black dotted line). *EC* extreme capsule, *MCA* middle cerebral artery, *SV* Sylvian vein

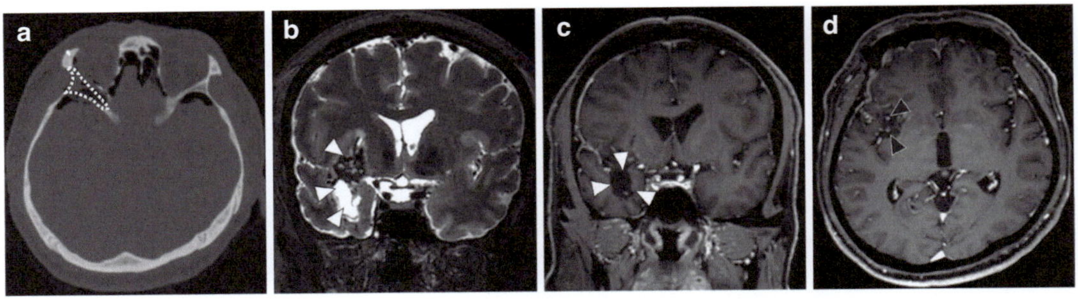

Fig. 19.7 Postoperative computed tomography (CT) scan and magnetic resonance imaging (MRI). (**a**) Axial view of CT scan demonstrates the extent of bony removal of the greater sphenoid wing. Postoperative MRI shows gross total removal of the tumor (white arrow heads) in the right insular and medial temporal lobe in immediate postoperatively (**b**) and 1 month after surgery (**c** and **d**). The middle cerebral artery branches that used to overlie the insular tumor are well preserved (black arrow heads)

The medial temporal pole was then partially removed until we reached and exposed the tumor. Neuro-navigation-guided localization was critical during the entire procedure. Tumor in the temporal lobe was removed in the same manner as in the insula. At the medial margin of the tumor, subpial dissection was performed not to violate the oculomotor nerve and adjacent vascular structures. After complete removal of the tumor, we further resected the temporal lobe in the lateral and posterior direction to maximize the extent of resection. The temporal horn of the lateral ventricle was opened and sealed with gelfoam and fibrin glue. After meticulous hemostasis, the dural layer was closed, and the lateral orbital wall was reconstructed. Complete removal of the insular tumor was verified with early postoperative MRI (Fig. 19.7). The patient showed no neurological deficits after surgery. The final diagnosis was WHO grade 4 astrocytoma IDH-wild type with TERT mutation. The patient underwent chemoradiotherapy with temozolomide and had been stable until the tumor recurred at 13 months after the initial surgery. Despite chemotherapy with temozolomide and bevacizumab, the patient expired 24 months after the initial surgery.

Tips and Pitfalls

Although ETOA has several potential advantages, not all insular gliomas are amenable to ETOA. We believe that anteriorly located small insular tumors are most suitable to ETOA. Using the Berger-Sanai classification scheme [5], tumors in Zone I (anterosuperior) and IV (inferolateral) are the best indications of ETOA, whereas tumors in Zone II (posterosuperior) and III (infero-posterior) may be more effectively accessed by a transcranial approach. Insular gliomas frequently extend to the frontal and temporal lobes. As in the case demonstrated, temporal lobe extension could be easily accessed through an ETOA as demonstrated by Park et al. [14]. However, depending on the frontal extension of the tumor, its extent and size should be carefully discussed before ETOA is attempted.

The posterior orbital gyrus is associated with executive behavior and cognition, where the inferior fronto-occipital fasciculus and uncinate fasciculus are located. In general, partial resection of the posterior orbital gyrus rarely results in significant neurological deficits [15, 16]. In our cases, all patients had insular gliomas in their nondominant hemispheres and thus were not at risk of any language deficit after surgery. However, it should be verified whether resection of the posterior orbital gyrus in the dominant side might lead to a neurological deficit. With more extensive orbital rim removal through an eyebrow incision [17], a retractor system could be inserted deep into surgical field, which helps to preserve posterior orbital gyrus to expose the insula.

During endoscopic procedures, safety should be a greatest concern because maneuverability of surgical instruments is generally limited. Fine dissection and bleeding control may not be comparable to those that can be achieved through classical transcranial approaches. Especially, in glioma resection, tectile sense delivered through the ultrasonic aspirator is extremely important to differentiate tumor tissue from normal brain parenchyma. It is critical to obtain maximal working space to overcome the inborn limitation of ETOA, and we believe lateral and even superior orbitotomy is critical, as has been demonstrated by many other groups [18, 19].

Presurgical vascular assessment is also essential for ETOA. Lateral lenticulostriate arteries arise from the proximal MCA, usually from the M1 segment and more rarely from the post-bifurcation or M2 segment. It is known that the most lateral lenticulostriate arteries are located about 15.3 mm medial to the limen insulae [20], which becomes more spacious in the presence of insular tumors and thus serves as a safe entry zone to the insular region. However, the presurgical assessment of the MCA anatomy is essential for ETOA. In cases in which early branches of the MCA significantly diminish accessibility to the insular region, ETOA may not be a good choice of approach. The sphenoparietal sinus is also one of the major vascular structures encountered during ETOA. The sphenoparietal is located inferior to the posterior aspect of the lesser wing of the sphenoid bone. It receives venous flow from the middle meningeal vein, Sylvian vein, and anterior temporal vein and ends in the anterior part of the cavernous sinus [21]. While the most indicated skull base tumors for ETOA such as a meningioma generally obliterate their underlying venous sinuses, the sphenoparietal sinus may be prominent, and its sacrifice under ETOA could also result in brain swelling. The presence of prominent sphenoparietal sinus should be evaluated by conventional angiography or MRI venography preoperatively.

Summary

ETOA is a potentially promising approach for accessing the insular region. Using this minimally invasive approach, an insular tumor was effectively accessed and removed without retraction of the frontal and temporal operculum. ETOA is the only surgical corridor through which the MCA and its branches are not directly violated in performing subpial dissection of the tumor and, thus, offers a unique advantage. Although not all insular tumors can be removed through the ETOA, it may serve as a good surgical route to reach the insula in selective cases. Careful case selection and meticulous presurgical evaluation are essential.

References

1. Uddin LQ, Nomi JS, Hebert-Seropian B, Ghaziri J, Boucher O. Structure and function of the human insula. J Clin Neurophysiol. 2017;34(4):300–6.
2. Tang Q, Lian Y, Yu J, Wang Y, Shi Z, Chen L. Anatomic mapping of molecular subtypes in diffuse glioma. BMC Neurol. 2017;17(1):183.
3. Roh TH, Park HH, Kang SG, Moon JH, Kim EH, Hong CK, et al. Long-term outcomes of concomitant chemoradiotherapy with temozolomide for newly diagnosed glioblastoma patients: a single-center analysis. Medicine (Baltimore). 2017;96(27):e7422.
4. Duffau H, Moritz-Gasser S, Gatignol P. Functional outcome after language mapping for insular World Health Organization Grade II gliomas in the dominant hemisphere: experience with 24 patients. Neurosurg Focus. 2009;27(2):E7.
5. Hervey-Jumper SL, Li J, Osorio JA, Lau D, Molinaro AM, Benet A, et al. Surgical assessment of the insula. Part 2: Validation of the Berger-Sanai zone classification system for predicting extent of glioma resection. J Neurosurg. 2016;124(2):482–8.
6. Moshel YA, Marcus JD, Parker EC, Kelly PJ. Resection of insular gliomas: the importance of lenticulostriate artery position. J Neurosurg. 2008;109(5):825–34.
7. Skrap M, Mondani M, Tomasino B, Weis L, Budai R, Pauletto G, et al. Surgery of insular nonenhancing gliomas: volumetric analysis of tumoral resection, clinical outcome, and survival in a consecutive series of 66 cases. Neurosurgery. 2012;70(5):1081–93; discussion 93–4.
8. Delion M, Mercier P. Microanatomical study of the insular perforating arteries. Acta Neurochir. 2014;156(10):1991–7; discussion 7–8.
9. Schaller C, Jung A, Clusmann H, Schramm J, Meyer B. Rate of vasospasm following the transsylvian versus transcortical approach for selective amygdalohippocampectomy. Neurol Res. 2004;26(6):666–70.
10. Schaller C, Zentner J. Vasospastic reactions in response to the transsylvian approach. Surg Neurol. 1998;49(2):170–5.
11. Kim EH, Yoo J, Jung I-H, Oh JW, Kim J-S, Yoon JS, et al. Endoscopic transorbital approach to the insular region: cadaveric feasibility study and clinical application (SevEN-005). J Neurosurg. 2021;135(4):1164–72.

12. Moe KS, Bergeron CM, Ellenbogen RG. Transorbital neuroendoscopic surgery. Neurosurgery. 2010;67(3 Suppl Operative):ons16–28.
13. Shiban E, Krieg SM, Haller B, Buchmann N, Obermueller T, Boeckh-Behrens T, et al. Intraoperative subcortical motor evoked potential stimulation: how close is the corticospinal tract? J Neurosurg. 2015;123(3):711–20.
14. Park HH, Roh TH, Choi S, Yoo J, Kim WH, Jung I-H, et al. Endoscopic transorbital approach to mesial temporal lobe for intra-axial lesions: cadaveric study and case series (SevEN-008). Oper Neurosurg. 2021;21(6):E506–15.
15. Burks JD, Conner AK, Bonney PA, Glenn CA, Baker CM, Boettcher LB, et al. Anatomy and white matter connections of the orbitofrontal gyrus. J Neurosurg. 2018;128(6):1865–72.
16. Conner AK, Briggs RG, Sali G, Rahimi M, Baker CM, Burks JD, et al. A connectomic atlas of the human cerebrum—Chapter 13: Tractographic description of the inferior fronto-occipital fasciculus. Oper Neurosurg (Hagerstown). 2018;15(Suppl_1):S436–S43.
17. Lim J, Sung KS, Kim W, Yoo J, Jung I-H, Choi S, et al. Extended endoscopic transorbital approach with superior-lateral orbital rim osteotomy: cadaveric feasibility study and clinical implications (SevEN-007). J Neurosurg. 2021;137(1):18–31.
18. Nagm A, Ogiwara T, Hirouchi T, Hongo K. Comparative analysis between lateral orbital rim preservation and osteotomy for transorbital endoscopic approaches to the cavernous sinus: an anatomic study. Oper Neurosurg. 2019;16(1):E37.
19. Noiphithak R, Yanez-Siller JC, Revuelta Barbero JM, Otto BA, Carrau RL, Prevedello DM. Comparative analysis between lateral orbital rim preservation and osteotomy for transorbital endoscopic approaches to the cavernous sinus: an anatomic study. Oper Neurosurg. 2019;16(1):86–93.
20. Tanriover N, Rhoton AL Jr, Kawashima M, Ulm AJ, Yasuda A. Microsurgical anatomy of the insula and the sylvian fissure. J Neurosurg. 2004;100(5):891–922.
21. Tubbs RS, Salter EG, Wellons JC III, Blount JP, Oakes WJ. The sphenoparietal sinus. Oper Neurosurg. 2007;60(Suppl_2):9–12.

Part VI

Skull Base Pathology: Anterior Fossa

Transorbital Neuroendoscopic Correction of Skull Base Trauma, CSF Leaks, and Abscesses

20

Kris S. Moe

Introduction

This chapter will discuss transorbital neuroendoscopic repair of anterior and middle cranial fossa trauma, as well as the treatment of causally related cerebrospinal fluid (CSF) leaks and infectious processes. As will be demonstrated, these conditions are interrelated anatomically and conceptually. Our approach to orbital fractures not involving the ACF has been described in detail in other sources [1, 2] and will not be discussed herein; likewise, temporal bone trauma is beyond the scope of this book.

There are a number of concerns in managing trauma in this region. The first, and most important, is damage to the frontal and temporal lobes of the brain. Surgical intervention in the regions of the brain adjacent to the skull base is less commonly undertaken for correction of subdural and epidural hemorrhages than in other locations. Damage to the brain parenchyma in these locations is, when indicated, typically treated by an open approach such as a frontal or pterional craniotomy or decompressive craniectomy. Another indication is for debridement and correction of herniation into the paranasal sinuses to prevent meningitis, abscess, and other sinus complications which are discussed below. An additional concern is pneumocephalus/CSF leak. While tension pneumocephalus can certainly be life-threatening and may require emergent treatment [3], the concern with non-tension pneumocephalus is related less to the presence of intracranial air than to the concomitant dural defect and CSF leak which raises the risk of meningitis. However, a large volume CSF leak also carries a risk of brainstem herniation into the foramen magnum. Vision-related issues are also common with trauma in this area. These can manifest as diplopia, visual loss, or blindness. Though these conditions may require surgical correction, they are not typically indications for emergent surgery.

It is often stated that skull base reconstruction is required for re-establishment of "compartmentalization" of the various structures involved. This may not always be the case. While dural defects exposed to the paranasal sinuses in the interorbital skull base require repair due to the risk of cerebritis, abscess, and CSF leak in a contaminated environment, dural lacerations overlying the orbital skull base (particularly those overlying orbital periosteum) may not need repair.

Another location in which the need for reconstruction may be controversial is frontal sinus fractures. Earlier policy was that posterior table fractures displaced greater than the thickness of the cortical bone should repaired due to the risk

K. S. Moe (✉)
Division of Facial Plastic Surgery, Departments of Otolaryngology and Neurological Surgery, University of Washington School of Medicine, Seattle, WA, USA
e-mail: krismoe@uw.edu

T. H. Schwartz et al. (eds.), *Endoscopic Transorbital Surgery of the Orbit, Skull Base and Brain*,
https://doi.org/10.1007/978-3-031-59504-2_20

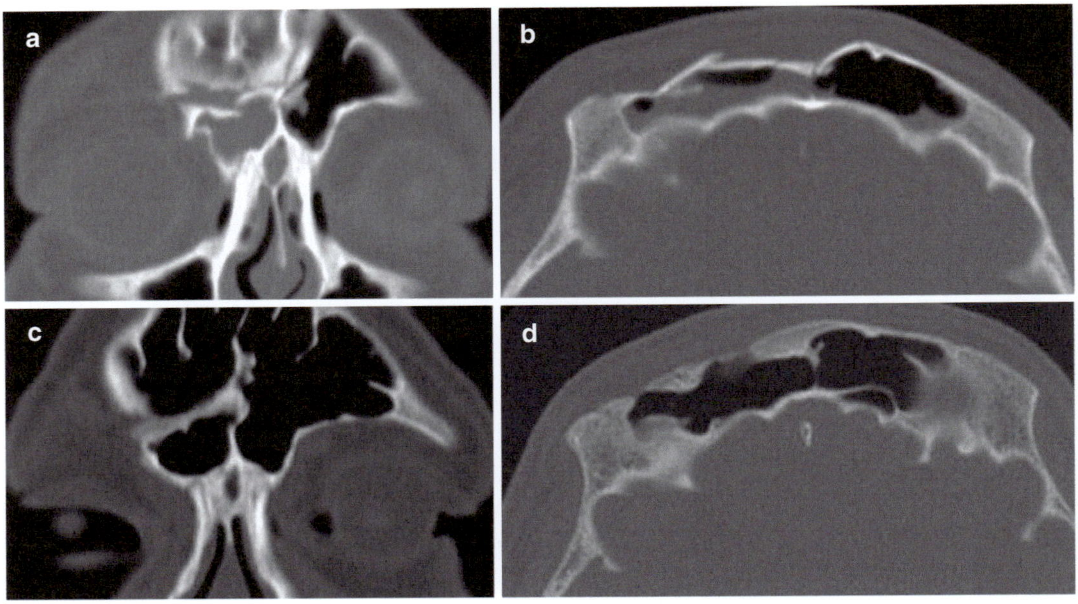

Fig. 20.1 CT scan: spontaneous remodeling of frontal sinus fractures. (**a**) Coronal image at time of injury. (**b**) Axial image at time of injury. Note anterior wall fracture with opacification of the right side. (**c**) Coronal image 3 months after injury. (**d**) Axial image 3 months after surgery. Note complete aeration of the frontal sinus bilaterally, with return of bone fragments to near-normal position

of intracranial mucocele formation. Similarly, classic teaching has been that displaced anterior table fractures should be repaired to prevent frontal sinus mucoceles. However, experience has shown that fractures not obstructing the frontal sinus outflow tract, including minimally displaced fractures of the tract itself, may be managed conservatively. Furthermore, mildly displaced anterior wall fractures may remodel spontaneously, particularly in young patients (Fig. 20.1) [4, 5].

There is also controversy regarding repairing or replacing the bone of the orbital roof when it has been removed due to trauma or tumor. Some surgeons are concerned that failure to reconstruct this area may result in permanent pulsatile exophthalmos. We have found, however, that the majority of the bone of the orbital roof or greater wing of the sphenoid can be removed without disturbance. Pulsatile exophthalmos, if it occurs, typically resolves in 1–2 weeks without residual sequelae. Thus, the need for "compartmentalization" is, in our experience, limited mostly to the requirement of repair of lacerated dura or major vasculature when exposed to the paranasal sinuses. We therefore favor a more nuanced consideration of the requirement for reconstruction, considering whether the defect will cause a functional or visually significant compromise.

Open vs. Endoscopic Repair

The choice of an open vs. endoscopic strategy for skull base trauma depends on many of the same factors that are considered in tumor surgery as discussed in Chap. 1. A primary issue is whether wide-field exposure is required. This may be the case with widespread damage with extensive dural laceration for which a large pericranial flap is needed. Another indication for an open approach is severe fractures with displaced, comminuted bone fragments requiring extensive elevation and repositioning with internal fixation. In some instances, fracture reduction may require moderate force in a vector that is challenging to provide endoscopically. In addition, placement of multiple craniofacial fixation plates can be challenging with an endoscopic approach. While titanium mesh fixation is possible endoscopically, this may require transcutaneous screw placement which is time- and labor-intensive and may provide little benefit over an open trichophytic or coronal approach.

An endoscopic approach is often the procedure of choice for more limited regions of trauma. From a technical perspective, endoscopy provides improved illumination, magnification, and viewing on multiple monitors for the entire surgical team to observe [2]. The reduced pathway volume requirements also allow less retraction of critical structures.

Transnasal endoscopic approaches have long been used to address fractures of the interorbital skull base with CSF leak when a locoregional flap or graft is deemed adequate for the repair. Transorbital approaches expand this domain to the remainder of the ACF and anterior regions of the MCF. They have an added advantage in their superiority of visualization and access for orbital trauma repair (Fig. 20.2).

An endoscopic repair is advantageous in that the approach creates little additional trauma; it may be less likely to propagate areas of dural injury that inadvertently expand during a craniotomy and thus allow a more limited repair; and the postoperative recovery may be more rapid, depending on the underlying injury. Details on the techniques and approaches of transorbital endoscopic surgery are covered in Chap. 1.

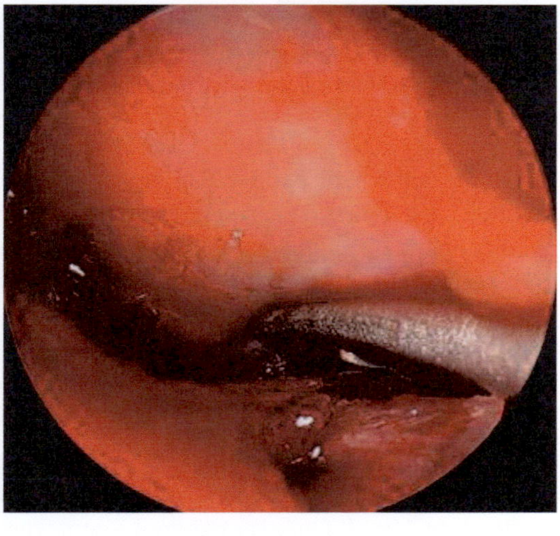

Fig. 20.2 Endoscopic photograph of fracture of the apex of the left orbital floor. Suction elevator raising periorbita at the posterior extent of the fracture. Note the large optical cavity and excellent retraction of orbital contents allowing full visualization of critical structures

Transorbital Endoscopic Ligation or Cauterization of the Ethmoid Arteries

Control of blood flow through the ethmoid arteries may be important before skull base tumor surgery or to control epistaxis related to trauma, anticoagulation, or other causes. While angiography with embolization can be very effective for occluding blood flow in many regions of the skull base, this cannot be performed on the ethmoid arteries. While transnasal endoscopic ligation of the ethmoid arteries is possible, this can be challenging due to their coverage by mucosa, as well as the need to access them in confined spaces at the skull base. Furthermore, tumors within the nasal cavity may obstruct access to these vessels. And if an ethmoid artery contracts into the orbit while working from a transnasal approach, it may continue to bleed and cause a vision-threatening retrobulbar hematoma/compartment syndrome.

For these reasons, a transorbital endoscopic approach may be a favorable alternative. There are actually usually three or more ethmoid arteries [6] (anterior, middle, and posterior), all of which can easily be accessed through a precaruncular medial transorbital approach [7]. They can also be approached through the medial aspect of a superior quadrant pathway (Chap. 1). The vessels are located in the fronto-ethmoid suture, which is typically visible as a linear indentation in the superior aspect of the lamina papyracea. When viewed in-line, they form a trajectory that points posteriorly toward the optic canal (Fig. 20.3).

Once the vessels are located, they can be cauterized with narrow bipolar forceps and divided, or a small clip can be placed across the pedicle. When addressing the posterior ethmoid artery, it is essential to dissect several millimeters behind the pedicle to visualize the optic nerve entering the canal. This is critical to ensure that cauterization is not performed near the optic nerve. Lower voltage cautery may be used posteriorly, and the

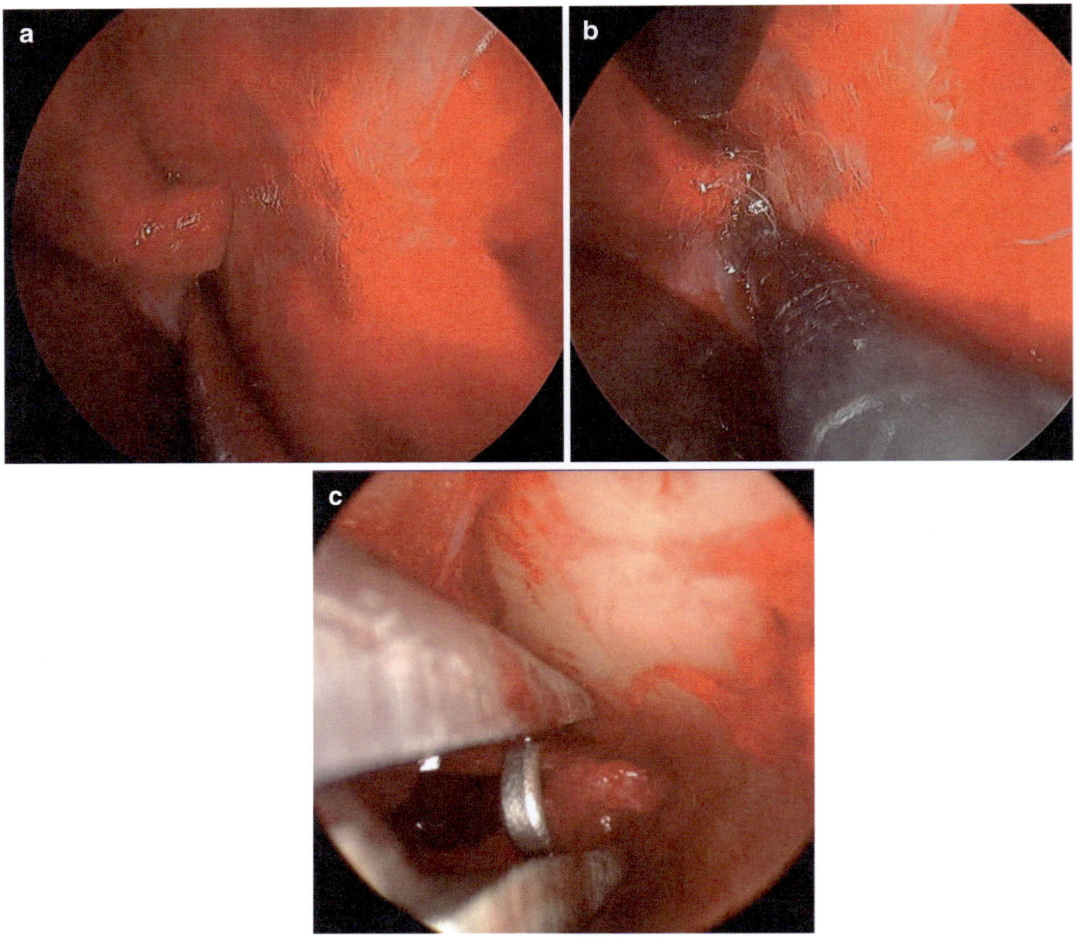

Fig. 20.3 Right anterior ethmoid neurovascular pedicled viewed through a medial transorbital approach. (**a**) Isolation of the pedicle with orbital contents displaced laterally using malleable retractor; (**b**) cauterization of pedicle with bipolar forceps; (**c**) alternative placement of vessel clip across pedicle

vessel can be grasped and retracted anteriorly before cauterizing. Once this aspect of the procedure is completed, there is usually no need for closure of the conjunctival incision.

Trauma of the Orbit and Optic Nerve

Penetrating trauma involving the orbit requires detailed cooperation with an ophthalmologist, and any persistent foreign body should be left in place until a full evaluation is performed and a plan is agreed upon. A detailed examination should be performed including the condition of the optic nerve and extraocular muscles when possible. A CT or CT/angiography scan should be obtained, with angiography as indicated. If the dura is likely to be involved, a neurological surgeon should be consulted.

When practical, the foreign body is removed under endoscopic visualization with standby capability of open craniotomy and immediate angiography available. The approach is chosen as outlined in Chap. 1. Once the material is removed, examination of the involved orbital/skull base bone is performed. Control of any hemorrhage or CSF leak is undertaken. Displaced orbital bone is usually removed rather than replaced, to prevent the risk of displacement during the healing period. Should disruption of the globe or extraocular muscles be noted, these are repaired by the ophthalmology service.

An orbital fracture involving the greater wing of the sphenoid or orbital roof is typically repaired only if the involved bone is displaced to the extent that it causes dysfunction of the extraocular muscles (diplopia) or significant globe displacement (exophthalmos more commonly than enophthalmos in this region). A variance of globe position of up to 2 mm is considered within the range of normal on exophthalmometry (Chap. 1), and displacement greater than this should be corrected if it is bothersome to the patient and the globe has not been damaged. We typically delay surgery for 1–2 weeks after injury to allow resolution of edema.

Surgical correction involves removal of the displaced bone through the appropriate approach. Typically, when bone is displaced enough to cause this degree of proptosis, it is removed rather than repositioned to prevent recurrence. However, if the bone is not fragmented and returns easily into normal position, it may be preserved (Fig. 20.4). With orbital roof fractures, great caution must be undertaken to be certain that the bone fragment is not attached to the optic nerve or internal carotid artery. If there is significant dural damage adjacent to the fracture, any herniating frontal lobe tissue should be gently debrided, and hematoma should be evacuated. A layer of dural substitute can then be placed over defects in the dura. If there is significant exposure of the underlying levator muscle, a layer of thin (0.25 mm) polydioxanone (PDS) sheet can be placed intra- or extracranially across the bone defect to prevent adherence.

Fractures of the greater wing of the sphenoid result only with very significant force due to the thickness of the bone. They are thus often associated with additional fractures of the temporal bone, zygomaticomaxillary complex, or other craniofacial regions. In addition, these injuries often cause considerable transfer of force to the orbital contents thereby risking injury to those structures. As with orbital roof fractures, these fractures are not treated unless there is a functional or significant esthetic compromise (proptosis). The treatment of these fractures varies depending on the presence of other fractures, as well as the comminution of the bone. Similar to orbital roof fractures, the goal is to remove the displaced bone and place a sheet of thin PDS across the defect if needed to prevent interference of function of the lateral rectus muscle that could occur with rough bone edges or abrupt contour changes. If the displaced bone fragment is immobile, the obstructing component may need to be drilled out with a coarse diamond drill or ultrasonic aspirator.

Retrobulbar hematoma One of the most severe complications of an orbital fracture is the formation of a retrobulbar hematoma causing orbital compartment syndrome. This presents with proptosis, retro-orbital pain and visual loss due to optic nerve compression or vascular occlusion. These findings are confirmed on physical examination, along with elevated intraocular pressure. The treatment of this, even if suspected but not proven by imaging, is emergent canthotomy and cantholysis, with consideration given to the use of agents such as carbonic anhydrase and acetazolamide to lower the intraocular pressure. It should be confirmed that the intraocular pressure drops with these measures and an emergent ophthalmology evaluation should be obtained. While imaging may be obtained afterward, treatment should not be delayed for this reason. Once the intraocular pressure is reduced, the ophthalmologist will determine whether to take the patient to the operating room for exploration or elect to carefully observe the patient in the hospital.

Optic nerve decompression is a somewhat controversial topic in the context of traumatic visual loss. Consideration of decompression typically arises when a patient presents with delayed visual loss after trauma, with findings on CT scan of optic nerve compression typically in the optic canal. However, the endoscopic surgical techniques studied in those investigations involved transnasal optic nerve decompression, which is limited to medial and inferior decompression

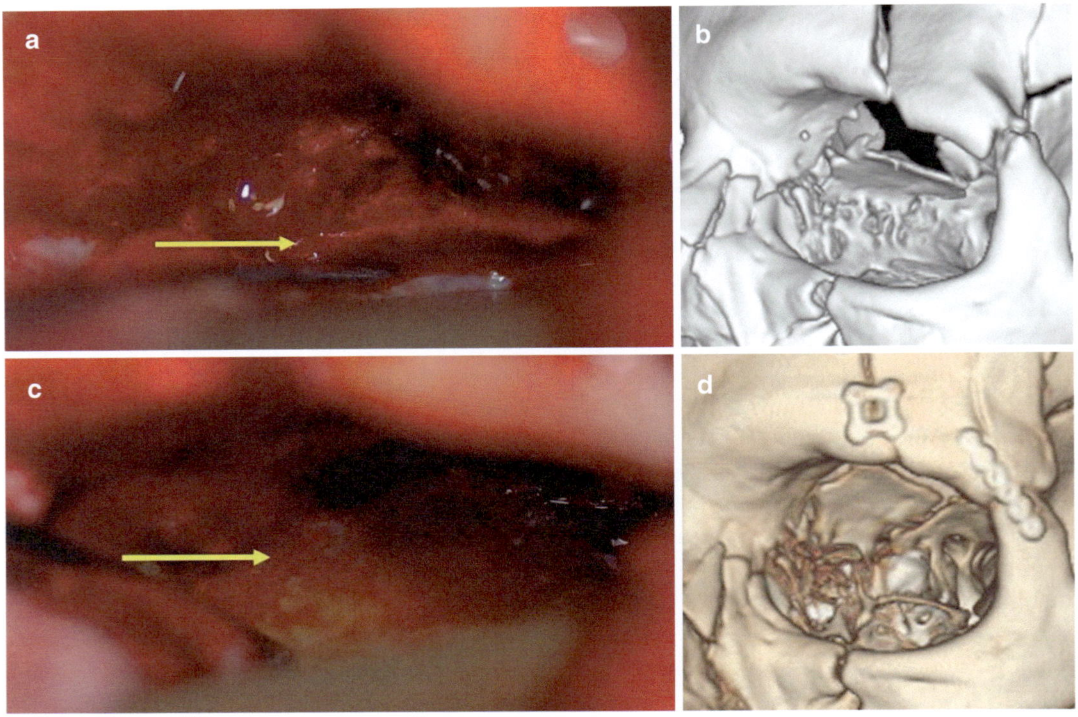

Fig. 20.4 Transorbital endoscopic repair of left orbit roof fracture. (**a**) Photo, arrow demonstrating inferiorly displaced orbital roof fragment. Note herniated brain superior to bone, orbital contents displaced with malleable retractor inferior to bone. (**b**) Coronal CT demonstrating orbital roof fracture. (**c**) Photo, arrow demonstrates repositioned orbital roof bone. (**d**) CT demonstrating postoperative appearance

(180° or less) using a drill. Though a prospective study has not been performed, transorbital endoscopic technique makes possible as much as a 360° decompression possible, opening the entire canal and following the nerve intracranially. Depending on the type of decompression desired, a superior quadrant approach may be undertaken which allows removal of the anterior clinoid, optic strut, roof, and medial and lateral walls of the canal (see Chap. 1, Figs. 1.10 and 1.11). To decompress the inferior canal, addition of an inferior or medial approach may be necessary depending on the location of the underlying fracture. The surgeon may want to add an orbital apex decompression [8] as well, again depending on the location and extent of the fracture(s), which may be done partially through a superior or completely through an inferior approach. Optic sheath fenestration is then undertaken at the discretion of the surgeon, with care to avoid injury to the ophthalmic artery (Fig. 20.5).

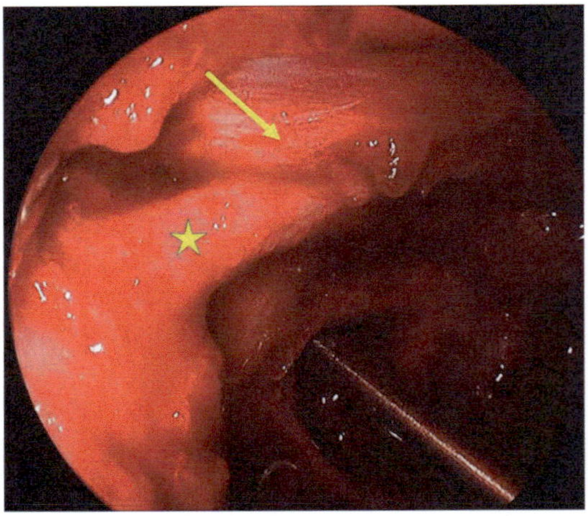

Fig. 20.5 Transorbital decompression of right orbital apex and optic nerve to dural entrance, viewed from contralateral precaruncular approach. Star, optic nerve; arrow, frontal dura. Note the removal of bone surrounding the optic nerve. Instrument points to internal carotid artery. (Decompression performed for oncologic indications)

Frontal Sinus Trauma

There are indications for transorbital repair of trauma of the frontal, ethmoid, and sphenoid fractures. Most ethmoid and sphenoid fractures do not require repair unless there is a CSF leak, and when this is required, it is usually performed with a transnasal endoscopic approach. In severe cases, discussed below in the section on repair of CSF leaks, sphenoethmoid trauma or CSF leak may be corrected transorbitally in order to access the area through a coplanar approach above the cranial base in that the reconstruction material can be placed intracranial-extradurally over a wider area for improved sealing and fixation (see discussion below).

Decision-making in the care of frontal sinus fractures is complex given the multitude of treatment options available. The primary goal of any therapy is to restore a safe frontal sinus that is unlikely to result in intracranial or infectious complications over the patient's remaining lifespan. In addition, the result must be cosmetically acceptable. The traditional management of frontal sinus cranialization (removing the posterior wall, all frontal sinus mucosa, and sealing off the outflow tracts) or obliteration (removing all sinus mucosa but preserving the bone, filling the sinus typically with fat, and obstructing the outflow tracts) has typically been considered to be the safest. However, experienced surgeons have all taken care of long-term complications occurring 20 or more years after these procedures, and thus considerable thought should be given to function-preserving procedures when possible [4, 5].

For minimally displaced anterior wall fractures, particularly in younger patients, a component of auto-reduction may occur as described above. In these cases, a highly satisfactory functional and cosmetic outcome may result without surgical intervention. More severe frontal sinus fractures, particularly those with entrapped bone fragments, may be appropriate for transorbital endoscopic repair. For acute fractures of the anterior sinus wall that are visibly depressed over a limited region, an upper quadrant approach through a blepharoplasty incision can be used to access the floor of the frontal sinus through the floor of the orbital roof. The supratrochlear nerve often courses through the desired surgical pathway. While this is preserved when convenient, it may be transected if it presents a technical challenge, and sensation will typically return to near normal over the ensuing 4–6 months. With the aid of navigation, the optimal location to enter the sinus is chosen, and the bone is drilled with a coarse diamond burr or removed with an ultrasonic aspirator. The sinus is entered, and the fracture is viewed with a 0- or 30° endoscope. Leaving the overlying periosteum intact, the bone fragment is elevated. The position can then be checked against a mirror-image surgical navigation plan using the contralateral normal side as a template (see Chap. 1). For small fractures, elevation may provide adequate therapy as long as the bone appears to remain in reduction. If the bone does not remain in the correct position, or if an element of support is desired, a resorbable sponge can be placed within the sinus to posterior to the displaced bone.

Acute fractures of the posterior wall of the frontal sinus are typically corrected in conjunction with repair of a dural laceration and CSF leak after a trial of nonsurgical therapy. In this case an ipsilateral (or bilateral for increased working space) approach is undertaken, and the frontal sinus is explored. With the aid of navigation as needed, the fractured bone is located. The mucosa is then removed from the fractured and adjacent bone, using radiofrequency aspiration, for full visualization. If the bone of the fracture site is free-floating, it is gently elevated from the underlying dura with a periosteal elevator and removed. If there is a crack but the bone is stable, no further bone is removed, but the adjacent bone is demucosalized (Fig. 20.6). The defect is then covered with a dural substitute if dural is widely exposed, or a dermal substitute. All wrinkles in the implant material are smoothed so that it lays flat. The construct is then covered with fibrin glue. If considerable pulsation is transmitted through the dura, the region is compressed with resorbable sponge for support. The wound is then closed with 5-0 resorbable suture through the orbicularis oculi muscle and 5-0 fast-absorbing interrupted sutures through the skin.

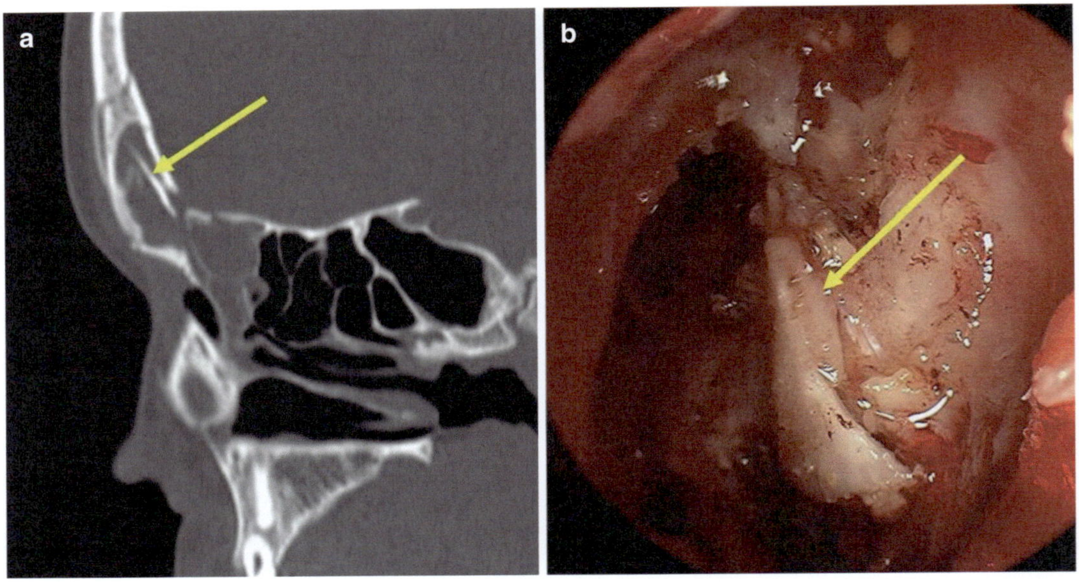

Fig. 20.6 Fracture, posterior table of frontal sinus. (**a**) Sagittal CT scan of fracture; yellow arrow depicts bone fragment seen in photograph. (**b**) Fracture demucosalized, dura exposed with CSF leak visible lateral to bone fragment (same orientation as CT). Photograph taken from left superior lid crease approach across the frontal sinus toward the midline

For acute fractures involving the frontal sinus outflow tract, a decision is made regarding the likelihood of healing with a patent drainage system. If uncertain, the frontal sinus function can be followed with serial CT scans, particularly if the posterior wall is intact. If the posterior wall is unstable and the outflow tract is obstructed, strong consideration should be given to an open repair of the sinus.

Healed fractures of the frontal sinus may also require endoscopic correction if the displaced bone fragments are causing obstruction of sinus drainage. In this situation the displaced bone is removed with a coarse diamond burr or ultrasonic aspirator. In addition, the intersinus septum can be removed with a curved drill to allow the sinus to drain through the contralateral unaffected side. This may be combined with an endoscopic transnasal procedure to widen or join the frontal outflow tracts.

There remain frontal sinus fractures that should be treated with a coronal incision and osteoplastic approach. These include large, comminuted anterior wall fractures that require plating for an acceptable cosmetic outcome. Similarly, extensive posterior wall fractures that are likely to allow mucocele formation with intracranial extension (Fig. 20.7) should be treated with cranialization or obliteration.

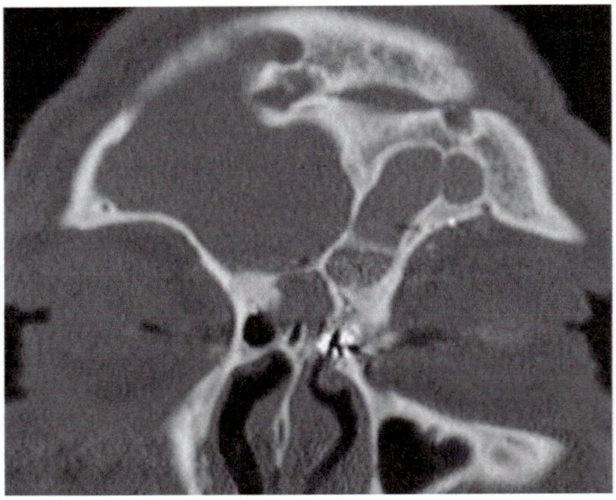

Fig. 20.7 Coronal CT scan demonstrating bilateral frontal sinus outflow obstruction due to trauma from a gunshot wound 35 years prior to presentation. Note the fractures and bullet fragments obstructing the frontal outflow tracts, with bilateral frontal sinus mucoceles and right-sided intracranial extension

Fractures involving the frontal outflow tracts bilaterally should also be treated in this fashion.

CSF Leak Repair

Repair of CSF leak is a common indication for the use of transorbital neuroendoscopic surgery, typically when due to frontal sinus fractures, iatrogenic injury during craniotomy, encephaloceles, and mucoceles. While these are most often used for pathology involving or adjacent to the frontal sinus, they are also applicable to the interorbital skull base—particularly extensive pathology that would be challenging to repair with a transnasal approach using a single septal mucosa flap, for locations that are unfavorable due to challenging visualization and/or working angles and for conditions in which coplanar surgery above and below the skull base is beneficial [3, 9]. In 2011 we presented our initial series of 12 consecutive cases we performed for CSF leaks 50% of which were revisions, with up to five prior procedures [10]. All cases were successful, though one recurred approximately 2 years later and was found to have intracranial hypertension which responded to a ventriculoperitoneal shunt.

To appreciate the applications of transorbital approaches in CSF leak repair, it is important to understand the unique role of the orbit in skull base topography. As can be seen in Fig. 20.8, the orbits relate to the cranial base and frontal sinus with significant curvature. On sagittal view, the anterior orbit ceiling is situated at a higher altitude than the orbital apex. Similarly, the central orbit roof occupies a higher altitude than the interorbital skull base. Furthermore, the orbit roof comprises the floor of the frontal sinus anteriorly. These differences in altitude relative to the skull base can be exploited to create favorable working angles to access regions of the adjacent skull base and brain.

Frontal sinus CSF leaks Transorbital access to CSF leaks related to the frontal sinus is gained through an upper blepharoplasty portal and a superior quadrant approach as described in Chap. 1. Navigation is used to plan the ideal trajectory to the pathology, and the incision is generally centered on that vector.

Once the defect has been identified and adequately exposed, the method of reconstruction is chosen. As these are typically low-pressure leaks, the repair need not be complex. An intradural

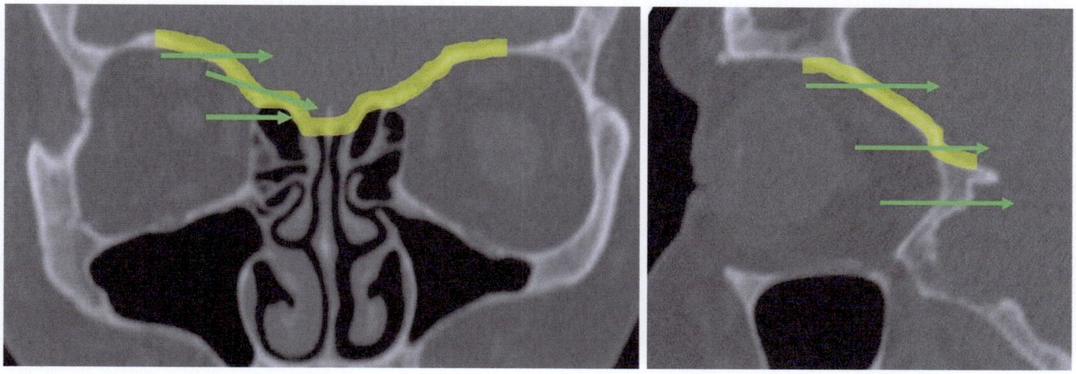

Fig. 20.8 Topography of the medial orbit roof and interorbital skull base, coronal and sagittal CT scan. Yellow highlights demonstrate the complex topography of the orbit roof. Green arrows demonstrate possible pathway vectors. These can be chosen to minimize brain retraction, shorten the approach, or provide synchronous access above and below the skull base

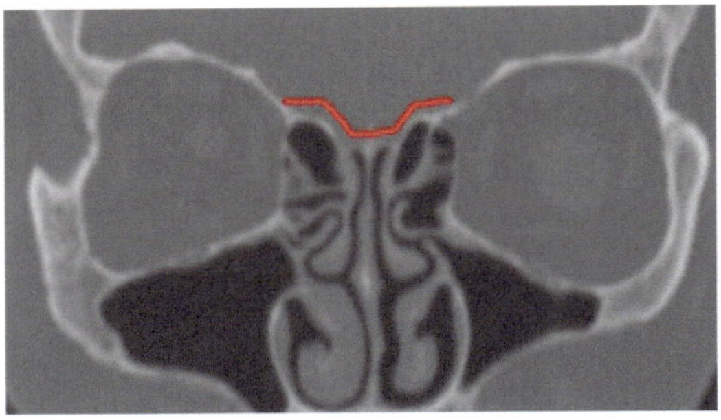

Fig. 20.9 Transorbital placement of dural repair material on the intracranial aspect of the interorbital skull base. Red line represents position of repair material. This can be intradural, extradural, or both, using vectors demonstrated in previous figure

layer of allogenic dura or synthetic graft may be placed, followed by a larger area onlay graft of similar material. This can then be covered with fibrin glue. If desired, a layer of resorbable sponge can be placed to support the construct during healing. For small- to medium-sized sinuses, the remainder of the sinus can be filled with fibrin glue for support.

It is important to consider ipsilateral frontal outflow patency when repairing the defect. Outflow obstruction may occur from chronic sinusitis or posttraumatic bone displacement. In this case, the outflow tract can be surgically enlarged, the intersinus septum can be removed with a diamond drill to allow the sinus to drain out the opposite outflow tract if it is patent, or both measures can be undertaken. It is also important to ensure that reconstruction material (other than resorbables) is not placed where it will obstruct sinus drainage.

Interorbital ethmoid and sphenoid sinus CSF leaks As described above, for large dural defects, particularly those that are bilateral and span the interorbital skull base, a mono- or biportal transorbital repair may be beneficial. Depending on the region of the leak, a medial or superior approach may be chosen based on navigation vector analysis. A craniectomy is then performed in the medial orbital roof superior to the fronto-ethmoid suture. The dura is then elevated off the skull base and the area of dural damage is located. A layer of allogenic dermal graft or dural substitute is then placed across the interorbital skull base and fixated with fibrin glue. The frontal lobes are then allowed to descend onto the construct where they aid in sealing the repair and holding it in place between the dura and bone (Fig. 20.9).

Mucoceles/Mucopyocele

Mucoceles can involve the orbit, frontal sinus, or both. Orbital mucoceles are usually posttraumatic in etiology, though frontal sinus mucoceles may be the result of trauma or other causes that obstruct the sinus outflow tract. When these enlarge, they may involve the adjacent craniofacial compartments (Fig. 20.7).

Orbitofrontal mucoceles may become quite large and erode through the anterior wall of the frontal sinus. They may become infected, becoming mucopyoceles which can then cause osteomyelitis and lead to spread either extra- and/or intracranially. These may expand intracranially to the point that they cause frontal lobe compression [11, 12] (Fig. 20.10).

The portal used for these mucoceles is typically an upper blepharoplasty incision, based on navigation vector analysis as described in Chap. 1 (Fig. 20.11).

When the superior orbit is involved, it is typically due to erosion through the bone of the floor of the frontal sinus. After endoscopic orbital exploration and evacuation and irrigation of the orbital abscess, the defect in the floor of the frontal sinus is enlarged, and the frontal sinus is entered. Purulence is evacuated from the frontal sinus in a similar manner. When an epidural or brain abscess is being treated, there

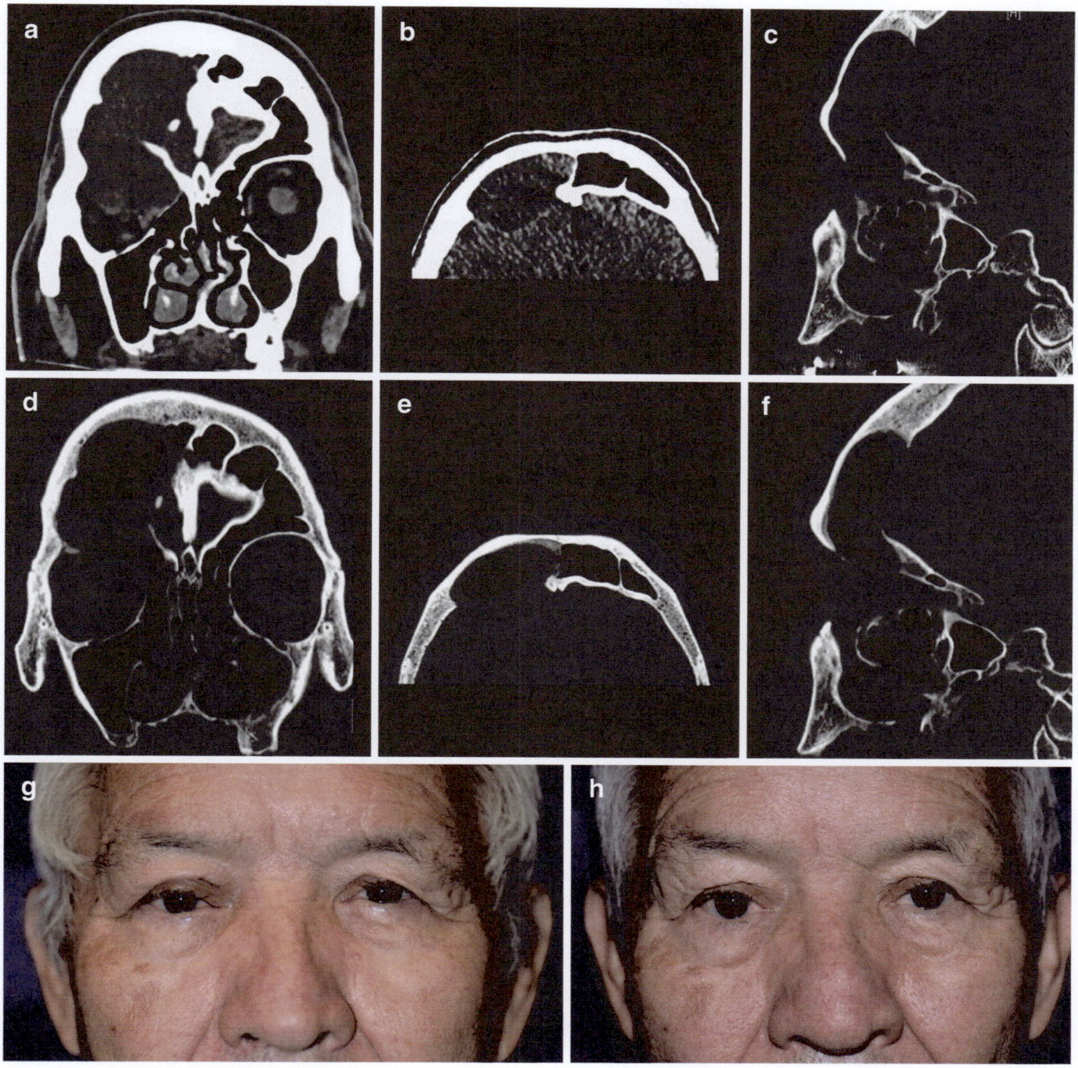

Fig. 20.10 Massive mucocele occupying right orbit and frontal sinus, extending into right frontal lobe. (**a**) Preoperative coronal CT. (**b**) Preoperative axial CT. (**c**) Preoperative sagittal CT. (**d**) Postoperative coronal CT. (**e**) Postoperative axial CT. (**f**) Postoperative sagittal CT. Note in **d** and **f** the resorbing fibrin glue and dissolving sponge. (**g**) Appearance 6 weeks and (**h**) 1.5 years after surgery

is typically a defect in the posterior wall of the frontal sinus. This may not be apparent without palpation of the bone or removal of the overlying mucosa. Once the defect is located, it is followed with the aid of navigation to the targeted pathology. Adequate cranial bone is removed to explore and irrigate the region, ensuring that no region of purulence remains. A small penrose drain may be placed if desired in cases in which there is no CSF leak; this may be externalized through the blepharoplasty incision or placed through the frontal outflow tract or ethmoid sinus into the nasal cavity whence it is eventually be removed.

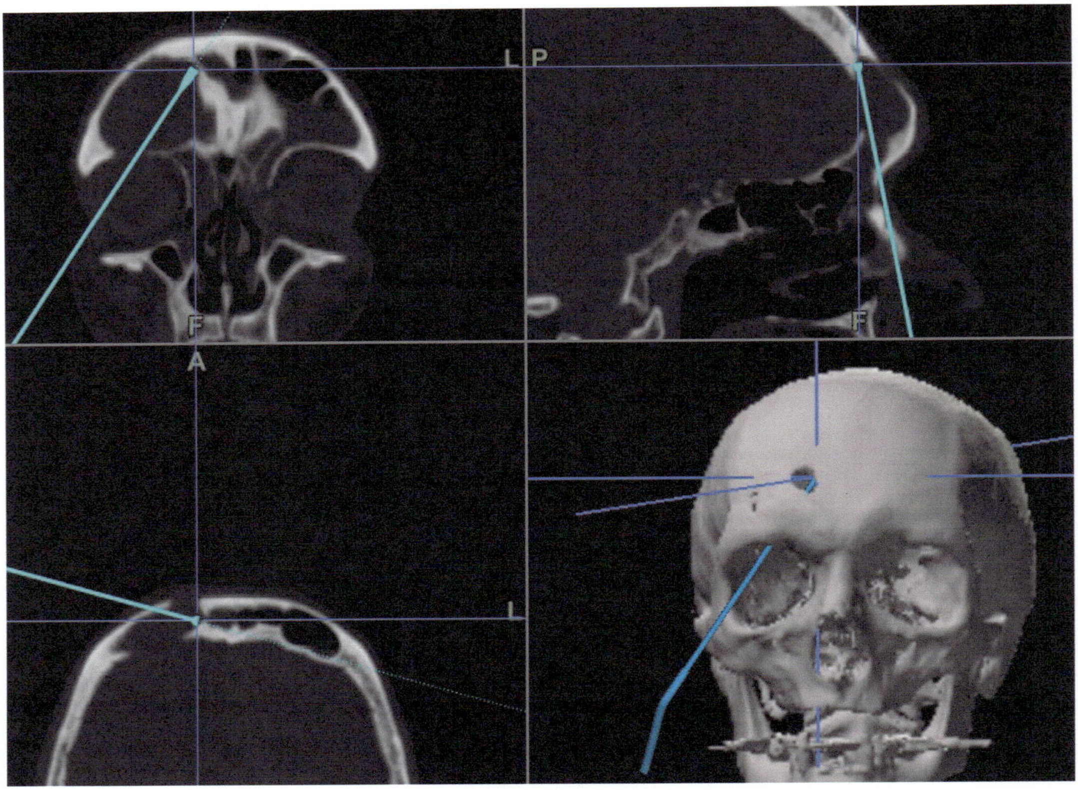

Fig. 20.11 Navigation approach analysis, right orbitofrontal mucocele. Superior transorbital vector is checked to confirm that pathway will allow drainage of orbital and frontal abscess and remove intersinus septum. Note axial CT, lower left, showing absent posterior wall of frontal sinus; lower right three-dimensional reconstruction showing erosion of anterior table of frontal sinus

Reconstruction after treatment of large intracranial mucoceles is a more complex issue. Some of these cause frontal lobe displacement and may push relatively sharp bone edges intracranially (Fig. 20.12). These cases may present with CSF leak due to dural tears from pulsation against the bone, and it is important to take down any concerning bone edges. For cases that do not present with CSF leak, the dura should be carefully inspected and tested with a Valsalva maneuver to rule out an occult leak. After evacuation or the mucocele, the frontal lobe will displace forward into its premorbid position. There have been anecdotal descriptions of hemorrhage thought to be due to vascular injury with frontal lobe migration; placement of a resorbable sponge against the frontal lobe may allow the frontal lobe to expand more gradually.

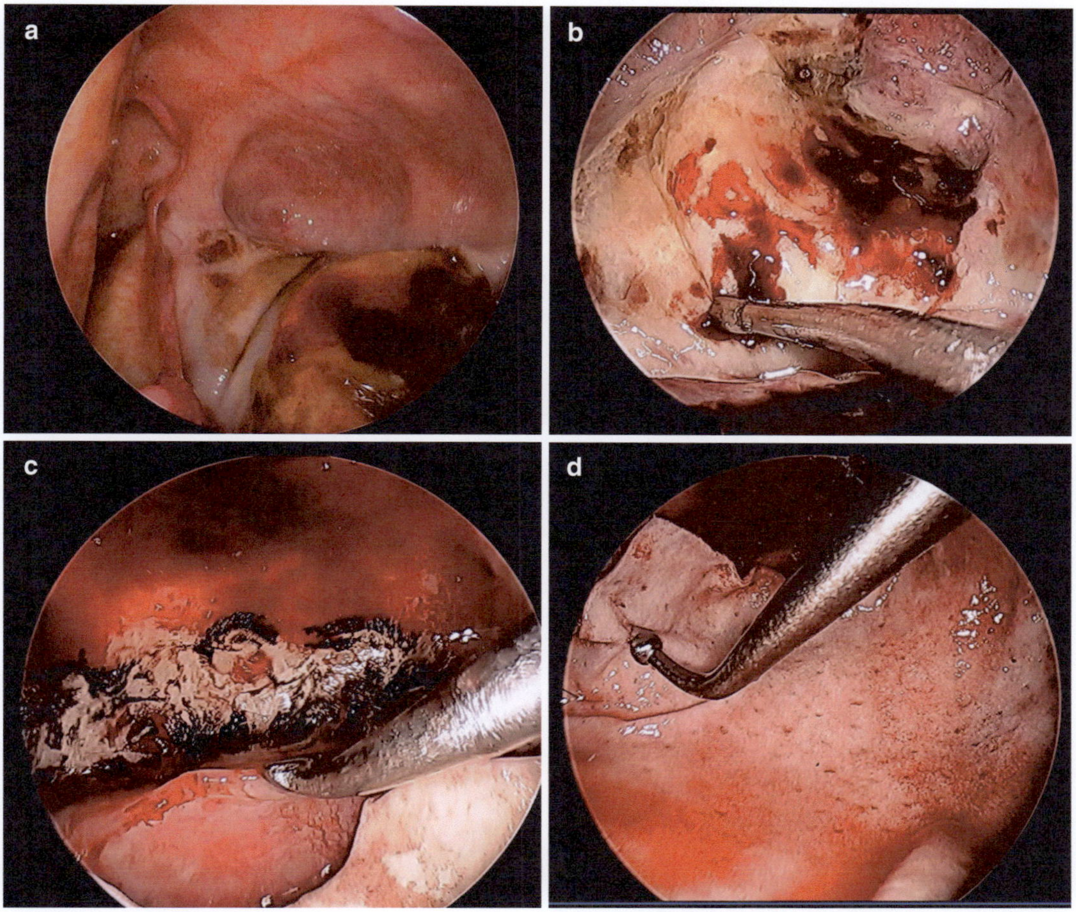

Fig. 20.12 Large right frontal/intracranial mucocele. (**a**) Lateral view through left frontal sinus looking into right frontal sinus. (**b**) Anterior view from ipsilateral superior approach. Note white dura (encephalocele) visible between mucosalized bone above and below. (**c**) Mobile edge of posterior sinus wall has lacerated dura, causing CSF leak. (**d**) Covering entire encephalocele and dural tear with allogenic dermis graft (positioning graft with probe). The graft is then secured with fibrin glue and resorbable sponge

Abscess

Abscesses involving the skull base and brain are usually sinogenic, with similar pathophysiology to that of mucopyoceles. In 2012 we presented a series of 13 patients with sinogenic complications including epidural and orbital abscess with orbital apex syndrome, all who underwent transorbital endoscopic treatment as described above [9]. All procedures were successful without complication or recurrence, and we have subsequently treated frontal lobe abscesses in the same fashion (Figs. 20.13, 20.14, and 20.15).

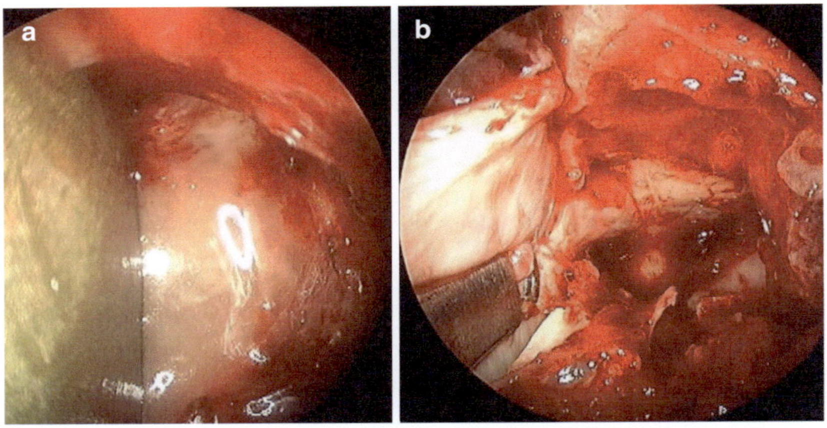

Fig. 20.13 Abscess right medial orbit apex, medial precaruncular approach, endoscopic view. (**a**) Malleable retractor retaining orbital contents, note purulence at apex. (**b**) View after orbit and optic nerve decompression, medial orbital bone removed. Suction freer elevator placed along periorbita points to posterior ethmoid artery and optic nerve

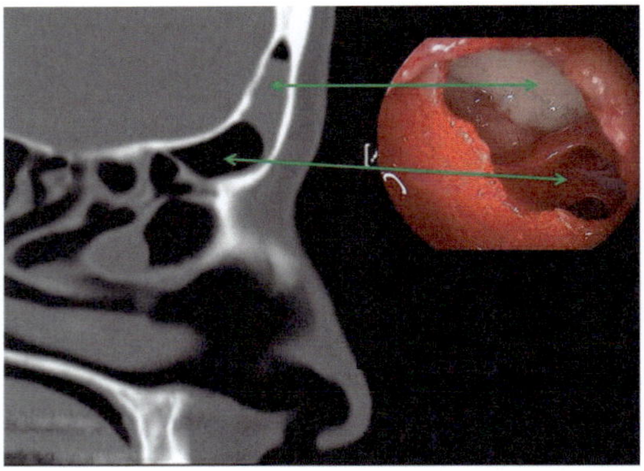

Fig. 20.14 Transorbital view of frontal sinus abscess. Left, CT scan with green arrows pointing to corresponding anatomy on right medial transorbital view of frontal sinus abscess

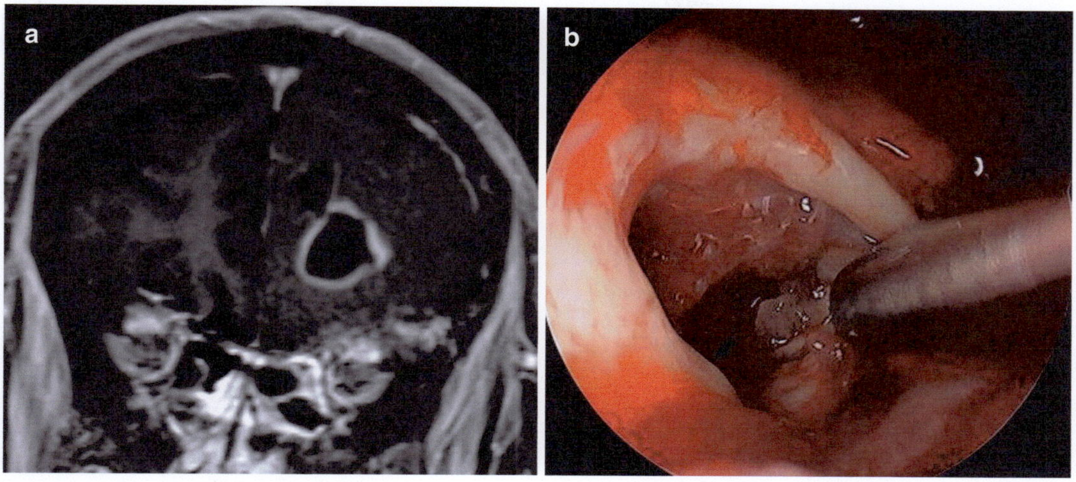

Fig. 20.15 Left frontal lobe abscess, sinogenic. (**a**) MRI demonstrating left frontal lobe abscess with peripheral enhancement. This began as a left frontal sinus abscess, which subsequently spread to the left orbit and brain. (**b**) A left superior transorbital approach was used to drain the orbital abscess and enter into the frontal sinus. Intraoperative photograph through posterior wall of frontal sinus shows defect in dura extending into the parenchyma of the frontal lobe

Prevention of Long-Term Sequelae in Skull Base Trauma

As discussed in this chapter, the management of ACF, MCF, and orbital trauma involves complex and nuanced decision-making, including when open or endoscopic management is in the patient's best interest. These decisions must be made not only regarding acute and life-saving management but also in view of the life-long prevention of complications and sequelae of the trauma. Among the most common of these complications are CSF leak, orbitofrontal mucocele, and intracranial abscess. It is thus critical for the surgeon to obtain complete MRI and CT imaging in complex trauma cases and evaluate potential sites of current and future sinus outflow obstruction and treat accordingly. Likewise, it is important to evaluate any fractures adjacent to dura for the possibility of future dural laceration from intracranial pulsation. Follow-up CT scans at 3 months and then a year later can be useful in determining whether normal paranasal sinus function has returned or whether there is ongoing mucosal thickening and trapping of secretions (Fig. 20.16). In equivocal cases, several years of annual imaging may be indicated for patients who are reliably able to participate in surveillance.

While the endoscopic transorbital and transnasal techniques used in skull base surgery have made possible the minimally disruptive management of selected craniofacial injuries and many of the potential delayed complications, every effort must be made at the time of initial treatment to ensure that these do not occur.

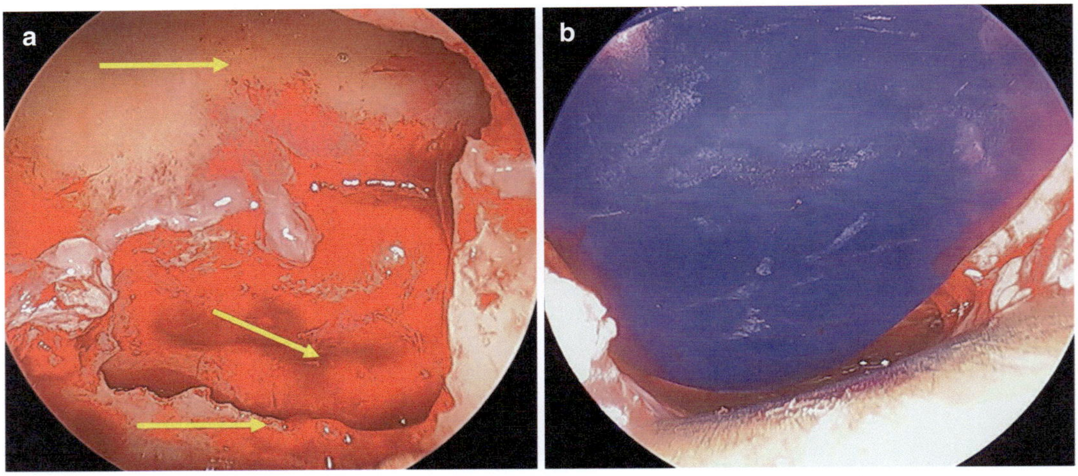

Fig. 20.16 Right orbitofrontal mucocele in patient with history of frontal sinus trauma 33 years earlier. (**a**) Superior transorbital view through orbital roof showing drained mucocele cavity (upper arrow); new drainage cavity into supraorbital ethmoid sinus and nasal cavity (middle arrow indicates drainage path); and edge of orbital roof defect that was created for access (lower arrow). (**b**) 0.25 mm PDS sheet placed across orbital roof defect to prevent orbital contents from obstructing frontal drainage tract. Malleable retractor retracting orbital contents inferiorly

References

1. Bly R, Liu J, Cjudekova M, Chang SH, Moe KS. Computer-guided orbital reconstruction improves surgical outcomes. JAMA Facial Plastic Surg. 2013;15(2):113–20.
2. Bevans S, Moe KS. Advances in orbital reconstruction. In: Moe KS, editor. Trauma in facial plastic surgery, Facial plastic surgery clinics of North America, vol. 25(4). Elsevier; 2017. p. 479–644.
3. Bly R, Morton R, Kim LJ, Moe KS. Tension pneumocephalus after endoscopic sinus surgery: a technical report of multiportal endoscopic skull. Otolaryngol Head Neck Surg. 2014;151(6):1081–3. PMID: 25139951
4. Patel S, Berens AM, Devarajan K, Whipple ME, Moe KS. Evaluation of a minimally disruptive treatment protocol for frontal sinus fracture. JAMA Facial Plast Surg. 2017;19(3):225–31. PMID: 28152148
5. Podolsky D, Moe KS. Frontal sinus fractures. Semin Plast Surg. 2021;35(04):274–83.
6. Berens AM, Davis GE, Moe KS. Transorbital endoscopic identification of supernumerary ethmoid arteries. Allerygy Rhinol. 2016;7(3):144–6. PMID: 28107146
7. Moe KS. The precaruncular approach to the medial orbit. JAMA Facial Plast Surg. 2003;5:483–7.
8. Balakrishnan K, Moe KS. Applications and outcomes of orbital and transorbital endoscopic surgery. Otolaryngol Head Neck Surg. 2011;144(5):815–20. PMID: 21493355
9. Moe KS, Kim LJ, Bergeron CM. Transorbital endoscopic repair of complex cerebrospinal fluid leaks. Laryngoscope. 2011;121:13–30.
10. Miller C, Berans A, Patel S, Humphreys I, Moe KS. Transorbital approach for improved access in the management of paranasal sinus mucoceles. J Neurol Surg B Skull Base. 2019;80(06):593–8. https://doi.org/10.1055/s-0038-1676982.
11. Miller C, Rly RA, Moe KS. Endoscopic orbital and periorbital approaches in minimally disruptive skull base surgery. J Neurol Surg B Skull Base. 2020;81(4):459–71. PMID: 33072486
12. Lim JH, Sardesai M, Ferreira M, Moe KS. Transorbital neuroendoscopic management of sinogenic complications involving the frontal sinus, orbit and anterior cranial fossa. J Neurol Surg. 2012;73(B6):394–400.

The Transorbital Approach for Repair of Lateral Sphenoid Sinus Encephaloceles

21

Dimitrios Mathios, Ernest Bobeff, Davide Longo, Kyle J. Godfrey, Kris S. Moe, and Theodore H. Schwartz

Introduction

The sphenoid sinus exhibits high intra- and inter-individual variation of pneumatization. At its extreme, an individual can have a hypoplastic sphenoid sinus on one side and a hyper-aerated sinus on the other side (Fig. 21.1a). This variation affects the patterns of CSF leaks in the sphenoid sinus. Patients with a well-aerated sphenoid sinus and idiopathic intracranial hypertension (IIH) have a higher chance of a spontaneous CSF leak in the lateral sphenoid sinus, unlike leaks in the central sphenoid sinus in non-well-aerated sphenoid sinuses where the etiology of a leak is usually traumatic or iatrogenic [1]. Many investigators have postulated that spontaneous sphenoid sinus CSF leaks derive from a persistent Sternberg's canal. This hypothesis has recently been disputed [2]. Depending on the location of the sphenoid sinus CSF leak, they are separated into type I if they are medial to the foramen rotundum (FR) and the vidian canal (VC), type II if they are medial to FR, type III if they are lateral to FR, and type IV if the encephalocele passes through the FR (Fig. 21.1b).

The first report of spontaneous cerebrospinal rhinorrhea was described by Charles Miller in 1826 [3], in a patient with hydrocephalus in whom communications were found at autopsy between the nasal and the cranial cavity. The first endonasal repair of CSF leak in the sphenoid sinus was described by Oscar Hirsch in 1952 [4]. Since then, the techniques for the endonasal repair of CSF leaks have been refined, and their applications have expanded to encompass the repair of lateral sphenoid sinus leaks.

The traditional minimally invasive approach for the repair of these leaks is an endoscopic endonasal approach (EEA). Depending on the pneumatization and the medio-lateral location of the leak in the sphenoid sinus, the repair can be achieved through a standard transsphenoidal approach with or without the use of angled scopes [5] and instruments or more frequently through a transpterygoid approach [6] to the lateral sphenoid sinus (Fig. 21.2a).

D. Mathios · D. Longo · T. H. Schwartz (✉)
Department of Neurosurgery, Weill Cornell Medicine, NewYork–Presbyterian Hospital, New York, NY, USA
e-mail: mathios@wustl.edu; davide.longo3@studio.unibo.it; schwarh@med.cornell.edu

E. Bobeff
Department of Neurosurgery, Weill Cornell Medicine, New York Presbyterian Hospital, New York, NY, USA

Department of Neurosurgery, Barlicki University Hospital, Lodz, Poland

Department of Sleep Medicine and Metabolic Disorders, Medical University of Lodz, Lodz, Poland
e-mail: ernest.bobeff@umed.lodz.pl

K. J. Godfrey
Department of Ophthalmology and Neurosurgery, Weill Cornell Medicine, New York, NY, USA
e-mail: kyg9004@med.cornell.edu

K. S. Moe
Division of Facial Plastic Surgery, Departments of Otolaryngology and Neurological Surgery, University of Washington School of Medicine, Seattle, WA, USA
e-mail: krismoe@uw.edu

T. H. Schwartz et al. (eds.), *Endoscopic Transorbital Surgery of the Orbit, Skull Base and Brain*,
https://doi.org/10.1007/978-3-031-59504-2_21

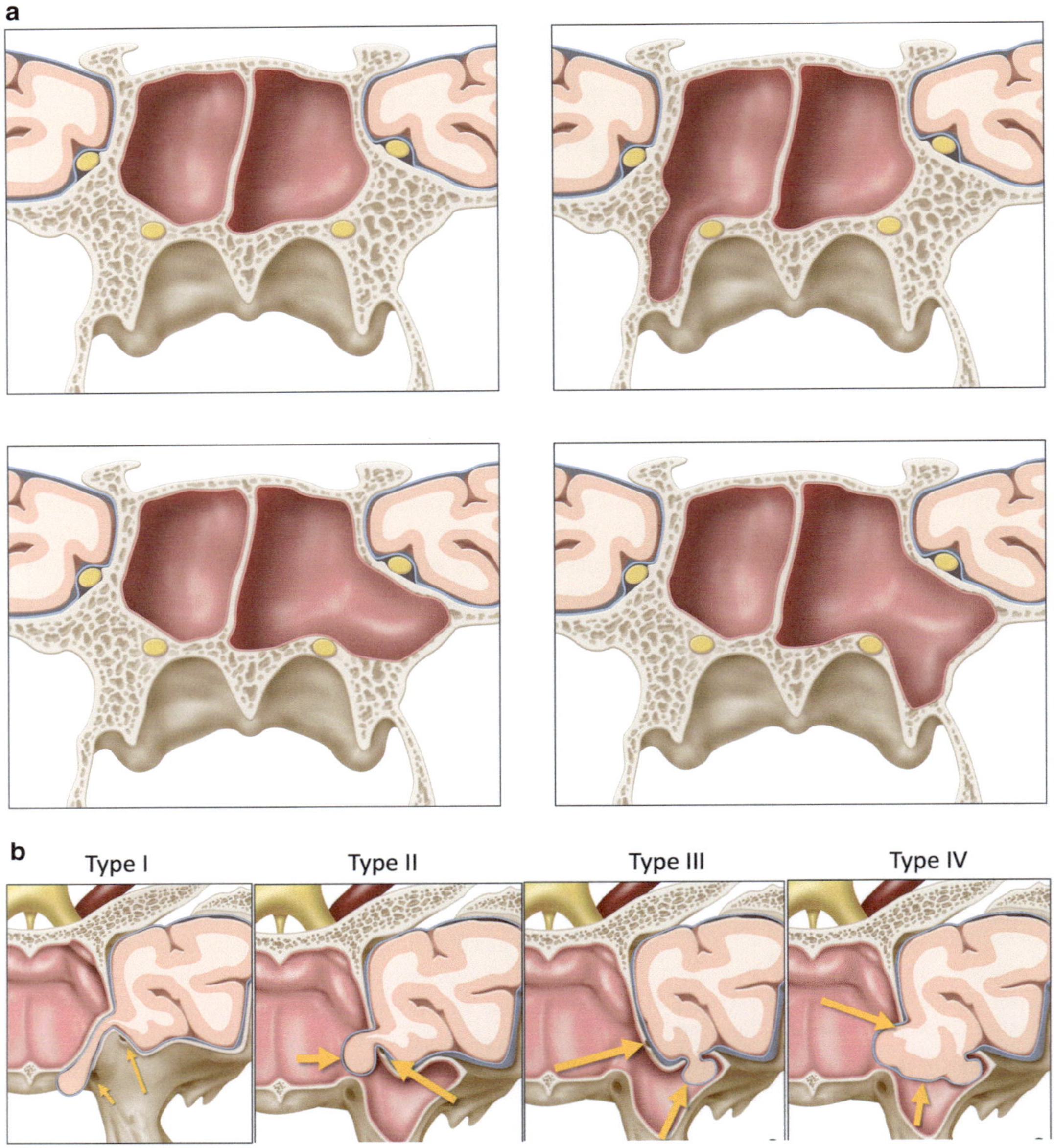

Fig. 21.1 (**a**) Patterns of sphenoid sinus aeration. (**b**) Types of lateral sphenoid sinus encephaloceles in relation to V2. (With permissions from Hanz et al., Low incidence of true Sternberg's canal defects among lateral sphenoid sinus encephaloceles, Acta Neurochirurgica, 2020)

Transmaxillary approaches (either ipsilateral or contralateral) [7, 8] have also been developed to provide a favorable angle to approach the lateral sphenoid sinus. However, encephaloceles lateral to FR (type III) can be challenging to reach. A recent paper with a multi-institutional experience has shown that type III leaks have a higher rate of facial numbness and dry eye from damage to the contents of the pterygopalatine fossa incurred during the transpterygoid approach [9].

More recently, the transorbital approaches (TOA) have provided another corridor to approach lesions in the middle fossa (Fig. 21.2a) [10]. Here, we present the first series of cases of a lateral to V2 sphenoid sinus encephalocele via an ipsilateral transorbital approach showing

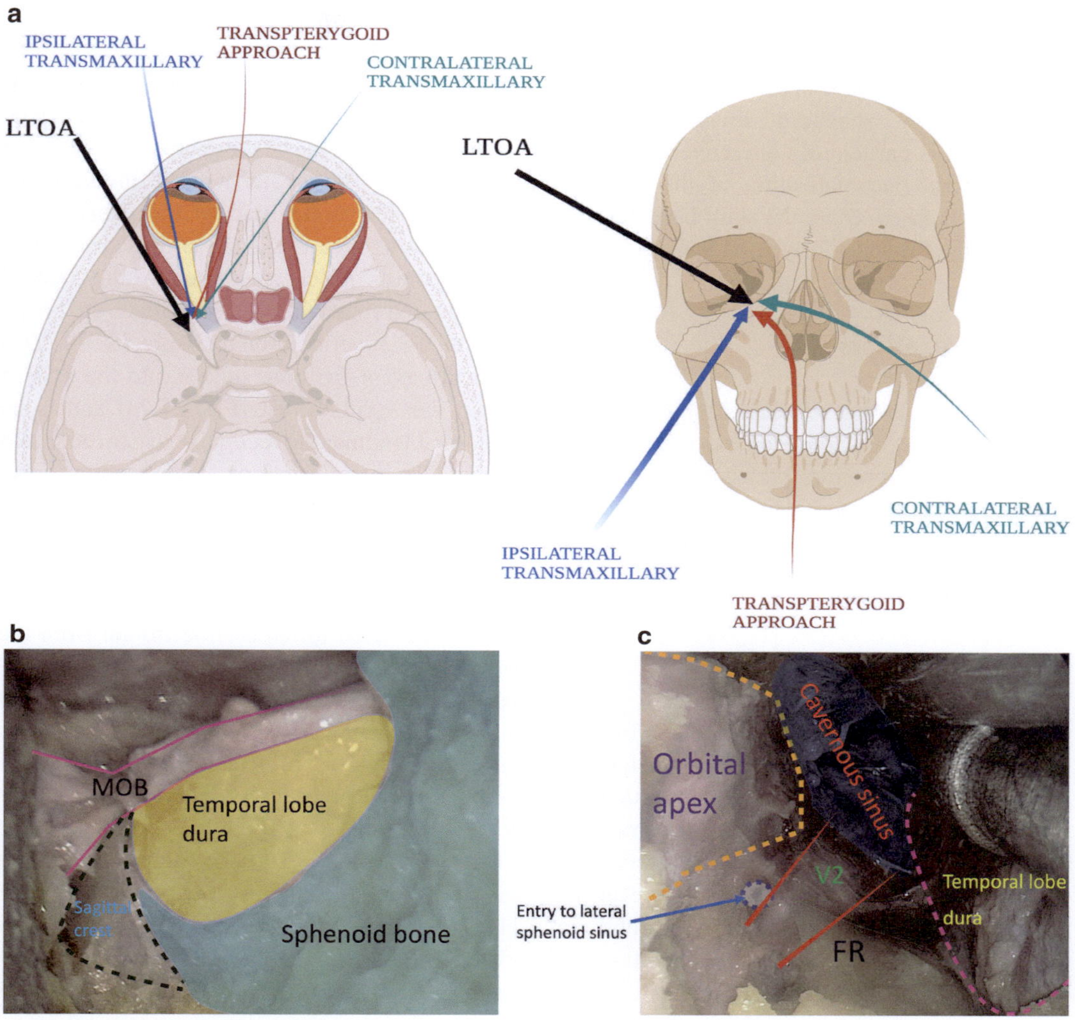

Fig. 21.2 (**a**) Cartoon illustration depicting the minimally invasive skull base approaches targeting the foramen rotundum. Created with BioRender.com. (**b**) Cadaveric dissection through a lateral transorbital approach depicting the relevant anatomy in the approach. In the picture the meningo-orbital band (MOB) has been partially cut and the sphenoid bone and the sagittal crest have been partially drilled. (**c**) After complete transection of the meningo-orbital band and subtemporal dissection, the lateral wall of the cavernous sinus is encountered, and V2 is seen emanating from its inferior aspect. Followed distally, V2 is visualized as it enters the foramen rotundum (FR). A small hole entering the lateral sphenoid sinus is visualized in the figure

durable leak repair. We have shown via cadaveric dissections that the TOA is a more direct approach than the endonasal approach to address pathology lateral to the FR, especially in lateral pneumatization of the sphenoid sinus [10]. This approach avoids transgressing the pterygopalatine fossa contents such as the vidian nerve, the pterygopalatine ganglion, the sphenopalatine artery, and manipulation of V2 at the FR.

Patient Selection and Indications

Patient Presentation

The patients usually present with the primary complaint of clear drainage from their nose, nasal congestion, positional headaches and rarely with evidence of meningitis at presentation.

Indications

The lateral transorbital approach is suitable for addressing any sphenoid sinus CSF leak. However, it is particularly attractive in cases of excess lateral pneumatization of the sphenoid sinus and in cases where the skull base defect is lateral to the FR and V2 (type III leaks).

Contraindications

There are no absolute contraindications; relative contraindications are active orbital infection, history of keloid formation, presence of significant ophthalmological comorbidities (glaucoma, retinal detachment), and intraorbital mass where orbital retraction can increase intraocular pressure.

Diagnostic Workup

The gold standard in the diagnosis of CSF leak is the collection of the nasal fluid and analysis for b2-transferin. If the rhinorrhea is intermittent and fluid cannot be collected, a CT cisternography or a pledget study can confirm the presence and point to the location of the leak. However, the diagnosis can often be made based on observation. If the patient leans forward in the office and drops of clear fluid running from their nose in association with a visualized encephalocele in the skull base, the evidence is often sufficient.

Imaging

A maxillofacial CT scan with thin cuts through the orbit and skull base and an MRI brain with thin cuts through the skull base and orbits are very useful for preoperative planning, decision on optimal trajectory to access the lesion, and intraoperative navigation.

Surgical Anatomy

The greater wing of the sphenoid is the bone most relevant to this surgical approach. A fundamental understanding of the anatomy of this bone is imperative. The greater wing of the sphenoid constitutes the largest part of the lateral orbit. Superficially, once this bone is drilled laterally, the temporalis muscle is exposed. At the depth of the orbit, the sphenoid bone constitutes the lateral wall of the superior orbital fissure (SOF). This vertical part of the bone adjacent to the SOF is called the sagittal crest (Fig. 21.2a) and is an important landmark to recognize to gain access to the middle fossa. Superior to the sagittal crest, the meningo-orbital band (Fig. 21.2b) is identified, a fold of the dura between the temporal and frontal lobe connecting these two lobes with the periosteum of the orbit. This structure can be safely transected to release the frontal from the temporal lobe and allow for the dissection to proceed subtemporally toward the cavernous sinus and Meckel's cave. Dissection toward Meckel's cave allows for proximal identification of the trigeminal nerve branches (Fig. 21.2c), especially V2, which can be traced distally to identify the FR from which V2 exits. The anteromedial and the anterolateral triangle, as defined by Dolenc [11], are exposed to ensure accurate localization of V2. The FR (Fig. 21.2c) is an anatomical landmark in the repair of lateral sphenoid sinus CSF leaks as it is the most relevant anatomical structure encountered in these cases, and many investigators classify the location of these leaks based on their relative position with this structure.

Surgical Technique

Equipment

Intraoperative navigation using preoperative CT and/or MRI is paramount to confirm landmarks and targets and help plan a trajectory before incision.

We prefer to fix the patient's head on the operating table using a Mayfield holder, but this is optional depending on the navigation platform used. Usually, the procedure can require as many as three operators: one to retract the globe, one to navigate the scope and the operating surgeon. The use of a scope holder is optional. When used, it can free up one person so that only two operators are required in the field.

Lubricated corneal protectors are used to cover the patient's eyes. Loop magnification is used in the first part of the approach. The eyelid crease incision and dissection down to the lateral orbital rim and superficial lateral orbital wall are done with overhead light illumination and loop magnification.

The use of 0° and angled scopes is paramount to achieve the best illumination at the depth of the orbit. A brain spatula is used as an orbital content retractor, and instruments adopted from endoscopic endonasal trays are used in combination with endoscopy.

Surgical Steps

1. A lumbar drain can be placed at the beginning of the case, and intrathecal fluorescein can be used to visualize the area of leak intraoperatively.
2. The approach can be made either through an upper eyelid crease incision through the following layers: skin and subcutaneous tissue, orbicularis oculi and dissection in a pre-septal plane down to the orbital rim or through a retrocanthal subconjunctival approach. See more details in the case presentations.
3. Dissect and retract the orbital contents from the orbital wall, taking extra care not to violate the periorbita. The orbit from the superior orbital fissure to the inferior orbital fissure is dissected free from the lateral orbital wall. Retraction is relieved every 20 min and the pupils are checked for symmetry during that time.
4. Drill the lateral orbital wall deep to the orbital rim to create room for the instruments to pass. The drilling proceeds towards the FR based on intraoperative navigation. Two variations in TOA have been described to access and repair lateral sphenoid encephalocele: (a) the transorbital middle fossa approach, which is an extradural intracranial approach, and (b) the transorbital transsphenoidal approach, which connects the orbit to the lateral sphenoid sinus to approach the lesion extracranially. We will describe each:

Lateral Transorbital Approach Through the Middle Fossa

The bone of the greater wing of the sphenoid is removed from SOF to IOF. Once the posterior orbital wall has been removed, the temporal lobe dura and the meningo-orbital band are exposed. The meningo-orbital band is cut to allow for subtemporal dissection to expose the area of proximal V2 and FR. The encephalocele and dural defect should be readily accessible in relation to FR. The encephalocele at this point is coagulated and excised, leaving the skull base defect to the lateral sphenoid sinus visible. Depending on the size of the defect either a button graft (intradural/extradural layer of acellular matrix sutured together) or an inlay acellular matrix graft only is designed and fashioned intradurally to cover the dural defect. An onlay layer of fat can be placed between the dura and bone and this can be covered with Tisseel fibrin glue. In this approach, the sphenoid sinus is never entered, and the repair is done purely within the middle fossa.

Transorbital Approach Through the Sphenoid Sinus

For the transorbital transsphenoidal approach, the bone removal is more inferior. The inferior orbital fissure can be transected to allow for superior displacement of the orbital contents, and drilling commences until the lateral sphenoid sinus is entered. Through the bone defect created, the encephalocele can be seen, the mucosa over the bony defect can be stripped, and the encephalocele can be coagulated and transected to prepare the skull base for reconstruction. Glue and fat can be fashioned over the skull base defect. The medial aspect of the skull base defect is visualized endonasally to ensure no egress of CSF.

At the end of the operation and after hemostasis has been obtained and the repair site has been inspected for good closure, the orbit is allowed to recoil back to its original position, and the skin is closed. Two- or three-layer closure is used to close the orbicularis muscle, the skin and/or the deeper periosteal layer. A piece of compressive gauze is used over the incision for extubation and in the immediate postoperative setting.

Postoperative Care

If the patient has a lumbar drain in place, it usually stays in for 2 days to continuously drain at a rate of about 5 cc/h. This can be helpful, especially in the case of idiopathic intracranial hypertension (IIH). An antibiotic/steroid ointment is prescribed for the first few days to be used over the incision to decrease swelling, and the patients are prescribed an optional 3-day taper of oral steroids. The patients are usually seen in a step-down unit or the ICU, where they get frequent neurological and eye checks and ensure good drainage of CSF through the lumbar drain. In cases of IIH, the patient is also prescribed acetazolamide for 2 weeks. After the lumbar drain is removed, the patient undergoes an MRI brain or a maxillofacial CT with thin cuts through the orbit as baseline imaging and to document the repair.

Complications

No large series of patients operated on through a transorbital approach for lateral sphenoid sinus CSF leak repair has been published and therefore there is no significant amount of data on complications. The theoretical complications from this procedure include numbness in the V2 distribution from dissection around V2, orbital hematoma, infection, and wound dehiscence as well as the development of pseudomeningocele and CSF leak either through the skin incision or through the nose.

Outcomes

In the three cases described above, all three patients did not have recurrent CSF leaks, with a median follow-up time of 2 years (6 months–10 years). Eyelid swelling and diplopia were transient for a few weeks after surgery; no clinically significant exophthalmos was observed in any of these patients.

Case Presentations

Case 1

A 50-year-old male with a history of IIH previously treated with a right frontal ventriculoperitoneal shunt presented with clear drainage through his right nostril. A head CT revealed a bony defect lateral (type III) to the FR with an associated encephalocele (Fig. 21.3a). The patient's shunt was evaluated for patency and was found to be functional [10].

Procedure

A lateral TOA middle fossa approach was done to expose the encephalocele (Fig. 21.3b).

The encephalocele was transected, and the dural defect was closed with an inlay synthetic collagen matrix (Fig. 21.5b). Abdominal fat was harvested and grafted at the area as an onlay between the dural and bone defects. Fibrin glue was applied to keep the fat in place. The incision was closed in three layers; the periosteal layer was closed with 5-0 Biosyn suture (Medtronic, USA), the orbicularis muscle was closed with 7-0 vicryl, and the skin was closed with running 6-0 plain gut suture (Medtronic, USA).

A Lumbar drain was not placed in this case as the patient already had a functional shunt. The shunt was dialed down to promote cerebrospinal fluid diversion away from the repair site. Postoperatively the patient's rhinorrhea ceased. He experienced transient, mild eyelid edema, mild transient ptosis and ecchymosis but experi-

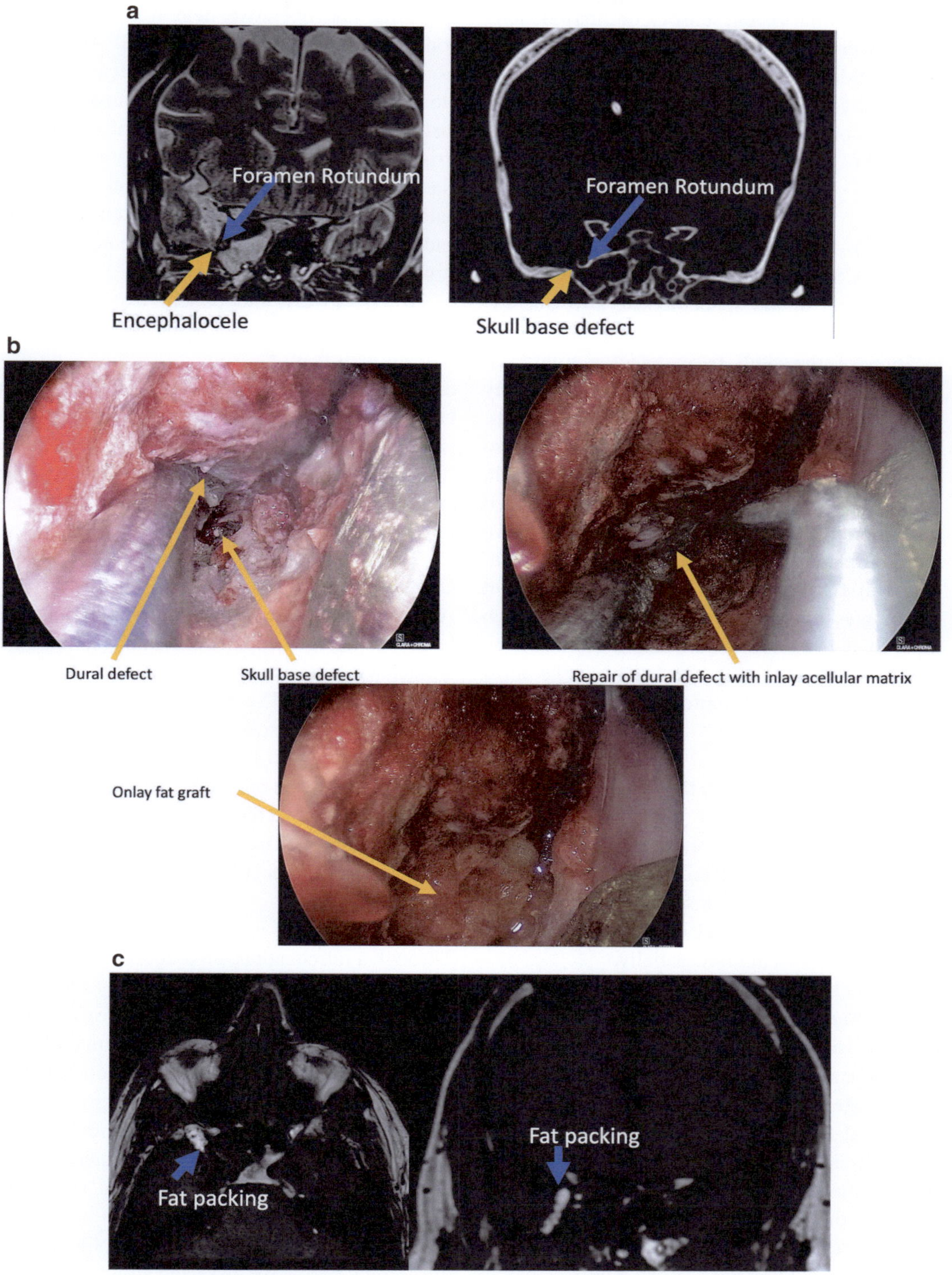

Fig. 21.3 (**a**) Preoperative coronal T2 sequence MRI and CT scan in case 1 indicating the area of the skull base defect and the associated encephalocele. Note the defect is lateral to the foramen rotundum. (**b**) Intraoperative pictures of the dural defect after inlay repair with a collagen matrix and placement of fat for repair of the skull base defect. (**c**) Postoperative axial and coronal T1 sequence indicating good placement of the fat graft and good closure of the skull base defect

enced no double vision, sensory, or motor deficits after surgery. The patient was discharged on postoperative day 3. MRI revealed proper closure of the skull base dehiscence (Fig. 21.3c). The patient was seen on a 10-month follow-up with no evidence of CSF leak.

Case 2

A 70-year-old male presented with a severe spontaneous CSF leak likely arising from the left greater wing of the sphenoid lateral to the FR (type III) (Fig. 21.4a). Due to the extreme lateral location of the skull base defect a transnasal approach would have been a very lengthy approach. With preoperative computer analysis, we measured this distance at 75 mm. We also investigated a suborbital transmaxillary approach, which measured 55 mm (Fig. 21.4b). While it was more direct, this approach would have required extensive dissection through the infratemporal fossa, which would cause significant bleeding. A transorbital transsphenoidal approach through a retrocanthal, subconjuctival incision measured 30 mm (Fig. 21.4c), was the most direct and efficacious approach to the lesion.

Procedure

A TOA approach through the sphenoid sinus was performed as described above (Fig. 21.4d). Through this opening, we attempted to localize the CSF leak. With a detailed exploration of the skull base using a 0° endoscope, we were able to localize the leak (Fig. 21.4e). The mucosa was then taken down circumferentially.

A small craniectomy was performed in the middle cranial fossa adjacent to the leak where the dura was exposed. An abdominal fat graft was harvested, and a small piece was placed medial to the leakage site to plug this egress point. A small amount of fibrin glue was placed directly on the middle cranial fossa defect, and another segment of abdominal fat was fashioned to fill the distal aspect of the defect, followed by the application of additional glue to keep the fat layers attached to the bone defect (Fig. 21.4f). The rest of the abdominal fat graft was placed into the lateral sphenoid sinus defect to obliterate this point of egress, making the lateral orbital wall surface flat. After the operative field was inspected to confirm no residual bleeding or CSF egress, the canthotomy and cantholysis incisions were closed with 5-0 caprosyn suture followed by 6-0 fast-absorbing gut suture. The patient's eyes were irrigated with a balanced salt solution. A single Nasopore was placed in the left nasal cavity. The patient was then allowed to awaken, extubate, and be taken to the recovery room in good condition.

Postoperatively, the patient experienced no diplopia or CSF leaking, nor did he have any significant pain from the surgery. He had a lumbar drain for 48 h. At a detailed follow-up visit 1 year later, he had no leak recurrence and no orbital issues, including pain, diplopia, or visual decline (Fig. 21.4g). He has been 10 years out from his surgery, and he has not had any evidence of recurrent leaks.

Case 3

A 59-year-old woman developed a severe CSF leak with pneumocephalus localizing on the right greater wing of the sphenoid, lateral to V2 (type III) (Fig. 21.5a). The patient had a very well-pneumatized right sphenoid sinus. We had previously performed an EEA, but the defect was so lateral that we were not able to adequately visualize it for repair. We therefore decided to proceed with a transorbital transsphenoidal approach for the repair of this encephalocele.

Procedure

Through a retrocanthal, subconjuctival approach, we took down the bone immediately above the inferior orbital fissure under endoscopic visualization. This continued until the temporal lobe dura was encountered. We then continued to work medially along the planned surgical course intracranially and extracranially, removing bone with ultrasonic aspiration until the lateral aspect of the highly pneumatized sphenoid sinus was encountered.

At this point we encountered the FR and the infraorbital nerve. We dissected around this intracranially to confirm the site. We then opened the lateral aspect of the sphenoid sinus widely and explored this further medially. We found a large

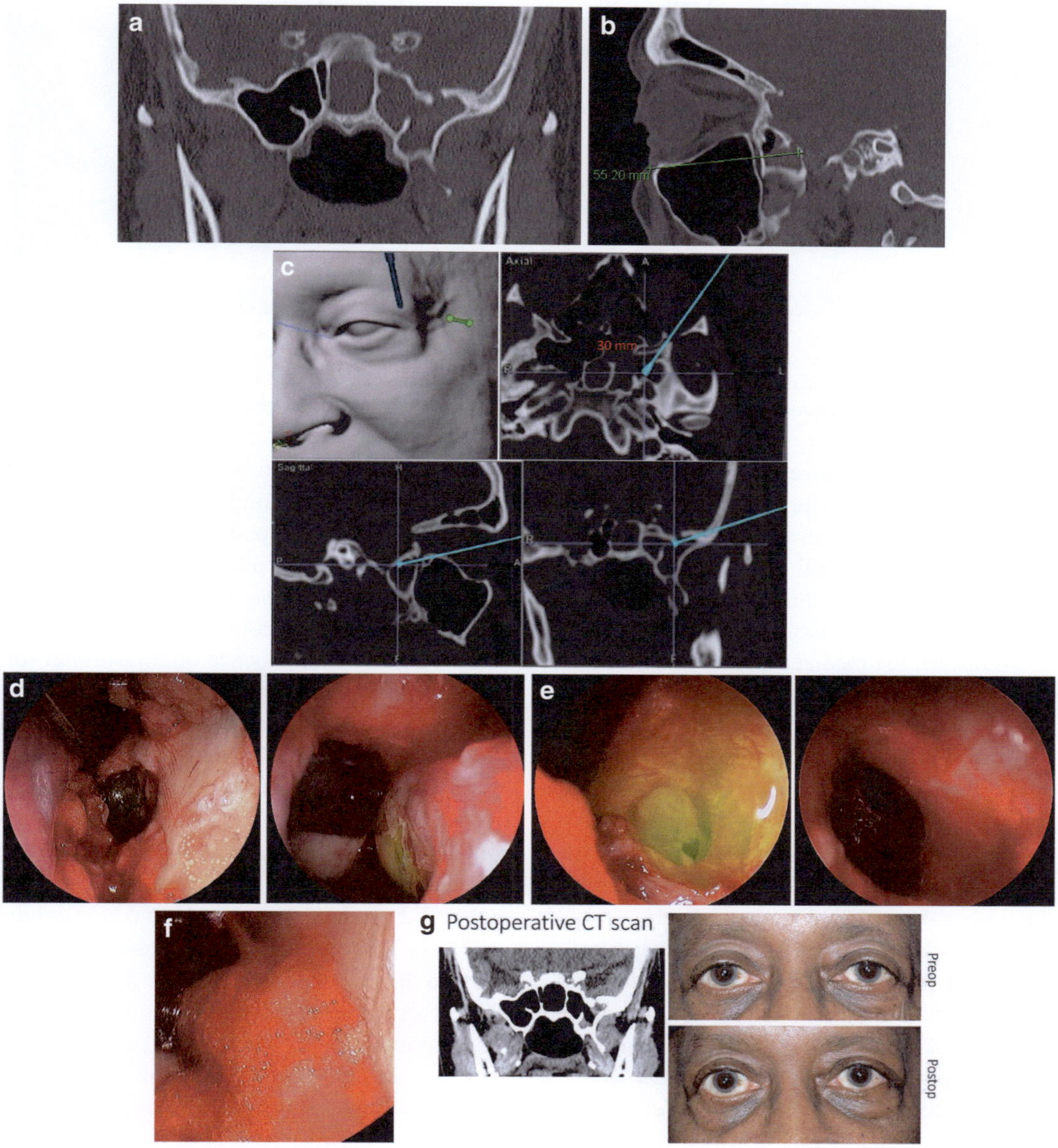

Fig. 21.4 (**a**) Case 2, Coronal CT scan showing a skull base defect lateral to V2 on the left with associated opacification of the left sphenoid sinus. (**b**) Infraorbital, transmaxillary route to the encephalocele. (**c**) 3D, as well as axial, coronal and sagittal reconstructions of the lateral transorbital approach trajectory to the target. (**d**) Intraoperative view at the inferior orbital fissure with a small opening to the lateral sphenoid sinus. The green fluorescence dye indicates an active CSF leak. (**e**) The area of the skull base defect is identified after transection of the encephalocele. (**f**) The closure of the skull base defect is shown with the use of an abdominal fat graft and glue. (**g**) The postoperative CT scan shows opacity in the area of the skull base defect, showing good placement of the fat graft. The patient's face looks almost identical preoperatively and postoperatively

vertical defect in the site that we had marked as a navigation target. CSF was emanating from this defect. We therefore removed the mucosa from the sphenoid cell circumferentially. We then injected fibrin glue into the sphenoid cell and placed a piece of fat graft harvested from the abdomen. We then injected further glue along the pathway created within the lateral sphenoid bone

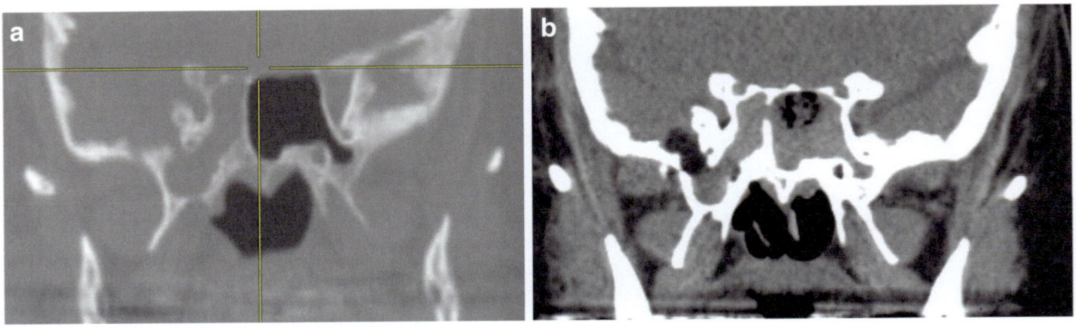

Fig. 21.5 (**a**) Preoperative coronal CT scan on case 3. Note the skull base defect on the right sphenoid wing associated with opacification of the ipsilateral sphenoid sinus. (**b**) Postoperative coronal CT scan revealed a lucency at the area of the skull base defect, indicating good placement of the fat graft

and placed another piece of fat graft. This filled out the defect in the lateral orbital wall to reconstruct the bony contour. Once the orbital reconstruction was confirmed so that no void existed and that the orbital volume was symmetric, the canthotomy incision was closed with 5-0 PDS.

To inspect the medial aspect of the defect, we debrided the nasal cavity in the region of the maxillary, ethmoid and sphenoid sinuses endoscopically. Upon inspection of the sphenoid sinus, there was no evidence of a CSF leak in the region. We injected this with fibrin glue to provide further support for the medial reconstruction. We then placed a Nasopore dressing within the nose and concluded the procedure.

The patient was then allowed to awaken and was taken to the recovery room in good condition. She had a lumbar drain for 2 days. Her vision remained at her baseline but did have a lateral diplopia in the far lateral gaze that resolved in a few weeks. She developed a corneal abrasion immediately after surgery, which was treated with a temporary tarsorrhaphy stitch. She had no recurrence of the CSF leak (Fig. 21.5b) until she expired 2 years later due to an unrelated disease.

Concluding Remarks

Lateral sphenoid sinus CSF leaks are frequently associated with idiopathic intracranial hypertension and a well-aerated sphenoid sinus. The standard of care for the repair of these lesions is currently an EEA. However, encephaloceles lateral to FR (type III) can be challenging to reach. A recent paper with a multi-institutional experience has shown that type III leaks have a higher rate of facial numbness and dry eye from damage to the contents of the pterygopalatine fossa incurred during the transpterygoid approach [9]. A growing body of evidence on transorbital surgery now shows these approaches provide an efficient and direct route to the paramedian skull base and middle fossa. Here, we describe the relevant imaging findings, indications, and operative technique for transorbital repair of lateral sphenoid sinus encephaloceles. We provide the first series of sphenoid sinus encephaloceles lateral to V2 treated via an ipsilateral transorbital approach. This approach provided durable results with no facial numbness and no dry eye. The TOA route has many advantages compared to the EEA for exposure of paramedian pathology; the orbit provides a sterile environment compared to the nose, and the repair is a direct one as it affords to place an inlay and onlay layer to close the dural defect and additional material, instead of relying on an extradural onlay, especially in cases of increased intracranial pressure. However, the EEA provides an in situ pedicled vascularized flap that has been shown to provide good long-term outcomes [12]. The orbit, however, can work as a buttress of the reconstruction and eliminates the empty space that inevitably exists in endonasal surgery. Finally, it remains to be seen whether CSF leaks medial to V2 can be repaired equally well with the lateral TOA as with the EEA.

References

1. Shetty PG, Shroff MM, Fatterpekar GM, Sahani DV, Kirtane MV. A retrospective analysis of spontaneous sphenoid sinus fistula: MR and CT findings. AJNR Am J Neuroradiol. 2000;21(2):337–42.
2. Hanz SZ, et al. Low incidence of true Sternberg's canal defects among lateral sphenoid sinus encephaloceles. Acta Neurochir (Wien). 2020;162(10):2413–20. https://doi.org/10.1007/s00701-020-04329-2.
3. Alph R. Mémoire sur la nature de l'écoulement a queux trés-abondant qui accompagne certains fractures de la base du crane. Arch Générales Méd. 1845;9(4):389–421.
4. Hirsch O. Successful closure of cerebrospinal fluid rhinorrhea by endonasal surgery. AMA Arch Otolaryngol. 1952;56(1):1–12. https://doi.org/10.1001/archotol.1952.00710020018001.
5. Maxfield AZ, et al. Endoscopic management of lateral sphenoid cerebrospinal fluid leaks: identifying a radiographic parameter for surgical planning. Laryngoscope Investig Otolaryngol. 2020;5(3):375–80. https://doi.org/10.1002/lio2.412.
6. Hofstetter CP, Singh A, Anand VK, Kacker A, Schwartz TH. The endoscopic, endonasal, transmaxillary transpterygoid approach to the pterygopalatine fossa, infratemporal fossa, petrous apex, and the Meckel cave. J Neurosurg. 2010;113(5):967–74. https://doi.org/10.3171/2009.10.JNS09157.
7. Patel CR, Wang EW, Fernandez-Miranda JC, Gardner PA, Snyderman CH. Contralateral transmaxillary corridor: an augmented endoscopic approach to the petrous apex. J Neurosurg. 2018;129(1):211–9. https://doi.org/10.3171/2017.4.JNS162483.
8. Wilson DA, Williamson RW, Preul MC, Little AS. Comparative analysis of surgical freedom and angle of attack of two minimal-access endoscopic transmaxillary approaches to the anterolateral skull base. World Neurosurg. 2014;82(3–4):e487–93. https://doi.org/10.1016/j.wneu.2013.02.003.
9. Tosi U, et al. Endoscopic endonasal repair of encephaloceles of the lateral sphenoid sinus: a multi-institution experience. J Neurosurg. 2023;140(3):705–11.
10. Mathios D, et al. Lateral transorbital approach for repair of lateral sphenoid sinus meningoencephaloceles in proximity to foramen rotundum: cadaveric study and case report. Oper Neurosurg. 2023;25(2):168–75.
11. Dolenc VV. Cavernous sinus tumors. In: Anatomy and surgery of the cavernous sinus. Vienna: Springer; 1989. p. 269–338.
12. Michael AP, et al. The critical importance of a vascularized flap in preventing recurrence after endoscopic repair of spontaneous cerebrospinal fluid leaks and meningoencephaloceles. J Neurosurg. 2021;137:79–86. https://doi.org/10.3171/2021.7.JNS211427.

Part VII

Skull Base Pathology: Posterior Fossa

Petrous Apex: Approach and Tumors

22

Alberto Di Somma, Giulia Guizzardi, Alejandra Mosteiro, Alberto Prats-Galino, and Joaquim Enseñat

Abbreviations

PA	Petrous apex
mm	Millimeters
IOF	Inferior orbital fissure
SOF	Superior orbital fissure
CSF	Cerebro-spinal fluid
GSPN	Greater superficial petrosal nerve
MRI	Magnetic resonance imaging
EANS	European Association of Neurosurgical Societies
ENT	Ear-nose-throat
WHO	World Health Organization
ICA	Internal carotid artery
3D	Tridimensional

The petrous apex (PA) is the anteromedial portion of the petrous part of the temporal bone. Being a deep-seated structure harboring important vascular and neural canals, it has always represented a complex surgical target. However, its rather frequent involvement in skull base lesions prompted the development of many surgical strategies to reach the PA and adjacent posterior fossa area.

Since the introduction of the middle fossa transpetrosal-transtentorial approach (Kawase's approach) to the PA in the mid-1980s, transcranial approaches have been considered the gold standard even when they are characterized by a high degree of technical complexity and a high risk of postoperative complications [1]. With the aim of minimizing this surgical morbidity and the need for brain retraction, novel minimally invasive approaches have been explored as an alternative. Among the various techniques, the endoscopic endonasal and transorbital approaches have encountered incredible evolutions over the last few years [2, 3].

This chapter provides a step-by-step explanation on how to approach the PA area with the superior eyelid transorbital approach. Anatomic reference points are given to guide the entire dissection, particularly while creating the working space to feasibly reach the PA, safely remove its upper portion, and access the posterior cranial fossa. Preliminary experience with the technique is reported with a set of clinical cases, and specific indications and limitations of the transorbital approach are discussed.

Relevant Surgical Anatomy of the Petrous Apex

The petrous apex (PA) is the pyramid-shaped anteromedial portion of the petrous part of the temporal bone. The petrous bone is obliquely posi-

A. Di Somma (✉) · G. Guizzardi · A. Mosteiro · J. Enseñat
Department of Neurological Surgery, Hospital Clínic de Barcelona, Barcelona, Spain

A. Prats-Galino
Laboratory of Surgical Neuroanatomy, Universitat de Barcelona, Barcelona, Spain
e-mail: aprats@ub.edu

T. H. Schwartz et al. (eds.), *Endoscopic Transorbital Surgery of the Orbit, Skull Base and Brain*,
https://doi.org/10.1007/978-3-031-59504-2_22

tioned within the skull base, with the apex located anteromedially and the base situated posterolaterally. Its anterosuperior surface forms the floor of the middle cranial fossa, while the posterosuperior face constitutes the anterior wall of the posterior cranial fossa. The PA is subdivided by the internal auditory canal into an anterior and a posterior portion. The larger anterior portion of the PA typically contains bone marrow, whereas the smaller posterior portion is denser in appearance [4, 5].

The PA houses important vascular and neuronal canals. The carotid canal and the internal auditory canal are the largest, whereas Dorello's singular and arcuate canals are markedly smaller and not always visualized. The internal auditory canal traverses the petrous bone from the inner ear to the posterior cranial fossa and contains the vestibulocochlear and facial nerves (cranial nerves VIII and VII, respectively) [6]. It runs in a coronal plane with reference to the skull but at an angle of approximately 45° in relation to the long axis of the petrous bone.

The petrous carotid canal, within the anterior portion of the PA, contains the horizontal portion of the internal carotid artery. The foramen lacerum is the fibrocartilaginous medial extension of the bony floor of the carotid canal. It is located in the sphenopetroclival junction, between the PA (temporal bone), the pterygoid process (sphenoid bone) and the clivus (occipital bone).

Dorello's canal extends through the medial portion of the PA, between the petrosphenoidal suture inferiorly and the petrosphenoidal ligament (Gruber's) superiorly. It contains the abducens nerve (cranial nerve VI) as it passes from the pontine cistern to the cavernous sinus. A marked depression is seen in the anterosuperior aspect of the PA that hosts the trigeminal root entering Meckel's cave. Meckel's cave contains the Gasserian ganglion that subsequently divides into the three branches of the trigeminal nerve (cranial nerve V).

Endoscopic Superior Eyelid Transorbital Approach to the Petrous Apex

Complex skull base tumors represent a great neurosurgical challenge, for which many different approaches have been designed for more than a century. The general evolution of surgical procedures towards minimally invasive alternatives has prompted a transition from the classic transcranial approaches to the endoscopic access through natural openings to access the skull base. In this context, the endonasal approach has been widely accepted as a ventral route to access the entire skull base [7, 8]. However, the lateral extension in the coronal plane is a well-known limitation of this approach. To overcome this restriction and to expand the surgical exposure in the coronal plane, another ventral route has been recently proposed and is gaining popularity in the skull base community: the endoscopic transorbital approach [9–12]. Initially devised to treat orbital pathology [13, 14], the transorbital route has been experiencing rapid evolution and is currently being used for both extra- [15, 16] and intradural skull base lesions [17, 18]. A classification of the technical difficulty according to the treated pathology has been depicted [19].

Indeed, many anatomical studies have been investigating the areas that can be reached by this route: potentially, the entire lateral skull base could be accessed from the transorbital corridor, including the anterior, middle and posterior cranial fossa [3, 11, 20–22].

We identify some steps during the transorbital endoscopic surgery to the PA [23], described as follows.

Skin Incision

The skin incision is made in the superior eyelid crease to minimize cosmetic defects (surgical wounds hidden with open eyes). It is advisable to mark the incision in the awake patient before undergoing the induction of anesthesia, as this may distort the wrinkle pattern in the eyelid. Alternatively, in the asleep patient, elevating the eyelid in a physiological manner can reveal the natural wrinkles and the same effect can be sought laterally to stress the lateral canthal lines. Usually, the selected wrinkle is usually located at 8–10 mm from the horizontal palpebral fissure in females and 6–8 mm in males. Local anesthesia with bupivacaine and epinephrine is injected under the skin of the superior eyelid.

Skin incision is performed using a monopolar Colorado microdissection needle, at very low intensity, directed to the lateral orbital canthus. The palpebral portion of the orbicularis oculi muscle is incised precisely at the junction between the pre-tarsal and pre-septal orbicularis, and its fibers spared, following a post-orbicularis and preseptal plane, in a superolateral direction towards the lateral orbital rim. Care must be taken in this phase not to transect the avascular "white plane" that includes the superior tarsus, the orbital septum, and the tendon of the elevator palpabrae muscle (elevator aponeurosis) to avoid the risk of postoperative ptosis. The lacrimal gland could be encountered during dissection: it must be preserved and mobilized supero-medially if needed.

Hence, the superior and lateral orbital rim can be palpated at the level of the frontozygomatic suture. At this point, some tack-up sutures can be placed at the corners of the surgical opening. The periosteum is cut straight down to the bone of the lateral orbital rim and then dissected towards the orbit, while preserving the periorbital fascia for close-up reconstruction at the end of the surgery. Dynamic retraction is applied to displace the orbit medially so the endoscope can be inserted at the superolateral corner of the surgical corridor. At this point, identification of the inferior (IOF) and superior (SOF) orbital fissures serves for anatomical orientation before removing the lateral orbital wall. The zygomaticofacial and zygomaticotemporal branches of the maxillary nerve entering the zygomatico-orbital foramina on the orbital surface of the zygomatic bone—together with the corresponding arteries—can be identified during the dissection; these must be coagulated and cut. A malleable retractor is now introduced to slightly separate the orbital contents medially. If an accidental breach opens the periorbita, careful coagulation of the intraorbital fat should be performed for retraction. Then, the endoscope can be inserted to proceed with the creation of a working space. A systematic check of the pupil size, every 20 min, is advisable throughout the surgery; in case a pupil change is noticed, it is advisable to wait until spontaneous reversal [24].

Working Space Creation

Working space creation is one of the most important phases of the transorbital approach: adequate exposure and bone removal are essential for the proper maneuverability and efficacy of the technique. Especially when reaching the PA region, a bigger working area must be created compared to a transorbital approach to the anterior of the middle fossa: this could be achieved also with the temporary removal of the lateral orbital rim [17]. The craniectomy starts by drilling the intraorbital portion of the zygomatic body, which delimits the lateral wall of the orbit until the temporalis deep fascia is exposed. Subsequently, drilling proceeds over the greater sphenoid wing, following the temporal fascia/muscle. After greater sphenoid wing removal, the temporal dura mater is seen. At this point, dedicated bone removal of different bone structures should be performed.

Sagittal Crest, Middle Fossa Dissection

Hence, to reach the PA from a transorbital perspective, it is crucial to remove several "bone pillars" of the transorbital route. In the medial portion of the surgical field, the sagittal crest and its base (the maxillary strut) need to be completely removed to clearly expose the foramen rotundum with the maxillary branch of the trigeminal nerve (Fig. 22.1c, d) [25]. When performing this part of the drilling, attention must be focused on the presence of a large lateral recess of the sphenoid sinus. If this anatomic variation is present, an opening of the sinus during the drilling may occur, and a postoperative careful reconstruction with an autologous fat graft would be needed to prevent a CSF leak. Otherwise, the base of the anterior clinoid, formed by the lesser sphenoid wing, needs to be drilled down (Fig. 22.1a). At this point, interdural dissection of the lateral wall of the cavernous sinus could be started, following the trajectory of V2. As the dissection continues upwards, a dura connection is encountered, the meningo-orbital band (MOB), which obstacles further interdural peeling and the

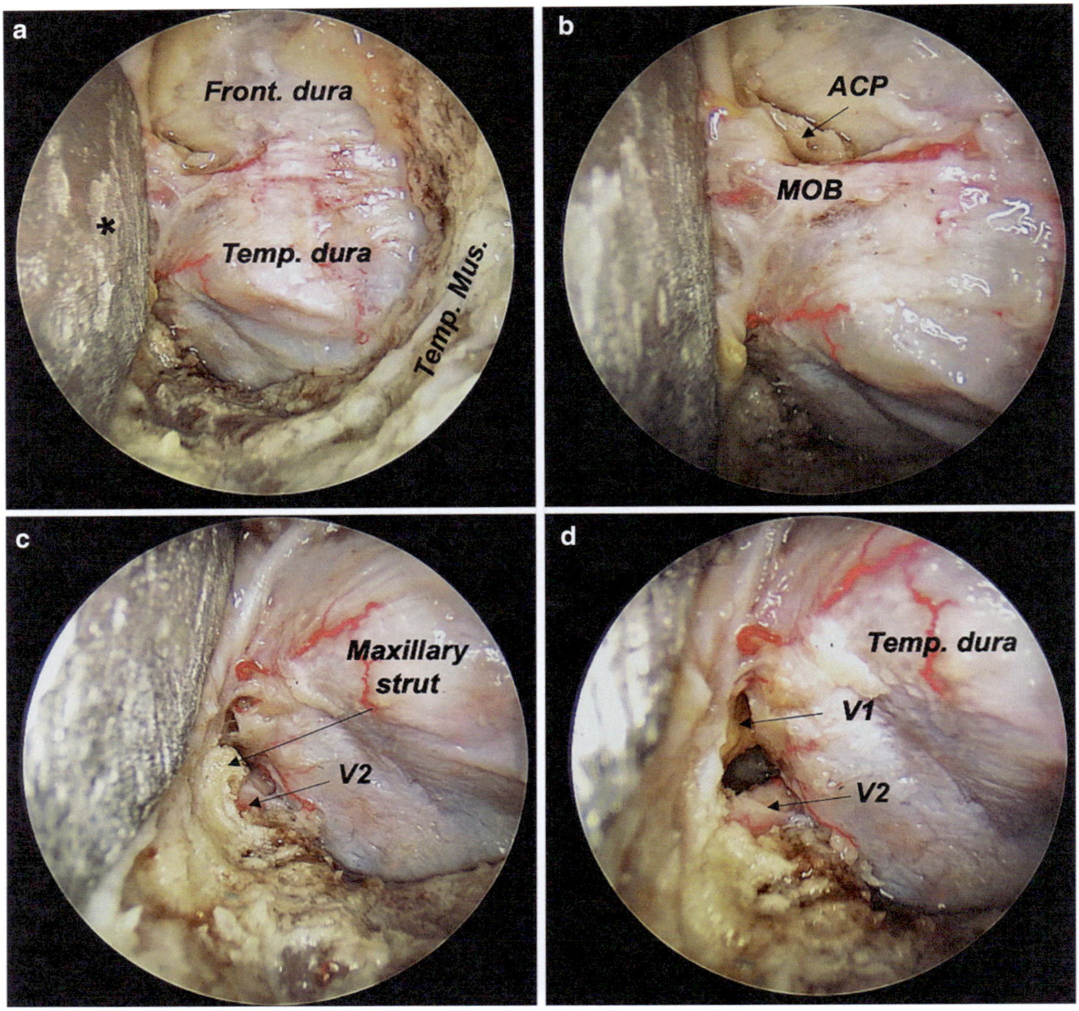

Fig. 22.1 Working space for TO approach to the petrous apex area. Cadaveric dissections (left side). (**a**) The endoscopic lateral orbital craniectomy and the opening of the superior orbital fissure exposes the dura, protecting the temporal pole. Further drilling of the lesser sphenoid wing and the base of the anterior cranial fossa floor exposes the frontal dura and the lateral attachment of the anterior clinoid process (ACP). A retractor (asterisk) maintains the periorbita medially and out of the field of view. (**b**) The meningo-orbital band (MOB) is seen extending from the frontal and temporal dura to the periorbita. The recurrent meningeal artery courses within the MOB. Adequate exposure of the MOB is essential, as cutting it will permit lateral retraction of the temporal lobe and subsequent access towards deep-seated middle and posterior fossa structures. (**c**) The inferomedial limit of bone exposure is the maxillary strut, i.e., the base of the sagittal crest. The maxillary strut impedes advancing further to the lateral wall of the cavernous sinus and needs to be removed. (**d**) Removing these two osseous structures exposes the maxillary (V2) and ophthalmic (V1) branches of the trigeminal nerve, running in the lateral wall of the cavernous sinus

mobilization of the temporal lobe. The meningo-orbital band should be coagulated and cut to achieve the adequate retraction of the temporal dura from the lateral cavernous sinus (Fig. 22.1b). The MOB can also be cut before starting the interdural dissection. Moreover, at this point the dissection can be extended in an extradural fashion to elevate the temporal dura and expose the entire floor of the middle cranial fossa. The floor of the middle fossa needs to be flattened down to get sufficient maneuverability at a depth of the surgical field [26, 27] (Fig. 22.2). The boundaries for a safe bone resection at this stage are: inferiorly, the lateral pterygoid muscle, covering the infratemporal fossa; medially, the lateral wall of the cavernous sinus; laterally, the limits with the squama temporalis; superiorly, the lesser sphenoid wing of the sphenoid bone; posteriorly, the greater superficial petrosal nerve, the petrous portion of the carotid artery and the anterior surface of the petrous segment of the temporal bone; anteriorly, the limits in between the ventral and vertical portion of the greater sphenoid wing and the horizontal portion of the greater sphenoid wing [26] (Fig. 22.2f).

Drilling of the Petrous Apex

Partial removal of the middle fossa floor and continuing with the extradural dissection of the temporal lobe unveils the petrous part of the temporal

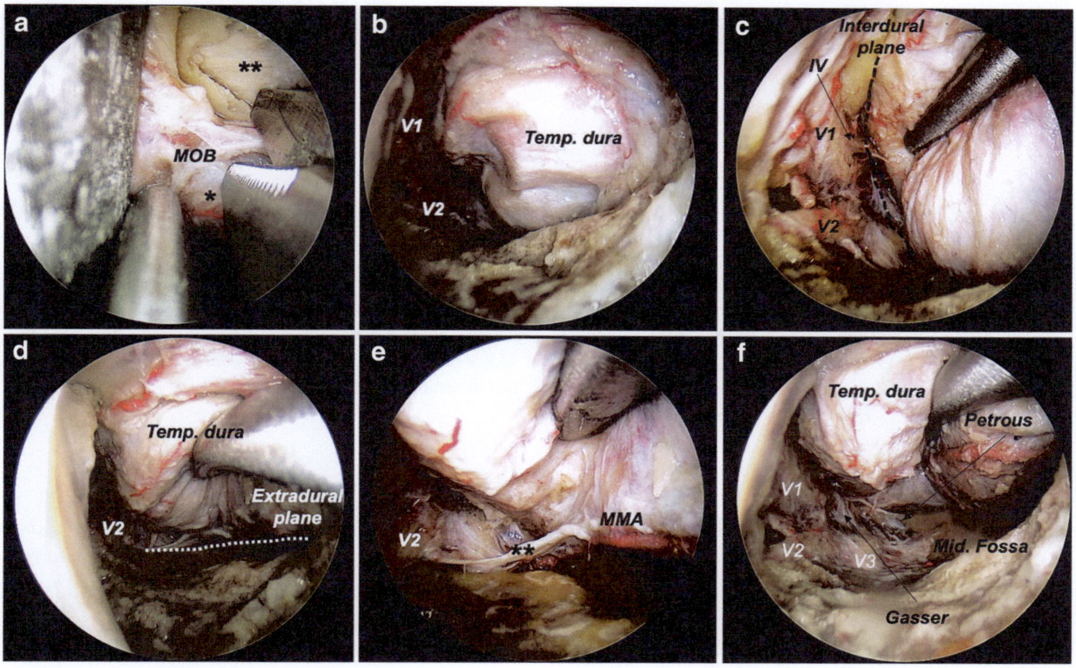

Fig. 22.2 Middle fossa dissection. Cadaveric dissections (left side). (**a**) The meningo-orbital band (MOB) extends from the temporal (asterisk) and frontal (double asterisk) dura to the periorbita. The MOB can be cut to facilitate the lateral retraction of the temporal lobe, which increases the exposure of the lateral wall of the cavernous sinus and eases the access toward deep-seated structures. (**b**) The lateral wall of the cavernous sinus comes into view. (**c**) An interdural peeling (black dashed line) is achieved by dissecting the virtual plane between the inner and outer dura layers, conforming to the lateral wall of the cavernous sinus. (**d**) An extradural peeling (white dotted line) is attained by dissecting the dura propria of the temporal lobe away from the middle fossa floor. (**e**) The point of union between the interdural and the extradural spaces is at the level of V2. Cutting off the dura attachment (double asterisk) at this point joins both spaces and increases the surgical exposure towards the petrous bone. Of note, the middle meningeal artery (MMA) is exposed with the extradural peeling. (**f**) Coagulating and cutting the MMA completes the dura dissection. The petrous bone, the petrous apex, the Gasserian ganglion and its three branches are now displayed

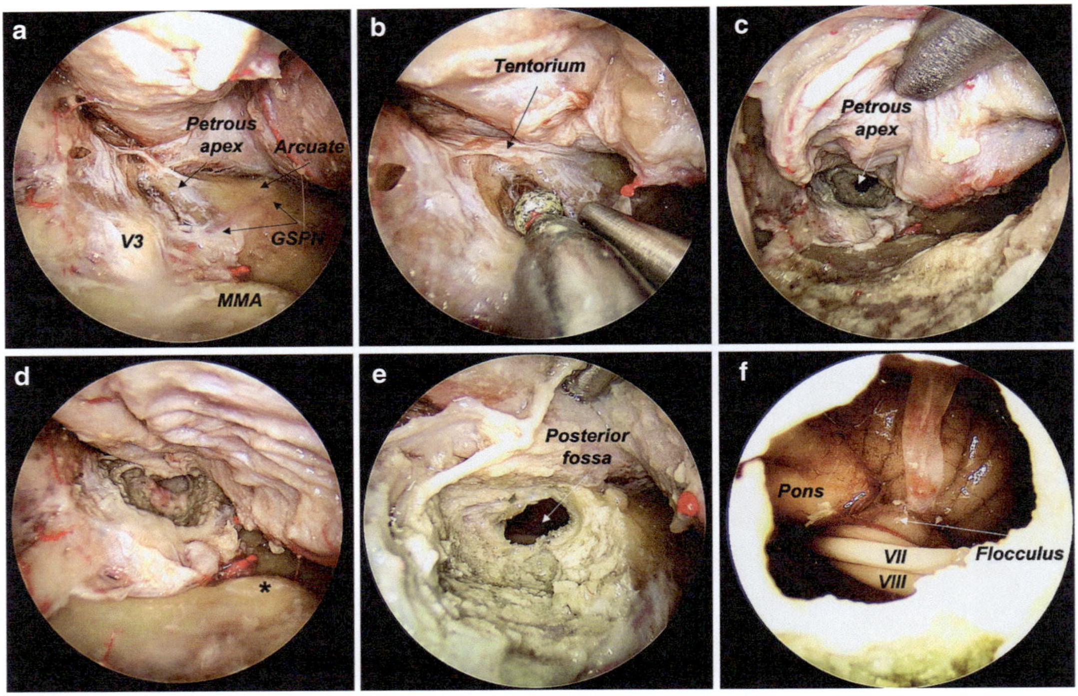

Fig. 22.3 Drilling of the petrous apex. Cadaveric dissections (left side). (**a**) The limits of petrous apex removal are shown: the great superficial petrosal nerve (GSPN), V3, arcuate eminence and the petrous ridge. (**b**) The petrous apex is removed. (**c**) Panoramic view of the middle cranial fossa after removal of the petrous apex and opening of the posterior fossa dura. (**d**, **e**) Close-up view after removing the petrous apex, before (**d**) and after (**e**) opening the posterior fossa dura. The mid-subtemporal ridge, at the floor of the middle fossa, is marked with (asterisk). (**f**) Accessing the posterior fossa through the petrous apex. The VII and VIII cranial nerves are seen coursing towards the internal acoustic meatus

bone and the PA. The corridor thus created permits performing an anterior petrous apex removal lateral to the mandibular branch (V3) of the trigeminal nerve. The anterior and inferior limit is represented by the petrous segment of internal carotid artery and the GSPN; the medial limit is represented by the Gasserian ganglion and the mandibular branch of the trigeminal nerve. This bone removal allows direct access to the structures of the posterior skull base [27] (Fig. 22.3).

After the drilling of the PA, the anterior edge of the tentorium cerebelli is exposed. Hence, after ligation/coagulation and cutting of the superior petrosal sinus, a wider access to the posterior fossa area can be obtained. The cranial fossa structures that can be visualized from this standing point are, from cranial to caudal, the midbrain and the IV cranial nerve, the pons, the cerebellum, and VII and VIII cranial nerves right before entering the internal acoustic canal, the trigeminal root (Fig. 22.4). If a 30° endoscope is introduced, it is possible to visualize the basilar artery, the III and VI cranial nerves, and the lower cranial nerves. A virtual three-dimensional model, created using Amira Visage Imaging software (Amira Visage Imaging Inc.), provides a visual 3D summary of the transorbital pathway to the petrous apex (Fig. 22.5).

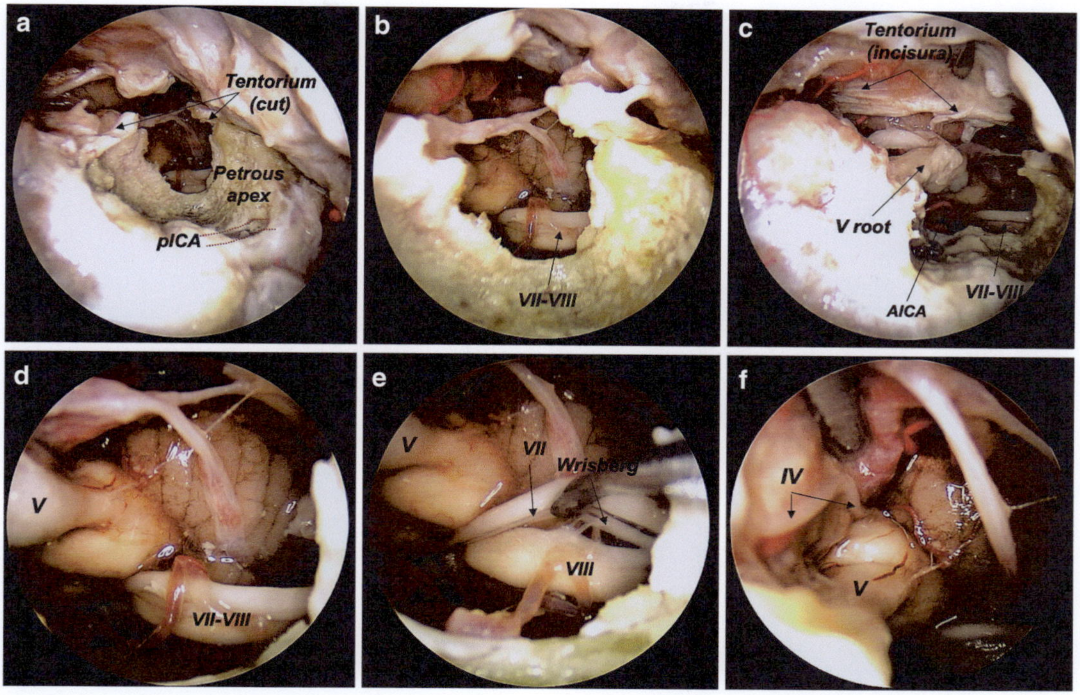

Fig. 22.4 Posterior fossa area exposure. Cadaveric dissections (left side). (**a–c**) Completing the drilling of the petrous apex medially facilitates the exposure of the trigeminal ganglion and V3. Particular care must be taken not to injure the petrous segment of the internal carotid artery (pICA). Cutting off the tentorium at its attachment in the petrous ridge significantly increases the surgical view towards the posterior fossa, particularly within the medial portion of the ponto-mesencephalic area. (**d–f**) Close-up view of the posterior fossa after the apex petrosectomy

Reconstruction

As learned from endoscopic endonasal surgery, a multilayer reconstruction with autologous materials represents the most useful technique [28, 29]. An autologous fat graft is used to fill the surgical corridor, and it is fixed with fibrin glue. Other heterologous materials may be used for bone reconstruction [23]. Most importantly, the periosteum overlying the lateral orbital rim must be consciously closed with running sutures. At the end, the orbicularis oculi muscle and the eyelid skin are closed with simple or continuous sutures. If, during the drilling of the middle fossa floor, the lateral recess of the sphenoidal sinus is accidentally opened, a fat graft should be used for reconstruction because of the high risk of postoperative CSF leak.

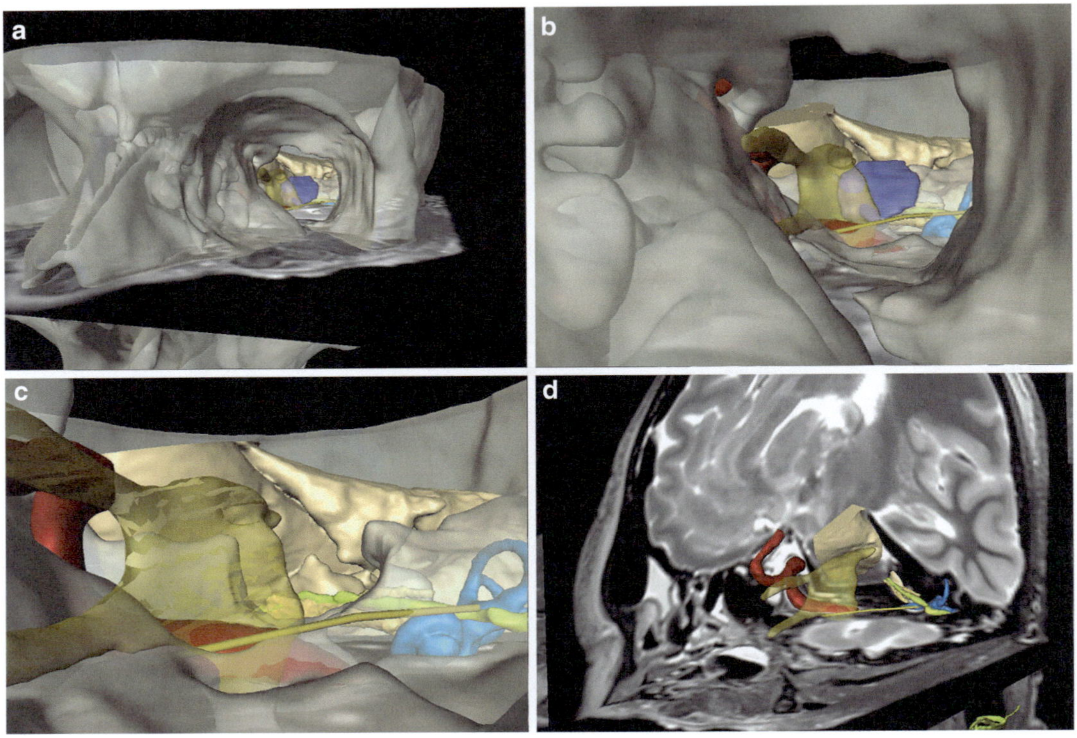

Fig. 22.5 3D Analysis of Transorbital Approach to the petrous apex. A virtual three-dimensional model was created using Amira Visage Imaging software (Amira Visage Imaging Inc.). (**a**) Ventral perspective showing the transorbital craniectomy and the location of the petrous apex (blue area). An axial MRI of the specimen is co-registered with the 3D CT scan to perform a dedicated reconstruction of the main neurovascular structures involved in the transorbital approach to the petrous apex. (**b**) Close-up view of the petrous apex via a transorbital ventral perspective. Note the greater superficial petrosal nerve (straight yellow line crossing the middle fossa floor) in close relation with the petrous internal carotid artery (red); note also that the Gasserian ganglion-V3 complex needs to be displaced medially to get more area of the petrous apex to be removal from a transorbital perspective. (**c**) Removal of the petrous apex area and exposure of the posterior fossa neurovascular structures. (**d**) Main neurovascular structures surrounding the petrous apex area

Lesion Removal: Illustrative Clinical Cases

Herein we report two illustrative cases of petroclival tumors resection that had been operated in our center through a combined endoscopic endonasal and transorbital approach.

Illustrative Case 1

A 34-year-old male presented with severe dizziness. The MRI revealed an extra-axial left-side hyper-enhancing lesion involving the middle and posterior cranial fossa, compatible with a preoperative diagnosis of petroclival meningioma (Fig. 22.6a–c). As demonstrated in the 3D reconstruction, the lesion contacted the internal carotid artery (ICA) and the basilar artery (BA), occupied the clivus and the petroclival area, and caused brainstem compression (Fig. 22.6d–f).

Following EANS guidelines about petroclival meningiomas [30], and after extensive discussion in our Skull Base Unit, a minimally invasive approach was chosen and a combined endoscopic endonasal and transorbital approach was performed [12].

With the assistance of our oculoplastic surgeon, a superior eyelid crease skin incision and a lateral orbital wall craniectomy were performed.

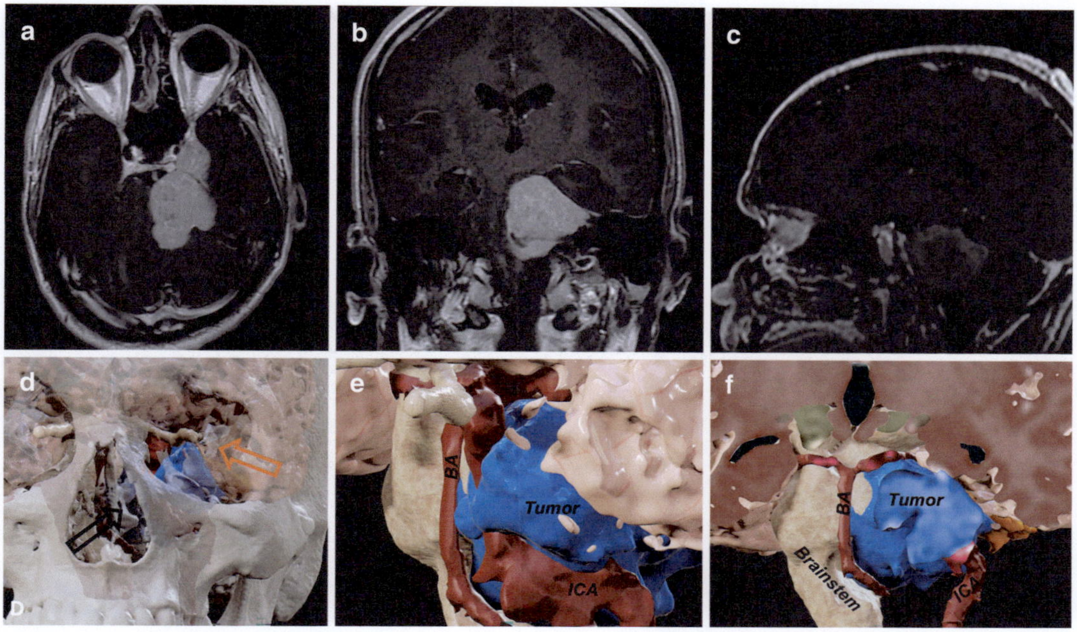

Fig. 22.6 Combined endoscopic endonasal and transorbital endoscopic approach for a petroclival meningioma (case presentation and preoperative planning). T1-weighted post-contrast preoperative MRI axial (**a**), coronal (**b**) and sagittal plane (**c**) shows a left sphenopetroclival lesion with homogenous post-contrast enhancement. Preoperative planning 3D reconstructions obtained with Brainlab workstation (**d–f**). In the external reconstruction (**d**), the endonasal (black arrow) and the transorbital perspective (orange arrow) are illustrated. The lesion (blue) is contacting the internal carotid artery (ICA) anteriorly and inferiorly, and with the basilar artery (BA) medially, and it is determining brainstem compression (**e**, **f**)

Drilling of the greater sphenoid wing exposed the temporal dura (Fig. 22.7a). After drilling of the middle fossa floor, the maxillary branch of the trigeminal nerve (V2) was identified (Fig. 22.7b); at this point, interdural peeling was started until the tumor was encountered (Fig. 22.7c): the anterior surface of the tumor was seen emerging in the interdural space. The tumor capsule was opened, and tumor debulking started. The portion of the lesion extending to the posterior fossa was accessed through the trigeminal pore and was removed in combination with the endonasal pathway (Fig. 22.7d).

Hence, at this zone, the endonasal midline transclival route and the transorbital approach were able to work simultaneously yet from opposite sides of the lesion until satisfactory decompression was achieved (Figs. 22.8 and 22.9).

Hemostasis was achieved by means of thrombin agents and mechanical compression. Transorbital reconstruction was performed with an autologous fat graft and a dura substitute. For endonasal reconstruction, an autologous fat graft and a naso-septal flap were used [31]. In the early postoperative period, the patient developed lateral gaze diplopia and upper eyelid edema, which progressively improved and solved within a few days. At the last follow-up, the patient presented V1–V2 hypoesthesia and slight left hypoacusia. The pathology report showed a clear cells meningioma (WHO grade 2 [32]). Early postoperative MRI showed a subtotal removal with an extent of resection of 80%; adjuvant radiotherapy treatment on the lesion remnant was indicated (54 Gray, 30 fractions). At the last radiological follow-up (2 years), the residual lesion was stable (Fig. 22.10).

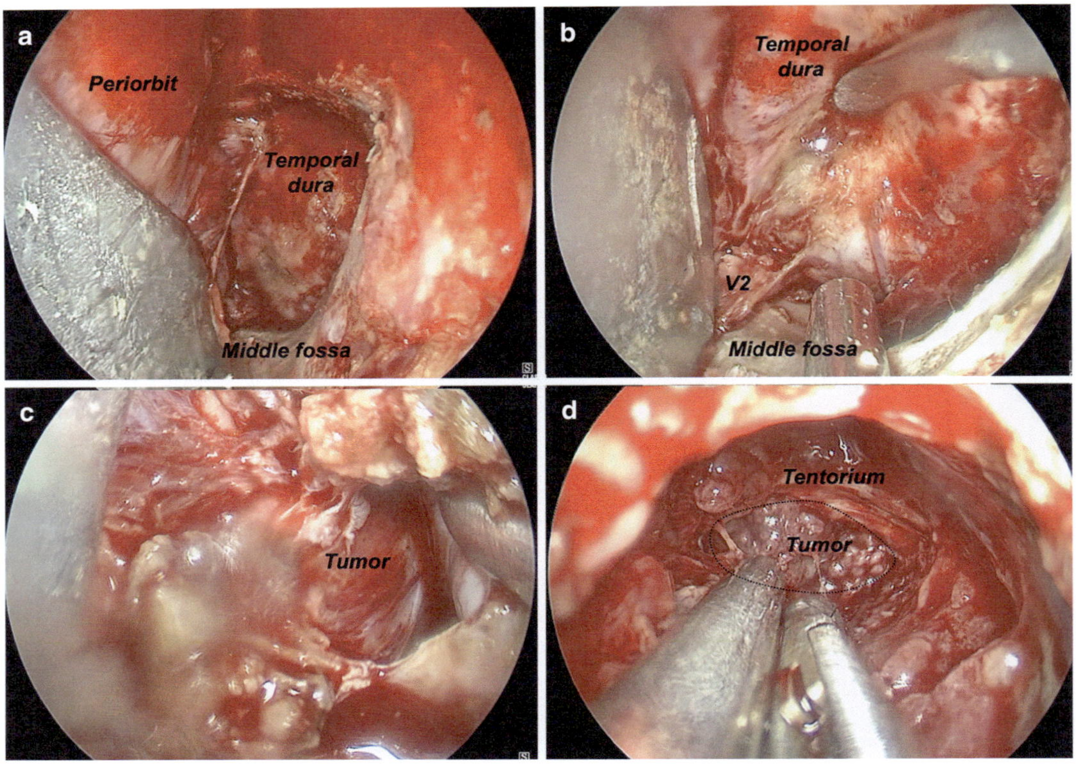

Fig. 22.7 Combined endoscopic endonasal and transorbital endoscopic approach to a petroclival meningioma (endoscopic transorbital approach intraoperative images). Drilling of the greater sphenoid wing was performed to expose temporal dura (**a**). After drilling of the middle fossa floor, the maxillary trigeminal branch (V2) was identified (**b**): at this point interdural peeling was started until encountering the tumor (**c**). The lesion was accessed through the trigeminal pore (dotted black line) and the anterior edge of the tentorium cerebelli (**d**)

Illustrative Case 2

A 73-year-old male presented with severe gait instability and dizziness. The MRI revealed an extra-axial left-side lesion with homogeneous enhancement involving the middle and posterior cranial fossa, compatible with a petroclival meningioma (Fig. 22.11a–c).

A combined endoscopic endonasal and transorbital approach was performed.

A superior eyelid crease incision and lateral orbital wall craniectomy were performed with the assistance of an oculoplastic surgeon. Drilling the greater sphenoid wing exposed the temporal dura, and the drilling of the middle fossa floor revealed the maxillary branch of the trigeminal nerve (V2) (Fig. 22.12a). An interdural peeling led to the tumor (Fig. 22.12b).

Tumor debulking and dissection were started from both corridors simultaneously (Fig. 22.12c) and continued until satisfactory brainstem decompression was achieved. Hemostasis was later achieved by means of thrombin agents and mechanical compression.

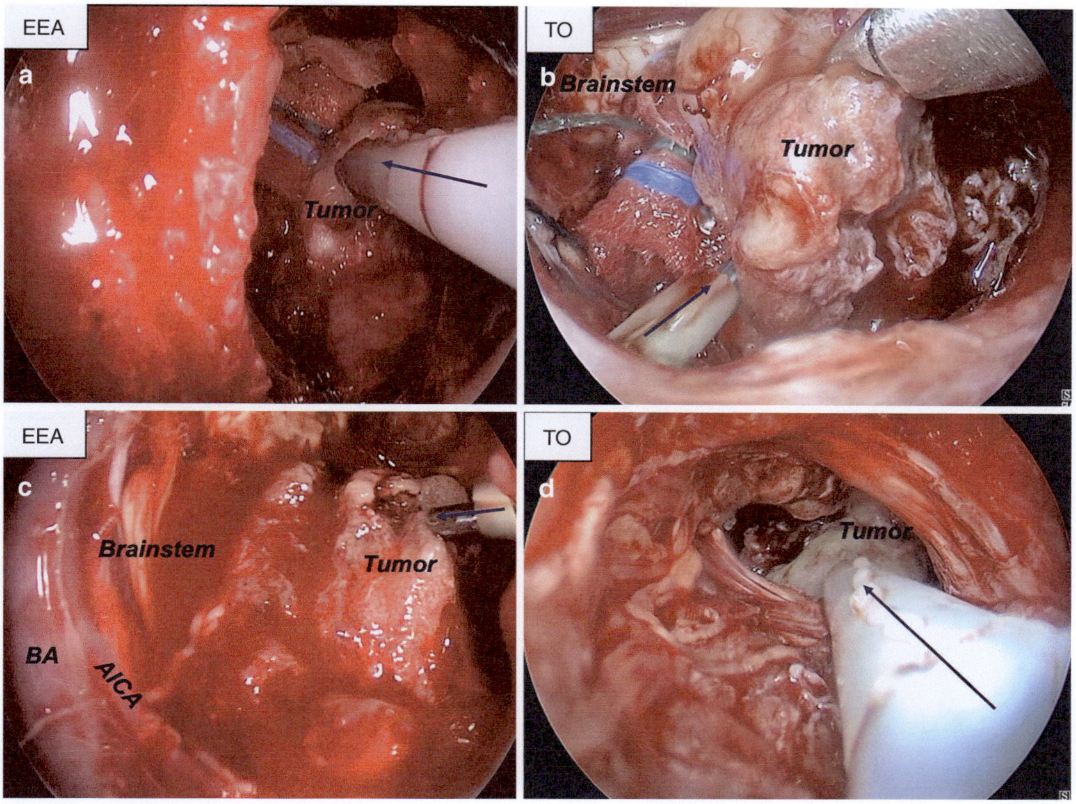

Fig. 22.8 Combined endoscopic endonasal and transorbital endoscopic approach to a petroclival meningioma (endoscopic endonasal and transorbital approach, intraoperative images). In this panel, simultaneous endonasal (EEA) and transorbital (TO) intraoperative views are offered (**a** and **b**, **c** and **d**). During a simultaneous combined approach is possible to work with instruments from both corridors at the same time. In fact, the ultrasonic aspirator, indicated with the blue arrow, used from the endonasal corridor (**a**) can be seen perfectly from the transorbital route (**b**). In the same manner, the ultrasonic aspirator indicated with the blue arrow is visualized from the endonasal perspective (**c**) when used from the transorbital corridor (**d**). During tumor dissection and debulking, basilar (BA), antero-inferior cerebellar artery (AICA) and the brainstem could be seen from endonasal and transorbital approach (**b**, **c**)

Transorbital reconstruction was performed with an autologous fat graft and a dura substitute (Fig. 22.12d).

For the endonasal reconstruction, an autologous fat graft and a naso-septal flap were used [31]. In the early postoperative period, the patient developed upper eyelid edema, which rapidly improved, and VI cranial nerve palsy, which remained up to the time of the last follow-up. The pathology report showed transitional meningioma (WHO grade 1 [32]). Early postoperative MRI showed a subtotal removal with an extent of resection of 90%; adjuvant treatments were not required. At the last radiological follow-up (2 years), the residual lesion was stable (Fig. 22.11d–f).

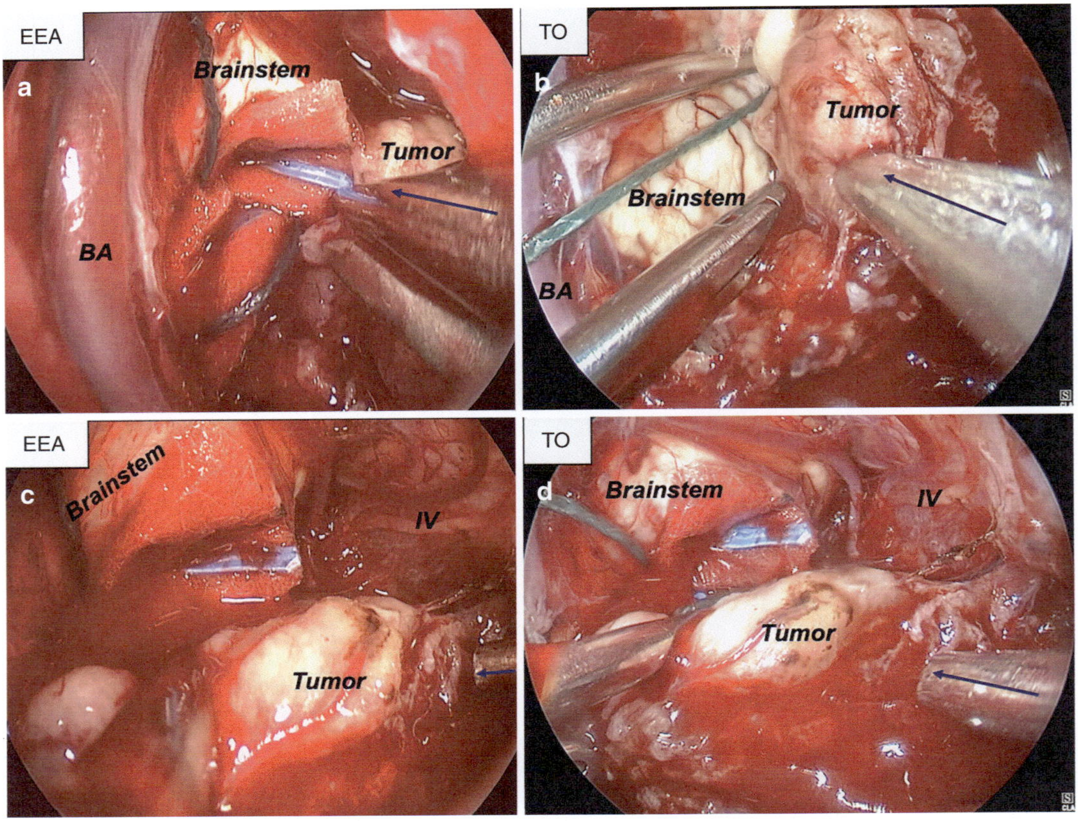

Fig. 22.9 Combined endoscopic endonasal and transorbital endoscopic approach to a petroclival meningioma (endoscopic endonasal and transorbital approach, intraoperative images). In this panel, simultaneous endonasal (EEA) and transorbital (TO) intraoperative views are offered (**a** and **b**, **c** and **d**). In fact, the aspirator indicated with the blue arrow can be seen from the endonasal corridor (**a**) when used from the transorbital route (**b**). In the same manner, the aspirator indicated with the blue arrow is visualized from the endonasal perspective (**c**) when used from the transorbital corridor (**d**). During tumor dissection and debulking, basilar (BA), the IV cranial nerve (IV) and the brainstem could be seen from endonasal and transorbital approach (**c**, **d**). Continuing with tumor removal, brainstem decompression could be achieved

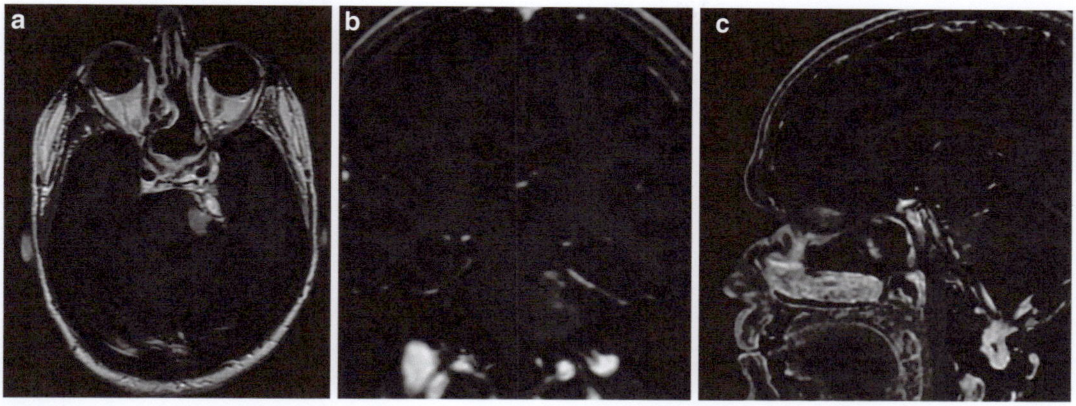

Fig. 22.10 Combined endoscopic endonasal and transorbital endoscopic approach to a petroclival meningioma (surgical outcome). (**a–c**) Two-year follow-up post-contrast cerebral MRI after radiotherapy treatment, showing stability of tumor residual lesion

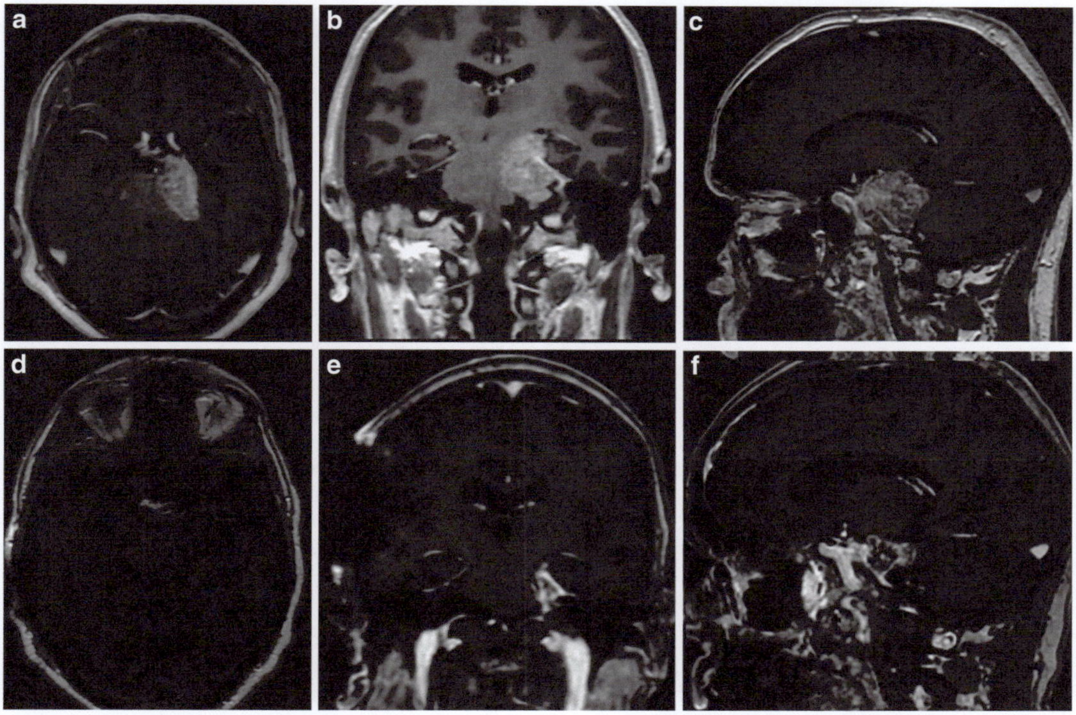

Fig. 22.11 Combined endoscopic endonasal and transorbital endoscopic approach to a petroclival meningioma (case presentation and surgical outcome). The preoperative T1-weighted post-contrast brain MRI (**a–c**) revealed an extra-axial left-side lesion with homogeneous enhancement involving the middle and posterior cranial fossa, compatible with a preoperative diagnosis of petroclival meningioma. At the 2 years postoperative follow-up, T1-weighted post-contrast brain MRI (**d–f**) shows the stability of residual tumor

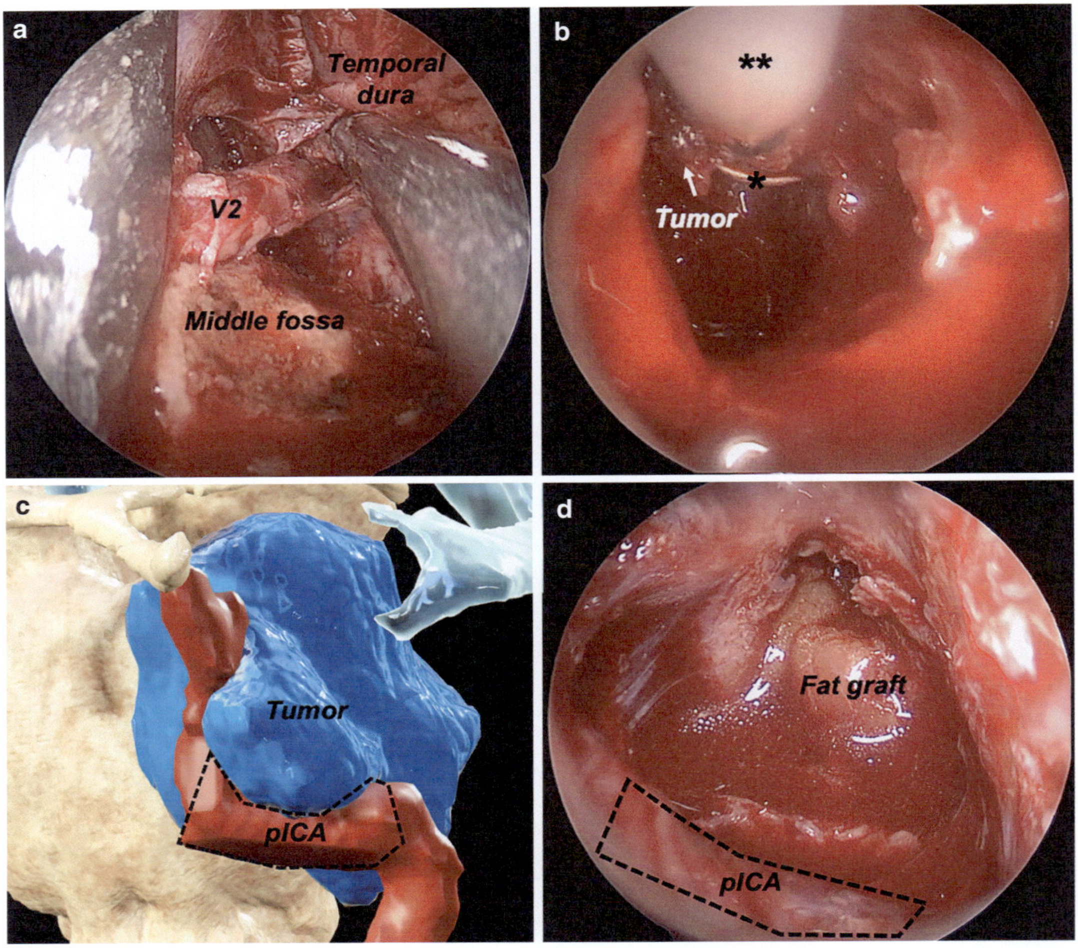

Fig. 22.12 Combined endoscopic endonasal and transorbital endoscopic approach to a petroclival meningioma (endoscopic transorbital approach intraoperative images and 3D reconstruction). After drilling of the middle fossa floor, the maxillary trigeminal branch (V2) was identified (**a**). At this point interdural peeling was started until encountering the tumor (**b**) that was dissected from both corridors. In fact, a curette (black asterisk) dissects the tumor from the endonasal approach while an ultrasonic aspirator (black double asterisk) is used from the transorbital corridor for tumor debulking, working simultaneously from both corridors (**b**). As seen in the preoperative 3D reconstruction obtained with Brainlab workstation (**c**), the tumor is strictly contacting the petrous segment of the internal carotid artery (pICA). Transorbital reconstruction was performed with a dural substitute and autologous fat graft (**d**)

Comparison with the Alternative Surgical Approaches

Transcranial Perspective

The PA is one of the most challenging areas in skull base surgery because it is surrounded by numerous critical neurovascular structures [33]. Multiple surgical approaches have been developed to address this complex zone over the years. All approaches to the petroclival region aim to acquire the best possible visualization of the important neural and vascular structures that could be compressed or encased by a lesion.

The petrous temporal bone is an obstacle in the approach to the petroclival region. Oftentimes neurosurgeons are unfamiliar with the anatomy of the petrous bone, prompting surgical approaches through more common suboccipital and pterional routes. Some authors have advocated using traditional neurosurgical approaches to these tumors [34–36]. The advantages of lateral skull base approaches include decreasing the operative distance to the tumor and neurovascular structures, improving visualization and lighting, and allowing access to the tumor with minimal brain retraction. Strategies to overcome the petrous bone as an obstacle have included resection of the PA with a middle fossa approach [37], resection of presigmoid retrolabyrinthine petrous bone with a posterior petrosal approach [38], and resection of the entire petrous bone with a complete petrosectomy [39].

Since the introduction of the middle fossa transpetrosal-transtentorial approach (Kawase's approach) to the PA in the mid-1980s, microscopic anterior petrosectomy has been recognized as a milestone pathway to various skull base lesions around the PA [1]. Kawase published an anterior petrosal approach to expose the posterior cranial fossa and to minimize retraction of the temporal lobe; to achieve this surgical target, a sufficient anterior petrosectomy should be performed [40]. The traditional Kawase approach provides an opening of the PA of the temporal bone between the V cranial nerve and the internal auditory canal. Due to its technical complexity [41], surgeons developed modified versions of this subtemporal approach in a multiplicity of variations and combinations during the following years. Noteworthy, a so-called modified Dolenc-Kawase approach, incorporating the surgical benefits of Dolenc's and Kawase's techniques, has been recently proven to achieve a larger area of exposure at the anterior PA [42]. This approach gives access to the prepontine area, Dorello's canal, anterior PA, and upper two-thirds of the clivus with better angulation and surgical flexibility [43]. It is a versatile approach for petroclival lesions that do not extend laterally and inferiorly to the internal auditory canal [44]. Some studies have favored transpetrosal approaches, including the presigmoid approach, due to the improved view of the tumor–brainstem cleavage, reduced retraction of brain tissue and the CNs, and the broader surgical field [45–47]; nevertheless, these approaches are more time-consuming, demanding, and morbid compared to other surgical routes, and require extensive training.

Another transcranial alternative is the retrosigmoid approach [48, 49]. Some surgeons prefer the retrosigmoid approach for its simplicity, remarkably useful for brainstem decompression, and the preservation of the petrous bone. The retrosigmoid intradural suprameatal approach was first introduced by Samii et al. [50], as a modification of the classic retrosigmoid approach intended to open Meckel's cave, exposing the trigeminal nerve and accessing the middle fossa. In this case the area of bone resected is similar to Kawase's approach. While the direction of drilling in Kawase's approach is from anterior and superior, the direction of drilling in Sami's approach is from posterior and inferior [51]. Despite its advantages, the retrosigmoid approach is mostly reserved for treating cerebello-pontine angle lesions [52].

In general, the need for cerebellum and temporal lobe retraction and the deep surgical corridors crossing the cranial nerves are the major disadvantages of the transcranial routes. As a matter of fact, despite all its variations, transcranial approaches report a huge rate of postoperative complications [53] and surgical morbidity remains high [3, 10, 32, 42], particularly with cranial nerve dysfunctions (66.8%). Postoperative complications include oculomotor nerve palsy (III, IV, and VI), dysfunction of the facial, trigeminal and cochlear and lower cranial nerves deficits, hemiparesis and ataxia.

Because none of the approaches have demonstrated superiority over the others, it is reasonable to say that satisfactory resections and outcomes can be anticipated when experienced surgeons utilize their familiar approaches and skillful microsurgical techniques [54].

Endonasal Perspective

To minimize surgical morbidity and brain retraction, ventral minimally invasive techniques have been explored: the endoscopic endonasal technique has been found to be a useful option for accessing the PA area and petroclival junction [2, 55, 56].

An extended endonasal transpterygoid and transclival approach associated with sphenoidectomy is performed to access the PA from the endonasal route [57]. At this point, several landmarks re exposed: the foramen lacerum and the paraclival internal carotid artery (ICA), including the vidian nerve and the soft tissue of pterygosphenoidal fissure [58]; at the level of the sphenoidal sinus floor, the lateral limit is represented by the Vidian nerve as it exits its canal at the vomerosphenoidal junction; this nerve leads to the horizontal segment of the ICA. Moreover, full skeletonization of the paraclival ICA and the exposure of the middle cranial fossa dura laterally is necessary to access PA area.

Dissecting the soft tissue surrounding the paraclival ICA to mobilize it is mandatory to obtain good exposure to the PA [58, 59]. Five main anatomical landmarks surrounding the anterior genu of the petrous ICA are identified as the posterior limit of the endoscopic endonasal transpterygoid approach: the end of the vidian canal (VC), the eustachian tube (ET), the foramen lacerum (FL), the petroclival fissure, and the pharyngobasilar fascia, the so-called "VELPPHA area" [60].

The boundaries of petrous bone removal from this perspective are: (a) inferiorly, the foramen lacerum and the floor of the sphenoid sinus; (b) laterally, the paraclival ICA that was previously lateralized; (c) medially, the lateral portion of the clivus; and (d) superiorly, the abducens nerve.

However, as a strict midline route [61], the endoscopic endonasal approach may be unable to properly manage lesions involving the most lateral aspects of the skull base.

Indications and Limitations of Endoscopic Transorbital Approach

The endoscopic superior eyelid transorbital approach can be used in several pathological scenarios with a progressive level of difficulty [19]. Extraconal and extradural lesions and bone pathologies (hyperostosis, fractures and bone defects) can be treated with this approach [9, 62, 63], as s well asintradural sphenoorbital meningiomas (involving or not the anterior clinoid process) [10, 64]. Furthermore, lesions of the middle cranial fossa, for example, in Meckel's cave or of the cavernous sinus areas, can be addressed through this route [21, 65–67]. Intracerebral lesions of the temporal lobe can also be treated through the transorbital path [68, 69].

For lesions involving the petroclival region the transorbital approach can be used alone or in combination with the endonasal or the transmaxillary route [33, 58, 70, 71]. New indications are still under investigation, and further clinical studies are needed to verify the reproducibility of anatomic studies and hypotheses.

The endoscopic transorbital approach requires a specific learning curve for the neurosurgeon: elaborate bimanual dissection and meticulous bleeding control could be hard to obtain with the endoscope in such a reduced space. Moreover, a comprehensive understanding of the neuroanatomy as seen via the transorbital approach is mandatory, which is not completely usual. Furthermore, interdisciplinary cooperation among other specialists (ENT surgeons, ophthalmologists, and anesthesiologists) is mandatory to obtain satisfactory results.

Due to the absence of specific orbital pressure control instruments, the intermittent release of the orbit content displacement should be used to avoid postoperative visual deficits and frequent control of the pupil size must be performed: this could lead to a larger surgical time. Although transient ocular dysfunction has been reported, permanent visual impairment or long-term ophthalmological alterations are rare, with satisfactory visual outcomes [72, 73]. Of note, cerebrospinal fluid leakage does not seem as frequent after transorbital surgery as it is in extended endonasal surgery [26, 74].

Conclusions

In this chapter, the current surgical approaches for treating petrous apex lesions have been resumed and contrasted.

We believe that the endoscopic transorbital approach represents a valid and feasible minimally invasive therapeutic option, alone or in combination with other surgical routes, to access selected petrous apex pathologies and even lesions extending towards the posterior fossa. It offers a different perspective, minimizing brain manipulation. More studies and clinical cases are necessary to develop its potential completely.

References

1. Kawase T, Shiobara R, Toya S. Anterior transpetrosal-transtentorial approach for sphenopetroclival meningiomas: surgical method and results in 10 patients. Neurosurgery. 1991;28(6):869–75; discussion 75–6.
2. Zanation AM, Snyderman CH, Carrau RL, Gardner PA, Prevedello DM, Kassam AB. Endoscopic endonasal surgery for petrous apex lesions. Laryngoscope. 2009;119(1):19–25.
3. Di Somma A, Andaluz N, Cavallo LM, Topczewski TE, Frio F, Gerardi RM, et al. Endoscopic transorbital route to the petrous apex: a feasibility anatomic study. Acta Neurochir. 2018;160(4):707–20.
4. Last RJ, McMinn RMH. Last's anatomy: regional and applied. Churchill Livingstone; 1994.
5. Matsushima T, Matsushima K, Kobayashi S, Lister JR, Morcos JJ. The microneurosurgical anatomy legacy of Albert L. Rhoton Jr., MD: an analysis of transition and evolution over 50 years. J Neurosurg. 2018;129(5):1331–41.
6. Chae R, Rodriguez Rubio R. Anatomy of petrous face. Handb Clin Neurol. 2020;170:143–56.
7. Kassam A, Snyderman CH, Mintz A, Gardner P, Carrau RL. Expanded endonasal approach: the rostrocaudal axis. Part I. Crista galli to the sella turcica. Neurosurg Focus. 2005;19(1):E3.
8. Kassam A, Snyderman CH, Mintz A, Gardner P, Carrau RL. Expanded endonasal approach: the rostrocaudal axis. Part II. Posterior clinoids to the foramen magnum. Neurosurg Focus. 2005;19(1):E4.
9. Almeida JP, Omay SB, Shetty SR, Chen YN, Ruiz-Treviño AS, Liang B, et al. Transorbital endoscopic eyelid approach for resection of sphenoorbital meningiomas with predominant hyperostosis: report of 2 cases. J Neurosurg. 2018;128(6):1885–95.
10. Dallan I, Sellari-Franceschini S, Turri-Zanoni M, de Notaris M, Fiacchini G, Fiorini FR, et al. Endoscopic transorbital superior eyelid approach for the management of selected spheno-orbital meningiomas: preliminary experience. Oper Neurosurg (Hagerstown). 2018;14(3):243–51.
11. Di Somma A, Andaluz N, Cavallo LM, de Notaris M, Dallan I, Solari D, et al. Endoscopic transorbital superior eyelid approach: anatomical study from a neurosurgical perspective. J Neurosurg. 2018;129(5):1203–16.
12. Di Somma A, Langdon C, de Notaris M, Reyes L, Ortiz-Perez S, Alobid I, et al. Combined and simultaneous endoscopic endonasal and transorbital surgery for a Meckel's cave schwannoma: technical nuances of a mini-invasive, multiportal approach. J Neurosurg. 2020;134(6):1836–45.
13. Moe KS, Bergeron CM, Ellenbogen RG. Transorbital neuroendoscopic surgery. Neurosurgery. 2010;67(3 Suppl Operative):ons16–28.
14. Ferrari M, Schreiber A, Mattavelli D, Belotti F, Rampinelli V, Lancini D, et al. The inferolateral transorbital endoscopic approach: a preclinical anatomic study. World Neurosurg. 2016;90:403–13.
15. Locatelli D, Restelli F, Alfiero T, Campione A, Pozzi F, Balbi S, et al. The role of the transorbital superior eyelid approach in the management of selected spheno-orbital meningiomas: in-depth analysis of indications, technique, and outcomes from the study of a cohort of 35 patients. J Neurol Surg B Skull Base. 2022;83(2):145–58.
16. Schwartz TH, Henderson F, Di Somma A, Kong DS, de Notaris M, Enseñat J, et al. Endoscopic transorbital surgery: another leap of faith? World Neurosurg. 2022;159:54–5.
17. Lim J, Sung KS, Kim W, Yoo J, Jung IH, Choi S, et al. Extended endoscopic transorbital approach with superior-lateral orbital rim osteotomy: cadaveric feasibility study and clinical implications (SevEN-007). J Neurosurg. 2021;137(1):18–31.
18. Park HH, Roh TH, Choi S, Yoo J, Kim WH, Jung IH, et al. Endoscopic transorbital approach to mesial temporal lobe for intra-axial lesions: cadaveric study and case series (SevEN-008). Oper Neurosurg (Hagerstown). 2021;21(6):E506–15.
19. Di Somma A, Kong D-S, de Notaris M, Moe K, Sanchez JC, Schwartz T, et al. Endoscopic transorbital surgery levels of difficulty. J Neurosurg. 2022;137(4):1187–90.
20. Gassner HG, Schwan F, Schebesch KM. Minimally invasive surgery of the anterior skull base: transorbital approaches. GMS Curr Top Otorhinolaryngol Head Neck Surg. 2015;14:Doc03.
21. Priddy BH, Nunes CF, Beer-Furlan A, Carrau R, Dallan I, Prevedello DM. A side door to Meckel's cave: anatomic feasibility study for the lateral transorbital approach. Oper Neurosurg (Hagerstown). 2017;13(5):614–21.
22. Alqahtani A, Padoan G, Segnini G, Lepera D, Fortunato S, Dallan I, et al. Transorbital transnasal endoscopic combined approach to the anterior and middle skull base: a laboratory investigation. Acta Otorhinolaryngol Ital. 2015;35(3):173–9.
23. Di Somma A, Sanchez España JC, Alobid I, Enseñat J. Endoscopic superior eyelid transorbital approach: how I do it. Acta Neurochir. 2022;164(7):1953–9.
24. Kong DS, Young SM, Hong CK, Kim YD, Hong SD, Choi JW, et al. Clinical and ophthalmological out-

come of endoscopic transorbital surgery for cranioorbital tumors. J Neurosurg. 2018;131(3):667–75.
25. Corrivetti F, de Notaris M, Di Somma A, Dallan I, Enseñat J, Topczewski T, et al. “Sagittal crest”: definition, stepwise dissection, and clinical implications from a transorbital perspective. Oper Neurosurg (Hagerstown). 2022;22(5):e206–12.
26. Guizzardi G, Mosteiro A, Hoyos J, Ferres A, Topczewski T, Reyes L, et al. Endoscopic transorbital approach to the middle fossa: qualitative and quantitative anatomic study. Oper Neurosurg (Hagerstown). 2022;23(4):e267–75.
27. Guizzardi G, Prats-Galino A, Mosteiro A, Santos C, Topczewski T, Torales J, et al. Multiportal combined endoscopic endonasal and transorbital pathways: qualitative and quantitative anatomic studies of the “connection” skull base areas. Oper Neurosurg (Hagerstown). 2023;24(5):e342–50.
28. Esposito F, Dusick JR, Fatemi N, Kelly DF. Graded repair of cranial base defects and cerebrospinal fluid leaks in transsphenoidal surgery. Oper Neurosurg (Hagerstown). 2007;60(4 Suppl 2):295–303; discussion 303–4.
29. Cavallo LM, Solari D, Somma T, Cappabianca P. The 3F (fat, flap, and flash) technique for skull base reconstruction after endoscopic endonasal suprasellar approach. World Neurosurg. 2019;126:439–46.
30. Giammattei L, di Russo P, Starnoni D, Passeri T, Bruneau M, Meling TR, et al. Petroclival meningiomas: update of current treatment and consensus by the EANS skull base section. Acta Neurochir. 2021;163(6):1639–63.
31. Hadad G, Bassagasteguy L, Carrau RL, Mataza JC, Kassam A, Snyderman CH, et al. A novel reconstructive technique after endoscopic expanded endonasal approaches: vascular pedicle nasoseptal flap. Laryngoscope. 2006;116(10):1882–6.
32. Louis DN, Perry A, Reifenberger G, von Deimling A, Figarella-Branger D, Cavenee WK, et al. The 2016 World Health Organization classification of tumors of the central nervous system: a summary. Acta Neuropathol. 2016;131(6):803–20.
33. Lee WJ, Hong SD, Woo KI, Seol HJ, Choi JW, Lee JI, et al. Endoscopic endonasal and transorbital approaches to petrous apex lesions. J Neurosurg. 2022;136(2):431–40.
34. Goel A, Muzumdar D. Conventional posterior fossa approach for surgery on petroclival meningiomas: a report on an experience with 28 cases. Surg Neurol. 2004;62(4):332–8; discussion 8–40.
35. Spallone A, Makhmudov UB, Mukhamedjanov DJ, Tcherekajev VA. Petroclival meningioma. An attempt to define the role of skull base approaches in their surgical management. Surg Neurol. 1999;51(4):412–9; discussion 9–20.
36. Shen T, Friedman RA, Brackmann DE, Slattery WH, Hitselberger WE, Schwartz MS, et al. The evolution of surgical approaches for posterior fossa meningiomas. Otol Neurotol. 2004;25(3):394–7.
37. Kusumi M, Fukushima T, Mehta AI, Cunningham CD, Friedman AH, Fujii K. Middle fossa approach for total resection of petrous apex cholesterol granulomas: use of vascularized galeofascial flap preventing recurrence. Neurosurgery. 2013;72(1 Suppl Operative):77–86; discussion.
38. Gross BA, Tavanaiepour D, Du R, Al-Mefty O, Dunn IF. Evolution of the posterior petrosal approach. Neurosurg Focus. 2012;33(2):E7.
39. Aversa A, Essayed WIBN, Al-Mefty O. Total petrosectomy for the total resection of sphenopetroclival meningioma: 2-dimensional operative video. Oper Neurosurg (Hagerstown). 2021;21(1):E22–E3.
40. Jung IH, Yoo J, Roh TH, Park HH, Hong CK. Importance of sufficient petrosectomy in an anterior petrosal approach: relightening of the Kawase pyramid. World Neurosurg. 2021;153:e11–e9.
41. Borghei-Razavi H, Tomio R, Fereshtehnejad SM, Shibao S, Schick U, Toda M, et al. Pathological location of cranial nerves in petroclival lesions: how to avoid their injury during anterior petrosal approach. J Neurol Surg B Skull Base. 2016;77(1):6–13.
42. Katiyar V, Sharma R, Bora SK, Suri A. Anterior petrous rhomboid approach for petroclival chondrosarcoma. World Neurosurg. 2022;164:348.
43. Tripathi M, Deo RC, Suri A, Srivastav V, Baby B, Kumar S, et al. Quantitative analysis of the Kawase versus the modified Dolenc-Kawase approach for middle cranial fossa lesions with variable anteroposterior extension. J Neurosurg. 2015;123(1):14–22.
44. Suri A, Sharma R, Katiyar V, Raheja A. Modified Dolenc-Kawase anterior petrous rhomboid approach for petroclival meningioma: surgical nuances and complication avoidance. Neurosurg Focus Video. 2022;6(2):V12.
45. Elhadi AM, Almefty KK, Mendes GA, Kalani MY, Nakaji P, Dru A, et al. Comparison of surgical freedom and area of exposure in three endoscopic transmaxillary approaches to the anterolateral cranial base. J Neurol Surg B Skull Base. 2014;75(5):346–53.
46. Al-Mefty O, Ayoubi S, Smith RR. The petrosal approach: indications, technique, and results. Acta Neurochir Suppl (Wien). 1991;53:166–70.
47. Erkmen K, Pravdenkova S, Al-Mefty O. Surgical management of petroclival meningiomas: factors determining the choice of approach. Neurosurg Focus. 2005;19(2):E7.
48. Cui H, Zhou CF, Bao YH, Wang MS, Wang Y. Extended suboccipital retrosigmoid surgical approach is effective for resection of petrous apex meningioma. J Craniofac Surg. 2016;27(5):e429–33.
49. de Souza DG, Ditzel Filho LF, Makonnen G, Zoli M, Naudy C, Muto J, et al. Retrosigmoid approach for resection of petrous apex meningioma. Neurosurg Focus. 2014;36(1 Suppl):1.
50. Samii M, Tatagiba M, Carvalho GA. Retrosigmoid intradural suprameatal approach to Meckel's cave and the middle fossa: surgical technique and outcome. J Neurosurg. 2000;92(2):235–41.

51. Munich SA, Morcos JJ. Petrous apex meningioma with extension into Meckel's cave: resection using a retrosigmoid intradural suprameatal approach. J Neurol Surg B Skull Base. 2019;80(Suppl 3):S300–S1.
52. Ali MS, Magill ST, McDermott MW. Petrous face meningiomas. Handb Clin Neurol. 2020;170:157–65.
53. Tomio R, Horiguchi T, Borghei-Razavi H, Tamura R, Yoshida K, Kawase T. Anterior transpetrosal approach: experiences in 274 cases over 33 years. Technical variations, operated patients, and approach-related complications. J Neurosurg. 2022;136(2):413–21.
54. Li D, Tang J, Ren C, Wu Z, Zhang LW, Zhang JT. Surgical management of medium and large petroclival meningiomas: a single institution's experience of 199 cases with long-term follow-up. Acta Neurochir. 2016;158(3):409–25; discussion 25.
55. Kasemsiri P, Solares CA, Carrau RL, Prosser JD, Prevedello DM, Otto BA, et al. Endoscopic endonasal transpterygoid approaches: anatomical landmarks for planning the surgical corridor. Laryngoscope. 2013;123(4):811–5.
56. Mehta GU, Raza SM. Endoscopic endonasal transpterygoid approach to petrous pathologies: technique, limitations and alternative approaches. J Neurosurg Sci. 2018;62(3):339–46.
57. Hardesty DA, Montaser AS, Carrau RL, Prevedello DM. Limits of endoscopic endonasal transpterygoid approach to cavernous sinus and Meckel's cave. J Neurosurg Sci. 2018;62(3):332–8.
58. Topczewski TE, Di Somma A, Pineda J, Ferres A, Torales J, Reyes L, et al. Endoscopic endonasal and transorbital routes to the petrous apex: anatomic comparative study of two pathways. Acta Neurochir. 2020;162(9):2097–109.
59. Freeman JL, Sampath R, Casey MA, Quattlebaum SC, Ramakrishnan VR, Youssef AS. Transposition of the paraclival carotid artery: a novel concept of self-retaining vascular retraction during endoscopic endonasal skull base surgery technical report. Acta Neurochir. 2016;158(8):1625–9.
60. Kaen A, Cárdenas Ruiz-Valdepeñas E, Di Somma A, Esteban F, Márquez Rivas J, Ambrosiani Fernandez J. Refining the anatomic boundaries of the endoscopic endonasal transpterygoid approach: the "VELPPHA area" concept. J Neurosurg. 2018;131(3):911–9.
61. Cavallo LM, Messina A, Cappabianca P, Esposito F, de Divitiis E, Gardner P, et al. Endoscopic endonasal surgery of the midline skull base: anatomical study and clinical considerations. Neurosurg Focus. 2005;19(1):E2.
62. Lim JH, Sardesai MG, Ferreira M, Moe KS. Transorbital neuroendoscopic management of sinogenic complications involving the frontal sinus, orbit, and anterior cranial fossa. J Neurol Surg B Skull Base. 2012;73(6):394–400.
63. Dallan I, Castelnuovo P, Turri-Zanoni M, Fiacchini G, Locatelli D, Battaglia P, et al. Transorbital endoscopic assisted management of intraorbital lesions: lessons learned from our first 9 cases. Rhinology. 2016;54(3):247–53.
64. Peron S, Cividini A, Santi L, Galante N, Castelnuovo P, Locatelli D. Spheno-orbital meningiomas: when the endoscopic approach is better. Acta Neurochir Suppl. 2017;124:123–8.
65. Jeon C, Hong CK, Woo KI, Hong SD, Nam DH, Lee JI, et al. Endoscopic transorbital surgery for Meckel's cave and middle cranial fossa tumors: surgical technique and early results. J Neurosurg. 2018;131(4):1126–35.
66. Bly RA, Ramakrishna R, Ferreira M, Moe KS. Lateral transorbital neuroendoscopic approach to the lateral cavernous sinus. J Neurol Surg B Skull Base. 2014;75(1):11–7.
67. Santos C, Guizzardi G, Di Somma A, Lopez P, Mato D, Ensenat J, et al. Comparison of accessibility to cavernous sinus areas throughout endonasal, transorbital, and transcranial approaches: anatomic study with quantitative analysis. Oper Neurosurg (Hagerstown). 2023;24(4):e271–80.
68. Chen HI, Bohman LE, Emery L, Martinez-Lage M, Richardson AG, Davis KA, et al. Lateral transorbital endoscopic access to the hippocampus, amygdala, and entorhinal cortex: initial clinical experience. ORL J Otorhinolaryngol Relat Spec. 2015;77(6):321–32.
69. Kim EH, Yoo J, Jung IH, Oh JW, Kim JS, Yoon JS, et al. Endoscopic transorbital approach to the insular region: cadaveric feasibility study and clinical application (SevEN-005). J Neurosurg. 2021;135(4):1164–72.
70. Park HH, Hong SD, Kim YH, Hong CK, Woo KI, Yun IS, et al. Endoscopic transorbital and endonasal approach for trigeminal schwannomas: a retrospective multicenter analysis (KOSEN-005). J Neurosurg. 2020;133(2):467–76.
71. Corvino S, Guizzardi G, Sacco M, Corrivetti F, Bove I, Enseñat J, et al. The feasibility of three port endonasal, transorbital, and sublabial approach to the petroclival region: neurosurgical audit and multiportal anatomic quantitative investigation. Acta Neurochir. 2023;165(7):1821–31.
72. Goncalves N, Lubbe DE. Transorbital endoscopic surgery for sphenoid wing meningioma: long-term outcomes and surgical technique. J Neurol Surg B Skull Base. 2020;81(4):357–68.
73. Yoo J, Park HH, Yun IS, Hong CK. Clinical applications of the endoscopic transorbital approach for various lesions. Acta Neurochir. 2021;163(8):2269–77.
74. Vural A, Carobbio ALC, Ferrari M, Rampinelli V, Schreiber A, Mattavelli D, et al. Transorbital endoscopic approaches to the skull base: a systematic literature review and anatomical description. Neurosurg Rev. 2021;44(5):2857–78.

Extended Endoscopic Transorbital Approach for the Posterior Cranial Fossa

23

Chang-Ki Hong and Dong-Won Shin

Introduction

In the modern neurosurgical era, the advancement of hemostatic agents and the illumination of cameras aid the progression of endoscopic neurosurgical procedures. Since Jho and Carrau reported the first case series of the endoscopic endonasal approach (EEA) for pituitary adenomas, the EEA is one of the most efficient approaches for the sellar or parasellar pathologies [1]. Conventional transcranial surgery and endoscopic surgery complement each other, as the former focuses on minimizing skin incisions for better cosmetic outcomes and shorter operation times, while the latter prioritizes maintaining a wide surgical view and expanding its surgical indications. Since Moe et al. reported the first clinical outcome of transorbital neuroendoscopic surgery, the transorbital approach broadened its application [2]. Endoscopic skullbase surgery is a subspecialty of endoscopic surgery that uses an endoscope to access and treat conditions of the skull base through small incisions or natural openings like the nose or orbit. This approach provides a minimally invasive alternative to traditional open craniotomy surgery, which requires the removal of a portion of the skull to access the brain.

The indications for endoscopic skullbase surgery have been expanding as technology and techniques have advanced. The use of endoscopic techniques allows for a more precise and focused surgery for the treatment of skull base disorders. Minimally invasive surgery via endoscope provides less damage to surrounding normal tissue and earlier recovery.

The endoscopic transorbital approach (ETOA) has been performed without orbital rim osteotomy [3–5]. It is adequate for extraconal lesions or orbital wall fractures. However, cutting the superior-lateral orbital rim is inevitable for manipulating instruments in a deeper field. Orbital rim osteotomy gives a wide surgical corridor that expands surgical indications [5, 6]. Extended ETOA (EETOA) is defined as ETOA accompanied by extending osteotomy, including superior and lateral orbital rims as well as a part of frontal bone to maximize the surgical corridor.

ETOA is one of the attempts to replace conventional craniotomy. As an EEA widens its usefulness through transpterygoid, transcavernous, transclival, or far medial approach, the ETOA also expands its application toward middle or

C.-K. Hong (✉)
Neurosurgery, Brain Tumor Center, Asan Medical Center, College of Medicine, Ulsan University, Seoul, South Korea
e-mail: changki.hong@amc.seoul.kr

D.-W. Shin
Department of Neurosurgery, Brain Tumor Center, Gil Medical Center, College of Medicine, Gachon University, Incheon, South Korea
e-mail: dwshinns@gilhospital.com

T. H. Schwartz et al. (eds.), *Endoscopic Transorbital Surgery of the Orbit, Skull Base and Brain*,
https://doi.org/10.1007/978-3-031-59504-2_23

posterior cranial fossa pathologies [7–9]. The earliest attempt is trigeminal schwannomas or spheno-orbital meningiomas [10–12]. The surgical outcome is satisfactory for those middle fossa lesions, however, petroclival meningiomas are still a no man's land for the endoscopic neurosurgical procedure. Only anatomical studies have been published to evaluate the feasibility of ETOA in petroclival lesions [13–17]. There are several obstacles that need to be overcome. First, we encounter a new perspective through the transorbital approach. Neurosurgeons are accustomed to the transcranial view, which is usually accessed from above or lateral to the patients, so the temporal lobe is mainly retracted to the surgeon's side. In contrast, we need to elevate the temporal lobe against gravity in ETOA. Second, we have difficulty manipulating instruments through a narrow surgical field. A rigid retractor should be brought to the field to elevate the temporal lobe throughout the procedure, which results in a more limited control of the surgical instruments. Herein, we introduced our surgical technique and tips to treat posterior fossa lesions by EETOA.

Indication

The EETOA can be applied to the following indications

- Cavernous sinus meningiomas
- Petroclival meningiomas (PCMs)
- Prepontine epidermoid cyst
- Brainstem cavernous malformation

ETOA poses several difficulties working on posterior fossa rather than middle fossa pathologies because of the limited surgical corridor made by the orbital cavity [2, 18–20]. The working distance is also longer than open craniotomies. Additionally, temporal lobe retraction is mandatory to expose the posterior fossa. Generally, in ETOA performed without the orbital rim osteotomy, the temporal lobe must be towed only using the sucker because the working space is narrow. Consequently, working on the petrous apex is limited by the narrow space [17, 21]. For this reason, although trigeminal schwannoma is one of the best indications for ETOA, Samii type D, which is mostly confined to the posterior fossa mass, is not a good surgical candidate for ETOA [10, 14]. ETOA has expanded its application by osteotomy of both superior and lateral orbital rims. Moreover, part of the frontal base and temporal bone are also drilled to maximize the surgical field, bringing a retractor to elevate the temporal lobe. Herein, EETOA maximizes surgical corridors to overcome the limitation of ETOA.

Kawase classified petroclival meningioma into four types according to tumor origin and growing direction, whereas Seifert demonstrated three types based on the tumor growth pattern [22, 23]. Among those types, the tumor that grows through porus trigeminus and invades the posterior fossa can be a surgical candidate for EETOA because it occupies the surgical space in the middle cranial fossa (Fig. 23.1). In contrast, clival-type PCM is difficult to remove via EETOA because it is limited in the posterior fossa. The surgical view of EETOA with anterior petrosectomy is like the pretemporal anterior petrosal approach (APA), which shows the surgical axis from the anterior to posterior direction. The best surgical indication for EETOA is tumors that grow along the cavernous sinus lateral wall toward the posterior fossa. The classic APA is the subtemporal route, which implies lateral to medial surgical direction. In this approach, the origin and terminal of the trigeminal nerve are horizontal in surgical view, whereas the trigeminal nerve in EETOA with anterior petrosectomy goes toward the surgeon's aspect.

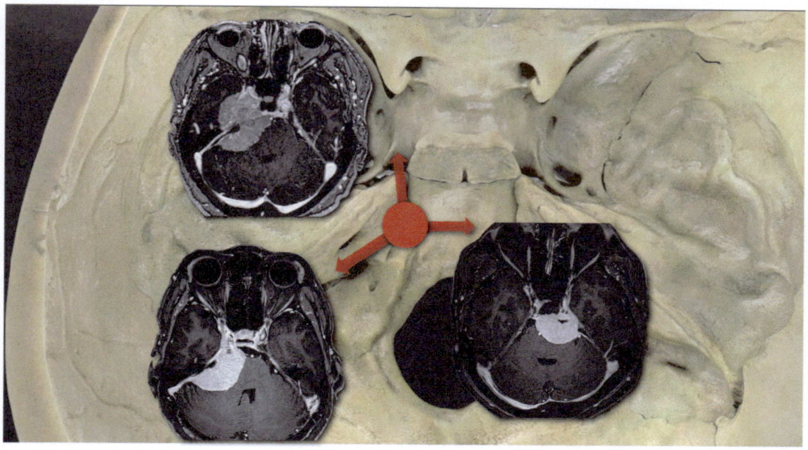

Fig. 23.1 Classification of petroclival meningioma, upper left: the cavernous type, right: the clivus type, lower left: the tentorium or the petrous type, an arrow is tumor growth direction

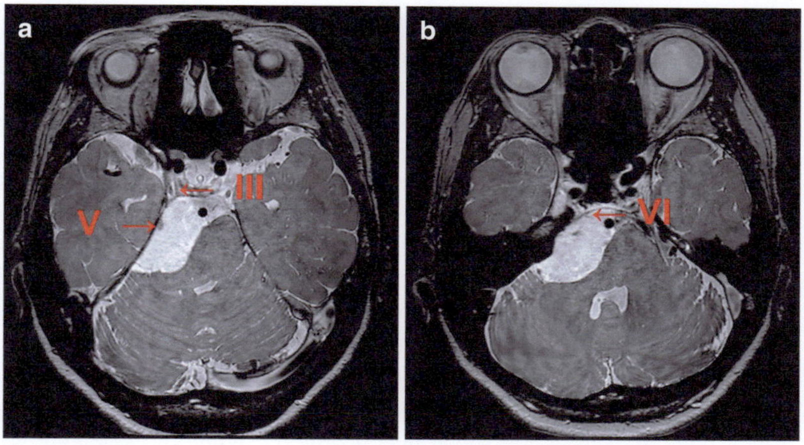

Fig. 23.2 Proton density MRI in a patient with petroclival meningioma. (**a**) Arrows indicate the oculomotor nerve in the oculomotor triangle and the trigeminal nerve compressed by the tumor. (**b**) The arrow points to the abducens nerve being compressed by the tumor and passing through Dorello's canal

Preoperative Evaluation

The basic imaging work-up for the EETOA includes brain magnetic resonance image (MRI), computed tomography (CT) angiography, facial bone CT, and temporal bone CT for anatomical aspects. The extent of the frontal sinus is also evaluated to avoid opening it if possible. Enhanced Proton density MRI helps to evaluate the relationship between the tumor and deviated cranial nerves (Fig. 23.2). T2-weighted images can help to predict the arachnoid interface between the brainstem and tumors. If brainstem invasion is suspected, subtotal resection without major neurologic deficit should be the goal for surgery. The bone thickness of the greater wing of the sphenoid bone is also considered. The route of the petrous internal carotid artery and greater superficial petrous nerve (GSPN) are evaluated through CT angiography. Evaluation of aeration of the mastoid air cells is done prior to surgery in order to determine the need for the use of bone wax or autologous abdominal fat graft during the procedure. Preoperative ophthalmologic evaluation is also requested, especially in elderly patients, to prevent ocular damage during surgery. If the patients have glaucoma or compromised retinal artery circulation, external compression of the eyeball with a rigid retractor can lead to devastating results.

Operation Technique

Patient Positioning and Skin Incision

The whole procedure is carried out above the patient's head, like in an open craniotomy. The patient is positioned supine, and the head is fixed using a three-pin head holder. The head is slightly rotated to the contralateral side and extended 10° to allow natural retraction by gravity on the frontal lobe. It is important to protect the cornea before draping the face by applying lubricating ophthalmic ointment with a tarsorrhaphy suture or corneal shield. Betadine solution should be diluted with normal saline (5:5 ratio) to minimize skin irritation and prevent corneal injury. The face is prepped and draped in a sterile fashion; the eyebrow is infiltrated with an anesthetic. An incision is made along the inferior margin of the eyebrow, which gives a better cosmetic result than an eyebrow or supra-eyebrow incision, and it is extended to the frontozygomatic suture over the superior-lateral orbital rim (Fig. 23.3). Eyelid incision requires cooperation with the ophthalmologic or plastic surgery department to achieve better cosmetic results, whereas infra-eyebrow incision is mostly performed by the neurosurgeon without consultation. It also secures the frontal bone as well as the superolateral orbital rim, which is to be removed. The medial limit of the incision is the supraorbital notch to prevent injury of the supraorbital nerve. The orbicularis muscle is incised and retracted on each side. Tagging the subcutaneous layer with 4-0 black silk is useful for retracting the skin in opposite directions. The temporalis muscle is dissected from the temporal bone using a monopolar coagulator and pulled away from the temporal bone. During this stage, caution is needed to avoid injuring the temporal branch of the facial nerve and the supraorbital nerve. Additionally, no pressure should be exerted on an eyeball by instruments or traction ties.

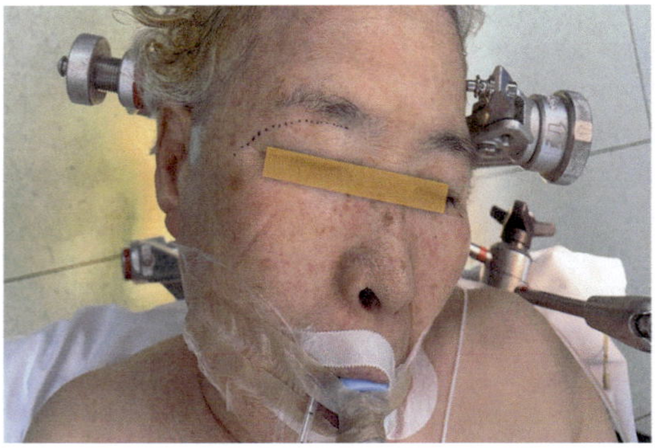

Fig. 23.3 Infra-eyebrow incision. An eyebrow incision is made along the inferior eyebrow which gives a better cosmetic result than an eyebrow or supra-eyebrow incision, and it is extended to the frontozygomatic suture over the superior-lateral orbital rim

Craniotomy and Anatomical Dissection

Initial bone work is performed through the inside of the orbital cavity like in other ETOAs. Orbital contents are retracted towards medial-inferior direction with a malleable retractor to avoid injury. Caution is needed because longstanding or high-force compression can lead to ocular injury, so intermittent decompression or flexible retraction is recommended. Once the frontal dura mater and temporalis muscle are exposed, the superior-lateral orbital rim is removed with an osteotome or B1 cutting drill. Drilling the greater wing of sphenoid bone as much as possible before osteotomy of the orbital rim is an easier way than removing the orbital rim immediately after a skin incision.

Removing the orbital rim is made easier by first drilling as much as possible of the greater wing of the sphenoid bone, leaving only the orbital rim intact, instead of removing it after making a skin incision (Fig. 23.4). The surgical view is like that in the fronto-temporo-orbito-zygomatic approach. It is an important step to maximal osteotomy, including the superior-lateral orbital rim, for several reasons. First, it gives a wide exposure to the temporal lobe. Second, extra space can bring the rigid retractor to elevate the temporal lobe. Third, the greater wing of the sphenoid bone is also fully exposed so the surgeon can maximize bone work, which gives additional space for the temporal skull base by retracting the temporalis muscle [5, 6, 24].

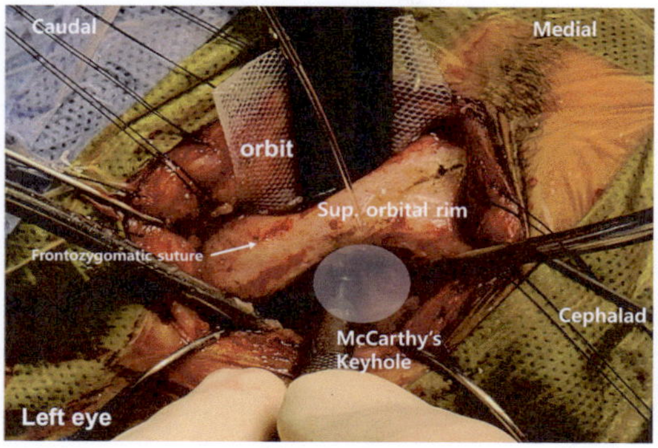

Fig. 23.4 The bone working area in EETOA is larger than conventional ETOA with lateral orbital rim osteotomy. *EETOA* extended endoscopic transorbital approach, *ETOA* endoscopic transorbital approach

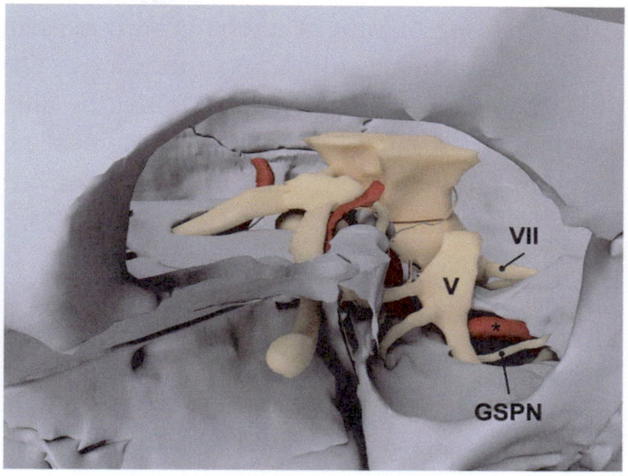

Fig. 23.5 A detailed computer-based 3D image shows the main neurovascular structures around the petrous apex region, which can be seen via the extended transorbital approach. *GSPN* greater superficial petrosal nerve. *V* trigeminal nerve, *VII* facial nerve, * petrous internal carotid artery

Anterior Petrosectomy

Maximal exposure of the temporal lobe by dissecting the temporalis muscle from the sphenoid bone medial to the lateral direction is one of the most important points of this approach. Extradural dissection and drilling of the lesser wing of the sphenoid bone as well as the orbital roof are carried out simultaneously until the meningo-orbital band (MOB) is identified [19]. Once the MOB is divided, the dura propria is carefully peeled off to expose the lateral wall of the cavernous sinus. After the dura propria of the temporal lobe is dissected, the margin of the anterior clinoid process is fully exposed. Extradural anterior clinoidectomy as well as optic nerve decompression can be performed case by case.

Venous bleeding from the cavernous sinus is controlled by gelatin-thrombin hemostatic agents. The middle meningeal artery (MMA) is subsequently coagulated and cut. GSPN is usually located at the posterior-medial side of MMA [25–28]. GSPN is dissected posterior to the anterior direction to minimize retraction injury. After exposure to the posteromedial triangle (i.e., Kawase triangle), drilling of the petrous apex is carried out until the posterior fossa dura mater is encountered. It is important to drill both premeatal and postmeatal triangles to maximize the surgical corridor [29–31]. The angle of attack in EETOA is narrower than in subtemporal anterior petrosectomy because it is anterior-to-posterior direction rather than a lateral-to-medial direction (Fig. 23.5). Removing the trigeminal impress after retracting the V3 toward the medial side is useful for fully securing the surgical view. Drilling begins at the anterior-medial area and extends toward the posterior-lateral side limited by the GSPN, cochlear, and arcuate eminence. A coarse diamond drill head is utilized to safely remove both cortical and cancellous bone of the petrous apex. A similar technique is well described by Labib et al. [32, 33]. Draining the cerebrospinal fluid (CSF) from the lumbar drain helps to decrease temporal lobe retraction. The extent of bone work is determined by tumor location and growing direction.

Durotomy and Tentorium Resection

We prefer a T-shape durotomy starting anterior to the posterior direction of the horizontal limb and extending toward the tentorial edge and posterior fossa dura. Each dura leaflet is reflected in the opposite direction. When the durotomy is performed, caution is needed at the entry point of the trochlear nerve at the tentorium as well as the vein of Labbe draining in the superior petrosal sinus (SPS). Cutting posterior to the entry point of the trochlear nerve and splitting SPS anterior to the draining of vein of Labbe is an important point to avoid catastrophic complications. The SPS should be clipped or ligated when the dura incision is crossing. Shooting the hemostatic agent toward the venous sinus can lead to devastating venous infarction.

Surgical View and Cranial Nerve Locations

APA via EETOA is similar to a pretemporal APA after orbtiozygomatic craniotomy. Compared to subtemporal APA, which exposes the lateral side of the brainstem, APA via EETOA can expose the anterior-lateral side of the brainstem (Fig. 23.6). The deviation of the angle gives the difference in cranial nerve locations as well as their routes in the operation field. In subtemporal APA, the trigeminal nerve is horizontal to the temporal base, whereas APA via EETOA shows the vertical direction toward operators in trigeminal, facial, and vestibulocochlear nerves (Fig. 23.6). Furthermore, the abducens nerve is easier to access via subtemporal APA than APA via EETOA, which requires drilling the posterior clinoid process or trigeminal impression. For this reason, APA via EETOA can be more effective for tumors growing anterior to the posterior direction along the petrous portion of the temporal bone than for tumors growing on the medial side toward the clivus or brainstem. Cavernous sinus meningioma occupying the posterior fossa is also one of the indications of this approach.

Closure

After the main procedure, primary dura closure is rarely possible, so an artificial dura substitute (Duragen) is placed in-lay manner and is made to approximate the dura as much as possible. The petrous part of the temporal bone is usually well-pneumatized, so dead space should be sealed with an autologous abdominal fat graft. Acellular dermal matrix (Megaderm) is used to cover the defect of the orbital roof, and the autologous abdominal fat graft packed the epidural dead space. Superior-lateral orbital rim is re-positioned with a microplate. The orbicularis muscle is approximated with vicryl 3-0, and skin closure is done with nylon 5-0 through simple or continuous suturing.

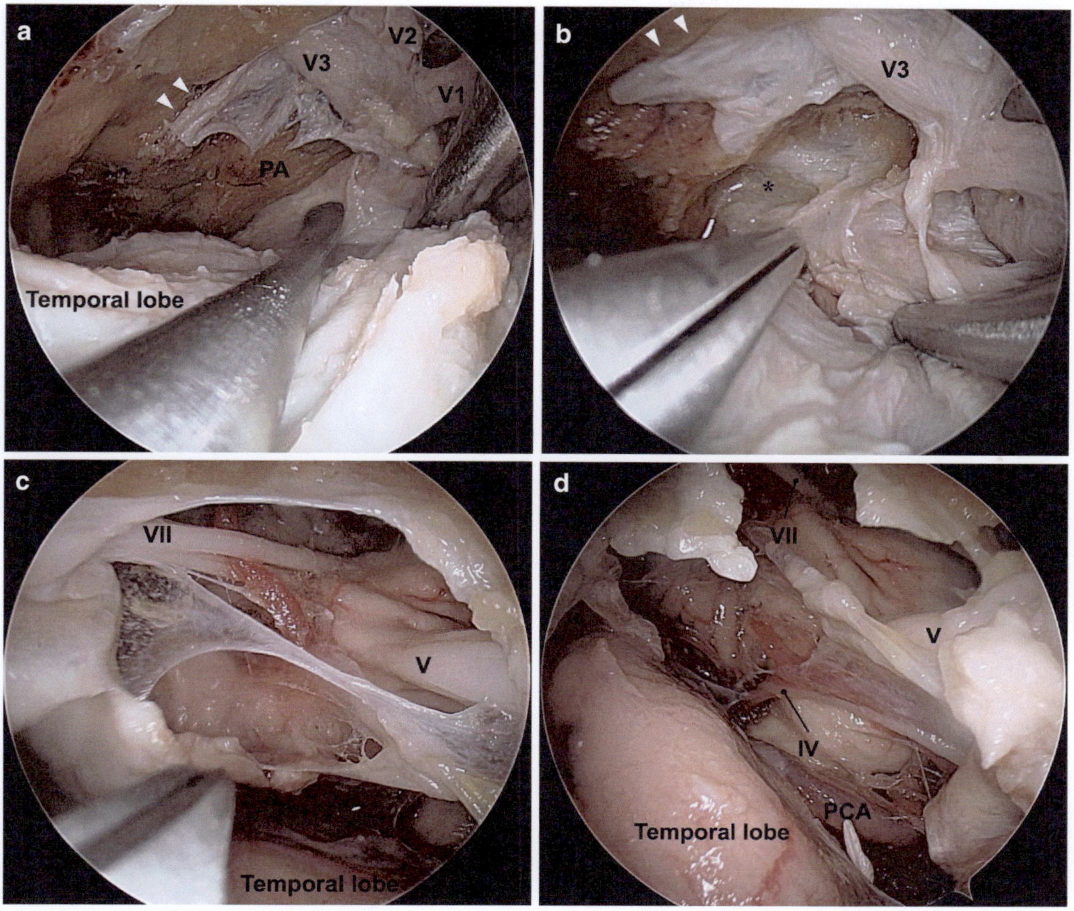

Fig. 23.6 Photographs of stepwise cadaveric dissection illustrating the EETOA. (**a**) Complete interdural exposition of the lateral wall of the cavernous sinus via an endoscopic transorbital approach, left orbit. (**b**) The posterior fossa dura (*) is identified after drilling the rhomboid fossa. (**c**) The prepontine cisternal space between V and VII–VIII complex is exposed. *V* trigeminal nerve, *VII* facial nerve. (**d**) The tentorium is divided while the trochlear nerve (IV) is preserved. The double arrowhead indicates a greater superficial petrosal nerve. *PA* petrous apex, *V1* ophthalmic nerve, *V2* maxillary branch of the trigeminal nerve, *V3* mandibular branch of the trigeminal nerve

Postoperative Management

An ophthalmologic check-up is usually requested during the early postoperative period. Periorbital swelling and ecchymosis are controlled by applying an ice pack. Artificial tears are recommended to prevent dry eyes. Early ambulation is encouraged for the patient. The eyebrow incision is cleaned daily, and ophthalmic antibiotic ointment is applied. Stitch-out is usually done after 5 postoperative days.

Complications

Intraocular pressure should be cautiously examined during the procedure because instrument compression can occur. Increased orbital pressure over 60–100 min can cause permanent visual complications [34, 35]. Therefore, it is necessary to consciously relieve the pressure on the orbit during transorbital surgery. CSF leakage does not occur as much as in EEA. However, careful dura mater closure and sealing air cells of the petrous

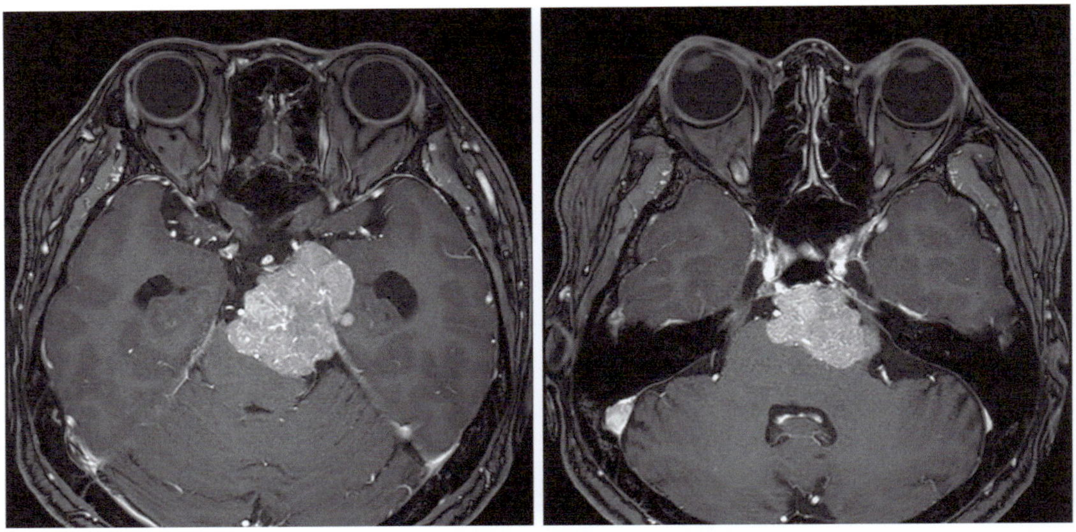

Fig. 23.7 Preoperative contrast-enhanced MRI in axial view, showing a meningioma originated from the petroclival junction, which grows along the clivus

apex or packing autologous abdomen fat graft are required. Forehead and periorbital numbness due to supraorbital nerve injury should be checked in the early postoperative period. The rate of other complications is comparable to that in open skull base surgery, including the injury of the vein of Labbe, facial nerve injury, or internal carotid artery injury. Enophthalmos can occur if rigid bone reconstruction or dead space is not appropriately managed because of the extensive removal of the lateral orbital.

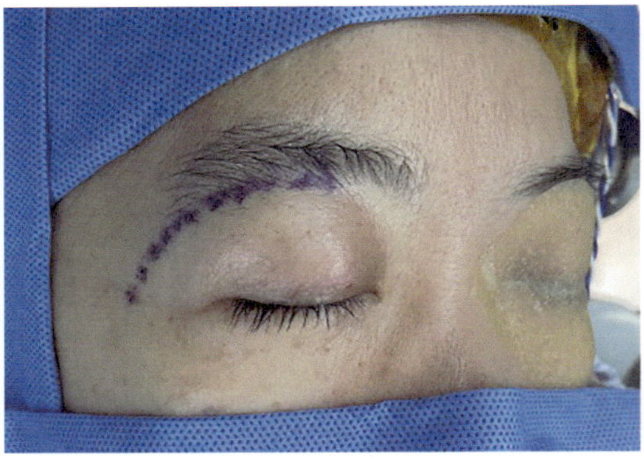

Fig. 23.8 The infra-eyebrow skin incision is designed for an endoscopic transorbital approach. An incision begins just lateral to the supraorbital notch and ends at the level of the lateral canthus

Illustrative Cases

A 43-year-old woman presented with right-side hemiparesis and diplopia. Her neurologic examination showed grade IV right hemiparesis and partial oculomotor nerve palsy on the left side. An MRI revealed a tumor originating from the petroclival junction, which grew along the clivus, and the upper margin was at the level of the third ventricle (Fig. 23.7). Proton-density gadolinium-enhanced MRI showed compression of the trigeminal and abducens nerves. The oculomotor nerve was not identified because it was severely deviated by the tumor. EETOA was performed through an infra-eyebrow incision (Fig. 23.8). After cutting the MOB, the dura propria of the temporal lobe was peeled off. GSPN and postero-medial triangle were identified. We drilled the petrous apex until the posterior fossa dura was encountered. The Dura incision was made in a T-shape and each dura leaflet was reflected on the opposite side. The trigeminal nerve deviated to the lateral side of the tumor as well as the trochlear nerve. The oculomotor nerve was identified at the top of the tumor, but it was not observed in the preoperative MRI. After gross total resection of the tumor, we identified the bilateral oculomotor nerves, ipsilateral trochlear nerve, ipsilateral trigeminal nerve, and bilateral PCAs. Stepwise dissection is shown in Fig. 23.9. Postoperative MRI showed no residual tumors (Fig. 23.10).

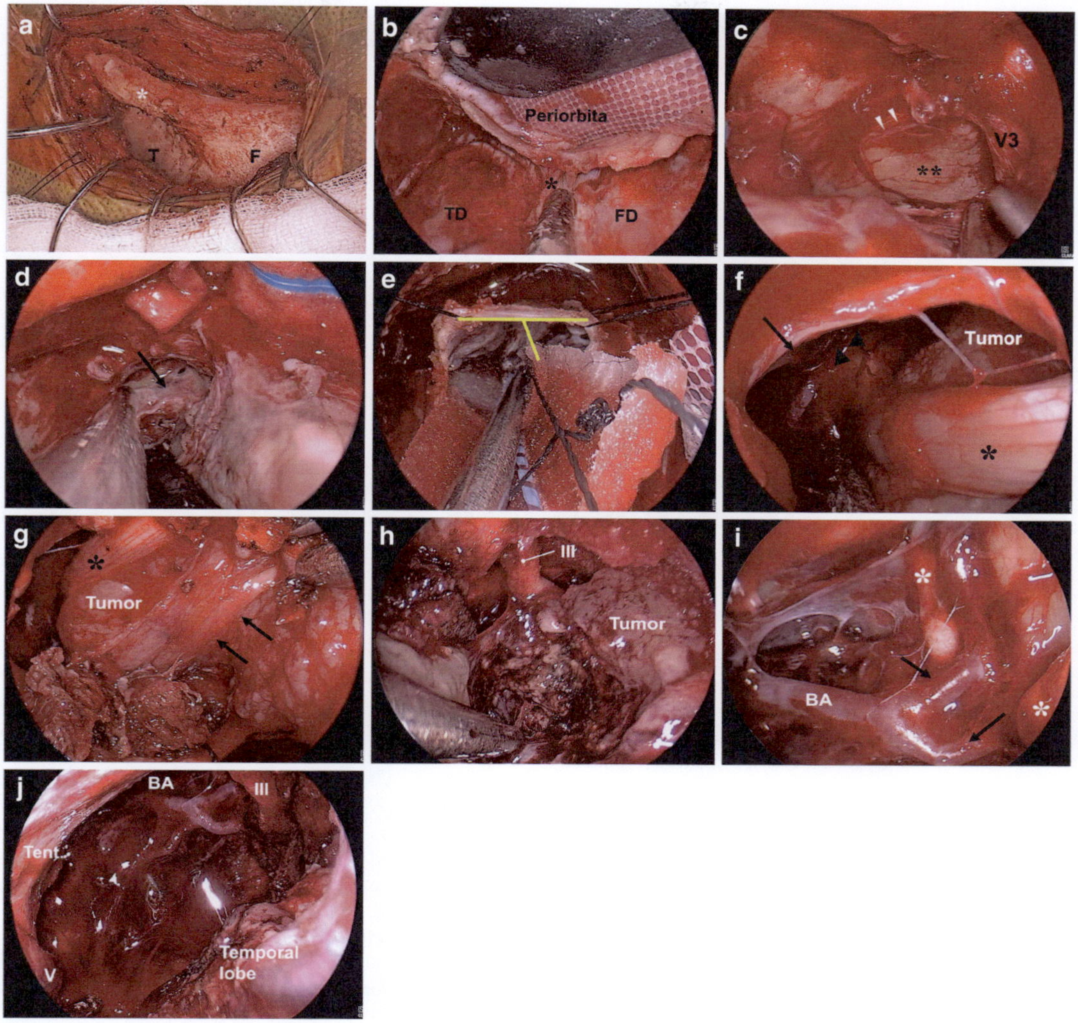

Fig. 23.9 Intraoperative view of the extended ETOA. (**a**) Orbital rim, frontal, and temporal bone exposure after infra-eyebrow skin incision. The temporalis muscle is retracted to the lateral side to achieve maximal exposure of the temporal bone. * orbital rim, *F* frontal bone, *T* temporal bone. (**b**) The meningo-orbital band (*) is identified after craniotomy and extended drilling. Periorbita is gently pushed away with the rigid retractor. Frontal and temporal bones are widely removed. (**c**) The posteromedial triangle (**) is exposed after peeling off the dura propria of the temporal lobe, V3, and GSPN (white arrowhead). (**d**) The posterior fossa dura (black arrow) is encountered after drilling of the petrous apex. (**e**) The first dura incision is made parallel to the temporal base. It is extended toward the dural fold of the tentorium and the posterior fossa dura. The superior petrosal sinus is carefully ligated or clipped before cutting. The trochlear nerve and vein of the Labbe should be protected during cutting tentorium. (**f**) The trigeminal nerve (*) deviated to the lateral side of the tumor. The brainstem (arrowhead) and the facial nerve complex (arrow) are identified. (**g**) The trigeminal nerve (*) and trochlear nerve (black arrow) are identified at the lateral side of the tumor. (**h**) The oculomotor nerve (*) is noted at the top of the tumor. (**i**) Bilateral oculomotor nerves (*) and posterior cerebral arteries (black arrow) are identified after the total removal of the tumor. *BA* basilar artery. (**j**) A wide view of the surgical field after tumor resection. Oculomotor nerve, trigeminal nerve, basilar artery, and posterior cerebral arteries are noted. *BA* basilar artery, *Tent* tentorium, *III* oculomotor nerve, *V* trigeminal nerve

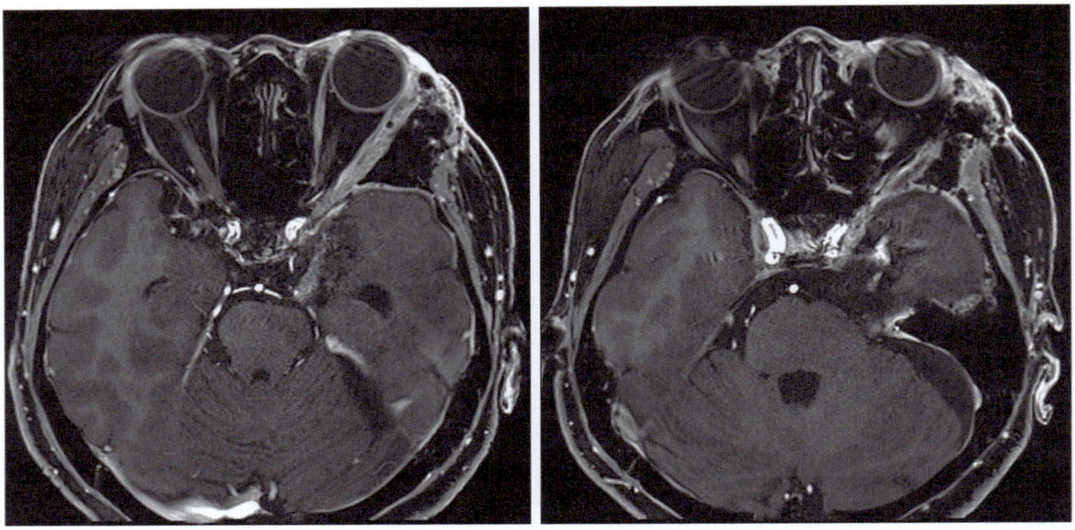

Fig. 23.10 The postoperative contrast-enhanced MRI in axial views shows total resection of the lesion. The transorbital surgical corridor used in this case is visible

References

1. Jho HD, Carrau RL. Endoscopic endonasal transsphenoidal surgery: experience with 50 patients. Neurosurg Focus. 1996;1(1):E4.
2. Moe KS, Bergeron CM, Ellenbogen RG. Transorbital neuroendoscopic surgery. Oper Neurosurg. 2010;67(3):ons16–28.
3. Noiphithak R, Yanez-Siller JC, Barbero JMR, Otto BA, Carrau RL, Prevedello DM. Quantitative analysis of the surgical exposure and surgical freedom between transcranial and transorbital endoscopic anterior petrosectomies to the posterior fossa. J Neurosurg. 2018;69(2):1–9.
4. Noiphithak R, Yanez-Siller JC, Barbero JMR, Otto BA, Carrau RL, Prevedello DM. Comparative analysis between lateral orbital rim preservation and osteotomy for transorbital endoscopic approaches to the cavernous sinus: an anatomic study. Oper Neurosurg. 2019;16(1):86–93.
5. Lim J, Sung KS, Kim W, Yoo J, Jung IH, Choi S, et al. Extended endoscopic transorbital approach with superior-lateral orbital rim osteotomy: cadaveric feasibility study and clinical implications (SevEN-007). J Neurosurg. 2021;137(1):18–31.
6. Lim J, Cho K. The modified lateral supraorbital approach for tumors of the petroclival junction extending into the anterior cerebellopontine area. J Neurooncol. 2016;127(3):541–50.
7. Cavallo LM, Messina A, Cappabianca P, Esposito F, de Divitiis E, Gardner P, et al. Endoscopic endonasal surgery of the midline skull base: anatomical study and clinical considerations. Neurosurg Focus. 2005;19(1):E2.
8. Carrau RL, Kassam AB, Snyderman CH, Duvvuri U, Mintz A, Gardner P. Endoscopic transnasal anterior skull base resection for the treatment of sinonasal malignancies. Oper Tech Otolaryngol Head Neck Surg. 2006;17(2):102–10.
9. Kassam AB, Gardner P, Snyderman C, Mintz A, Carrau R. Expanded endonasal approach: fully endoscopic, completely transnasal approach to the middle third of the clivus, petrous bone, middle cranial fossa, and infratemporal fossa. Neurosurg Focus. 2005;19(1):1–10.
10. Park HH, Hong SD, Kim YH, Hong CK, Woo KI, Yun IS, et al. Endoscopic transorbital and endonasal approach for trigeminal schwannomas: a retrospective multicenter analysis (KOSEN-005). J Neurosurg. 2020;133(2):467–76.
11. Dallan I, Locatelli D, Turri-Zanoni M, Battaglia P, Lepera D, Galante N, et al. Transorbital endoscopic assisted resection of a superior orbital fissure cavernous haemangioma: a technical case report. Eur Arch Otorhinol. 2015;272(12):3851–6.
12. Jeon C, Hong CK, Woo KI, Hong SD, Nam DH, Lee JI, et al. Endoscopic transorbital surgery for Meckel's cave and middle cranial fossa tumors: surgical technique and early results. J Neurosurg. 2018;131(4):1126–35.
13. Lee WJ, Hong SD, Woo KI, Seol HJ, Choi JW, Lee JI, et al. Endoscopic endonasal and transorbital approaches to petrous apex lesions. J Neurosurg. 2021;136(2):431–40.
14. Priddy BH, Nunes CF, Beer-Furlan A, Carrau R, Dallan I, Prevedello DMS. A side door to Meckel's cave: anatomic feasibility study for the lateral transorbital approach. Oper Neurosurg. 2017;13(5):614–21.

15. Somma AD, Andaluz N, Cavallo LM, Topczewski TE, Frio F, Gerardi RM, et al. Endoscopic transorbital route to the petrous apex: a feasibility anatomic study. Acta Neurochir. 2018;160(4):707–20.
16. Somma AD, Kong DS, de Notaris M, Moe KS, España JCS, Schwartz TH, et al. Endoscopic transorbital surgery levels of difficulty. J Neurosurg. 2022;137(4):1187–90.
17. Topczewski TE, Somma AD, Pineda J, Ferres A, Torales J, Reyes L, et al. Endoscopic endonasal and transorbital routes to the petrous apex: anatomic comparative study of two pathways. Acta Neurochir. 2020;162(9):1–13.
18. Bly R, Ramakrishna R, Ferreira M, Moe K. Lateral transorbital neuroendoscopic approach to the lateral cavernous sinus. J Neurol Surg B Skull Base. 2014;75(01):011–7.
19. Dallan I, Somma AD, Prats-Galino A, Solari D, Alobid I, Turri-Zanoni M, et al. Endoscopic transorbital route to the cavernous sinus through the meningo-orbital band: a descriptive anatomical study. J Neurosurg. 2017;127(3):1–8.
20. Locatelli D, Pozzi F, Turri-Zanoni M, Battaglia P, Santi L, Dallan I, et al. Transorbital endoscopic approaches to the skull base: current concepts and future perspectives. J Neurosurg Sci. 2016;60(4):514–25.
21. Koutourousiou M, Fernandez-Miranda JC, Filho FVG, de Almeida JR, Wang EW, Snyderman CH, et al. Outcomes of endonasal and lateral approaches to petroclival meningiomas. World Neurosurg. 2017;99:500–17.
22. Ichimura S, Kawase T, Onozuka S, Yoshida K, Ohira T. Four subtypes of petroclival meningiomas: differences in symptoms and operative findings using the anterior transpetrosal approach. Acta Neurochir. 2008;150(7):637–45.
23. Seifert V. Clinical management of petroclival meningiomas and the eternal quest for preservation of quality of life. Acta Neurochir. 2010;152(7):1099–116.
24. Lim J, Roh TH, Kim W, Kim JS, Hong JB, Sung KS, et al. Biportal endoscopic transorbital approach: a quantitative anatomical study and clinical application. Acta Neurochir. 2020;162(9):2119–28.
25. Day JD, Fukushima T, Giannotta SL. Microanatomical study of the extradural middle fossa approach to the petroclival and posterior cavernous sinus region. Neurosurgery. 1994;34(6):1009–10016.
26. Fava A, di Russo P, Passeri T, Camara B, Paglia F, Matano F, et al. The mini-combined transpetrosal approach: an anatomical study and comparison with the combined transpetrosal approach. Acta Neurochir. 2022;164(4):1079–93.
27. Kawase T. Technique of anterior transpetrosal approach. Oper Tech Neurosurg. 1999;2(1):10–7.
28. Kim SM, Lee HY, Kim HK, Zabramski JM. Cochlear line: a novel landmark for hearing preservation using the anterior petrosal approach. J Neurosurg. 2015;123(1):9–13.
29. Froelich S, Dunn IF, Youssef AS, Bambakidis NC. Petroclival meningiomas. Neurosurg Focus Video. 2022;6(2):V1.
30. Giammattei L, Passeri T, Abbritti R, Lieber S, Matano F, Van TL, et al. Surgical morbidity of the extradural anterior petrosal approach: the Lariboisière experience. J Neurosurg. 2022;138(1):276–86.
31. Giammattei L, di Russo P, Starnoni D, Passeri T, Bruneau M, Meling TR, et al. Petroclival meningiomas: update of current treatment and consensus by the EANS skull base section. Acta Neurochir. 2021;163(6):1639–63.
32. Labib MA, Zhao X, Houlihan LM, Abramov I, Catapano JS, Naeem K, et al. Comparative analysis of the combined petrosal and the pretemporal transcavernous anterior petrosal approach to the petroclival region. J Neurosurg. 2021;136(3):905–16.
33. Liao CH, Wang JT, Lin CF, Chen SC, Lin CJ, Hsu SPC, et al. Pretemporal trans-Meckel's cave transtentorial approach for large petroclival meningiomas. Neurosurg Focus. 2018;44(4):E10.
34. Lima V, Burt B, Leibovitch I, Prabhakaran V, Goldberg RA, Selva D. Orbital compartment syndrome: the ophthalmic surgical emergency. Surv Ophthalmol. 2009;54(4):441–9.
35. Kim W, Moon JH, Kim EH, Hong CK, Han J, Hong JB. Optimization of orbital retraction during endoscopic transorbital approach via quantitative measurement of the intraocular pressure—[SevEN 006]. BMC Ophthalmol. 2020;21(1):76.

Part VIII

Vascular Pathology

24 Transorbital Endoscopic Approach to the Sylvian Fissure

Diana C. Alvarez Caicedo, Theodore H. Schwartz, and Joao Paulo Almeida

Abbreviations

AChA	Anterior choroidal arteries
ACP	Anterior clinoid process
P2a	Anterior part of the perimesencephalic segment of the posterior cerebral artery
CSF	Cerebro-spinal fluid
M4	Cortical segment of the middle cerebral artery
EEAs	Endoscopic endonasal approaches
M2	Insular segment of the middle cerebral artery
ICA	Internal carotid artery
LSO	Lateral supraorbital
MOB	Meningo orbital band
MCA	Middle cerebral artery
M3	Opercular segment of the middle cerebral artery
OS	Optical strut
P2	Perimesencephalic segment of the posterior cerebral artery
PComA	Posterior communicating artery
A1	Pre-communicating segment of the anterior cerebral artery
M1	Sphenoidal segment of the middle cerebral artery
SCA	Superior cerebellar artery
TM	Temporal muscle
IOF	The inferior orbital fissures
SOF	The superior orbital fissures
TONES	Transorbital neuroendoscopic surgery

Introduction

Minimally invasive surgical approaches play a significant role in the current neurosurgical management of skull base and vascular pathology [1–11]. The basic principles of open skull base surgery traditionally involve the removal of more bone to avoid brain retraction, while the basic principles of minimally invasive surgery involve well-placed small openings and endoscopes to avoid brain retraction. The evolution of endoscopic endonasal approaches (EEAs) has markedly improved the instrumentation and neurosurgical facility of endoscope-assisted procedures [2, 6, 12–18]. Median and paramedian lesions, such as pituitary tumors and selected meningiomas and chordomas, are successfully resected through endoscopic approaches, with similar or better rates of gross total resection and complications than transcranial approaches [19–21]. The supraorbital eyelid incision has also

D. C. Alvarez Caicedo · J. P. Almeida (✉)
Department of Neurological Surgery, Mayo Clinic, Jacksonville, FL, USA
e-mail: almeida.joao@mayo.edu

T. H. Schwartz
Department of Neurosurgery, Weill Cornell Medicine, NewYork–Presbyterian Hospital, New York, NY, USA
e-mail: schwarh@med.cornell.edu

T. H. Schwartz et al. (eds.), *Endoscopic Transorbital Surgery of the Orbit, Skull Base and Brain*,
https://doi.org/10.1007/978-3-031-59504-2_24

gained popularity as a minimally invasive alternative to a pterional craniotomy for skull base pathology as well as for aneurysms with endoscopic assistance [22–28]. However, the supraorbital approach is limited inferiorly by the roof of the orbit, which, unless it is removed, limits access to the anatomic area directly behind the greater and lesser wings of the sphenoid, preventing ideal access to the proximal sylvian fissure and its contents. Using the orbit as an alternative option for surgical approaches led to the development of transorbital endoscopic surgery, also called TONES (transorbital neuroendoscopic surgery) [4, 29, 30].

Through a superolateral eyelid corridor, lesions in the lateral skull base can be treated via a transorbital endoscopic approach, representing a minimally invasive alternative to transcranial surgery in selected cases [4, 29, 30]. While the supraorbital approach has been widely applied to a variety of skull base and vascular pathologies, the transorbital neuroendoscopic approach has had much more limited applications [26, 28, 31–35]. So far, only very selected cases have been considered for transorbital endoscopic surgery for the management of intra-axial tumors or cerebral vascular lesions [4, 36–39].

The sylvian fissure and its contents, namely the middle cerebral artery, the surface of the insula as well as the uncus are frequent sites of neurosurgical pathology, more commonly aneurysms. Reaching these areas generally involves a pterional craniotomy, or some variation thereof, with dissection of the sylvian fissure and some degree of brain retraction, to achieve exposure of the ICA, M1 and more distal branches. However, the proximal part of the sylvian fissure lies just behind the orbit. Therefore, a more direct approach would be to use the corridor provided by the orbit as a more direct approach to the sylvian fissure. In this chapter, we describe the surgical anatomy and techniques for approaching the sylvian fissure via a transorbital endoscopic approach and its potential applications.

Anatomy and Surgical Technique

We divide the transorbital endoscopic approach into five steps for didactic reasons: (1) skin incision and periorbita dissection, (2) craniectomy, (3) dural opening, (4) intradural dissection, and (5) dural repair.

Skin Incision and Periorbital Dissection

Transorbital dissection is done via a superior eyelid incision (Fig. 24.1). The orbicularis layer is opened along the length of the incision to expose the periosteum of the lateral orbital rim, and dissection follows in a preseptal orbital plane. The orbital septum is a connective tissue structure that attaches peripherally at the periosteum of the orbital margin and merges centrally with the lid retractor structures. Careful dissection is performed to avoid transgressing this plane to avoid injuries to the elevator muscle and aponeurosis. The periorbita is gently elevated, from lateral to medial and superior to inferior, using a Freer elevator along the inner aspect of the lateral orbital rim toward the posterior wall of the orbit. Further dissection exposes the lateral aspect of the superior (SOF) and inferior orbital fissure (IOF) (Fig. 24.2), the main anatomical references for the transorbital craniectomy. Successful transorbital dissection followed by retraction of the orbit will create a surgical corridor of approximately 1.5 cm.

Craniectomy

The orbital roof, greater sphenoid wing and part of the orbital floor are exposed after adequate dissection. The extent of the transorbital craniectomy may vary according to the location and size of the lesion to be treated, but wide drilling of the orbital roof and greater sphenoidal wing is recommended to enlarge the surgical field and facilitate the use of instruments during the intradural stage. The superior and inferior orbital fissures are important anatomical references in the posterior wall of the orbit (Fig. 24.2). The orbital roof and basal frontal lobe are located superior to the SOF; the sphenoidal segment of the sylvian fissure, posterior orbital gyri and superior part of the temporal pole are lateral to the SOF and IOF, posterior to the greater and lesser sphenoidal

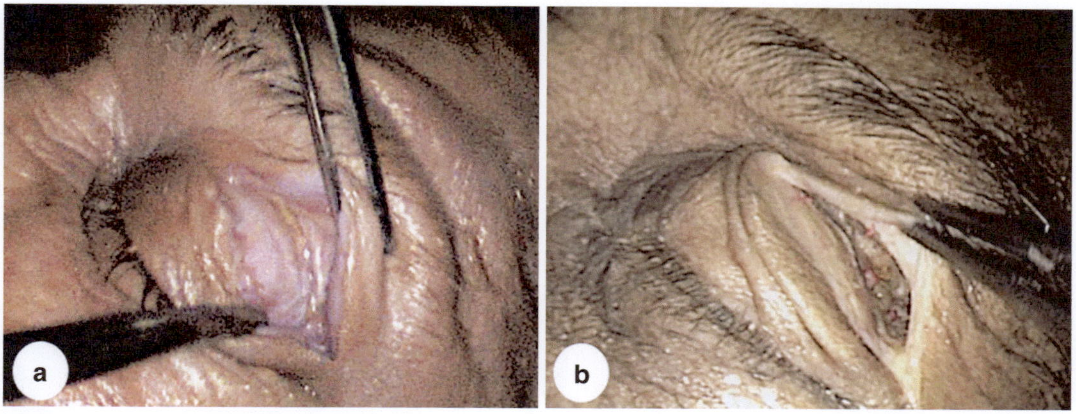

Fig. 24.1 Superior eyelid approach. (**a**) A skin incision is made over the superior eyelid. The supraorbital nerve represents the medial extent of the incision, which extends infero-laterally to the lateral canthus. (**b**) After opening the orbital muscle layer, dissection is done following the preseptal plane to prevent injury to the levator muscle and aponeurosis. Retraction of the periorbital tissue will expose the orbital roof and lateral orbital wall

wings; the temporal pole is fully exposed after extensive drilling of the greater sphenoidal wing, lateral to the IOF.

Drilling is initiated with a cutting-bit high-speed drill to remove the orbital roof and lateral portion of the greater sphenoidal wing. As the drilling progresses laterally, the temporal muscle in the temporal fossa is exposed and represents the lateral limit of the craniectomy. The initial drilling in the lateral and superior parts of the posterior wall of the orbit gives more space for bimanual work and facilitates further removal of the medial part of the greater sphenoidal wing. A diamond bit is used to drill the medial part of the greater sphenoidal wing because of the proximity to the SOF and IOF.

Once the orbital roof and greater sphenoid wing have been removed, the lesser sphenoid wing is exposed and removed (Figs. 24.3, 24.4, and 24.5). Penfield N.1 and angle endoscopic dissectors are used to detach the dura overlying the lesser sphenoidal wing prior to its removal using Kerrison rongeurs and drilling. Lesions located in the lateral aspect of the sphenoid segment of the sylvian fissure will require more extensive lateral drilling, which can be extended until the inner aspect of the pterion cranial point (Fig. 24.4). The mesial temporal lobe, carotid cistern and proximal sylvian fissure lesions benefit from an extradural removal of the anterior clinoid process (Fig. 24.5). After a successful craniectomy, exposure of the dura over the basal frontal lobe, temporal pole and sylvian fissure is achieved (Fig. 24.6).

Dural Opening

A wide dura opening is recommended to achieve an optimal surgical window for intradural dissection. Although a single linear incision over the sylvian fissure can be attempted, this might be insufficient for adequate exposure and mobilization of the frontal and temporal lobes. Therefore, we recommend performing three incisions over the dura, carried out in an "H" format, which will lead to a final square-shaped dural opening, exposing the basal frontal lobe, sylvian fissure and temporal lobe. The initial incision is performed over the sylvian fissure, running from medial to lateral. Two perpendicular incisions are then performed at the medial and lateral limits of the sylvian incision, running from inferior to superior over the frontal lobe and from superior to inferior over the temporal lobe. Kerrison rongeurs are then used to remove the dura and make the final square-shaped opening (Figs. 24.6and 24.7).

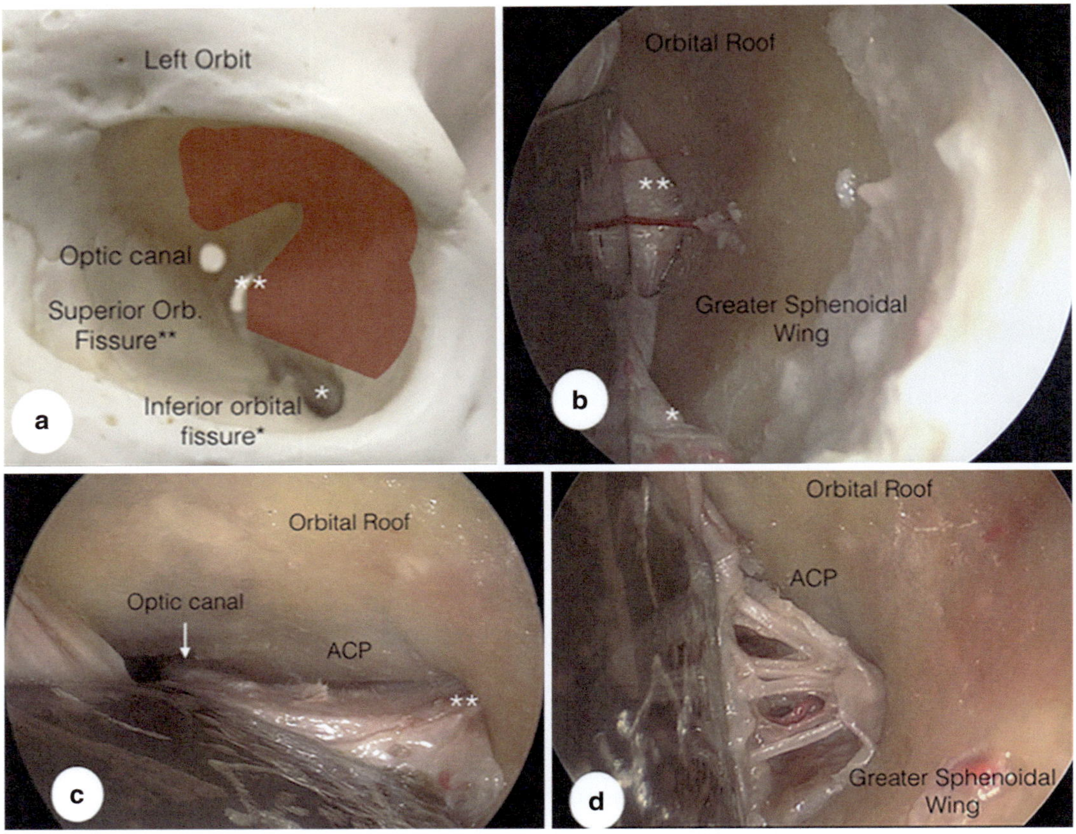

Fig. 24.2 Landmarks for the endoscopic transorbital approach to the skull base and sylvian fissure. The superior and inferior orbital fissures are the main anatomical references to the approach through the posterior wall of the orbit. Lesions in the orbital roof and basal frontal lobe require removal of the orbital roof superior to the SOF; removal of the greater sphenoidal wing lateral to the SOF and IOF exposes the sphenoidal segment of the sylvian fissure, posterior orbital gyri and superior part of the temporal pole; extensive drilling lateral to the greater sphenoidal wing lateral to the IOF exposes the temporal lobe and bone removal inferior to the IOF leads to the infratemporal fossa. (**a**) Left orbit showing the area of the craniectomy (marked area) used for the endoscopic transorbital approach to the sylvian region. Although the sylvian fissure might be exposed with smaller bone removal, extensive drilling is recommended to improve the surgical corridor during the intradural phase of the procedure. (**b**) Craniectomy is only performed after identification of the SOF and IOF and exposure of the orbital roof and greater sphenoidal wing. (**c**) Exposure of the optic canal and anterior clinoid process (ACP) is achieved after inferior retraction of the orbit. Removal of the ACP improves the exposure of the carotid cistern and allows exposure of the carotid bifurcation and middle cerebral artery origin. (**d**) Opening of the SOF. The endoscopic transorbital approach allows direct access to the SOF and its contents. *ACP* anterior clinoid process. * Inferior orbital fissure (IOF), ** superior orbital fissure (SOF)

Intradural Dissection

The Sylvian Fissure

The sylvian fissure is composed of a superficial and a deep part. The superficial part presents a stem and three rami: the anterior horizontal, anterior ascending, and posterior rami. The deep (cisternal) part is divided into an anterior part, the sphenoidal compartment, and a posterior part, the operculoinsular compartment (Figs. 24.8, 24.9, 24.10, 24.11, and 24.12). The sphenoidal compartment arises in the region of the limen insulae at the lateral margin of the anterior perforated substance. The sphenoidal compartment is a narrow space posterior to the sphenoid ridge, between the frontal and the temporal lobes, that

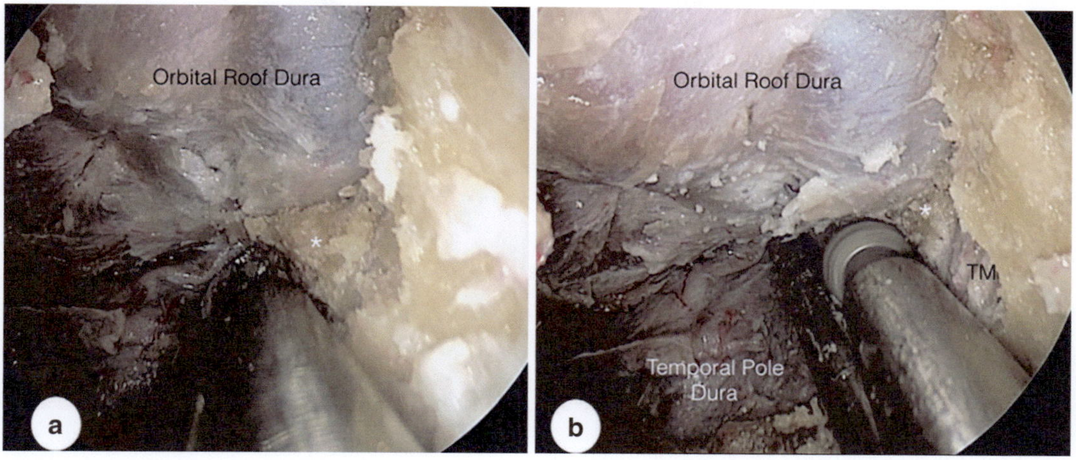

Fig. 24.3 Removal of the lateral portion of the lesser sphenoidal wing. Exposure of the sylvian fissure benefits from wide resection of the sphenoid ridge. Kerrison rongeurs (**a**) and high-speed drills (**b**) are used to remove the most lateral aspect of the lesser sphenoidal wing. * Intracranial projection of the pterion point

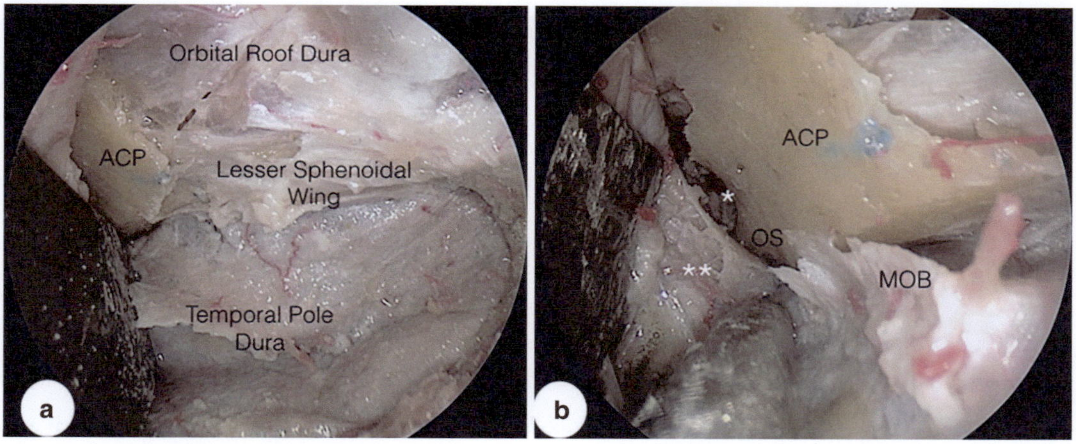

Fig. 24.4 Anterior clinoid process and approaches to the sylvian fissure and carotid cistern. (**a**) Exposure of the medial portion of the sylvian and carotid cisterns is improved after extradural removal of the anterior clinoid process. This bone projection is attached to the anterior fossa in three points: planum sphenoidale medially, lesser sphenoid wing laterally, and optic strut (OS) inferiorly. It composes the anterior part of the roof of the cavernous sinus and is superior to the SOF. (**b**) The meningo-orbital band (MOB) contains the meningo-orbital artery and is located medial to the SOF (**). It should be dissected and cut prior to drilling of the ACP. Complete anatomical detachment of the ACP may not be performed because of the projection of the optic strut inferiorly to the optic canal (*). *ACP* anterior clinoid process, *MOB* meningo-orbital band, *OS* optic strut. * Optic canal, ** superior orbital fissure (SOF)

communicates medially with the carotid cistern. The operculoinsular compartment is formed by two narrow clefts, the opercular cleft, between the opposing lips of the frontoparietal and the temporal opercula and the insular cleft, between the insula cortex and the opercula.

Although the lateral superficial part of the sylvian fissure cannot be adequately exposed via an endoscopic transorbital approach, the sphenoidal segment is a suitable region for this technique. A successful dura opening exposes the posterior orbital gyri, the temporal pole and the superficial

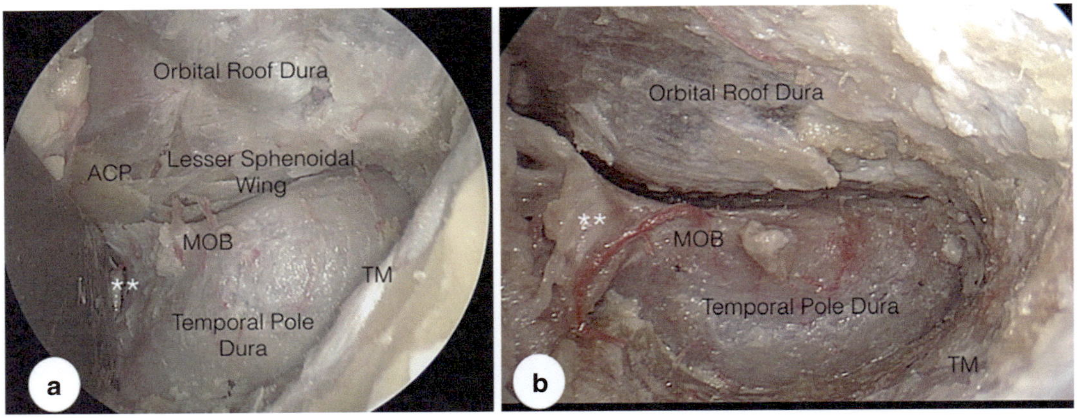

Fig. 24.5 Dural exposure. (**a**) Dural exposure prior to resection of the medial (ACP) and lateral limits of the lesser sphenoidal wing. (**b**) Wide drilling of the orbital roof and sphenoidal wings allows exposure of the dura over the basal frontal lobe, temporal pole and sylvian fissure. *ACP* anterior clinoid process, *MOB* meningo-orbital band, *TM* temporal muscle. ** Superior orbital fissure (SOF)

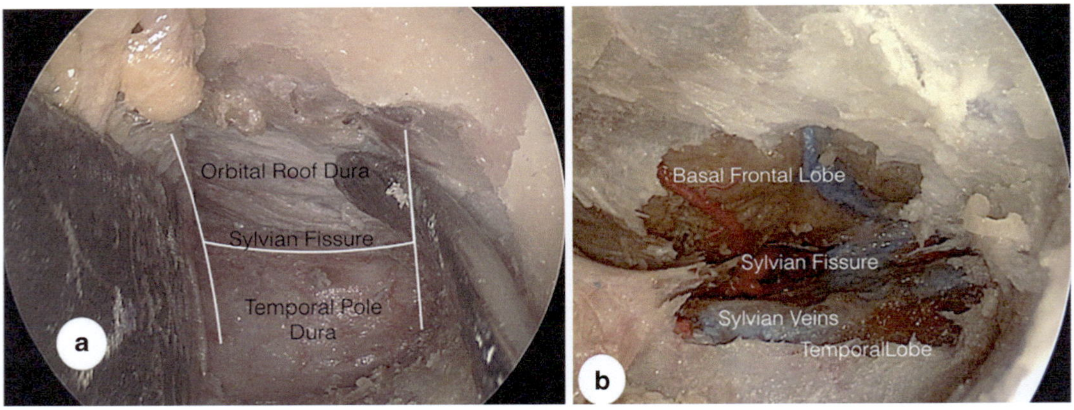

Fig. 24.6 Dural opening. (**a**) Three dural cuts are made in an "H" orientation, followed by dural removal using scissors and Kerrison rongeurs. (**b**) A square-shaped dural opening is achieved, exposing the posterior orbital gyri, sylvian fissure and temporal pole

part of the sphenoidal segment of the sylvian fissure (Fig. 24.8). Dissection proceeds with the opening of the arachnoid membranes over the anterior aspect of the sylvian fissure with endoscopic knives and microscissors. Dissection is carefully done to separate the arachnoid from the temporal branches of the MCA and deep sylvian fissure veins. This venous complex is connected medially to the sphenoparietal sinus and laterally to the superficial sylvian veins, and its extension may limit the approach. A large deep sylvian vein complex may limit the mobilization of the temporal lobe and the opening of the sylvian fissure, while a small venous complex (Fig. 24.9) allows direct exposure of the sphenoid segment. Small veins crossing the sylvian fissure between the frontal and temporal lobe may be ligated and cut, as performed in transcranial approaches.

Middle Cerebral Artery

The MCA originates in the carotid cistern at the medial end of the deep portion of the sylvian fissure, lateral to the optic chiasm and posterior to the olfactory tract division into medial and lateral

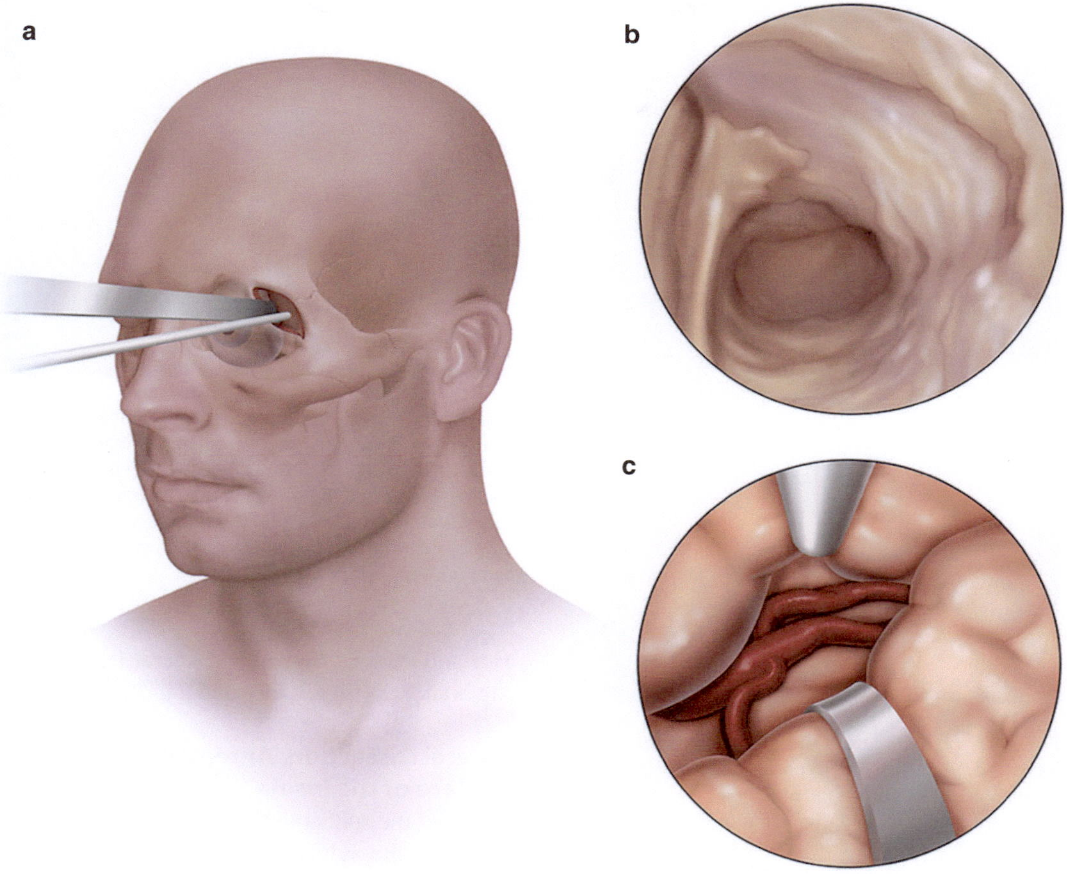

Fig. 24.7 The endoscopic transorbital approach to the sylvian fissure. (**a**) Position of the endoscope in the superior-lateral part of the orbit. (**b**) Dural exposure. (**c**) View of the sylvian fissure and middle cerebral artery branches and frontal and temporal lobes

olfactory striae. It can be divided into four segments: sphenoidal (M1), insular (M2), opercular (M3) and cortical (M4). The M1 segment runs laterally from its origin, parallel to the lesser sphenoid wing and approximately 1 cm posterior to the sphenoidal ridge. Anterior to the limen insula, the MCA turns posteriorly (genu of the MCA), originating the M2 segment. It runs over the lateral insular surface, usually as two main trunks (superior and inferior), which will originate other branches, cross the circular sulcus of the insula (M3 segment), and reach the cortical surface of the frontal, temporal and parietal lobes (M4 branches). The proximity of the M1 segment to the sphenoidal ridge makes it a good candidate for transorbital endoscopic approaches. The careful wide opening of the sphenoidal segment of the sylvian fissure allows exposure of the limen insula and identification of the M2 branches at the lateral insular surface.

Endoscopic transorbital identification of the MCA is possible after opening the sylvian fissure and identifying the temporopolar and anterior temporal branches of the MCA, which run over the anterior part of the temporal lobe (Figs. 24.7 and 24.8). These branches will lead the surgeon to the main trunk of the MCA in the sylvian cistern. This cistern extends medially along the sylvian fissure and over the insula to the carotid cistern. It contains the middle cerebral artery, its

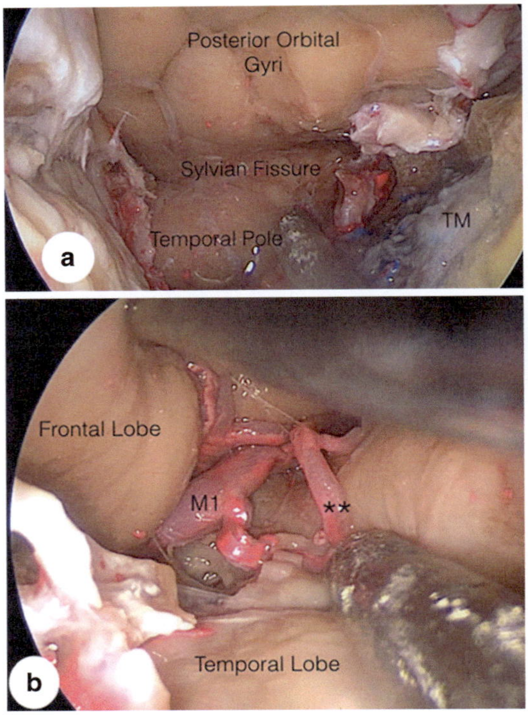

Fig. 24.8 (**a**) Initial exposure of the frontal and temporal lobes and sylvian fissure. Exposure of the posterior orbital gyri and superior part of the temporal pole is required for successful exposure and dissection of the sylvian fissure. Initial intradural dissection is performed with a 0° endoscope supported by an endoscope holder. This allows the application of bimanual microsurgical techniques using aspirators and microscissors. (**b**) Dissection starts with the identification of the superficial MCA branches, such as the anterior temporal arteries (**), which guide the surgeon toward the main trunk of the M1 segment. M1: sphenoidal segment of the middle cerebral artery (MCA), ** Anterior temporal branch

bifurcation and major branches, anterior perforating arteries, temporopolar and anterior temporal arteries (Figs. 24.10 and 24.11). Once the main trunk of the M1 segment has been found, dissection can be carried medially toward the carotid cistern, with exposure of the carotid bifurcation as well as the site of origin of M1 and A1. The medial lenticulostriate branches originate from the superior-posterior wall of the M1 and are observed during its course toward the anterior perforated substance (Fig. 24.10). Lateral dissection exposes the MCA bifurcation, limen insula and genu of the MCA, M2 segment and its superior and inferior trunks, and lateral lenticulostriate branches (Figs. 24.10 and 24.12).

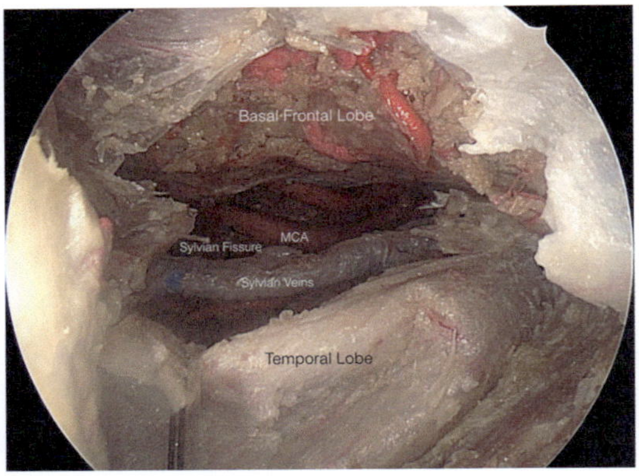

Fig. 24.9 Sylvian fissure and sylvian veins. Large sylvian veins draining into the sphenoparietal sinus may obstruct the surgical corridor and block visualization of the sylvian fissure. Small veins may be ligated; however, large draining vessels should be preserved, if possible, through careful dissection and mobilization toward the temporal lobe

Lateral Dissection: Anterolateral Surface of the Insula

Opening the sphenoidal and operculoinsular segments of the sylvian fissure allows exposure of the limen insula and anterior and lateral insular surface (Figs. 24.10 and 24.12). Mobilization of the frontal and temporal operculum allows visualization of the inferior circular sulcus and M2 branches in the anterior-inferior aspect of the insula. Perforating branches, originating from M2, enter the lateral insula surface perpendicularly and may be visualized after lateral mobilization of the M2 trunks. The superior-posterior part of the lateral insular surface may not be adequately exposed through this approach since it is hidden deeply below the posterior part of the frontotemporoparietal operculum.

Medial Dissection: Carotid, Crural and Ambiens Cistern

Dissection toward the medial aspect of the sylvian cistern will lead to the carotid cistern (Fig. 24.13). It is located between the sylvian and chiasmatic cisterns and contains the supraclinoid

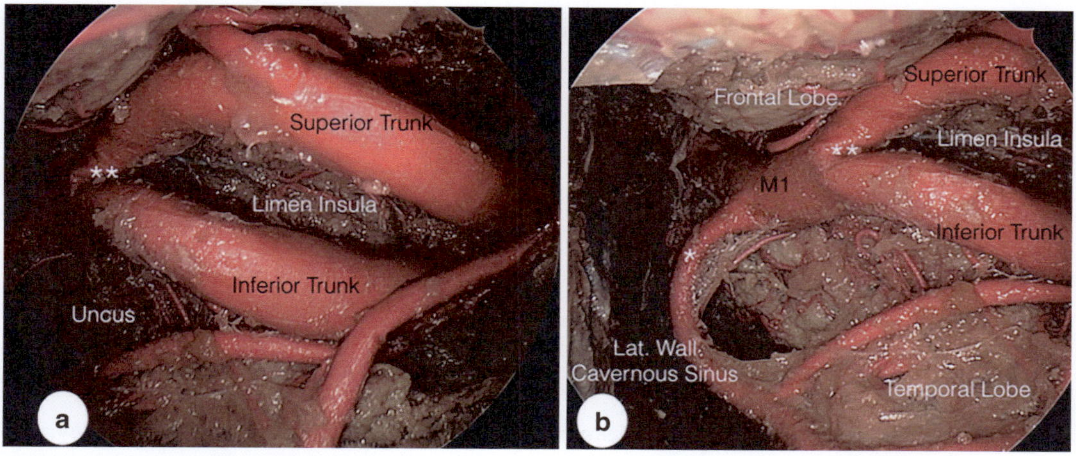

Fig. 24.10 Middle cerebral artery. (**a**) Dissection of the sylvian fissure leads to exposure of the distal portion of the M1 segment, MCA bifurcation and superior and inferior trunks of the MCA. The limen insula is shown at the site of the genu of the MCA (**), and the uncus is observed inferior to M1. (**b**) Further dissection with a 30° endoscope demonstrates the proximal segment of M1 exiting the carotid cistern and early temporal branches (*). * Early temporal branch, ** genu of the middle cerebral artery

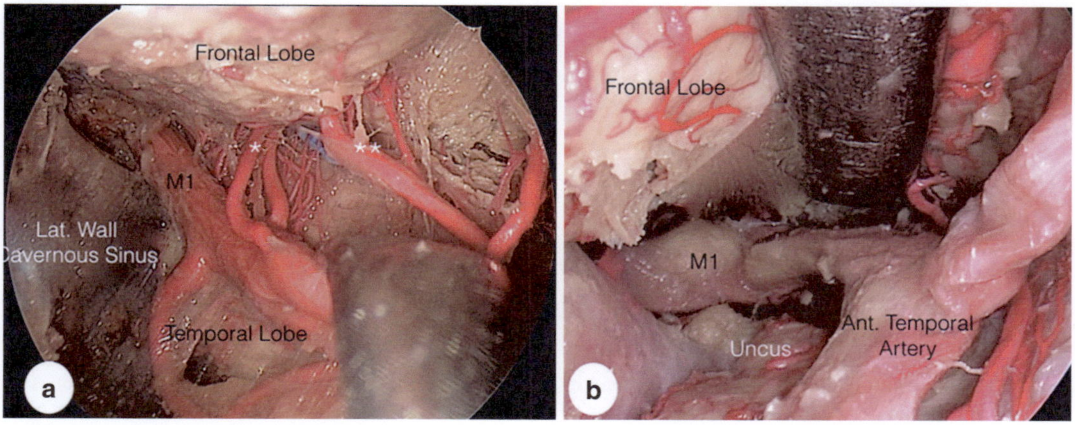

Fig. 24.11 The sphenoid segment of the MCA (M1 segment). (**a**) Exposure of the medial portion of the sylvian cistern and its contents, with a 30° endoscope. The medial (*) and lateral (**) lenticulostriate branches exit the superior and posterior walls of the MCA and run toward the anterior perforated substance to supply the internal capsule and deep nuclei. (**b**) The uncus is observed at the medial aspect of the temporal lobe, inferior to the M1 segment and closely related to the lateral wall of the cavernous sinus. Through an endoscopic transorbital transuncus approach, the amygdala and hippocampus may be resected. * Medial lenticulostriate branches, ** lateral lenticulostriate branches

portion of the internal carotid artery, the origins of the ophthalmic, posterior communicating (PcomA) and anterior choroidal arteries (AChA), the carotid bifurcation, initial portions of the A1 and M1 segments, and the perforating branches from the carotid artery. Posteriorly, this cistern communicates with the crural and ambiens cistern, which can also be visualized using 30° endoscopes and lateral retraction of the temporal lobe or after an anterior temporal lobectomy.

Dura Repair

Closure of the dura defect can be done using fascia temporalis grafts or artificial dura grafts inserted in two layers as inlay and outlay grafts. These can be sutured together in the middle as a "button" graft [40]. As in endoscopic endonasal surgery, the grafts must be larger than the dural defect and cover its borders entirely. The pressure of the orbit over the dura reconstruction keeps the grafts in place.

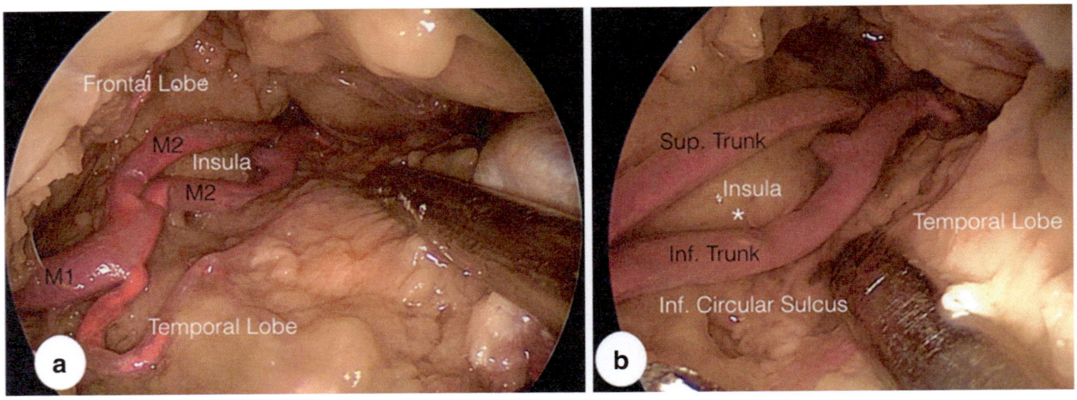

Fig. 24.12 Insular segment of the MCA (M2 segment). (**a**) Lateral dissection of sylvian fissure leads to exposure of its operculoinsular segment. The MCA bifurcates at the distal part of the M1 and turns around the limen insula, originating the genu of the MCA. (**b**) The superior and inferior trunks of the MCA run close to the inferior circular sulcus toward the posterior part of the operculoinsular segment of the sylvian fissure. In their trajectory, they develop perforating branches that cross perpendicularly to irrigate the insula

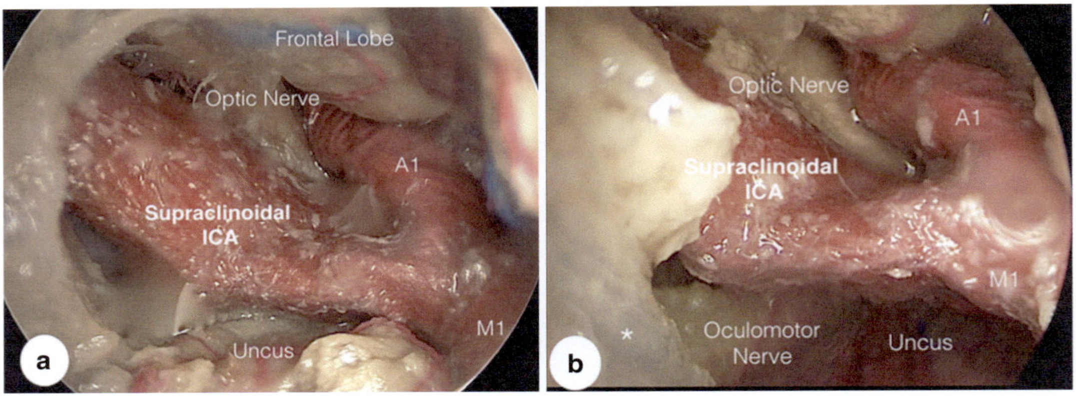

Fig. 24.13 Carotid cistern. Exposure of the carotid cistern with a 30° endoscope. (**a**) The carotid bifurcation and origin of A1 and M1 are shown. It is possible to visualize the trajectory of A1 above the left optic nerve. (**b**) The uncus is observed in its typical location medial to the supraclinoidal ICA and inferior to the M1 segment. After exiting the interpeduncular fossa, the oculomotor nerve runs medial to the uncus on its way to the roof of the cavernous sinus

The Evolution of Tones and Potential Applications of Transorbital Approaches to the Sylvian Fissure

Surgical approaches through and around the orbit have been implemented since the early twentieth century. In 1913, Frazier described the orbital roof craniotomy technique [41], which was later modified and performed via an eyebrow incision [22, 25, 28, 42, 43]. More recently, eyelid approaches to the anterior cranial base have also been proposed but generally in an "upward" trajectory toward the roof of the orbit and basal frontal lobe [31, 44].

The concept of pure transorbital endoscopic approaches to a variety of locations around the skull base was only proposed in 2010 by Moe et al. [29]. Without the need to remove the orbital rim, this might be considered the first description of a "true" transorbital approach [45]. As proposed by the authors, the orbit can be divided into four different quadrants, each with its specific approach: medial (precaruncular approach), superior (superior eyelid approach), lateral (lateral retrocanthal approach) and inferior (preseptal lower eyelid). Superior and lateral approaches allow exposure of the anterior and middle cranial fossae and superior orbital fissures [29, 46].

The transorbital endoscopic approach was initially developed as an alternative route for endoscopic treatment of skull base lesions [29, 47, 48]. As a natural corridor, the orbits have been used as an additional route to different skull base regions. Previous anatomical studies have demonstrated the utility of these approaches to reach multiple skull base structures, including the lateral wall of the cavernous sinus [37, 46, 49], Meckel's cave [39], the petrous carotid [39] and optic nerve [38]. We expand the previously described targets to include the sylvian fissure, middle cerebral artery and the crural cistern and its contents.

Intradural Dissection via the Transorbital Endoscopic Approach

The sylvian fissure is also readily accessible via a transorbital endoscopic approach. Guided by anatomical landmarks, such as the SOF and IOF, tailored bone resection and dural opening can be performed. Using an endoscope holder, bimanual dissection and careful dissection of the arachnoid membranes allow the opening of the sylvian cistern. Unlike transcortical approaches, transcisternal dissection requires manipulation of veins and arterial branches that may cross from one side to the other as well as eventual coagulation and ligation of those vessels. Dissection should be performed following standard microsurgical principles using knives, microscissors and aspirators; classic endoscopic endonasal maneuvers, such as the two-aspirator technique and retraction using curettes may be implemented for resection of intra-axial lesions but should be avoided during transcisternal dissection to reduce trauma to the normal surrounding parenchyma.

Potential Benefits and Clinical Applications

As demonstrated, the sylvian fissure and its surroundings, including the basal frontal lobe and temporal lobe, are adequately exposed via a transorbital endoscopic approach. Benefits of this approach include improved cosmetic results, lack of temporalis muscle dissection and the resulting atrophy, reduced brain retraction and excellent visualization. Using an oculoplastic surgeon for the opening and closing may further improve the cosmetic results.

Unlike classic lateral craniotomies, the transorbital endoscopic approach does not require scalp incisions or manipulations of the temporalis muscle. Those approaches to the sylvian region require temporalis muscle dissection, which may lead to muscle atrophy and cosmetic deformities [50]. Additionally, frontalis muscle palsy due to injury of the frontotemporal branches of the facial nerve may follow after lateral craniotomies [51]. Minimally invasive microsurgical approaches, such as eyelid [31] and supraorbital eyebrow [52] craniotomies, share the cosmetic benefits of the transorbital endoscopic approach and also result in superior cosmetic outcomes when compared to classic approaches [4, 31, 53].

The anterior view of the sphenoid segment of the sylvian fissure and frontal and temporal lobes achieved via the transorbital approach allows adequate exposure of this region with reduced brain retraction. If the surgical target is located in the frontal lobe or temporal pole, surgery may proceed with almost no brain manipulation; however, successful dissection of the sylvian fissure will require careful retraction of the surrounding parenchyma. The frontoorbitozygomatic approach allows similar visualization of the anterior and lateral aspects of the frontal and temporal lobes but requires a large craniotomy followed by extensive drilling of the skull base, which may lead to postoperative deformities if not adequately performed.

Potential candidates for transorbital endoscopic surgery include not only extradural tumors with intradural extension and intradural lesions but also vascular lesions in the sylvian region, such as

MCA aneurysms. Resection of spheno-orbital meningiomas via this approach has already been reported with successful results and no major complications [4, 29, 30]. Intradural lesions, such as frontobasal, temporal and insular gliomas and mesial temporal sclerosis, may be approached through this technique. A previous study reported the use of endoscopic-guided transorbital surgery for amydalahyppocampectomy in two patients [36]. Although the authors report the use of microscopes in the initial part of the procedure, this report demonstrates the clinical feasibility of the resection of intra-axial lesions through transorbital endoscopic-guided approaches.

Vascular lesions are special challenges for endoscopic approaches. Despite this, previous reports demonstrated the effectiveness of different endoscopic approaches in selected cases. Transcranial endoscopic-assisted microneurosurgery, through supraorbital craniotomies [24, 26, 54], has been reported as an effective option for surgical clipping of anterior circulation aneurysms. Additionally, an endoscopic endonasal approach for clipping of aneurysms [8, 55–57] and resection of cavernomas [58–61] has been advocated by groups with extensive experience in endoscopic skull base surgery, with successful results in selected cases. The experience of those groups reinforces the potential of transorbital endoscopic surgery. As shown in our anatomical study, the transorbital endoscopic approach is a feasible option for exposure of the sylvian fissure, supraclinoidal ICA, ICA bifurcation and middle cerebral artery and its branches. Therefore, through careful dissection, exposure and clipping of MCA bifurcation aneurysms may be feasible via this technique, and the proximal to distal exposure provides excellent proximal control. Aneurysms originating in other locations, such as the ICA bifurcation and the origin of the AChA and PcomA, may be reached but may demand larger craniectomies and more complex intradural dissection. Moreover, distal MCA aneurysms may be more easily exposed through a lateral craniotomy. Cavernomas located in the basal frontal lobe, anterior part of the insula, superior anterolateral brainstem or temporal pole are potential candidates for transorbital resection due to their superficial location and adequate exposure after a successful approach.

Limitations of the Technique

Common concerns related to the transorbital endoscopic approach are postoperative CSF leaks and orbital damage. Clinical results are limited, and it is difficult to draw definitive conclusions regarding these complications. So far, however, CSF leaks have not been reported as a major complication [4, 62–64]. The presence of the orbit and its contents keeps the skull base reconstruction in place and may justify the lower CSF rates of transorbital compared to extended endoscopic approaches.

Significant orbital damage and visual loss are rare after transorbital endoscopic surgery [4, 62, 64].

Intradural transorbital endoscopic dissection adds a significant challenge to the surgeon, who must be aware of the limitations of this technique. More common "minimally invasive" transcranial approaches, such as the lateral supraorbital (LSO), may be used to reach similar anatomical targets. First, the transorbital endoscopic approach requires comprehensive knowledge of skull base anatomy through a new surgical perspective. Second, the cisternal dissection and mobilization of arteries and veins are performed in a limited corridor. This demands previous experience with endoscopic skull base techniques and training in an anatomical laboratory. Lastly, intradural vascular complications may be troublesome. Although easily performed in an anatomical study, manipulation of intracranial vessels during surgery may lead to intraoperative hemorrhages secondary to arterial or venous damage that may be hard to control. As in endoscopic endonasal surgery, coordination with an assistant surgeon to keep the endoscope lens clean during hemostasis is paramount. The surgical corridor obtained with the approach should be adequate for the application of temporary clipping, compression with cotton balls and coagulation with bipolar electrocautery whenever necessary.

Conclusions

The transorbital endoscopic approach allows successful exposure of the sphenoidal portion of the sylvian fissure and M1 and M2 segments of the middle cerebral artery. The carotid cistern and its components, including the ICA bifurcation, A1 and M1 origin and perforating branches, can be exposed. In addition to the usual concerns related to the transorbital endoscopic approach, a limited surgical window for intradural bimanual dissection, potentially hard-to-control hemorrhages, and lack of adequate surgical tools are some of the limitations of the technique.

References

1. Banu MA, Guerrero-Maldonado A, McCrea HJ, Garcia-Navarro V, Souweidane MM, Anand VK, et al. Impact of skull base development on endonasal endoscopic surgical corridors: clinical article. J Neurosurg Pediatr. 2014;13(2):155–69. https://doi.org/10.3171/2013.10.peds13303.
2. Cappabianca P, Schwartz TH, Jane JA Jr, Zada G. Introduction: endoscopic endonasal skull base surgery. Neurosurg Focus. 2014;37(4):Introduction. https://doi.org/10.3171/2014.7.FOCUS14459.
3. Cavallo LM, Messina A, Gardner P, Esposito F, Kassam AB, Cappabianca P, et al. Extended endoscopic endonasal approach to the pterygopalatine fossa: anatomical study and clinical considerations. Neurosurg Focus. 2005;19:E5.
4. Dallan I, Castelnuovo P, Locatelli D, Turri-Zanoni M, Alqahtani A, Battaglia P, et al. Multiportal combined transorbital transnasal endoscopic approach for the management of selected skull base lesions: preliminary experience. World Neurosurg. 2015;84:97–107.
5. Ditzel Filho LF, Prevedello DM, Jamshidi AO, Dolci RL, Kerr EE, Campbell R, et al. Endoscopic endonasal approach for removal of tuberculum sellae meningiomas. Neurosurg Clin N Am. 2015;26:349–61.
6. Fernandez-Miranda JC, Prevedello DM, Gardner P, Carrau R, Snyderman CH, Kassam AB. Endonasal endoscopic pituitary surgery: is it a matter of fashion? Acta Neurochir. 2010;152(8):1281–2; author reply 1282.
7. Gardner PA, Prevedello DM, Kassam AB, Snyderman CH, Carrau RL, Mintz AH. The evolution of the endonasal approach for craniopharyngiomas: historical vignette. J Neurosurg. 2008;108(5):1043–7. https://doi.org/10.3171/JNS/2008/108/5/1043.
8. Gardner PA, Vaz-Guimaraes F, Jankowitz B, Koutourousiou M, Fernandez-Miranda JC, Wang EW, et al. Endoscopic endonasal clipping of intracranial aneurysms: surgical technique and results. World Neurosurg. 2015;84(5):1380–93. https://doi.org/10.1016/j.wneu.2015.06.032.
9. Komotar RJ, Starke RM, Raper DMS, Anand VK, Schwartz TH. Endoscopic endonasal compared with anterior craniofacial and combined cranionasal resection of esthesioneuroblastomas. World Neurosurg. 2013;80(1–2):148–59. https://doi.org/10.1016/j.wneu.2012.12.003.
10. Lee DL, Mccoul ED, Anand VK, Schwartz TH. Endoscopic endonasal access to the jugular foramen: defining the surgical approach. J Neurol Surg B. 2012;73:342–51.
11. Patel KS, Komotar RJ, Szentirmai O, Moussazadeh N, Raper DM, Starke RM, et al. Case-specific protocol to reduce cerebrospinal fluid leakage after endonasal endoscopic surgery: clinical article. J Neurosurg. 2013;119(3):661–8. https://doi.org/10.3171/2013.4.JNS13124.
12. Banu MA, Kim J-H, Shin BJ, Woodworth GF, Anand VK, Schwartz TH. Low-dose intrathecal fluorescein and etiology-based graft choice in endoscopic endonasal closure of CSF leaks. Clin Neurol Neurosurg. 2014;116:28–34. https://doi.org/10.1016/j.clineuro.2013.11.006.
13. Khan OH, Anand VK, Schwartz TH. Endoscopic endonasal resection of skull base meningiomas: the significance of a "cortical cuff" and brain edema compared with careful case selection and surgical experience in predicting morbidity and extent of resection. Neurosurg Focus. 2014;37:E7.
14. Ottenhausen M, Banu MA, Placantonakis DG, Tsiouris AJ, Khan OH, Anand VK, et al. Endoscopic endonasal resection of suprasellar meningiomas: the importance of case selection and experience in determining extent of resection, visual improvement, and complications. World Neurosurg. 2014;82:442–9.
15. Prevedello DM, Ditzel Filho LFS, Solari D, Carrau RL, Kassam AB. Expanded endonasal approaches to middle cranial fossa and posterior fossa tumors. Neurosurg Clin N Am. 2010;21(4):621–35., vi. https://doi.org/10.1016/j.nec.2010.07.003.
16. Snyderman CH, Carrau RL, Kassam AB, Zanation A, Prevedello D, Gardner P, et al. Endoscopic skull base surgery: principles of endonasal oncological surgery. J Surg Oncol. 2008;97:658–64.
17. Snyderman CH, Pant H, Carrau RL, Prevedello DM, Gardner P, Kassam AB. What are the limits of endoscopic sinus surgery?: the expanded endonasal approach to the skull base. Keio J Med. 2009;58:152–60.
18. Zhang M, Singh H, Almodovar-Mercado GJ, Anand VK, Schwartz TH. Required reading: the most impactful articles in endoscopic endonasal skull base surgery. World Neurosurg. 2016;92:499–512.e2.
19. Cappabianca P, Cavallo LM, Esposito F, De Divitiis O, Messina A, De Divitiis E. Extended endoscopic endonasal approach to the midline skull base: the evolving role of transsphenoidal surgery. Adv Tech

Stand Neurosurg. 2008;33:151–99. https://doi.org/10.1007/978-3-211-72283-1_4.
20. Castelnuovo P, Dallan I, Battaglia P, Bignami M. Endoscopic endonasal skull base surgery: past, present, and future. Eur Arch Otorhinolaryngol. 2010;267(5):649–63. https://doi.org/10.1007/s00405-009-1196-0.
21. Kasemsiri P, Carrau RL, Ditzel Filho LFS, Prevedello DM, Otto BA, Old M, et al. Advantages and limitations of endoscopic endonasal approaches to the skull base. World Neurosurg. 2014;82(6 Suppl):S12–21. https://doi.org/10.1016/j.wneu.2014.07.022.
22. Al-Mefty O. Supraorbital-pterional approach to skull base lesions. Neurosurgery. 1987;21(4):474–7.
23. Delashaw JB, Tedeschi H, Rhoton AL. Modified supraorbital craniotomy: technical note. Neurosurgery. 1992;30:954–6.
24. Ho CL, Hwang PY. Endoscope-assisted transorbital keyhole surgical approach to ruptured supratentorial aneurysms. J Neurol Surg A Cent Eur Neurosurg. 2015;76(5):376–83. https://doi.org/10.1055/s-0035-1547358.
25. Jane JA, Park TS, Pobereskin LH, Winn RH, Butler AB. The supraorbital approach: technical note. Neurosurgery. 1982;11(4):537–42. https://doi.org/10.1227/00006123-198210000-00016.
26. Reisch R, Fischer G, Stadie A, Kockro R, Cesnulis E, Hopf N. The supraorbital endoscopic approach for aneurysms. World Neurosurg. 2014;82(6 Suppl):S130–7. https://doi.org/10.1016/j.wneu.2014.07.038.
27. Srinivasan VM, Kan P, Germanwala AV, Pelargos P, Bohnen A, Choy W, et al. Key perspectives on woven EndoBridge device for wide-necked bifurcation aneurysms, endoscopic endonasal clipping of intracranial aneurysms, retrosigmoid versus translabyrinthine approaches for acoustic neuromas, and impact of local intraoperative steroid administration on postoperative dysphagia following anterior cervical discectomy and fusion. Surg Neurol Int. 2016;7:S720–4.
28. Van Lindert E, Perneczky A, Fries G, Pierangeli E. The supraorbital keyhole approach to supratentorial aneurysms: concept and technique. Surg Neurol. 1998;49(5):481–9; discussion 489–90. https://doi.org/10.1016/s0090-3019(96)00539-3.
29. Moe KS, Bergeron CM, Ellenbogen RG. Transorbital neuroendoscopic surgery. Neurosurgery. 2010;67(3 Suppl Operative):ons16–28. https://doi.org/10.1227/01.NEU.0000373431.08464.43.
30. Ramakrishna R, Kim LJ, Bly RA, Moe K, Ferreira M. Transorbital neuroendoscopic surgery for the treatment of skull base lesions. J Clin Neurosci. 2016;24:99–104.
31. Andaluz N, Romano A, Reddy LV, Zuccarello M. Eyelid approach to the anterior cranial base: technical note. J Neurosurg. 2008;109(2):341–6. https://doi.org/10.3171/JNS/2008/109/8/0341.
32. Andaluz N, Zuccarello M. Supraorbital and transorbital minicraniotomies. Response. J Neurosurg. 2014;121(5):1291–3.
33. Dlouhy BJ, Chae MP, Teo C. The supraorbital eyebrow approach in children: clinical outcomes, cosmetic results, and complications. J Neurosurg Pediatr. 2015;15:12–9.
34. Wilson DA, Duong H, Teo C, Kelly DF. The supraorbital endoscopic approach for tumors. World Neurosurg. 2014;82(1–2):e243–56. https://doi.org/10.1016/j.wneu.2013.02.002.
35. Zada G. Editorial: The endoscopic keyhole supraorbital approach. Neurosurg Focus. 2014;37:E21.
36. Chen HI, Bohman LE, Emery L, Martinez-Lage M, Richardson AG, Davis KA, et al. Lateral transorbital endoscopic access to the hippocampus, amygdala, and entorhinal cortex: initial clinical experience. ORL J Otorhinolaryngol Relat Spec. 2015;77:321–32.
37. Dallan I, Di Somma A, Prats-Galino A, Solari D, Alobid I, Turri-Zanoni M, et al. Endoscopic transorbital route to the cavernous sinus through the meningo-orbital band: a descriptive anatomical study. J Neurosurg. 2017;127(3):622–9. https://doi.org/10.3171/2016.8.JNS16465.
38. Di Somma A, Cavallo A, De Notaris LM, Solari M, Topczewski D, Bernal-Sprekelsen TE, et al. Endoscopic endonasal medial-to-lateral and transorbital lateral-to-medial optic nerve decompression: an anatomical study with surgical implications. J Neurosurg. 2017;127:199–208.
39. Ferrari M, Schreiber A, Mattavelli D, Belotti F, Rampinelli V, Lancini D, et al. The inferolateral transorbital endoscopic approach: a preclinical anatomic study. World Neurosurg. 2016;90:403–13.
40. Luginbuhl AJ, Campbell PG, Evans J, Rosen M. Endoscopic repair of high-flow cranial base defects using a bilayer button. Laryngoscope. 2010;120(5):876–80. https://doi.org/10.1002/lary.20861.
41. Frazier CH. I. An approach to the hypophysis through the anterior cranial fossa. Ann Surg. 1913;57(2):145–50. https://doi.org/10.1097/00000658-191302000-00001.
42. Delashaw JB Jr, Jane JA, Kassell NF, Luce C. Supraorbital craniotomy by fracture of the anterior orbital roof. Technical note. J Neurosurg. 1993;79(4):615–8. https://doi.org/10.3171/jns.1993.79.4.0615.
43. Reisch R, Perneczky A, Filippi R. Surgical technique of the supraorbital key-hole craniotomy. Surg Neurol. 2003;59(3):223–7. https://doi.org/10.1016/s0090-3019(02)01037-6.
44. Raza SM, Quinones-Hinojosa A, Lim M, Boahene KDO. The transconjunctival transorbital approach: a keyhole approach to the midline anterior skull base. World Neurosurg. 2013;80(6):864–71. https://doi.org/10.1016/j.wneu.2012.06.027.
45. Sonig A, Nanda A. Transorbital approach to the anterior cranial skull base. World Neurosurg. 2013;80(6):810–2. https://doi.org/10.1016/j.wneu.2012.07.024.
46. Bly RA, Ramakrishna R, Ferreira M, Moe KS. Lateral transorbital neuroendoscopic approach to the lateral cavernous sinus. J Neurol Surg B. 2014;75:11–7.

47. Dallan I, Locatelli D, Turri-Zanoni M, Battaglia P, Lepera D, Galante N, et al. Transorbital endoscopic assisted resection of a superior orbital fissure cavernous haemangioma: a technical case report. Eur Arch Otorrinolaringol. 2015;272:3851–6.
48. Locatelli D, Pozzi F, Turri-Zanoni M, Battaglia P, Santi L, Dallan I, et al. Transorbital endoscopic approaches to the skull base: current concepts and future perspectives. J Neurosurg Sci. 2016;60(4):514–25.
49. Alqahtani A, Padoan G, Segnini G, Lepera D, Fortunato S, Dallan I, et al. Transorbital transnasal endoscopic combined approach to the anterior and middle skull base: a laboratory investigation. Acta Otorhinolaryngol Ital. 2015;35(3):173–9.
50. Yasuda CL, Costa ALF, Franca M Jr, Pereira FRS, Tedeschi H, de Oliveira E, et al. Postcraniotomy temporalis muscle atrophy: a clinical, magnetic resonance imaging volumetry and electromyographic investigation. J Orofac Pain. 2010;24(4):391–7.
51. Youssef AS, Ahmadian A, Ramos E, Vale F, van Loveren HR. Combined subgaleal/myocutaneous technique for temporalis muscle dissection. J Neurol Surg B Skull Base. 2012;73(6):387–93. https://doi.org/10.1055/s-0032-1326778.
52. Jho HD. Orbital roof craniotomy via an eyebrow incision: a simplified anterior skull base approach. Minim Invasive Neurosurg. 1997;40:91–7.
53. Dallan I, Castelnuovo P, Turri-Zanoni M, Fiacchini G, Locatelli D, Battaglia P, et al. Transorbital endoscopic assisted management of intraorbital lesions: lessons learned from our first 9 cases. Rhinology. 2016;54(3):247–53. https://doi.org/10.4193/Rhino15.237.
54. Fischer G, Stadie A, Reisch R, Hopf NJ, Fries G, Böcher-Schwarz H, et al. The keyhole concept in aneurysm surgery: results of the past 20 years. Neurosurgery. 2011;68(1 Suppl Operative):45–51; discussion 51. https://doi.org/10.1227/NEU.0b013e31820934ca.
55. Heiferman DM, Somasundaram A, Alvarado AJ, Zanation AM, Pittman AL, Germanwala AV. The endonasal approach for treatment of cerebral aneurysms: a critical review of the literature. Clin Neurol Neurosurg. 2015;134:91–7. https://doi.org/10.1016/j.clineuro.2015.04.018.
56. Peris-Celda M, Da Roz L, Monroy-Sosa A, Morishita T, Rhoton AL Jr. Surgical anatomy of endoscope-assisted approaches to common aneurysm sites. Neurosurgery. 2014;10 Suppl 1(1):121–44; discussion 144. https://doi.org/10.1227/NEU.0000000000000205.
57. Szentirmai O, Hong Y, Mascarenhas L, Salek AA, Stieg PE, Anand VK, et al. Endoscopic endonasal clip ligation of cerebral aneurysms: an anatomical feasibility study and future directions. J Neurosurg. 2016;124(2):463–8. https://doi.org/10.3171/2015.1.jns142650.
58. Dallan I, Battaglia P, De Notaris M, Caniglia M, Turri-Zanoni M. Endoscopic endonasal transclival approach to a pontine cavernous malformation: case report. Int J Pediatr Otorhinolaryngol. 2015;79:1584–8.
59. He S-M, Wang Y, Zhao T-Z, Zheng T, Lv W-H, Zhao L-F, et al. Endoscopic endonasal approach to mesencephalic cavernous malformations. World Neurosurg. 2016;90:701.e7–701.e10. https://doi.org/10.1016/j.wneu.2016.02.064.
60. Kimball MM, Lewis SB, Werning JW, Mocco JD. Resection of a pontine cavernous malformation via an endoscopic endonasal approach: a case report. Neurosurgery. 2012;71(1 Suppl Operative):186–93; discussion 193–4. https://doi.org/10.1227/NEU.0b013e31824cabb1.
61. Nayak NR, Thawani JP, Sanborn MR, Storm PB, Lee JYK. Endoscopic approaches to brainstem cavernous malformations: case series and review of the literature. Surg Neurol Int. 2015;6(1):68. https://doi.org/10.4103/2152-7806.155807.
62. Bly RA, Morton RP, Kim LJ, Moe KS. Tension pneumocephalus after endoscopic sinus surgery: a technical report of multiportal endoscopic skull base repair. Otolaryngol Head Neck Surg. 2014;151:1081–3.
63. Koutourousiou M, Gardner PA, Stefko ST, Paluzzi A, Fernandez-Miranda JC, Snyderman CH, et al. Combined endoscopic endonasal transorbital approach with transconjunctival-medial orbitotomy for excisional biopsy of the optic nerve: technical note. J Neurol Surg Rep. 2012;73:52–6.
64. Schaberg M, Murchison AP, Rosen MR, Evans JJ, Bilyk JR. Transorbital and transnasal endoscopic repair of a meningoencephalocele. Orbit. 2011;30(5):221–5. https://doi.org/10.3109/01676830.2011.579686.

Lateral Transorbital Approach for Intracranial Aneurysm Surgery

25

Murat Ulutas

Problems in the natural sciences are solved through observation and experiments. Derived hypotheses are either transformed into concrete knowledge through repeated verification by experimentation and observation or are falsified and cast aside. A hypothesis that is verified through repeated tests and maintains its validity despite efforts to falsify it turns into law over time. In the natural sciences, old laws give rise to new and more complicated layers of new laws which, in turn, build upon their predecessors. Each layer complements the prior, allowing new layers to emerge. Thus, laws maintain their validity until they are falsified, allowing new knowledge and scientific methods to develop and existing laws to evolve into better ones. The key factor that has enabled the development of contemporary medical and scientific knowledge is the addition of layers of knowledge or law over existing layers as a result of experiments and observations.

A body of knowledge obtained through experiments and observations has gradually accumulated for approximately 4700 years, from identifying peripheral arterial dilation to developing current modern treatment methods for intracranial aneurysms [1]. This process, which started with the identification of aneurysms, turned into the search for treatment methods, and the knowledge obtained through the outcomes of treatment methods led to the production of new hypotheses; thus, the search for new treatment methods and surgical techniques has continued uninterrupted.

A Brief History of Intracranial Aneurysms and Surgical Treatment Methods

Peripheral arterial aneurysms were first described as arterial dilation in the Ebers Papyrus, which is estimated to have been written in 2725 BC by Imhotep, who is known as the founder of ancient Egyptian medicine. The term aneurysm was coined to describe the arterial dilation by Galen of Pergamon (129–210 BC). However, intracranial aneurysms could not be discovered and demonstrated until the end of the eighteenth century. Morgagni (1682–1771) described an unruptured carotid aneurysm during an autopsy in 1761, but it was John Blackall (1771–1860) who contributed the most important layer of knowledge by revealing the relationship between a ruptured intracranial aneurysm and the clinical properties of subarachnoid hemorrhage [2]. After the source of the hemorrhage had been detected through observation only, without any diagnostic method, a new scientific layer was created as a result of attempts to develop treatment methods to prevent

M. Ulutas (✉)
Department of Neurosurgery, Sanko University School of Medicine, Konukoglu Hospital, Gaziantep, Turkey

T. H. Schwartz et al. (eds.), *Endoscopic Transorbital Surgery of the Orbit, Skull Base and Brain*,
https://doi.org/10.1007/978-3-031-59504-2_25

intracranial aneurysm rupture. As the first method, attempts were made to prevent the aneurysm from being filled through ligation of the artery proximal to the aneurysm. Treatment of an intracranial aneurysm through ligation of the proximal carotid artery was first described by Victor Horsley (1857–1916) [1]. However, Harvey Cushing (1869–1939) was not convinced of treating intracranial aneurysms through carotid artery ligation due to the high morbidity and mortality rates following carotid artery occlusion. Cushing tried to treat aneurysms by wrapping them with muscle, but the first person to isolate an aneurysm from normal circulation was Norman Dott (1897–1973), who had previously received training with Cushing. Dott closed the aneurysm neck through suture ligation, which is quite dangerous and difficult [1]. The realization that the aneurysm neck needed to be closed to isolate it from normal circulation led to the creation of a new layer of knowledge in the treatment of aneurysms. Thus, proximal ligation was falsified, and the necessity to develop and test a new method arose. The silver clips designed by Cushing to control deep bleeding during tumor surgery were never used by Cushing in aneurysm surgery. However, these clips were used by Walter Dandy (1886–1946), who successfully performed the first-ever aneurysm clipping in 1937, thus giving rise to modern vascular neurosurgery [3]. After being tested and verified numerous times, the clipping method was, for many years, the gold standard in the treatment of aneurysms. The search for new surgical methods that would enable aneurysm clipping to be performed in a safe and less invasive manner with low complication rates soon followed.

During the years of intracranial aneurysm clipping, surgery required a fairly large skin incision and a large craniotomy bone flap. A wide exposure was required because the exact anatomical location of the lesion was not precisely known, the illumination was poor, there was little ability for magnification, and a lack of microsurgical tools and techniques that necessitated large surgical teams [4, 5]. The introduction of surgical microscopes in neurosurgical operations solved both the illumination and magnification issues [6]. With the development of bipolar coagulation and microsurgical techniques and instruments, the incorporation of neuroendoscopy into neurosurgery, and the introduction of intraoperative diagnostic methods, the size of the skin incisions and craniotomies gradually decreased. It became possible to surgically treat complicated cranial pathologies with smaller craniotomies, and surgical treatments became even less invasive [4, 5]. As new knowledge and modern technologies emerged, due to the gradually increasing anatomical knowledge and experience obtained through conventional surgery over time, minimally invasive interventions developed.

Pterional craniotomy was first described by Yasargil in 1975 and became the main approach in aneurysm surgery [7]. Orbitozygomatic craniotomy added removal of the lateral wall of the orbit and zygomatic arc to pterional craniotomy to reduce the need for brain retraction and to gain a larger surgical working area and a wider perspective [8]. Although these craniotomies provided significant benefits in terms of controlling the intracranial space, they also introduced certain disadvantages and morbidities. With increasing experience and knowledge, new minimally invasive interventions emerged such as the keyhole craniotomies, each of which marches closer to the orbital cavity over time (Fig. 25.1); supraorbital [5, 9, 10], lateral supraorbital [11], minipterional [12], and lateral transorbital [13, 14]. While these approaches were initially used in the surgical treatment of unruptured and anterior communicating artery aneurysms and selected tumors, they have recently begun to be used successfully in the surgical treatment of ruptured aneurysms as well [5, 9–11, 14].

One of the following three options is usually used, depending on a case-by-case evaluation, to avoid excessive brain retraction and complications during surgery for pathologies affecting the skull base or base of the brain: (1) wide bone resection with craniectomy toward the skull base until an appropriate and adequate field of view is achieved following craniotomy; (2) minimally

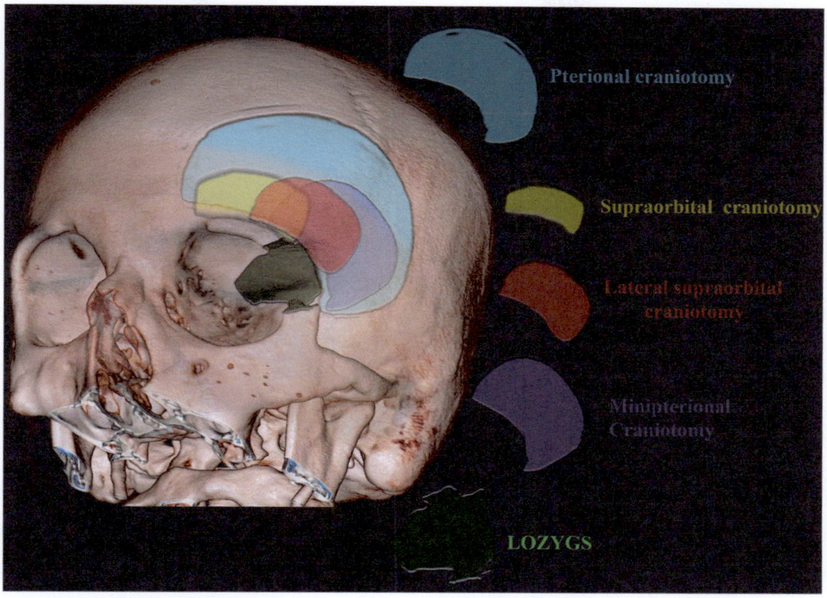

Fig. 25.1 Approaches used for aneurysm surgery have become closer to the orbital cavity by evolving over time into keyhole craniotomies. Finally, a direct view of the base of the brain over a short distance has been achieved by incorporating the orbital cavity in the approach through the lateral transorbital approach. *LOZYGS* lateral orbito-zygoma-sphenotomy

invasive intervention in appropriate cases; or (3) craniotomy or minimally invasive intervention supported by endoscopy or fully endoscopic intervention. With the equipment introduced by modern technology, including the expanded use of endoscopy in particular, neurosurgical interventions became less invasive.

Aneurysm Surgery via Endoscope-Assisted Microneurosurgery

The surgical treatment of an aneurysm is intended to safely and completely close off the connection between the aneurysm and the parent artery from which it originated. While doing this, care should be taken so as not to damage the neurovascular structures and ensure the passage of blood flow distal to the arteries. To perform this procedure, besides microsurgical skills, perfect visualization of regional anatomical structures, including the aneurysm and the surrounding arteries before, during and after clipping, is required to prevent possible complications [15–19]. Minimally invasive techniques that aim to completely occlude aneurysms are as safe as open surgery, offer much better cosmetic outcomes and result in less tissue damage [4, 5, 9–12, 14, 18].

Although the occlusion rate of microsurgical clipping is much higher than that of endovascular treatments, the number of open aneurysm surgeries is decreasing around the world. The most important reason for this is that endovascular treatment is less invasive than open surgical interventions. Therefore, the rates of complications associated with open surgical approaches and clipping need to be minimized. On the other hand, to reduce complications associated with clipping, it is necessary to fully expose and observe the morphology of the aneurysm, protect the parent arteries, their branches, and perforating arteries, and reduce the need for manipulation before, during and after clipping. Intraoperative issues with aneurysm surgery usually arise from excessive vascular dissection, manipulation or aneurysm retraction performed to expose blind spots that cannot be visualized with the direct view provided by the surgical microscope.

In minimally invasive interventions, endoscopic imaging is the best way to reveal blind spots, prevent complications associated with clipping, and avoid the need for manipulation for neurovascular control following clipping [15–19]. During the evolution of surgical approaches into minimally invasive interventions, the area of surgical access has gradually decreased, and the use of an endoscope has become necessary for the surgery to be safely performed. The term "endoscope-assisted microneurosurgery" (EAM) was introduced into the neurosurgical lexicon by Hopf and Pernecsky, and it was Perneczky who made the greatest contribution to developing the use of endoscopy during aneurysm surgery [20].

In minimally invasive aneurysm surgery, as the craniotomy becomes smaller, the surgical working area for manipulating the aneurysm and the viewing angle also become narrower. The maneuverability and working angles of conventional microsurgical instruments are especially decreased if the craniotomy is <15 mm in diameter [16]. Therefore, in aneurysm surgery with EAM, an endoscope is inserted into the surgical area in the following three stages: (1) evaluation of the aneurysm and neurovascular structures before clipping; (2) clipping of the aneurysm accompanied by an endoscope; and (3) evaluation of the aneurysm, parent arteries, their branches and perforating arteries after clipping [15, 17, 18]. During post-clipping endoscopic visualization, the rate of clip rearrangement due to incomplete occlusion of the aneurysm has been found to be 15%, while the rate of clip rearrangement due to the occlusion of parent arteries, their branches or perforating arteries has been found to be 6.1% [15]. In another study, suboptimal or incorrect clip positioning was detected at a rate of 19.1% and corrected via endoscopy [18]. A meta-analysis of aneurysm surgery with EAM has shown that endoscope-assisted aneurysm surgery significantly reduces the rates of intraoperative and postoperative complications and thus morbidity [19]. However, endoscopy alone is not adequate for displaying blood flow in real time. This issue has been resolved by adapting the endoscopic system to allow the real-time visualization of blood flow with indocyanine green (ICG) and sodium fluorescein [21, 22]. In this way, endoscopy ensures that blind spots can be revealed, blood flow can be controlled, and the aneurysm can be observed to determine whether complete occlusion has been achieved. As endoscopy is used more and more in aneurysm surgery, the transformation to fully endoscopic aneurysm surgery will become possible in the future.

Transorbital Approach for Aneurysm Surgery

With the shift from open surgery to keyhole craniotomies, less invasive methods evolved to approach the orbital cavity (Fig. 25.1). In this process, with the involvement of the orbital cavity in the intervention, transorbital approaches have entered the neurosurgical armamentarium in recent years. Due to the proximity of the orbital cavity to the anterior and middle fossa, it is possible to directly access the base of the skull and cerebrum with transorbital approaches; in this way, safe anatomical control can be achieved in a short distance (Fig. 25.2). Although transorbital endoscopic approaches have grown in popularity in certain tumor surgeries due to the advantages associated with the natural depth of the orbital cavity, because the limitations of endoscopic dissection may cause vascular complications and undesirable consequences, transorbital endoscopic approaches have not been developed for clinical application in aneurysm surgery. Some authors have written that the transorbital approach could only be used to treat middle cerebral artery (MCA) aneurysms [23, 24]. However, endoscopic dissection was easily performed in cadaveric studies, as the feared risk is that of intraoperative aneurysm rupture [23].

The lateral transorbital approach (LTOA), created by using the lateral orbito-zygoma-sphenotomy (LOZYGS), has been published as an alternative approach for aneurysm surgery, and the surgical technique was described in detail [14]. It has been shown that the LTOA can be

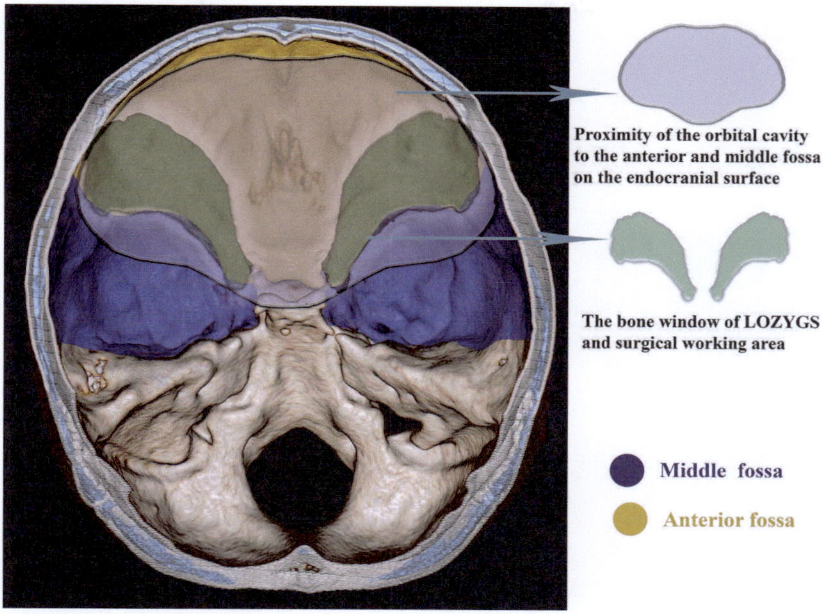

Fig. 25.2 Illustration of the large endocranial surface adjacency of the orbital cavity to the anterior and middle fossa and bone window which is created through LOZYGS. *LOZYGS* lateral orbito-zygoma-sphenotomy

safely used in the surgical treatment of ruptured and unruptured aneurysms and is different from other keyhole approaches. The LOZYGS is based on the principle of gaining direct access to the carotid, chiasmatic, and sylviàn cisterns and lamina terminalis, and surgical corridors after removing parts of the frontal, zygomatic, and sphenoid bones that compose the lateral orbital wall following lateral orbitotomy. In the LOZYGS technique, vascular and cisternal dissection can be safely performed using an anatomical orientation that surgeons are familiar with in open surgery.

In pterional-based aneurysm surgery, microsurgical manipulations are performed through a corridor created in the skull base via craniectomy and drilling of the sphenoid ridge following frontotemporal craniotomy. However, in the LOZYGS technique, the main surgical working area is obtained by drilling the lesser sphenoid wing, including the anterior clinoid process, directly after lateral orbitotomy without craniotomy. This bone window, which is created in the exocranium and is slightly larger than the burr hole, can be achieved with less bone loss than is created by the pterional approach (Fig. 25.3).

In aneurysm surgery, opening the sphenoidal and insular compartments of the Sylvian fissure increases the surgical field of view and reduces the need for retraction [7, 12, 25]. However, the least disruptive technique is to clip the aneurysm without Sylvian fissure dissection or with only as little as is needed. This is because while Sylvian fissure dissection has benefits, it also poses certain risks, such as damage to the Sylvian vein, parenchyma, MCA, and its branches. The fact that the brain is fragile and prone to damage, especially in cases of subarachnoid hemorrhage, makes it more difficult to open the Sylvian fissure. In the LOZYGS technique, it is usually sufficient to limit Sylvian fissure dissection to the sphenoidal compartment, except in cases of MCA aneurysms. In the LOZYGS technique, as reported by Figueiredo et al. [25], it has been shown that even restricted Sylvian fissure dissection is sufficient for MCA bifurcation aneurysms (Fig. 25.4).

With the increased viewing angle, which is possible via LOZYGS, control of the base of the cerebrum can be achieved (Fig. 25.5). As the internal carotid artery (ICA) and bifurcation are

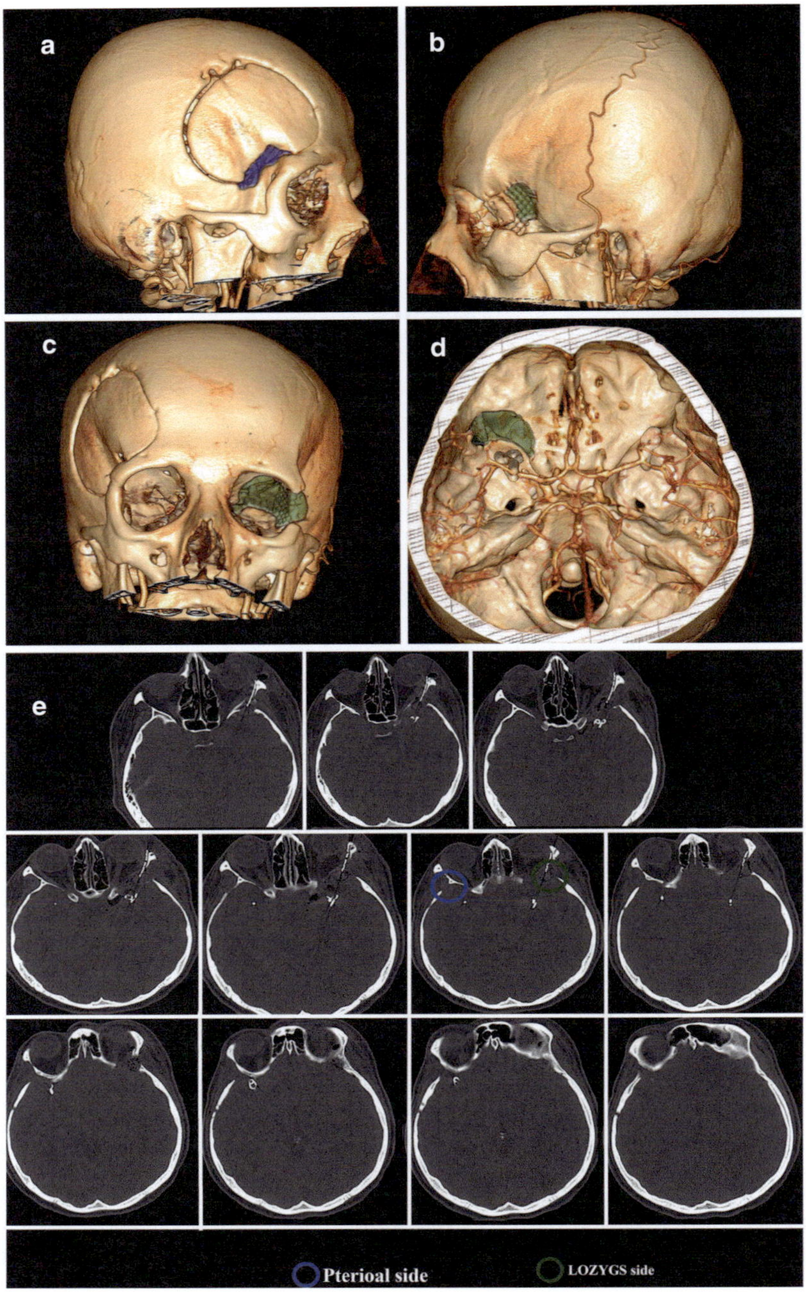

Fig. 25.3 A case of bilateral MCA aneurysms. Surgery for the ruptured aneurysm on the right side was performed with pterional craniotomy because aneurysm surgery with LOZYGS had not yet begun to be used. Surgery for the aneurysm on the left side was performed through LOZYGS per the patient's request due to the temporal muscle atrophy on the right side. Titanium mesh was used for reconstruction of the orbital lateral wall in the first cases. This is a unique sample case for comparing the bone defect in the skull base resulting from pterional approach and the LOZYGS (**a**–**d**). Comparison of the bone defects in the skull base on axial computed tomography sections in pterional and LOZYGS approaches (**e**). *MCA* middle cerebral artery, *LOZYGS* lateral orbito-zygoma-sphenotomy

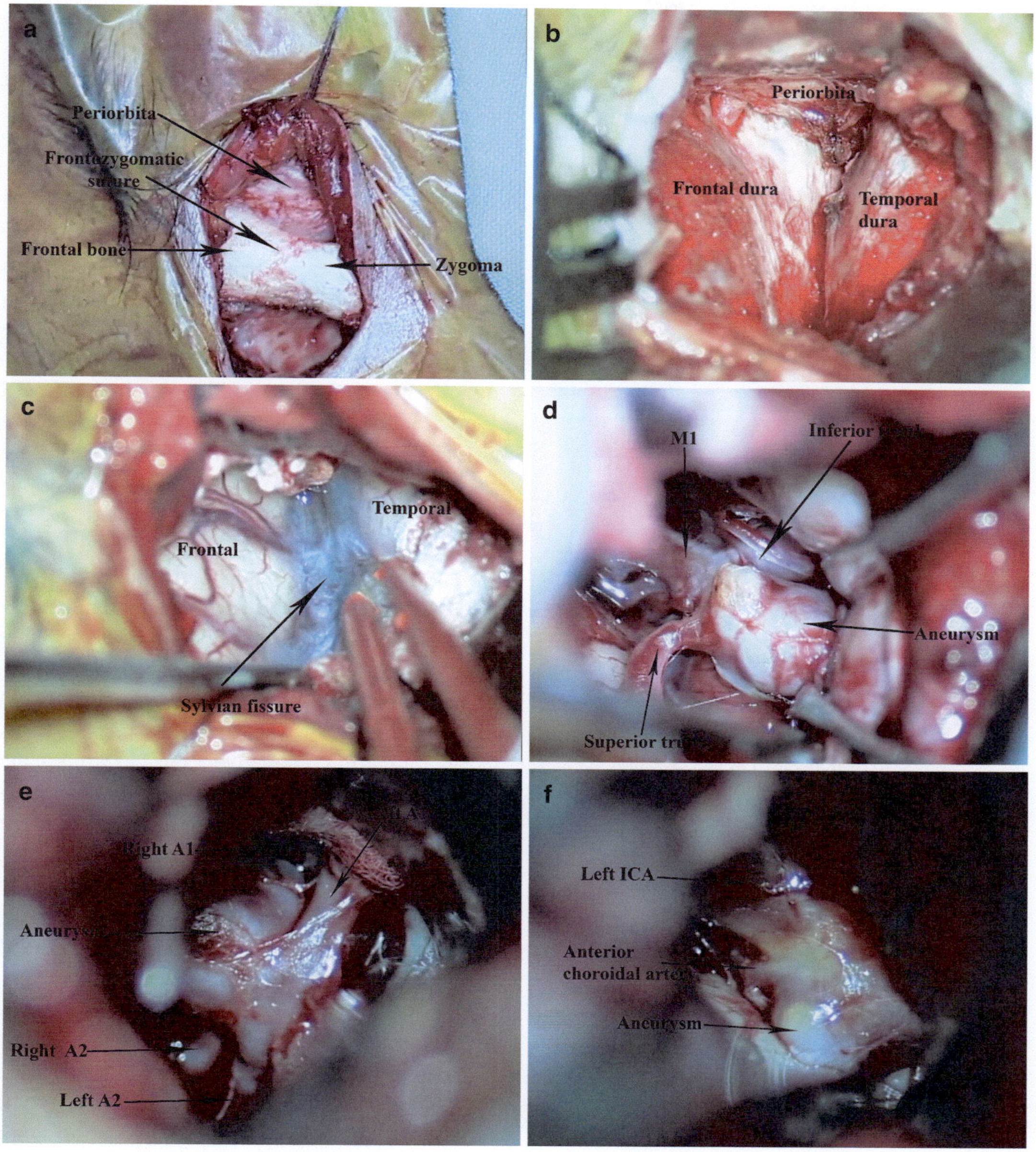

Fig. 25.4 (**a**) The appearance of the right lateral transorbital approach before LOZYGS after periorbita and temporal muscle dissection. (**b**) Apperance of the frontal and temporal dura which are adjacent to the lateral wall of the orbital cavity, after LOZYGS completed. (**c**) The appearance of the Silvian fissure after the dura is opened. Surgical microscope views of right middle cerebral artery (**d**), anterior communicating artery (**e**) and left ICA (**f**) aneurysms. *LOZYGS* lateral orbito-zygoma-sphenotomy, *ICA* internal carotid artery

revealed within a short distance, it is possible to perform dissection toward the aneurysm by setting the direction of dissection according to the location of the aneurysm. Revealing A1 first, especially in anterior communicating artery aneurysms, gives confidence to the surgeon by providing proximal control. In MCA aneurysms, the Sylvian fissure can be comfortably dissected until the limen insula, and the horizontal segment, bifurcation and inferior-superior trunks of

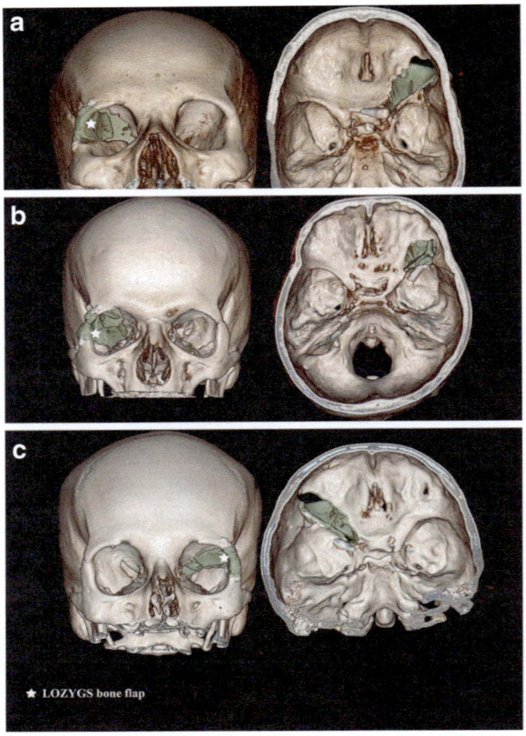

Fig. 25.5 Endocranial surface and anteroposterior exocranial apperance of the bone window and working areas created through LOZYGS in anterior communicating artery (**a**), middle cerebral artery (**b**) and internal carotid artery aneurysms operated via lateral transorbital approach. (**c**) Internal carotid artery aneurysms operated via lateral transorbital approach

the MCA can be revealed. In ICA aneurysms, anterior clinoidectomy also creates a very important additional surgical working area for proximal control. In the case of temporary clipping of the ICA, another key advantage is the fact that the temporary clip is positioned away from the aneurysm, making it easier to dissect the aneurysm, anterior choroidal artery, and posterior communicating artery, and does not interfere with proper positioning of the permanent clip. In the LTOA, LOZYGS facilitates the exposure of blind spots by providing a wide angle of view thanks to the orbital cavity, and the clinoidectomy creates an additional working area so that microsurgical dissection and manipulation of neurovascular structures can be safely performed. The most important advantage of the LOZYGS approach over keyhole craniotomies is that it allows blind spots to be revealed through microsurgical methods, which surgeons are familiar with from open surgery; additionally, it provides a larger working area and early proximal control. On the other hand, its disadvantage is that it requires anterior clinoidectomy.

In keyhole craniotomies, the area of surgical access created is as large as the small bone window that is opened. Therefore, an endoscope is needed to examine any blind spots. In contrast, with the LTOA, a larger area of access and working area can be obtained as the native orbital cavity joins the surgical area following the LOZYGS (Figs. 25.4 and 25.5). Thus, microsurgical dissection can be performed to expose blind spots and check the aneurysm, parent artery and perforating arteries following clipping. As is the case in open surgery, dissection may be needed to perform these checks on the neurovascular structures. Since it has been reported that endoscopy reduces the rate of complications even in open aneurysm surgery [17], it is certain that endoscopy will provide key information in endoscope-assisted LTOA. The fact that endoscopy reduces extra dissection maneuvers to examine the patency of local neurovascular structures is a sufficient reason to believe that endoscopy will be useful in the LTOA.

Endoscopy was not used in our clinical study [14] because the microsurgical manipulations required for aneurysm surgery were performed through LOZYGS, which provided a wide exposure and a certain level of experience first had to be achieved. The results had to be observed, and a learning curve was overcome. However, we fully believe that 'endoscope-assisted LTOA' will provide benefits for revealing blind spots with less dissection and maneuvering. Endoscopy will be particularly important if it can eliminate the need for anterior clinoidectomy as this will reduce the invasiveness of the intervention. Additionally, the visualization enabled by tilting the endoscope toward the orbital cavity for a more lateral field of view in cases of MCA aneurysms with a long M1 segment will make it easier to clip aneurysms in this region. Furthermore, it is also believed that endoscope-assisted LTOA will help make it easier to approach basilar artery aneurysms. With the application of endoscopic systems adapted for use with ICG and sodium fluorescein filters, arteries and aneurysms can be evaluated through inspection, and the blood flow and occlusion of the aneurysm can be observed.

Clipping has maintained its position as the gold standard since 1937, when the surgical clipping of cerebral aneurysms was first performed, due to its high occlusion and clinical success rate. On the other hand, endovascular intervention has not yet reached the same occlusion rate and is still under development with a high recanalization rate. Despite these handicaps, the field is shifting toward endovascular treatment as first-line therapy for many aneurysms that are suitable for surgery, since endovascular treatment is less invasive. In order not to fall behind in this competition, minimally invasive surgical interventions need to be further developed, facilitated and widely used clinically. Aneurysm surgical approaches and clipping techniques should be developed, and innovative interventions should continue to be explored.

We propose the following hypothesis: based on the anatomic adjacency of the anterior and middle fossa to the orbital cavity, it is possible for endoscope-assisted LTOA to compete with endovascular treatment by evolving into a less invasive intervention. This hypothesis will need first to be verified through anatomical studies and then tested in a controlled manner through clinical studies. As the role of endoscopy in LTOA increases, LOZYGS may become the primary step of the transformation into a transconjunctival-subconjunctival transorbital approach without orbitotomy with the help of technological innovations such as robotic surgery.

References

1. Milinis K, Thapar A, O'Neill K, Davies AH. History of aneurysmal spontaneous subarachnoid hemorrhage. Stroke. 2017;48(10):e280–3. https://doi.org/10.1161/STROKEAHA.117.017282.
2. Blackall J. Observations on the nature and cure of dropsies. London: Longman; 1814.
3. Dandy WE. Intracranial aneurysm of the internal carotid artery: cured by operation. Ann Surg. 1938;107(5):654–9. https://doi.org/10.1097/00000658-193805000-00003.
4. Perneczky A, Kindel S, Kanno T, Tschabitscher M, Reisch R. Keyhole approaches in neurosurgery: volume 1: concept and surgical technique. Cham: Springer; 2009.
5. Reisch R, Perneczky A. Ten-year experience with the supraorbital subfrontal approach through an eyebrow skin incision. Neurosurgery. 2005;57(4):242–55. https://doi.org/10.1227/01.neu.0000178353.42777.2c.
6. Rand R, Jannetta P. Microneurosurgery: application of the binocular surgical microscope in brain tumors, intracranial aneurysms, spinal cord disease, and nerve reconstruction. Clin Neurosurg. 1968;15:319–42. https://doi.org/10.1093/neurosurgery/15.cn_suppl_1.319.
7. Yasargil M, Fox J. The microsurgical approach to intracranial aneurysms. Surg Neurol. 1975;3(1):7.
8. Hakuba A, Liu S, Nishimura S. The orbitozygomatic infratemporal approach: a new surgical technique. Surg Neurol. 1986;26(3):271–6. https://doi.org/10.1016/0090-3019(86)90161-8.
9. Fischer G, Stadie A, Reisch R, Hopf NJ, Fries G, Bocher-Schwarz H, et al. The keyhole concept in aneurysm surgery: results of the past 20 years. Neurosurgery. 2011;68(1):45–51; discussion. https://doi.org/10.1227/NEU.0b013e31820934ca.
10. van Lindert E, Perneczky A, Fries G, Pierangeli E. The supraorbital keyhole approach to supratentorial aneurysms: concept and technique. Surg Neurol. 1998;49(5):481–9; discussion 9-90. https://doi.org/10.1016/s0090-3019(96)00539-3.
11. Hernesniemi J, Ishii K, Niemelä M, Smrcka M, Kivipelto L, Fujiki M, et al. Lateral supraorbital approach as an alternative to the classical pterional approach. Acta Neurochir Suppl. 2005;94:17–21. https://doi.org/10.1007/3-211-27911-3_4.
12. Figueiredo EG, Deshmukh P, Nakaji P, Crusius MU, Crawford N, Spetzler RF, et al. The minipterional craniotomy: technical description and anatomic assessment. Neurosurgery. 2007;61(5):256–64; discussion 64-5. https://doi.org/10.1227/01.neu.0000303978.11752.45.
13. Ulutas M, Boyaci S, Akakin A, Kilic T, Aksoy K. Surgical anatomy of the cavernous sinus, superior orbital fissure, and orbital apex via a lateral orbitotomy approach: a cadaveric anatomical study. Acta Neurochir. 2016;158(11):2135–48. https://doi.org/10.1007/s00701-016-2940-z.
14. Ulutas M, Çinar K, Dogan I, Secer M, Isik S, Aksoy K. Lateral transorbital approach: an alternative microsurgical route for supratentorial cerebral aneurysms. J Neurosurg. 2021;134(1):72–83. https://doi.org/10.3171/2019.9.Jns191683.
15. Fischer G, Oertel J, Perneczky A. Endoscopy in aneurysm surgery. Neurosurgery. 2012;70(2):184–90; discussion 90–1. https://doi.org/10.1227/NEU.0b013e3182376a36.

16. Gallieni M, Del Maestro M, Luzzi S, Trovarelli D, Ricci A, Galzio R. Endoscope-assisted microneurosurgery for intracranial aneurysms: operative technique, reliability, and feasibility based on 14 years of personal experience. Acta Neurochir Suppl. 2018;129:19–24. https://doi.org/10.1007/978-3-319-73739-3_3.
17. Kalavakonda C, Sekhar LN, Ramachandran P, Hechl P. Endoscope-assisted microsurgery for intracranial aneurysms. Neurosurgery. 2002;51(5):1119–26; discussion 26–7. https://doi.org/10.1097/00006123-200211000-00004.
18. Reisch R, Fischer G, Stadie A, Kockro R, Cesnulis E, Hopf N. The supraorbital endoscopic approach for aneurysms. World Neurosurg. 2014;82(6):130–7. https://doi.org/10.1016/j.wneu.2014.07.038.
19. Shao D, Li Y, Zhang B, Wu J, Xie S, Zheng X, et al. Endoscope-assisted microneurosurgery for intracranial aneurysms: a systematic review and meta-analysis. J Clin Neurosci. 2022;103:62–71. https://doi.org/10.1016/j.jocn.2022.06.029.
20. Hopf NJ, Perneczky A. Endoscopic neurosurgery and endoscope-assisted microneurosurgery for the treatment of intracranial cysts. Neurosurgery. 1998;43(6):1330–6; discussion 6–7. https://doi.org/10.1097/00006123-199812000-00037.
21. Hashimoto K, Kinouchi H, Yoshioka H, Kanemaru K, Ogiwara M, Yagi T, et al. Efficacy of endoscopic fluorescein video angiography in aneurysm surgery-novel and innovative assessment of vascular blood flow in the dead angles of the microscope. Oper Neurosurg. 2017;13(4):471–81. https://doi.org/10.1093/ons/opw042.
22. Nishiyama Y, Kinouchi H, Senbokuya N, Kato T, Kanemaru K, Yoshioka H, et al. Endoscopic indocyanine green video angiography in aneurysm surgery: an innovative method for intraoperative assessment of blood flow in vasculature hidden from microscopic view. J Neurosurg. 2012;117(2):302–8. https://doi.org/10.3171/2012.5.Jns112300.
23. Almeida JP, Ruiz-Trevino AS, Shetty SR, Omay SB, Anand VK, Schwartz TH. Transorbital endoscopic approach for exposure of the sylvian fissure, middle cerebral artery and crural cistern: an anatomical study. Acta Neurochir. 2017;159(10):1893–907. https://doi.org/10.1007/s00701-017-3296-8.
24. Di Somma A, Andaluz N, Cavallo LM, de Notaris M, Dallan I, Solari D, et al. Endoscopic transorbital superior eyelid approach: anatomical study from a neurosurgical perspective. J Neurosurg. 2017;129(5):1203–16. https://doi.org/10.3171/2017.4.jns162749.
25. Figueiredo EG, Deshmukh P, Zabramski JM, Preul MC, Crawford NR, Spetzler RF. The pterional-transsylvian approach: an analytical study. Neurosurgery. 2006;59(4):ONS263–9; discussion ONS9. https://doi.org/10.1227/01.Neu.0000233691.23208.9c.

Carotid Cavernous Fistulas

26

Maximilian Linxweiler and Umut Yilmaz

Anatomy and Classification of Carotid Cavernous Fistulas

Carotid cavernous fistulas (CCF; also referred to as cavernous sinus arterio-venous malformations (CS-AVM)) are vascular malformations with a non-physiological connection between branches of the internal (ICA) and/or external carotid artery (ECA) and the cavernous sinus (CS, [1–4]) and represent approximately 12% of all cerebral arterio-venous fistulas [1]. According to the classification described by Barrow et al. [5], one can distinguish between four CCF subtypes (see Table 26.1): (1) direct fistulas which represent high-flow connections between the ICA and the CS (Barrow Type A; most common subtype) and frequently originate from a penetrating or blunt trauma with rupture of the vessel wall; (2) indirect (syn. dural; less frequent subtype), non-traumatic, low-flow fistulas (Barrow Type B to D) with a small shunt volume that are often a result of sinus vein thrombosis or a dilatation of

Table 26.1 Barrow classification of CCFs

Barrow type	Feeder vessels		Characteristics
A	ICA		Direct, high-flow
B	Dural ICA branches to CS	Meningohypophyseal trunk (2/3)	Indirect, low-flow
		Inferolateral trunk (1/3)	
C	Dural ECA branches to CS	Maxillary artery (50%)	Indirect, low-flow
		Middle meningeal artery (30%)	
		Ascending pharyngeal artery (20%)	
D	Dural ICA and ECA branches to CS		Indirect, low-flow

ICA internal carotid artery, *ECA* external carotid artery, *CS* cavernous sinus

M. Linxweiler (✉)
Department of Otorhinolaryngology, Head and Neck Surgery, Saarland University Medical Center, Homburg, Saar, Germany
e-mail: maximilian.linxweiler@uks.eu

U. Yilmaz
Department of Neuroradiology, Saarland University Medical Center, Homburg, Saar, Germany
e-mail: umut.yilmaz@uks.eu

T. H. Schwartz et al. (eds.), *Endoscopic Transorbital Surgery of the Orbit, Skull Base and Brain*,
https://doi.org/10.1007/978-3-031-59504-2_26

pre-existing dural-arterial anastomoses [1, 2, 4, 6–8]. Indirect CCFs can further be divided into three subtypes depending on the pathological arterio-venous connections: Type B CCFs are dural shunts between the CS and branches of the ICA (meningohypophyseal trunk or inferolateral trunk), Type C CCFs are dural shunts between the CS and branches of the ECA (maxillary artery or middle meningeal artery or ascending pharyngeal artery) and Type D CCFs show pathological connections between the cavernous sinus and branches of both the internal and external carotid artery [1, 5].

While direct CCFs, in most cases, show acute-onset and severe symptoms, indirect CCFs are frequently indolent and can also be asymptomatic over a long time [8]. In most cases, CCFs become clinically apparent through eye-related symptoms: ocular motility disorder with diplopia, exophthalmos, conjunctival chemosis, eyelid ptosis, and visual impairment [1]. Other common symptoms are pulsatile tinnitus [1, 9] and headache. As a consequence of the fistula-associated high blood flow in the venous system, the highest risk for affected patients associated with CCFs is cerebral hemorrhage [1]. For the confirmation of clinical diagnosis and correct classification of CCF subtype, neuroimaging including digital subtraction angiography (DSA), magnetic resonance angiography (MRA) and/or computed tomographic angiography (CTA) is required [8]. Additionally, a careful analysis of imaging with identification of the CCF localization as well as feeding arterial and draining venous structures is essential for therapeutic management.

Endovascular Approaches for CCF Embolization

Treatment options for CCFs largely depend on the fistula subtype according to Barrow, blood flow velocity (high-flow vs. low-flow), the number and location of shunted pouches [10], the arterial supply, and the venous drainage. In direct AVMs an interventional treatment using preferably a transarterial or also a transvenous approach (via the inferior petrous sinus or superior/inferior ophthalmic vein) is often indicated due to severe and acute-onset clinical symptoms [1, 2, 11]. In contrast, the management of indirect CCFs is slightly different, as clinical symptoms are predominately mild or even nonexistent. Hence, observation is possible if patients are asymptomatic, and if the CCF shows no high-risk features, e.g., a sign of previous bleeding or high blood flow. In those patients, up to 70% of indirect CCFs spontaneously occlude over time following a local venous thrombosis [8]. Approaches to stimulate thrombosis of an indirect CCF if no spontaneous occlusion is observed include a repeated compression of the ipsilateral carotid artery [12] or the ipsilateral superior ophthalmic vein (SOV) [13] with reported success rates of 35% to 100% for selected cases. If patients show persistent symptoms and no spontaneous or manually provoked thrombosis is observed, interventional endovascular treatment is also indicated in indirect CCFs.

Traditional techniques for occlusion of indirect CCFs include either rarely indicated transarterial or preferably used transvenous embolization using platinum coils, Onyx, and/or acrylic glue [14, 15]. Standard transvenous approaches use the inferior petrous sinus, facial vein, pterygoid venous plexus, and/or the superior petrous sinus for endovascular access to the CCF [16, 17]. Independent of the chosen approach, the success rate remains significantly lower compared to direct CCFs [8, 16] mostly due to anatomical variations that hinder effective access to the fistulous connections. Nonetheless, up to 86% of cases can successfully be treated using the aforementioned endovascular techniques [16].

Transorbital Routes for Interventional CCF Treatment

When a complete embolization of indirect CCFs using traditional transarterial and/or transvenous routes is not possible due to insufficient visual-

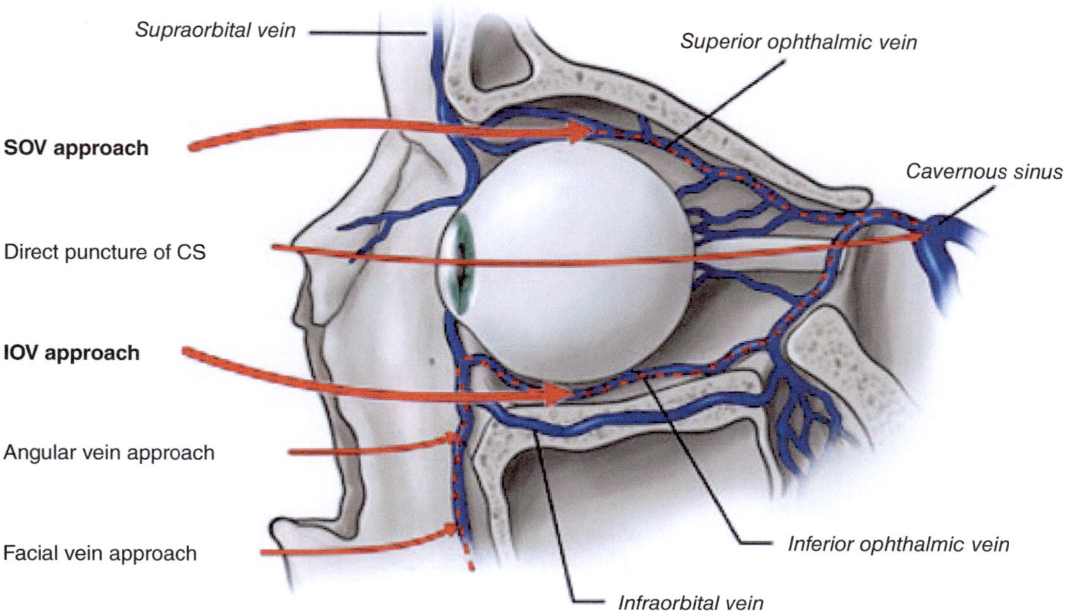

Fig. 26.1 Illustration of transorbital approaches to the cavernous sinus for embolization of carotid cavernous fistulas. *SOV* superior ophthalmic vein, *IOV* inferior ophthalmic vein, *CS* cavernous sinus (illustrations by medicalgraphics.de)

ization or an aberrant anatomy of the inferior petrosal sinus with a tortuous vessel conformation or discontinuity with the proximal jugular system [11], transorbital approaches may be used as an alternative. Those cases represent an anatomically and physiologically challenging disease that require the input of multidisciplinary teams for successful therapeutic management. In principle, several routes through the orbit cavity can be used to create access to the cavernous sinus for subsequent embolization (see Fig. 26.1): the superior ophthalmic vein (SOV) [4, 6, 7, 14, 18–30], the inferior ophthalmic vein (IOV) [3, 22, 29, 31], or the angular vein [32] can either be surgically exposed and cannulated or be accessed via direct percutaneous puncture.

Additionally, a direct transorbital puncture of the cavernous sinus through the superior orbital fissure was described [33–38]. All of these transorbital approaches reported success rates of up to 100% in predominately small case series with a maximum of 25 cases, which underlines the rare indication of these challenging procedures. Radiological images illustrating the aforementioned approaches in a clinical case are shown in Fig. 26.2.

While all of these approaches are technically feasible in experienced hands, most authors prefer surgical exposure and cannulation of the SOV for subsequent embolization as the first choice for transorbital access. As the SOV of the affected side is dilated in nearly all cases of indirect CCFs [39], this peripheral vein represents an easily accessible route to the cavernous sinus for endovascular interventions in most patients. Even if the SOV shows no dilatation or even thrombosis in pre-interventional imaging, a transorbital approach can still be successful [14].

In 1988, Teng et al. first described an occlusion of arteriovenous malformations of the cavernous sinus via the superior ophthalmic vein in 5 patients [22]. Over the following years, several groups described either a direct puncture [3, 22, 31] or a surgical exposure and catheterization of

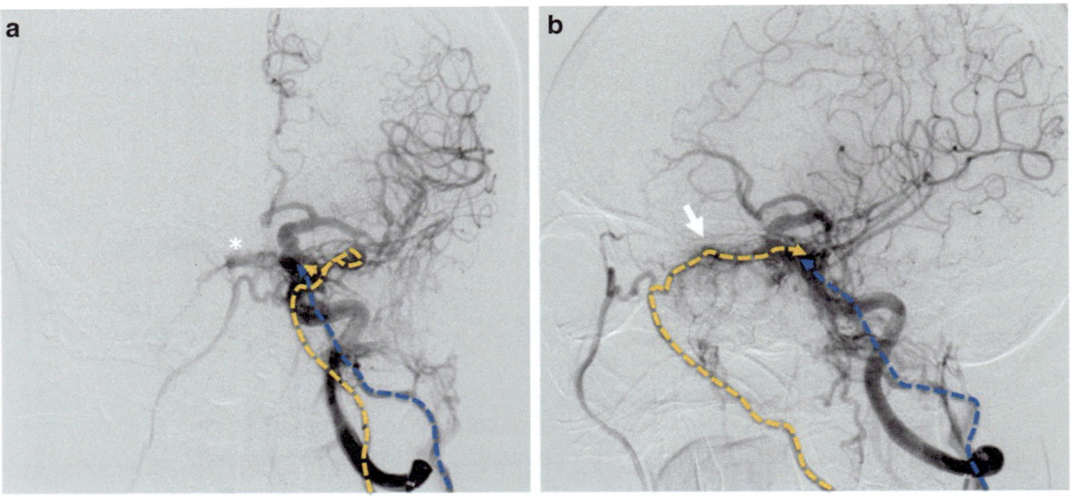

Fig. 26.2 Transvenous endovascular routes to the cavernous sinus. Digital subtraction angiography of the left internal carotid artery in the frontal head view (**a**) and oblique view (**b**) showing early venous drainage into the cavernous sinus (asterisk). Endovascular routes into the cavernous sinus include the route via the inferior petrous sinus (blue line), which drains into the jugular bulb and the route via the facial vein (yellow line). The white arrow shows the access point for the approach via the superior ophthalmic vein

the superior ophthalmic vein [4, 7, 19, 20, 23, 26–28] for endovascular treatment of indirect and also few cases of direct CCFs (see Table 26.2). Thereby, most authors preferred a surgical exposure of the SOV after an upper eyelid incision. In all of the aforementioned studies only sporadic minor complications were reported, including severe bleeding, especially if deep preparation was necessary, silk granuloma, palsy of the oculomotor and abducens nerve, transient diplopia, proptosis and chemosis [6, 19, 20, 31]. Success rates using this approach ranged from 67% to 100%. As an alternative to this open surgical approach, a direct transcutaneous puncture of the SOV may be possible and successful [3, 22, 29, 31, 33] but carries a relevant risk of hard-to-control intraoperative and postoperative complications.

In some cases, vein exposure can be difficult, especially when the vessel is porous or thin, and the SOV is not markedly dilatated due to low-pressure fistulas. Additionally, thrombosis of the SOV markedly complicates a successful cannulation, which is nonetheless possible in such cases [14]. If, due to the aforementioned or other reasons, an SOV approach is not feasible and/or not successful, a direct percutaneous puncture of the inferior orbital vein (IOV) or angular vein represents alternative techniques that can be considered. However, the evidence in literature is limited to less than 10 cases [3, 22, 29, 31, 32]. If neither the SOV nor the IOV or angular vein can be accessed due to small vessel size, thrombosis or anatomical variation, a direct transcutaneous puncture of the cavernous sinus through the orbit and the superior orbital fissure is a salvage option [33–38]. These procedures should be performed under intraprocedural fluoroscopic and/or computed tomography guidance to avoid injury of the at-risk structures.

Table 26.2 Published studies on transorbital approaches for embolization of carotid cavernous fistulas

Study	Year	No. of patients	Access to cavernous sinus	CCF type	Conclusions/recommendations	Success rate
Miller et al. [18]	1995	12	Surgical exposure + cannulation of the SOV	Direct (Barrow A), $n = 2$; indirect/dural (Barrow C + D), $n = 10$	Safe and effective treatment of both direct and dural CCFs that are not amenable to transarterial or other transvenous approaches	100% (12/12)
Goldberg et al. [19]	1996	9		Indirect/dural (Barrow B – D)	Technically straightforward, safe, and effective treatment for CCF	78% (7/9)
Quiñones et al. [20]	1997	13		Indirect/dural (Barrow B + D)	Direct, safe, and efficient way to occlude dural CCFs, indicated when (1) decreased visual acuity is associated with venous hypertension in the orbit; (2) a large SOV is seen on MR/CT; (3) the predominant arterial supply is from the ICA D); (4) the ECA feeders are dangerous to embolize because they anastomose with the ICA; and (5) the transvenous jugular route fails	92% (12/13)
Baldauf et al. [7]	2004	2		Indirect/dural (Barrow D)	Safe and effective technique; indicated when standard neuroradiological procedures do not succeed	100% (2/2)
Leibovitch et al. [6]	2006	25		Indirect/dural (Barrow B – D)	SOV is a useful route for CCF embolization; however, the presence of fragile or clotted veins can preclude successful cannulation; higher risk of uncontrolled bleeding when deeper orbital dissections is necessary	80% (20/25)
Wolfe et al. [23]	2010	10		Indirect/dural (Barrow B – D)	Excellent and definitive alternative treatment when traditional endovenous routes are inaccessible	90% (9/10)
Chalouhi et al. [24]	2012	10		Direct (Barrow A), $n = 1$; indirect/dural (Barrow B + D), $n = 9$	Treatment option in patients with CCF when all other endovascular approaches have been exhausted	100% (10/10)
Pansara et al. [25]	2013	1		Indirect/dural (Barrow D)	Indicated in cases where conventional transvenous accesses are not possible	100% (1/1)
Güven Yilmaz et al. [14]	2013	4		Indirect/dural (Barrow B + D)	Successful treatment via the SOV is possible, even when the vein is thrombosed	75% (3/4)
El-Hindy et al. [26]	2014	3		Indirect/dural (no information on Barrow type)	The SOV approach is indicated in cases where conventional access to the cavernous sinus may not be possible due to local variations of anatomy	67% (2/3)
Haider et al. [4]	2017	1		Indirect/dural (Barrow D)	Indicated in indirect CCF cases when accessing the CS is not possible due to venous outflow occlusion, stenosis, or marked tortuosity, as well as compartmentalization of the CS	100% (1/1)
Brenna et al. [21]	2020	2		Direct (Barrow A)	Indicated in cases where individual vascular anatomy is not amenable to transarterial or transvenous access or embolization	100% (2/2)
Arcuri et al. [27]	2021	3		Direct (Barrow A), $n = 1$; indirect/dural (no information on Barrow type), $n = 2$	SOV approach as a feasible and safe salvage procedure, which can find indication after other endovascular access failures	100% (3/3)
Trennheuser et al. [28]	2022	14		Indirect/dural (Barrow B – D)	Excellent success rate with no therapy-associated major complications	100% (14/14)

Table 26.2 (continued)

Study	Year	No. of patients	Access to cavernous sinus	CCF type	Conclusions/recommendations	Success rate
Mehrzad et al. [30]	2011	1	Direct percutaneous puncture of the SOV	Indirect/dural (Barrow D)	A useful method of treating indirect CCF when the inferior petrosal sinus is occluded and the transfacial vein approach is tortuous	100% (1/1)
Cecchini et al. [3]	2012	1	Direct percutaneous puncture of the IOV	Indirect/dural (Barrow D)	Safe route for CCF access and embolization when SOV and IPS are inaccessible	100% (1/1)
Chen et al. [31]	2017	1		Indirect/dural (Barrow B)	The SOV approach is a viable alternative to conventional transvenous methods for appropriately selected CCF cases	100% (1/1)
Dashti et al. [29]	2011	2	Direct percutaneous puncture of the IOV/SOV	Indirect/dural (Barrow B + D)	Indicated when more conventional endovascular approaches have been exhausted	100% (2/2)
Teng et al. [22]	1988	5	Direct percutaneous puncture of the IOV [4]; surgical exposure + cannulation of the SOV [1]	Indirect/dural (Barrow B + D)	Indicated when the SOV is enlarged and (1) dural AVMs of the CS are fed by small branches of the ICA or direct CCF with small tears, (2) dural AVMs of the CS are fed by multiple branches from both the ICA and ECA, one or both sides, (3) dural AVMs of the CS or direct CCF recur after trapping of the ICA	100% (5/5)
Iaccarino et al. [32]	1993	1	Direct percutaneous puncture of the angular vein	Indirect/dural (Barrow D)	Trans-orbital approach may be considered when the openings are in the antero-inferior compartment and the SOV is enlarged	100% (1/1)
Teng et al. [33]	1995	11	Direct percutaneous puncture of the CS through the superior orbital fissure	No information on Barrow type	Direct transorbital puncture through the superior orbital fissure as an alternate treatment for CCF, especially when the ipsilateral ICA has been occluded	100% (11/11)
Workman et al. [34]	2002	1		Indirect/dural (Barrow D)	Indicated when an alternative transarterial or transvenous route is not available	100% (1/1)
Satchi et al. [35]	2009	1		Indirect/dural (Barrow D)	In cases of dural CCF where standard endovascular treatment has failed and orbital venous channels are not sufficiently dilated to allow their surgical isolation in the anterior orbit, a transorbital puncture is a useful approach	100% (1/1)
Elhammady et al. [36]	2011	1		Indirect/dural (Barrow B)	Percutaneous transorbital puncture of CCFs is a feasible alternative to accessing the cavernous sinus when traditional transfemoral transvenous catheterization or direct SOV cutdown is not possible	100% (1/1)
Coumou et al. [37]	2014	1		Indirect/dural (Barrow D)	indicated if attempts at transvenous embolization are not successful	100% (1/1)
Puffer et al. [38]	2014	1		Indirect/dural (Barrow B)	In case of tortuosity and occlusion of venous access points to the cavernous sinus, this approach can be useful	100% (1/1)

CCF carotid cavernous fistula, *ICA* internal carotid artery, *IPS* inferior petrous sinus, *SOV* superior ophthalmic vein, *ECA* external carotid artery, *IOV* inferior ophthalmic vein, *CS* cavernous sinus

Surgical Technique and Recommendations for Clinical Practice

In general, transorbital approaches represent safe and efficient treatment options, especially for patients with indirect CCFs. Though successful transorbital embolization of direct CCFs has been reported in the literature [18, 21, 24, 27], these fistula types can efficiently be treated via transarterial approaches and are at much higher risk for complications when using transorbital access due to high fistula flow. Hence, we would only recommend these approaches for endovascular treatment of direct CCFs if all other alternative therapy options failed. In patients with indirect/dural CCF, transorbital approaches are safe and efficient treatment options with excellent therapeutic results. We indicate this surgical procedure under the following circumstances: (1) when patients are symptomatic or asymptomatic and show uncontrolled intraorbital hypertension, (2) when DSA reveals the diagnosis of Barrow Type C or D CCF with predominantly anterior venous drainage and (3) when embolization via the inferior petrous sinus fails. As a salvage option a transorbital approach can also be considered when (4) DSA shows a Barrow Typ B CCF and a transarterial embolization via the ECA is not successful.

Considering the various modifications of transorbital approaches (see Fig. 26.1), we prefer a surgical exposure and cannulation of the SOV as we have observed the highest success rate in our cohort using this approach with only minor complications in individual patients. As complications of this nonetheless challenging procedure can potentially lead to life-threatening situations (e.g., excessive intraorbital and/or intracranial bleeding), we prefer a surgical exposure of the SOV rather than a direct percutaneous puncture. The open technique ensures excellent visibility and fixation of the vein and thus minimizes the risk of uncontrolled bleeding. Even if severe bleeding occurs during preparation, branches of the SOV can be coagulated or the SOV can be ligated. Therefore, we recommend open exposure to the SOV. For the surgical procedure, we recommend using surgical loupes or the operating microscope for intraorbital dissection as important vascular and neural structures including the optic nerve, oculomotor nerve and abducens nerve are close to the operation field.

However, as all of the aforementioned structures are located inside the myofascial cone while the SOV lies in the extraconal space, precise operative technique should enable the preservation of these structures and prevent severe complications. All patients that are treated with a transorbital approach should undergo a pre- and postoperative ophthalmologic examination. We strongly recommend performing the procedure under general anesthesia in accordance with all published studies as listed in Table 26.2. Constant communication with the anesthesiology team is important during the orbital dissection, as (1) the dissection can elicit a vagal response, which we observed in nearly half of the patients, and (2) especially high-flow fistulas can create strong and hard-to-control bleeding, resulting in a blood loss of up to 500 ml [28]. Details of the surgical and interventional procedure using an open SOV approach are shown in Fig. 26.3.

First, the patient is positioned on the table of a C-arm X-ray in a neuroradiological intervention room and general anesthesia is induced by an anesthesiologist. The surgical procedure starts with a 1–2 cm incision in the medial sub-brow area of the upper eyelid at the affected side (Fig. 26.3a). After the incision of the orbicularis oculi muscle blunt dissection continues through the orbital fat until a prominent arch of the SOV can be exposed at a depth of 0.5–1.5 cm (Fig. 26.3b). Usually, the SOV shows a medial and a lateral branch. Next, the SOV is secured by placing a vessel loop and a ligation suture around the vein without tying the knot of the suture (Fig. 26.3c). Then, a venotomy is performed using either a delicate scissor or a scalpel followed by vessel cannulation with a (minimum 3F) catheter valve introducer that is fixed with a suture (Fig. 26.3d). Alternatively, the vessel can directly be punctured with a trocar introducer system, or a Seldinger technique can be applied using a sharp canule and guidewire. One important step at this point is to choose the right branch

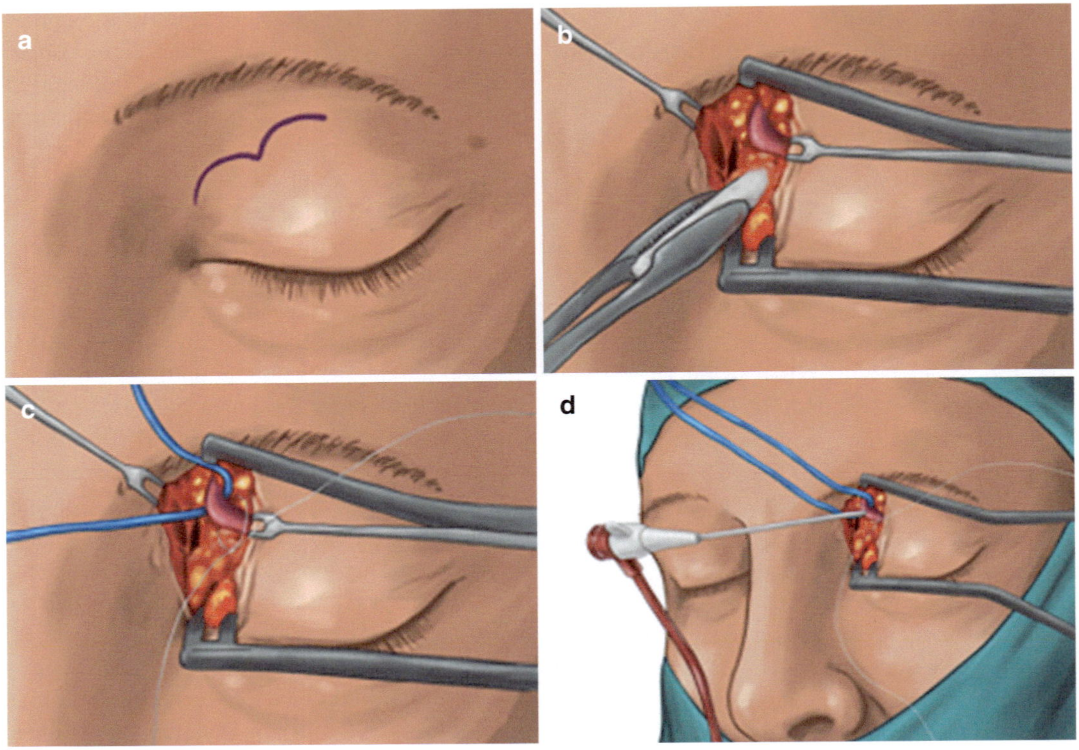

Fig. 26.3 Illustration of surgical technique for exposure and cannulation of the superior ophthalmic vein. (**a**) Incision line in the medial part of the upper eyelid; (**b**) intraorbital blunt preparation and exposure of the superior ophthalmic vein; (**c**) positioning of a vessel loop and ligation suture to secure the vein; (**d**) opening of the vein and cannulation with a 3F catheter valve introducer that is secured by tightening the ligation suture (illustrations by medicalgraphics.de)

of the arch-like SOV. Here, performing an Acland test can be helpful in identifying the branch with a higher venous backflow that is more suitable for cannulation (medial branch in 70% of cases, according to our experience). Once the catheter valve introducer is placed and secured with a suture, the eye should be protected with wet sterile compresses. All metal instruments, including wound retractors, must be removed so as not to interfere with X-ray imaging. Subsequently, the neuroradiologist starts with a transarterial angiography via the groin in order to evaluate the exact localization of the fistula(s) and the ideal site for embolization. Then, closure of the fistula can be performed by placing e. g. platinum coils or Onyx under continuous fluoroscopy guidance via the introducer placed in the SOV until no residual fistula flow is observed. A clinical example of a successful transorbital embolization via the SOV approach is shown in Fig. 26.4.

As a final step, the catheter is removed, both SOV branches are ligated, and the orbital wound is closed with careful suture of the orbicularis oculi muscle and the skin. Sutures can be removed on day 7 after surgery. In our view, perioperative antibiotics are not necessary and we observed no postoperative wound infection in our cohort so far. In most patients, a transient hematoma, chemosis and upper eyelid elevation weakness are observed and completely regress within the first 2–3 days after surgery.

While surgical exposure and cannulation of the SOV (open SOV approach) is feasible in the majority of patients with indirect CCFs, there are some situations when alternative transorbital approaches have to be considered. Occasionally,

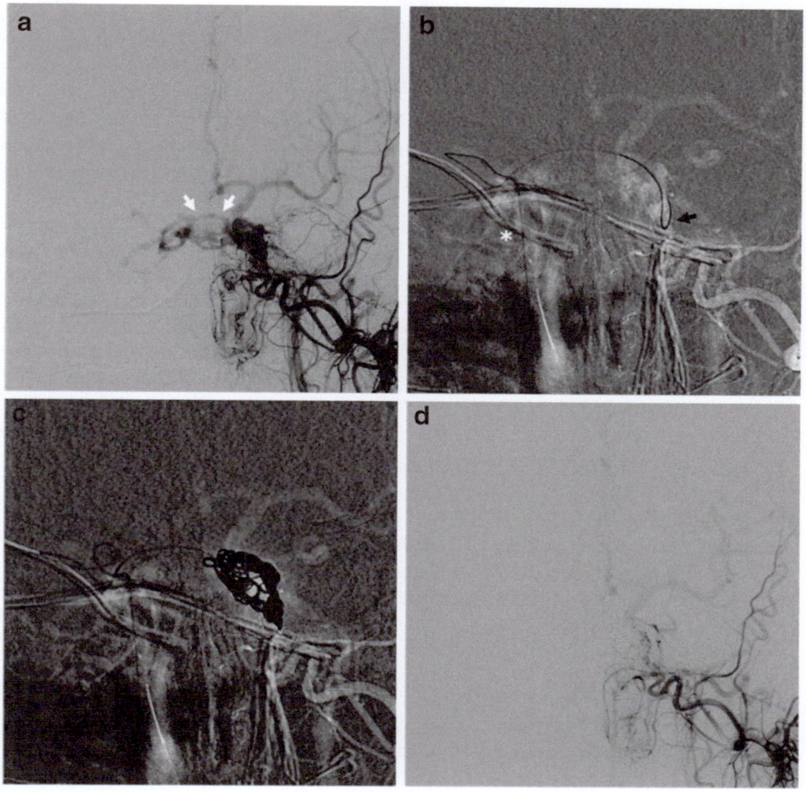

Fig. 26.4 Transorbital embolization of a carotid cavernous fistula. (**a**) Digital subtraction angiography of the left carotid artery in the frontal head view showing early venous drainage into the cavernous sinus via branches of the maxillary artery. (**b**) After cannulation of the right superior ophthalmic vein (SOV), a microcatheter (asterisk at the distal marker) is introduced and guided into the left cavernous sinus by passing the intercavernous sinus (white arrows in (**a**)) with a loop-shaped microwire (black arrow). (**c**) The cavernous sinus is filled with coils until early drainage ceases (**d**)

the SOV can be occluded due to thrombosis, which can hinder successful cannulation [14]. Additionally, the SOV can intraoperatively show as not sufficiently dilated to allow its surgical isolation in the anterior orbit [35]. In other cases, the vein can show a tortuous configuration, so cannulation is not possible [38]. These cases are extremely rare but have been described in the literature, so alternative transorbital routes may be required. In those situations, we recommend using a direct percutaneous puncture of the facial or angular vein, as their comparably wide diameter usually allows a smooth insertion of an introducer for subsequent embolization. A direct puncture of the IOV may be used but is technically more challenging as, in most cases, this vein is not or only minimally dilated in indirect CCF patients. In our view, a direct transorbital puncture of the cavernous sinus represents a salvage procedure if all of the aforementioned approaches fail and should be avoided due to the relevant risk of severe complications. A careful review of pre-interventional imaging can help to choose the most suitable and promising transorbital approach as a dilation, tortuosity, stenosis and/or thrombosis of the intraorbital veins can be anticipated. However, the surgeon and neuroradiologist must decide on the most appropriate based on a case-by-case discussion depending on anatomy, fistula type, and surgical experience. While some authors recommend the use of the open SOV approach only when pre-interventional imaging shows an enlarged SOV [19, 20, 22, 29, 32] other groups state that even a vascular stenosis or thrombosis are no contraindications for using this technique [18, 27]. Ultimately, it is important to have a salvage plan for each procedure in case of a failure of the initial approach whatever transorbital route one choses first.

Taken together, transorbital approaches represent effective and safe methods for endovascular treatment of mainly indirect CCFs with growing evidence in the literature on clinical success rates, management of complications and surgical technique. Nonetheless, transorbital approaches will largely remain salvage options for cases where conventional transvenous and/or transarterial procedures are not feasible due to functional or anatomical reasons, or are ultimately not successful. Adding this technique to the repertoire of physicians involved in the therapeutic management of CCF patients can improve the efficacy and safety of interventional and surgical treatment of this disease.

References

1. Andres RH, Remonda L, Do DD, Spreng A, Reinert M, Schroth G. Diagnosis and treatment of carotid cavernous fistulas. Röfo. 2008;180(7):604–13.
2. Phan K, Xu J, Leung V, Teng I, Sheik-Ali S, Maharaj M, et al. Orbital approaches for treatment of carotid cavernous fistulas: a systematic review. World Neurosurg. 2016;96:243–51.
3. Cecchini MM, Levitt MR, Taneja M, Hallam DK, Ghodke BV. Embolization of carotid-cavernous fistula via direct percutaneous puncture of the inferior ophthalmic vein. J Neuroradiol. 2012;39(3):181–5.
4. Haider AS, Garg P, Leonard D, Osumah T, Khan U, Vayalumkal S, et al. Superior ophthalmic vein access for embolization of an indirect carotid cavernous fistula. Cureus. 2017;9(9):e1639.
5. Barrow DL, Spector RH, Braun IF, Landman JA, Tindall SC, Tindall GT. Classification and treatment of spontaneous carotid-cavernous sinus fistulas. J Neurosurg. 1985;62(2):248–56.
6. Leibovitch I, Modjtahedi S, Duckwiler GR, Goldberg RA. Lessons learned from difficult or unsuccessful cannulations of the superior ophthalmic vein in the treatment of cavernous sinus dural fistulas. Ophthalmology. 2006;113(7):1220–6.
7. Baldauf J, Spuler A, Hoch HH, Molsen HP, Kiwit JC, Synowitz M. Embolization of indirect carotid-cavernous sinus fistulas using the superior ophthalmic vein approach. Acta Neurol Scand. 2004;110(3):200–4.
8. Henderson AD, Miller NR. Carotid-cavernous fistula: current concepts in aetiology, investigation, and management. Eye. 2018;32(2):164–72.
9. Waldvogel D, Mattle HP, Sturzenegger M, Schroth G. Pulsatile tinnitus–a review of 84 patients. J Neurol. 1998;245(3):137–42.
10. Kiyosue H, Tanoue S, Hori Y, Hongo N, Mori H. Shunted pouches of cavernous sinus dural AVFs: evaluation by 3D rotational angiography. Neuroradiology. 2015;57(3):283–90.
11. Shah A, Patel BC. Superior ophthalmic vein cannulation for carotid cavernous fistula. In: StatPearls. Treasure Island: StatPearls Publishing; 2021.
12. Kai Y, Hamada J, Morioka M, Yano S, Kuratsu J. Treatment of cavernous sinus dural arteriovenous fistulae by external manual carotid compression. Neurosurgery. 2007;60(2):253–7; discussion 7–8.
13. Cruz JP, van Dijk R, Krings T, Agid R. Ophthalmic vein compression for selected benign low-flow cavernous sinus dural arteriovenous fistulas. J Neurosurg. 2013;119(1):239–42.
14. Güven Yilmaz S, Yazici B, Çetinkaya A, Yağci A. Embolization of dural carotid-cavernous fistulas via the thrombosed superior ophthalmic vein. Ophthalmic Plast Reconstr Surg. 2013;29(4):272–6.
15. Arat A, Cekirge S, Saatci I, Ozgen B. Transvenous injection of Onyx for casting of the cavernous sinus for the treatment of a carotid-cavernous fistula. Neuroradiology. 2004;46(12):1012–5.
16. Texakalidis P, Tzoumas A, Xenos D, Rivet DJ, Reavey-Cantwell J. Carotid cavernous fistula (CCF) treatment approaches: a systematic literature review and meta-analysis of transarterial and transvenous embolization for direct and indirect CCFs. Clin Neurol Neurosurg. 2021;204:106601.
17. Gemmete JJ, Ansari SA, Gandhi DM. Endovascular techniques for treatment of carotid-cavernous fistula. J Neuroophthalmol. 2009;29(1):62–71.
18. Miller NR, Monsein LH, Debrun GM, Tamargo RJ, Nauta HJ. Treatment of carotid-cavernous sinus fistulas using a superior ophthalmic vein approach. J Neurosurg. 1995;83(5):838–42.
19. Goldberg RA, Goldey SH, Duckwiler G, Vinuela F. Management of cavernous sinus-dural fistulas. Indications and techniques for primary embolization via the superior ophthalmic vein. Arch Ophthalmol. 1996;114(6):707–14.
20. Quiñones D, Duckwiler G, Gobin PY, Goldberg RA, Viñuela F. Embolization of dural cavernous fistulas via superior ophthalmic vein approach. AJNR Am J Neuroradiol. 1997;18(5):921–8.
21. Brenna CTA, Priola SM, Pasarikovski CR, Ku JC, Daigle P, Gill HS, et al. Surgical sparing and pairing endovascular interventions for carotid-cavernous fistula: case series and review of the literature. World Neurosurg. 2020;140:18–25.
22. Teng MM, Guo WY, Huang CI, Wu CC, Chang T. Occlusion of arteriovenous malformations of the cavernous sinus via the superior ophthalmic vein. AJNR Am J Neuroradiol. 1988;9(3):539–46.
23. Wolfe SQ, Cumberbatch NM, Aziz-Sultan MA, Tummala R, Morcos JJ. Operative approach via the superior ophthalmic vein for the endovascular treatment of carotid cavernous fistulas that fail traditional endovascular access. Neurosurgery. 2010;66(6):293–9; discussion 9.
24. Chalouhi N, Dumont AS, Tjoumakaris S, Gonzalez LF, Bilyk JR, Randazzo C, et al. The superior ophthalmic vein approach for the treatment of carotid-cavernous fistulas: a novel technique using Onyx. Neurosurg Focus. 2012;32(5):E13.

25. Pansara A, Milburn JM, Perry M, Eubanks B. Clinical images - a quarterly column: transorbital coil embolization of a carotid cavernous fistula. Ochsner J. 2013;13(3):295–7.
26. El-Hindy N, Kalantzis G, Patankar T, Georgalas I, Jyothi S, Goddard T, et al. Difficult indirect carotid-cavernous fistulas–alternative techniques to gaining access for treatment. Clin Interv Aging. 2014;9:1687–90.
27. Arcuri F, Agostini T, Limbucci N, Laiso A, Mangiafico S, Spinelli G, et al. Salvage transorbital approach for the endovascular treatment of carotid cavernous fistulas. Oral Maxillofac Surg. 2021;26(1):45–51.
28. Trennheuser S, Reith W, Kühn JP, Morris LGT, Bozzato A, Naumann A, et al. Transorbital embolization of cavernous sinus dural arterio-venous malformations with surgical exposure and catheterization of the superior ophthalmic vein. Interv Neuroradiol. 2022;29(6):715–24.
29. Dashti SR, Fiorella D, Spetzler RF, Albuquerque FC, McDougall CG. Transorbital endovascular embolization of dural carotid-cavernous fistula: access to cavernous sinus through direct puncture: case examples and technical report. Neurosurgery. 2011;68(1):75–83; discussion.
30. Mehrzad H, Alam K, Rennie A. The treatment of a dural carotid cavernous fistula (CCF) using Onyx via a transorbital approach: a technical note. Neuroradiology. 2011;53(11):895–8.
31. Chen CJ, Mastorakos P, Caruso JP, Ding D, Schmitt PJ, Buell TJ, et al. Transorbital approach for endovascular occlusion of carotid-cavernous fistulas: technical note and review of the literature. Cureus. 2017;9(1):e976.
32. Iaccarino V, Spaziante R, Bonavolontà G, Cirillo S, De Divitiis E. Treatment of carotid-cavernous fistula by trans-venous anterior (trans-orbital) approach. Case report and review of previous report. J Neurosurg Sci. 1993;37(2):103–12.
33. Teng MM, Lirng JF, Chang T, Chen SS, Guo WY, Cheng CC, et al. Embolization of carotid cavernous fistula by means of direct puncture through the superior orbital fissure. Radiology. 1995;194(3):705–11.
34. Workman MJ, Dion JE, Tong FC, Cloft HJ. Treatment of trapped CCF by direct puncture of the cavernous sinus by infraocular trans-SOF approach. Case report and anatomical basis. Interv Neuroradiol. 2002;8(3):299–304.
35. Satchi K, Mitchell PJ, McNab AA. Transorbital puncture of the cavernous sinus to treat a dural carotid-cavernous sinus fistula. Ophthalmic Plast Reconstr Surg. 2009;25(1):54–6.
36. Elhammady MS, Peterson EC, Aziz-Sultan MA. Onyx embolization of a carotid cavernous fistula via direct transorbital puncture. J Neurosurg. 2011;114(1):129–32.
37. Coumou AD, van den Berg R, Bot JC, Beetsma DB, Saeed P. Direct orbital puncture of the cavernous sinus for the treatment of a carotid-cavernous dural AV fistula with a concomitant venous/lymphatic malformation. Orbit. 2014;33(1):68–71.
38. Puffer RC, Lanzino G, Cloft HJ. Using XperGuide planning software to safely guide catheter access to the cavernous sinus via transorbital puncture: a case report. Neurosurgery. 2014;10(2):E370–3; discussion E3.
39. Adam CR, Shields CL, Gutman J, Kim HJ, Hayek B, Shore JW, et al. Dilated superior ophthalmic vein: clinical and radiographic features of 113 cases. Ophthalmic Plast Reconstr Surg. 2018;34(1):68–73.

Transorbital Endoscopic Ligation of the Middle Meningeal Artery

27

Basit A. Jawad, Kittichai Mongkolkul, Daniel M. Prevedello, and Ricardo L. Carrau

Introduction

The middle meningeal artery (MMA) is an important vascular structure implicated in numerous intracranial pathologies, including intracranial hemorrhage, dural arteriovenous fistula (DAVF), aneurysms, pseudoaneurysms, traumatic arteriovenous fistula (AVF), and not uncommonly, migraines [1, 2]. Increasing evidence suggests that control of the middle meningeal artery is a successful treatment for chronic subdural hematomas [2, 3]. Furthermore, one may consider ligation of the MMA when attempting devascularization of a dural-based intracranial tumor such as a meningioma.

Historically, MMA ligation either involved a transcranial corridor for distal intracranial control or a trans-facial/infratemporal fossa approach for proximal extracranial control, most commonly as part of an oncologic exenteration [4–6]. Advancements in neuroendovascular techniques have burgeoned a new age of interventions capable of addressing middle meningeal artery pathology, and understandably, this minimally invasive technique currently represents the first-line approach for vessel embolization [4, 5]. Nevertheless, in situations where endovascular interventions are contraindicated, or where endovascular capabilities are not available, direct vessel control may be the best option.

Transorbital neuroendoscopic surgery (TONES) is an emerging technique in the armamentarium of the skull base surgeon [6, 7]. Transorbital corridors allow alternative access to select pathologies arising in the paranasal sinuses, intracranial and infratemporal fossae, as well as direct exposure to intra- and extraconal lesions [6]. As clinical experience increases, the indications of TONES may extend to the identification and control of skull base neurovascular structures.

In this chapter, we describe the anatomic intricacies and surgical steps for a transorbital corridor to access the middle meningeal artery. In general, transorbital endoscopic approaches offer a high degree of flexibility using various incisions and corridors that may be used in isolation or in combination with other approaches to tailor access to the target pathology. The four traditional transorbital corridors include the superior eyelid crease incision for a superior orbitotomy, precaruncular incision for medial access, a lateral retro-canthal incision for a lateral orbitotomy and the inferior pre-septal incision for an inferior orbitotomy. Access to the middle meningeal

B. A. Jawad (✉) · K. Mongkolkul
Department of Otolaryngology-Head & Neck Surgery, Ohio State University, Columbus, OH, USA

D. M. Prevedello · R. L. Carrau
Department of Otolaryngology-Head & Neck Surgery, Ohio State University, Columbus, OH, USA

Department of Neurosurgery, Ohio State University, Columbus, OH, USA

T. H. Schwartz et al. (eds.), *Endoscopic Transorbital Surgery of the Orbit, Skull Base and Brain*, https://doi.org/10.1007/978-3-031-59504-2_27

artery via an endoscopic assisted orbitotomy requires maneuverability in the inferolateral direction; thus, one may consider either the lateral retro-canthal approach or the inferior preseptal incision.

Anatomic Considerations

A detailed risk profile for transorbital surgery is documented in the *Surgical Risks* chapter of this textbook. With appropriate patient selection and correct technique, these procedures can be performed with a high degree of surgical safety [8]. Nevertheless, risks may include cosmetic deformities, ocular injury, injury to cranial nerves (CN2, CN3, CN4, V2, CN6), injury to extraocular muscles, retrobulbar hematoma, intracranial complications, orbital pain, and infection. Specific to a middle meningeal artery ligation, the surgeon should be mindful of neurovascular implications and counsel patients accordingly.

The middle meningeal artery typically arises from the 2nd portion of the external carotid's maxillary artery (muscular segment). As this vessel travels superiorly within the infratemporal fossa, it will pass through the neural ring of the auriculotemporal nerve before entering the foramen spinosum to supply the middle cranial fossa dura. Less frequently, however, it may aberrantly originate from the internal carotid artery, ophthalmic artery, ascending pharyngeal artery or vertebrobasilar system [2]. In such cases, it would not be uncommon to find an absent or hypoplastic foramen spinosum.

Furthermore, one should consider important neurovascular contributions from the middle meningeal artery, especially in patients with vasculopathy. The ophthalmic artery may be directly supplied by or receive indirect contributions via anastomoses between the sphenoid division and the recurrent branch of the ophthalmic artery. One should be judicious here to avoid inadvertently risk optic nerve ischemia and visual compromise [2, 9]. Additionally, the petrous branch supplies segments of the seventh cranial nerve and its sacrifice can potentially cause transient or permanent facial paresis [2].

Surgical Steps

Once the patient has been appropriately positioned, diluted betadine solution is used to sterilize the skin of the face, including the eyelids. A corneal shield protects the anterior globe. Intraoperative navigation may be considered and can be helpful. A lateral retrocanthal incision provides excellent access, but one could use an inferior preseptal approach only or, in select cases, a combination of both incisions. For the lateral retrocanthal approach, a conjunctival incision is placed just posterior to the insertion of the lateral canthus and directly towards the lateral bony orbit. Once the periosteum is exposed, it is sharply incised to allow sub-periorbital tissue elevation. For the inferior pre-septal approach, an incision is performed on the conjunctival surface of the lower eyelid roughly 2 mm anterior to the sclera. The incision proceeds until the orbicularis oculi muscle is identified, and the dissection proceeds along its posterior surface, anterior to the orbital septum. The orbital septum is protected to prevent herniation of orbital fat into the surgical field. The preseptal dissection plane is extended toward the orbital rim and overlying periosteum. The periosteum is incised sharply or with electrocautery. At this point, the periorbita is carefully elevated from medial to lateral and in a posterior direction until the inferior orbital fissure (IOF) is identified. The infraorbital fissure (IOF) is an important landmark in identifying the relationship between the maxilla (inferomedial), zygoma (inferolateral) and greater wing of the sphenoid (GWS) bone (superolateral) (Fig. 27.1).

At this point, one may begin to drill the lateral wall of the orbit to expose the temporalis muscle. This expands the working space and allows further insertion of surgical instruments. The zygomaticotemporal nerve (a terminal branch of the zygomatic nerve from the maxillary division of the trigeminal nerve) and associated vessels may be encountered in this step and occasionally require transection for expanded surgical access. Continued drilling in a posterior direction will eventually lead to the greater wing of the sphe-

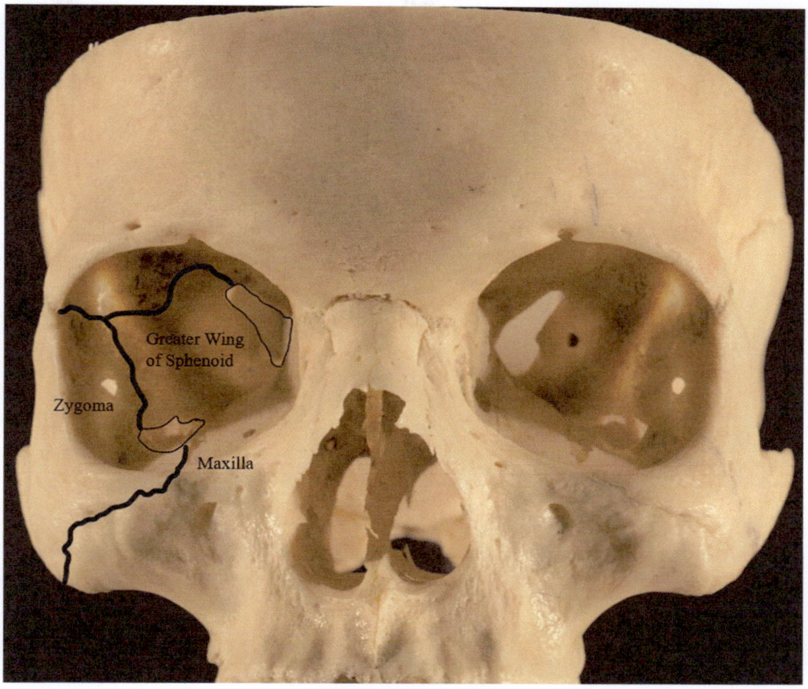

Fig. 27.1 Anatomic relationship of the IOF to the maxilla, zygoma and GWS

noid. Drilling of the greater wing of the sphenoid proceeds until the posteromedial segment of the infraorbital fissure is exposed.

Targeted removal of bone at this point can grant access to foramen ovale, foramen spinosum, sphenoid spine, foramen rotundum and lateral pterygoid plate. The surgeon should be cognizant of the close relationship to the temporal lobe in this region. Further superior drilling will expose the middle fossa dura while inferior drilling creates a passageway to the infratemporal fossa contents. To expose the infratemporal fossa, the underlying periosteum must be opened and the origin of the upper head of the lateral pterygoid muscle should be transected. We recommend drilling of the middle fossa floor superiorly to sequentially allow exposure of foramen ovale followed by foramen spinosum. The middle meningeal artery may be controlled with either clip ligation or bipolar electrocautery.

If the periorbita is not violated, it is unnecessary to plate or reline the bony dissection cavity. Any sharp or rough bony edges should be smoothed using a diamond drill bit. The conjunctival incision can be closed loosely using a 6-0 absorbable suture in a buried fashion. We place minimum suture material here so as not to cause irritation to the globe. A forced duction test should be performed. Postoperatively, the patient should be observed closely for orbital and cranial complications. An ice pack may be provided to assist with any swelling or bruising that may occur. As needed, artificial tears and nightly ophthalmic ointment will aid in healing and augment patient comfort (Figs. 27.2 and 27.3).

Step-by-Step Procedure

1. Conjunctival incision of choice (inferior eyelid preseptal and/or lateral retrocanthal approach)
   (a) Identification of the surgical plane between the orbicularis oculi and orbital septum
   (b) Preseptal dissection to expose the orbital rim
2. Subperiosteal elevation of the periorbita from the orbital floor and lateral orbit
3. Identification of the inferior orbital fissure
4. Drilling of the lateral orbital wall and greater wing of the sphenoid bone

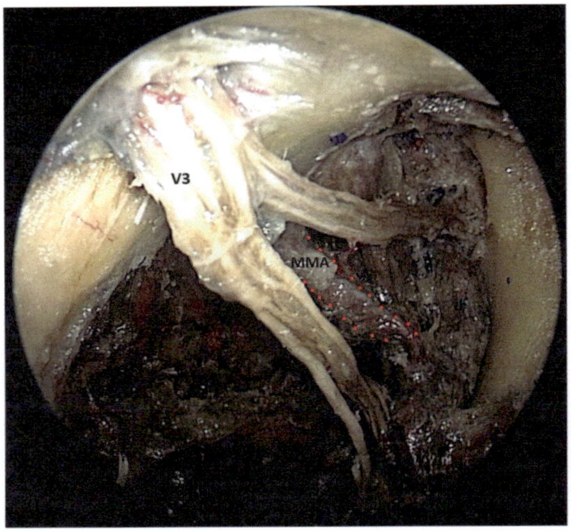

Fig. 27.2 Transorbital endoscopic dissection of the left infratemporal fossa with dissection of the mandibular division of the trigeminal nerve (V3) and middle meningeal artery (MMA)

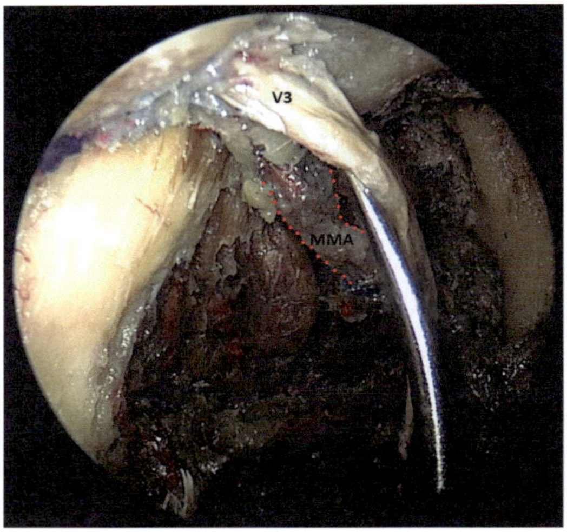

Fig. 27.3 Transorbital endoscopic dissection of the left infratemporal fossa. V3 reflected forward to allow identification of the middle meningeal artery

5. Opening of the periosteum of the infratemporal fossa
6. Transection of the upper head of the lateral pterygoid muscle
7. Middle fossa floor drilling superiorly and posteriorly to expose foramen ovale and middle meningeal artery passing through foramen spinosum
8. Ligation of the middle meningeal artery
9. Forced duction test
10. Conjunctival closure

Conclusion

Increasingly, a middle meningeal artery ligation is used in a wide range of clinical scenarios. The endoscopic transorbital approach offers a novel corridor for vascular control when endovascular methods may be contraindicated or unavailable. Careful patient selection and thorough patient counseling are necessary to optimize patient results. As surgical experience with transorbital corridors grows, transorbital endoscopic approaches may find greater utility in addressing skull base neurovascular structures.

Acknowledgements None.

Financial Support and Scholarship None.

Conflict of Interests None.

Funding Source None.

References

1. Yu J, Guo Y, Xu B, Xu K. Clinical importance of the middle meningeal artery: a review of the literature. Int J Med Sci. 2016;13(10):790–9. https://doi.org/10.7150/ijms.16489.
2. Martínez JL, Domingo RA, Sattur M, Porto G, Rivas GA, Al Kasab S, Spiotta. The middle meningeal artery: branches, dangerous anastomoses, and implications in neurosurgery and neuroendovascular surgery. Oper Neurosurg. 2022;22(1):1–13. https://doi.org/10.1227/ONS.0000000000000010.
3. Link TW, Boddu S, Paine SM, Kamel H, Knopman J. Middle meningeal artery embolization for chronic subdural hematoma: a series of 60 cases. Neurosurgery. 2019;85(6):801–7. https://doi.org/10.1093/neuros/nyy521.
4. Khorasanizadeh MH, Salih M, Harris D, Ogilvy CS. Technique to “trap” a segment of the middle meningeal artery for embolization of a carotid cavernous fistula: 2-dimensional operative video. Oper Neurosurg. 2021;21(5):E444. https://doi.org/10.1093/ons/opab273.

5. Lin NB, Mokin M, et al. Direct access to the middle meningeal artery for embolization of complex dural arteriovenous fistula: a hybrid treatment approach. J NeuroInterv Surg. 2015;7:e24.
6. Vural A, Carobbio AL, Ferrari M, et al. Transorbital endoscopic approaches to the skull base: a systematic literature review and anatomical description. Neurosurg Rev. 2021;44:2857–78. https://doi.org/10.1007/s10143-020-01470-5.
7. Lieber S, Fernandez-Miranda J. Anatomy of the orbit. J Neurol Surg B Skull Base. 2020;81(4):319–32. https://doi.org/10.1055/s-0040-1715096.
8. Balakrishnan K, Moe KS. Applications and outcomes of orbital and transorbital endoscopic surgery. Otolaryngol Head Neck Surg. 2011;144(5):815–20.
9. Hayashi N, Kubo M, Tsuboi Y, Nishimura S, Nishijima M, Ahmed A-AM, et al. Impact of anomalous origin of the ophthalmic artery from the middle meningeal artery on selection of surgical approach to skull base meningioma. Surg Neurol. 2007;68:568–71; discussion 71–2.

Part IX

Technical Nuances

Endoscopic Transorbital Anterior Clinoidectomy

28

Alberto Di Somma, Andrea De Rosa, Luis Reyes, and Joaquim Enseñat

Anatomy Review

Anterior Clinoid Process

The anterior clinoid process represents the medial end of the lesser wing of the sphenoid bone [1]. It has a triangular shape, composed of a body and three roots attaching it to the lesser sphenoid wing and sphenoid bone. The lateral root is represented by the medial end of the lesser sphenoid wing, the anterior root is represented by the roof of the optic canal, and the posterior root is represented by the optic strut, which is a bony pillar extending latero-medially from the inferior surface of the anterior clinoid process to the lateral wall of the sphenoid body, and which forms the floor of the optic canal, dividing it from the superior orbital fissure. The clinoidal segment of the internal carotid artery [2] runs along the posterior margin of the optic strut, inferiorly to the anterior clinoid process, and it is limited by two leaflets of dura mater emerging from the inferior and superior surfaces of the anterior clinoid process, the proximal and distal dural rings, respectively. Inferior and lateral to the anterior clinoid process, the oculomotor nerve exits from the cavernous sinus to enter the superior orbital fissure.

Endoscopic Transorbital Bone Anatomy

Anatomical knowledge of the bony anatomy from a transorbital perspective is mandatory to recognize all the landmarks that serve as a guide for a safe procedure. The lateral wall of the orbit represents the lateral limit of the corridor. Externally, it is formed by the frontal process of the zygomatic bone and the zygomatic process of the frontal bone, which join at the level of the fronto-zygomatic suture. The deep portion of the lateral wall is formed by the orbital surface of the zygomatic bone and the greater sphenoid wing. The roof of the orbit, composed anteriorly by the frontal bone, and posteriorly by the lesser sphenoid wing, represents the upper limit of the corridor. The superior orbital fissure is bounded superiorly by the sphenoid ridge and inferiorly by the greater sphenoid wing is a useful landmark for recognizing the limits of the anterior and middle cranial fossa. At the junction of the floor and

A. Di Somma (✉) · L. Reyes
Department of Neurological Surgery, Hospital Clínic de Barcelona, Barcelona, Spain
e-mail: LAREYES@CLINIC.CAT

A. De Rosa
Division of Neurosurgery, Department of Neurosciences, Reproductive and Odontostomatological Sciences, Università degli Studi di Napoli "Federico II", Naples, Italy

J. Enseñat
Department of Neurological Surgery, Hospital Clínic de Barcelona, University of Barcelona, Barcelona, Spain
e-mail: JENSENAT@clinic.cat

T. H. Schwartz et al. (eds.), *Endoscopic Transorbital Surgery of the Orbit, Skull Base and Brain*,
https://doi.org/10.1007/978-3-031-59504-2_28

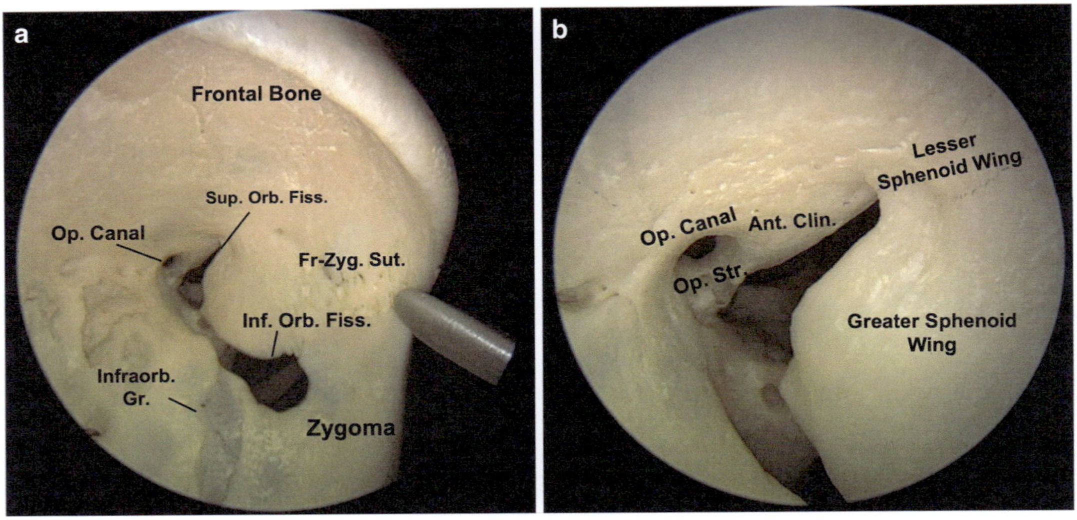

Fig. 28.1 Bone anatomy: Pictures from an endoscopic transorbital perspective of a dry skull (left orbit). The main bony anatomic landmarks of the transorbital corridor are shown in a panoramic fashion (**a**). A closer view (**b**) of the clinoidal area is shown. *Ant. Clin* anterior clinoid process, *Fr-Zyg Sut* fronto-zygomatic suture, *Inf. Orb.Fiss* inferior orbital fissure, *Infraorb. Gr* infraorbital groove, *Op. Can* optic canal, *Op. str* optic strut, *sup. orb. fiss* superior orbital fissure

lateral wall of the orbit, the inferior orbital fissure is recognized at the beginning of the approach. Moving in a medial direction, the superior orbital fissure is divided from the optic canal by the optic strut, which forms the floor of the canal, while the medial end of the lesser sphenoid wing continues with the roof of the optic canal. From the transorbital latero-ventral perspective, the base of the anterior clinoid process is visualized in the middle of its three roots, representing one of the bony pillars of the endoscopic transorbital approach [3] (Fig. 28.1).

Cadaveric Stepwise Dissection

In this section, we describe the step-by-step technique to perform an anterior clinoidectomy using the endoscopic transorbital corridor. All the data taken from anatomical dissections performed at the Laboratory of Surgical Neuroanatomy of Barcelona.

The specimen is positioned in line with the patient's position during an endoscopic transorbital approach, i.e., with the head in a neutral position, with a slight rotation of 5–10° towards the contralateral side, so that the lateral orbital wall is oriented in a plane parallel to the direction of the approach. Each step of the approach has been well described in previous publications [4–8].

The incision is made along a crease of the superior eyelid and extended laterally to a maximum of 1.5 cm beyond the lateral canthus, thus avoiding the risk of injuries to the branches of the facial nerve [9]. The skin and subcutaneous tissue are separated with blunt dissection until thorbicularis muscle fibers are reached and divided. The white plane, formed by the orbital septum, superiorly, and the superior tarsus, inferiorly, is then identified; this plane must be preserved as it represents the site of insertion of the *levator palpebrae* muscle. Dissection continues laterally until the periosteum covering the lateral orbital rim is reached and incised. After complete skeletonization of the lateral orbital rim, the dissection proceeds in a subperiosteal-subperiorbital fashion to reach the orbital cavity (Fig. 28.2).

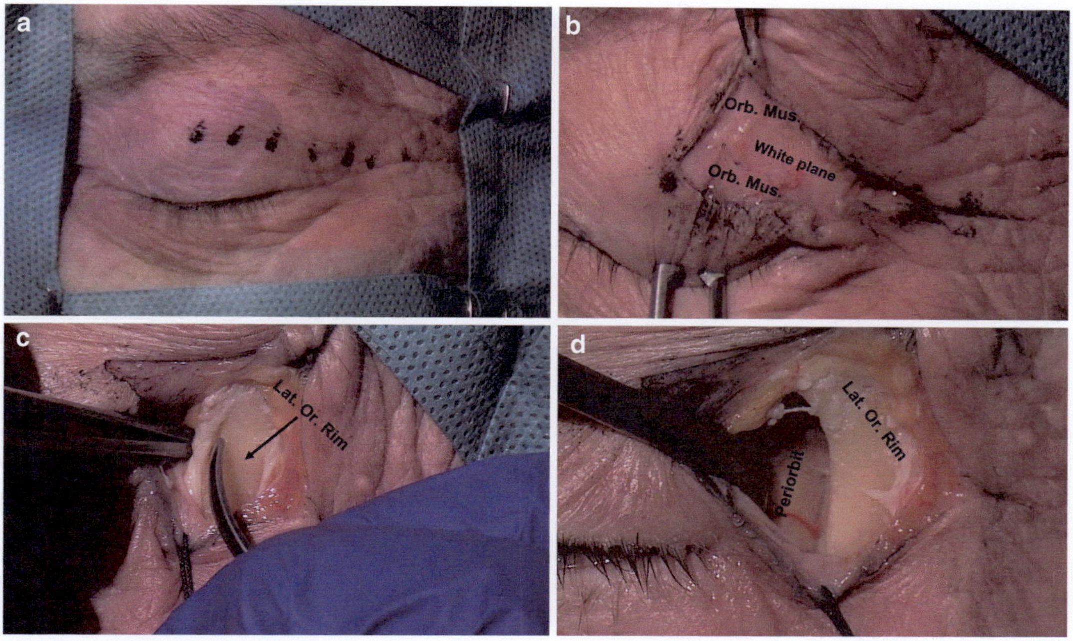

Fig. 28.2 Skin phase (left orbit). The initial phase of the approach, the "skin phase", begins with a linear incision of the upper eyelid, extended laterally for 1.5 cm (**a**). After the incision of the skin and subcutaneous tissue, the orbicularis muscle can be divided along its fibers and the white plane, formed by the superior tarsus and orbital septum, can be visualized and preserved (**b**). After exposure and incision of the periosteum covering the lateral orbital rim (**c**), the bone can be fully skeletonized. The dissection proceeds in a subperiosteal-subperiorbital fashion to create available space for the introduction of the endoscope (**d**). *Orb. Mus.* orbicularis muscle, *Lat. Orb. Rim* lateral orbital rim

At this phase, the endoscope can be inserted into the surgical field. To obtain maximum maneuverability, the surgical field should be figured out as a triangle, whose superior vertex is occupied by the endoscope, allowing the instruments to be inserted underneath. Progressive detachment of the periorbit reveals the lateral orbital wall along with the landmarks that must be recognized, such as the fronto-zygomatic fissure the superior and the inferior orbital fissure. The next step of the procedure, the "working-space creation" phase, begins with the drilling of the lateral wall of the orbit. In this phase, identification of the temporalis muscle fascia is mandatory; indeed, it provides a useful guide for the orientation of further drilling. As more lateral space is created, a retractor can be positioned parallel to the long axis of the inferior orbital fissure to allow gentle medialization and protection of the periorbit. The greater sphenoid wing is drilled until a "V" shape appears (with the vertex pointing toward the inferior orbital fissure). The base of the "V" is represented by the lesser sphenoid wing, and it is an extremely useful landmark since it should be drilled out and followed in a medial direction to reach the lateral root of the anterior clinoid process (the base of the anterior clinoid from a transorbital perspective). Bone removal proceeds at the center of the "V" to expose the dura of the temporal pole and above the base of the "V" to expose the basal frontal dura. The medial side of the "V" is represented by the *sagittal crest*, another bony pillar of the transorbital approach, which must be removed in its upper part to free the contents of the superior orbital fissure and to expose the meningo-orbital band [10] (Fig. 28.3).

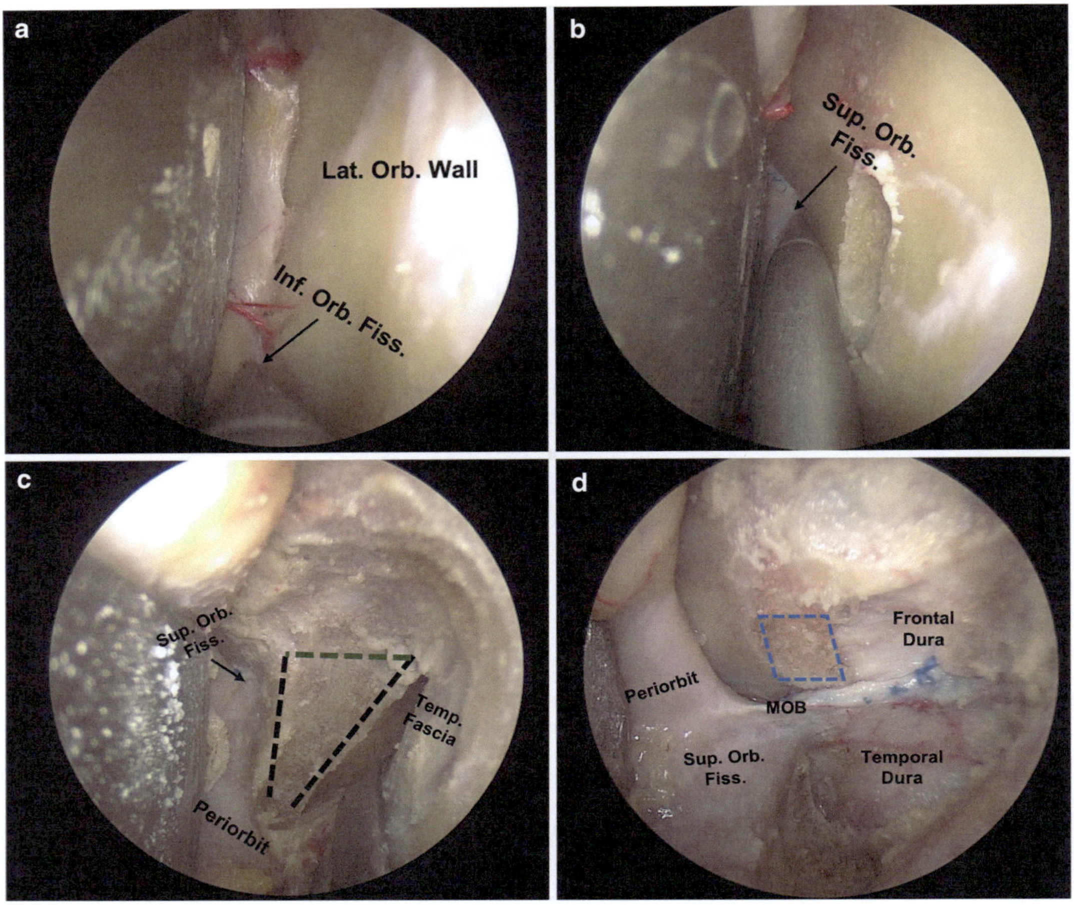

Fig. 28.3 Working space phase. Once the endoscope is inserted into the surgical field, the inferior orbital fissure (**a**) and the superior orbital fissure (**b**) must be identified to delimit the area of drilling of the greater sphenoid wing. The temporalis fascia represents the lateral limit of the approach. A triangular area (green and dark dotted lines) appears during the drilling of the greater sphenoid wing. The medial margin of this area is represented by the sagittal crest, the lateral margin corresponds to the outer surface of the sphenoid bone, and the superior base corresponds to the sphenoid ridge, which divides the anterior cranial fossa superiorly from the middle cranial fossa, inferiorly (**c**). The meningo-orbital band is exposed, along with the dura of the anterior and middle cranial fossa (**d**). The blue dotted area represents the base of the anterior clinoid process, which is reached after drilling of the sphenoid ridge in a lateral to medial direction (**d**). *Inf. Orb. Fis.* inferior orbital fissure, *Lat.Orb.Wall.* lateral orbital wall, *MOB* meningo-orbital band, *Sup.Orb.Fis.* superior orbital fissure, *Temp.fascia* fascia of the temporalis muscle

The meningo-orbital band, extending from the periorbita to the temporal dura, is then cut. This allows for medial and inferior dissection of the periorbita from the roof of the orbital cavity, exposing the optic canal . The base of the anterior clinoid process can be now identified between the superior orbital fissure and the optic canal. Anterior clinoidectomy starts at this point with removal of the lateral root of the clinoid by drilling the most medial aspect of the lesser sphenoid wing. Then, proceeding medially and superiorly, the anterior root of the anterior clinoid process is removed by unroofing the supero-lateral aspect of the optic canal. At this step, the anterior clinoid process is only attached by its posterior root, the optic strut, and its removal can be accomplished either by fracturing it from the optic strut with a lateral-directed rotation, procedure made safer by the direct visual control of the optic nerve, or by progressive drilling towards its base, whose margins are enveloped in surrounding dura mater, with the so-called "egg-shell" technique. Drilling of the cancellous bone ends with the identification and removal of the tip of the anterior clinoid, which is finally removed (Fig. 28.4).

At the end of the procedure, the optic nerve sheath, the proximal and distal dural rings enveloping the clinoidal segment of the internal carotid artery, and the superior orbital fissure are exposed extradurally. Opening of the dura reveals the optic nerve, the supra-clinoid portion of the carotid artery, just before its bifurcation, and the oculomotor nerve, which lies infero-laterally. Lateral to the oculomotor nerve, the uncus can also be appreciated (Fig. 28.5).

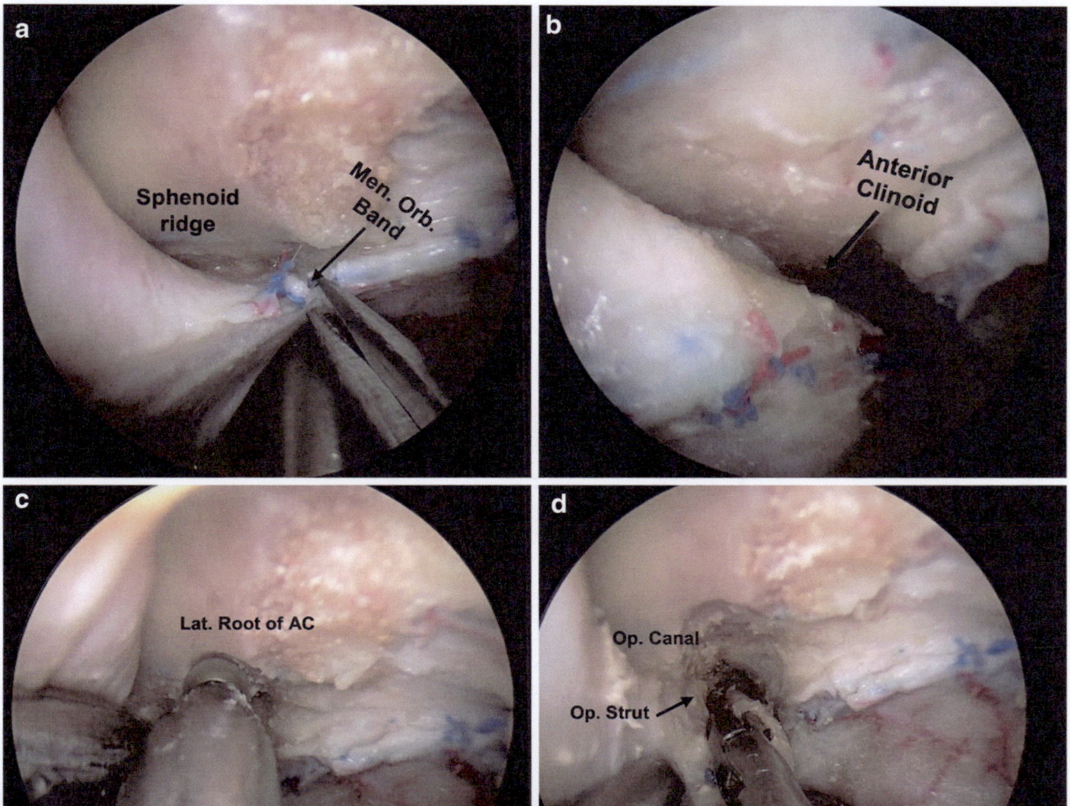

Fig. 28.4 Anterior clinoidectomy. The meningo-orbital band is cut (**a**) to fully expose the anterior clinoid process (**b**), which is detached from its roots, starting from the lateral roots, and proceeding with its anterior and posterior attachments, the roof of the optic canal and the optic strut, respectively (**c**). The anterior clinoid process can be then removed en bloc (**d**). *Lat. Root. Of AC* the lateral root of the anterior clinoid process, *Men. Orb. Band* meningo-orbital band, *Op. Canal* optic canal, *Op. Strut* optic strut

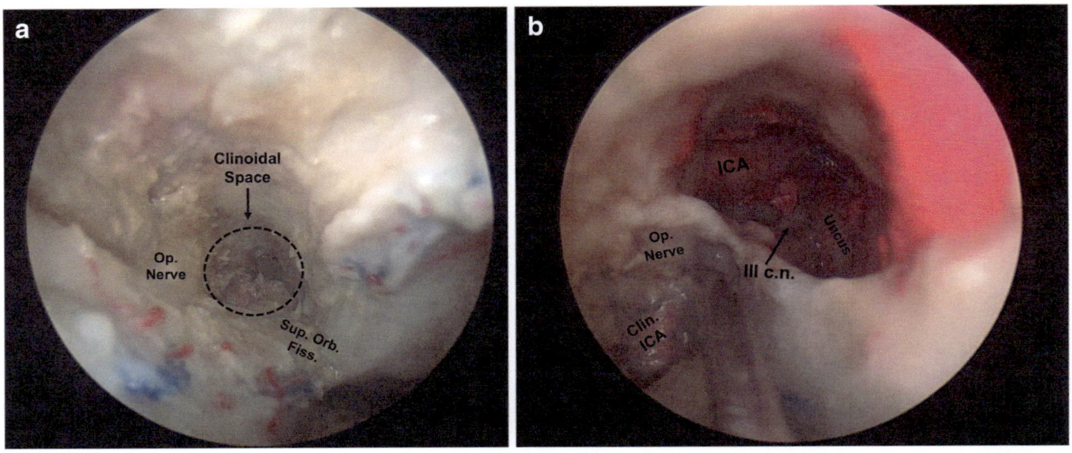

Fig. 28.5 Extra-intradural exposure. Once the anterior clinoid process is removed, the extradural compartment of the clinoidal triangle (dotted circle) can be exposed (**a**). (**b**) After the opening of the dura mater, the supraclinoidal region, along with the carotid cistern and the oculomotor membrane, can be visualized from a transorbital perspective. *III n.c.* oculomotor nerve, *Clin. ICA* clinoidal segment of the internal carotid artery, *ICA* terminal segment of the internal carotid artery, *Op. nerve* canalicular segment of the optic nerve, *Sup. Orb. Fiss* superior orbital fissure

Discussion

Anterior clinoidectomy is one of the fundamental procedures during neurovascular and skull base surgeries [11–16]. Even though many technical nuances and variations of the technique have been proposed [17–24], the principles to perform the anterior clinoidectomy mainly rely on detaching it from the three roots and the two main modalities to achieve this goal are represented by the extradural and intradural approach [25, 26]. The intradural approach has been introduced by Hauser and Gass [27], and its main principles rely on opening the dura mater, splitting the sylvian fissure and performing the anterior clinoidectomy under direct visualization of the critical neurovascular structures surrounding the anterior clinoid process. The key steps of the extradural technique, popularized by Dolenc et al. [28], are represented by the elevation of the frontotemporal dura from the sphenoid ridge, identification and cut of the meningo-orbital band, peeling of the middle fossa dura and exposure of the anterior clinoid process. During the extradural clinoidectomy, the intradural structures are protected by the dura mater, but the main drawbacks are the lack of direct control of the neurovascular structures and the risk of damaging the cranial nerve running through the superior orbital fissure and the lateral wall of the cavernous sinus during the peeling of the middle fossa dura.

With the introduction of the endoscopic skull base surgery, the main goal was to translate open skull base approaches' principles to minimally invasive corridors as represented by the endonasal route, whereas lateral extension among the clinoidal region has always represented a limitation of this strategy. With the evolution of instrumentation and techniques, even challenging maneuvers such as anterior clinoidectomy have been performed during the endoscopic endonasal approach [29–31]. In a recent paper by Xiao et al., the main steps and possible indications of endoscopic endonasal anterior clinoidectomy have been reported [30].

With the more recent application of the endoscopic transorbital approach to the neurosurgical armamentarium, many regions of the skull base have been reached, both in anatomical and clinical settings [8, 32–39]. Of particular interest is the possibility to reach the supero-lateral portion of the optic canal by means of the transorbital route [40]. As neurosurgeons became more familiar with the ventral perspective given by this approach, it followed that anterior clinoidectomy was also successfully executed during the endoscopic transorbital route [4, 41]. In this case, the anterior clinoid process is addressed in a lateral to medial direction, firstly detaching its lateral root, the lesser sphenoid wing, and then proceeding with the anterior and posterior roots, namely the roof of the optic canal and the optic strut. The transorbital approach provides several advantages in performing an anterior clinoidectomy. First, the direction of the dissection follows the projection of the anterior clinoid process, which extends in a postero-medial direction. The drilling process is thus made easier and can be performed even without a complete peeling of the lateral wall of the cavernous sinus. The ventral perspective of the clinoid region provided by the transorbital corridor is of particular interest as it allows the visual control of the optic nerve and contents of the superior orbital fissure during the execution of delicate steps of the procedure, such as the unroofing of the optic canal. Furthermore, it must be underlined that transorbital anterior clinoidectomy is performed in a purely extradural fashion. The main limitations of the technique are represented by the poor familiarity with the anatomy offered by the orbital corridor and the limited maneuverability; extensive and dedicated bone work during the "working space" phase is essential to overcome this drawback. Of primary concern is also the control of the clinoidal segment of the internal carotid artery located in the posterior/deep portion of the surgical field from a transorbital perspective. Concerning clinical applications, only a few cases in which transorbital anterior clinoidectomy was performed have been described [41] (Figs. 28.6, 28.7, and 28.8).

Due to their location and the pathological modification of the bone due to tumoral infiltration, spheno-orbital and clinoidal meningiomas could represent two possible indications of anterior clinoidectomy. In particular, the hyperostotic bone associated with these lesions could serve both as a pathway created by the tumor itself and as a barrier between the surgical field and the surrounding neurovascular structures.

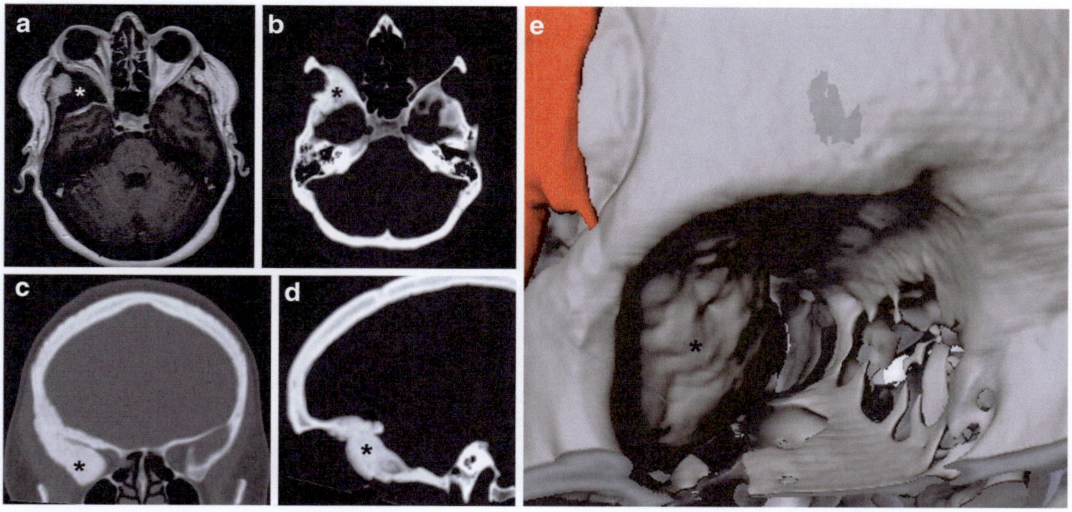

Fig. 28.6 Clinical case. Preoperative axial contrast-enhanced MRI (**a**), and axial (**b**), coronal (**c**) and sagittal (**d**) CT scan showing a right spheno-orbital meningioma (*) with a globular portion infiltrating the temporalis muscle and causing hyperostosis of the middle cranial fossa floor, lateral wall of the orbit and involving medially to the anterior clinoid process. The amount of hyperostosis abutting the orbital cavity is better appreciated by a BrainLab® 3D reconstruction (**e**). The patient complained of right proptosis. Results from the ophthalmometry showed a Hertel base 100: 27 (OD)–23 (OS)

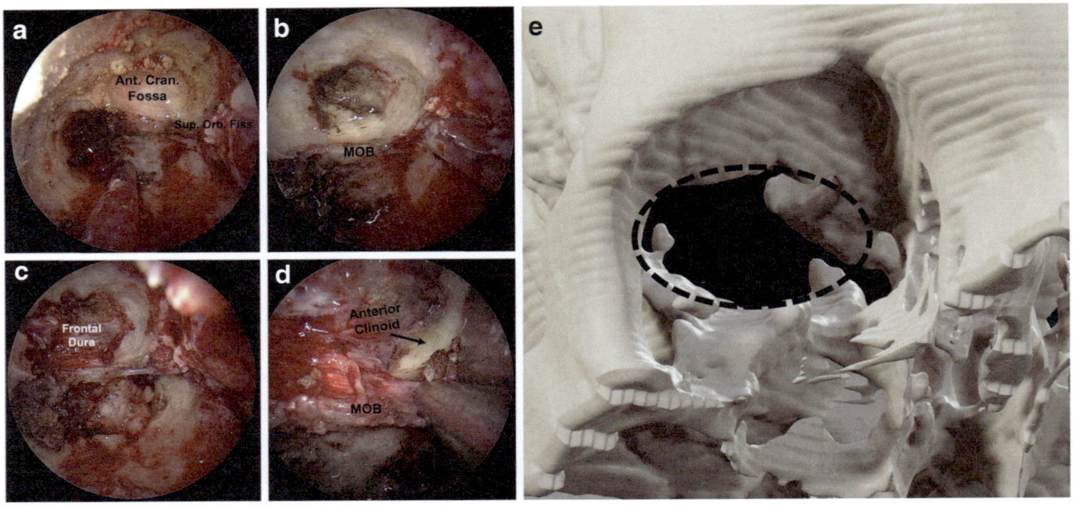

Fig. 28.7 Clinical case. An endoscopic transorbital approach was indicated to remove the hyperostotic bone and relieve patients' symptoms. After the removal of the hyperostotic bone infiltrating the lateral wall of the orbit (**a**), the dura of the anterior and posterior cranial fossa, along with the meningo-orbital band, were exposed (**b**). The dura of the temporal pole was opened to expose and remove the globular portion of the tumor (**c**). In this case, drilling of the hyperostotic bone continued until the base of the anterior clinoid process was reached (**d**). A complete anterior clinoidectomy was not indicated in this case. 3D BrainLab® reconstruction demonstrated the amount of bone removed (dotted circle) and the decompression of the orbital cavity (**e**). *Ant.Cran.Fossa* anterior cranial fossa, *MOB* meningo-orbital band, *Sph. Ridge* sphenoid ridge, *Sup.Orb.Fiss.* superior orbital fissure; black arrow indicates the base of the anterior clinoid reached in this case

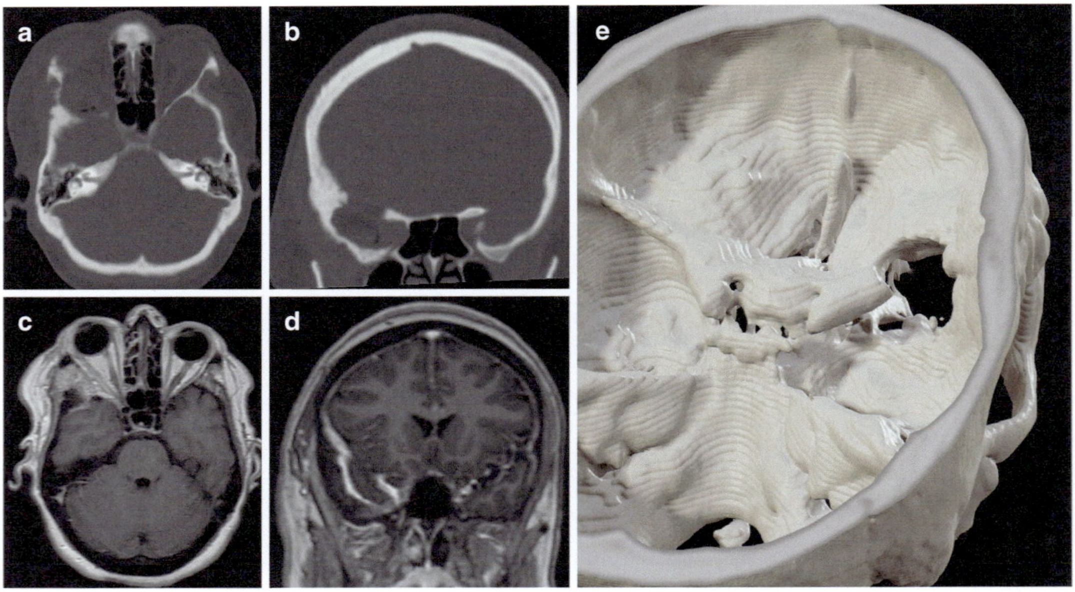

Fig. 28.8 Clinical case. Postoperative axial (**a**) and coronal (**b**) CT scans showing the adequate removal of the hyperostotic bone. Axial (**c**) and coronal (**d**) contrast-enhanced postoperative MRI confirming the total removal of the globular portion of the tumor; the surgical field was reconstructed by means of an autologous fat graft. 3D BrainLab® reconstruction clearly shows the limits of bone removal, such as the lateral root of the anterior clinoid process. The patient recovered from the proptosis, also confirmed by the subsequent ophthalmologic evaluation (Hertel base 100: 21.5 (OD)–23 (OS) in the early postoperative period; Hertel base 104. 18 (OD)–16 (OS) at 5-months follow-up)

Conclusions

With the technique's evolution and widespread application, the endoscopic transorbital approach has now entered the skull base neurosurgeon's armamentarium. The possibility of translating the main principles of the microscopic transcranial surgery to the evolving minimally invasive endoscopic approach is of paramount importance. The anterior clinoidectomy, one of the most important and useful strategies used in skull base surgery, can be effectively performed during an endoscopic transorbital approach. Anatomic knowledge and surgical experience are mandatory for the proper execution of this delicate procedure.

References

1. Rhoton ALJ. The supratentorial cranial space: microsurgical anatomy and surgical approaches. Neurosurgery. 2002;51(4):S1-iii–S-vi.
2. Bouthillier A, van Loveren HR, Keller JT. Segments of the internal carotid artery: a new classification. Neurosurgery. 1996;38(3):425–32; discussion 32–3.
3. Di Somma A, Kong DS, de Notaris M, Moe KS, Sánchez España JC, Schwartz TH, et al. Endoscopic transorbital surgery levels of difficulty. J Neurosurg. 2022;137:1187–90.
4. López CB, Di Somma A, Cepeda S, Arrese I, Sarabia R, Agustín JH, et al. Extradural anterior clinoidectomy through endoscopic transorbital approach: laboratory investigation for surgical perspective. Acta Neurochir. 2021;163(8):2177–88.
5. Di Somma A, Sanchez España JC, Alobid I, Enseñat J. Endoscopic superior eyelid transorbital approach: how I do it. Acta Neurochir. 2022;164:1953–9.
6. Jeon C, Hong CK, Woo KI, Hong SD, Nam DH, Lee JI, et al. Endoscopic transorbital surgery for Meckel's cave and middle cranial fossa tumors: surgical technique and early results. J Neurosurg. 2018;131(4):1126–35.
7. Almeida JP, Ruiz-Treviño AS, Shetty SR, Omay SB, Anand VK, Schwartz TH. Transorbital endoscopic approach for exposure of the sylvian fissure, middle cerebral artery and crural cistern: an anatomical study. Acta Neurochir. 2017;159(10):1893–907.
8. Moe KS, Bergeron CM, Ellenbogen RG. Transorbital neuroendoscopic surgery. Neurosurgery. 2010;67(3 Suppl Operative):ons16-28.
9. Abdel Aziz KM, Bhatia S, Tantawy MH, Sekula R, Keller JT, Froelich S, et al. Minimally invasive transpalpebral "eyelid" approach to the anterior cranial base. Neurosurgery. 2011;69(2 Suppl Operative):ons195-206; discussion -7.
10. Dallan I, Di Somma A, Prats-Galino A, Solari D, Alobid I, Turri-Zanoni M, et al. Endoscopic transorbital route to the cavernous sinus through the meningo-orbital band: a descriptive anatomical study. J Neurosurg. 2017;127(3):622–9.
11. Day AL. Aneurysms of the ophthalmic segment. A clinical and anatomical analysis. J Neurosurg. 1990;72(5):677–91.
12. Heros RC, Nelson PB, Ojemann RG, Crowell RM, DeBrun G. Large and giant paraclinoid aneurysms: surgical techniques, complications, and results. Neurosurgery. 1983;12(2):153–63.
13. Martinez-Perez R, Joswig H, Tsimpas A, Poblete T, Albiña P, Perales I, et al. The extradural minipterional approach for the treatment of paraclinoid aneurysms: a cadaver stepwise dissection and clinical case series. Neurosurg Rev. 2020;43(1):361–70.
14. Lee JH, Sade B, Park BJ. A surgical technique for the removal of clinoidal meningiomas. Neurosurgery. 2006;59(1 Suppl 1):ONS108-14; discussion ONS-14.
15. Day JD. Cranial base surgical techniques for large sphenocavernous meningiomas: technical note. Neurosurgery. 2000;46(3):754–9; discussion 9–60.
16. Sayyahmelli S, Sun Z, Avci E, Başkaya MK. Role of extradural clinoidectomy and optic unroofing in resection of an anterior clinoidal meningioma with encasement of the internal carotid artery and its branches. J Neurol Surg B Skull Base. 2022;83(Suppl 3):e650–2.
17. Tayebi Meybodi A, Lawton MT, Yousef S, Guo X, González Sánchez JJ, Tabani H, et al. Anterior clinoidectomy using an extradural and intradural 2-step hybrid technique. J Neurosurg. 2018;130(1):238–47.
18. Froelich SC, Aziz KM, Levine NB, Theodosopoulos PV, van Loveren HR, Keller JT. Refinement of the extradural anterior clinoidectomy: surgical anatomy of the orbitotemporal periosteal fold. Neurosurgery. 2007;61(5 Suppl 2):179–85; discussion 85–6.
19. Sai Kiran NA, Furtado SV, Hegde AS. How I do it: anterior clinoidectomy and optic canal unroofing for microneurosurgical management of ophthalmic segment aneurysms. Acta Neurochir. 2013;155(6):1025–9.
20. Alejandro SA, Carrasco-Hernández JP, da Costa MDS, Ferreira DS, Lima JVF, de Amorim BL, et al. Anterior clinoidectomy: intradural step-by-step en bloc removal technique. World Neurosurg. 2021;146:217–31.
21. Chang DJ. The "no-drill" technique of anterior clinoidectomy: a cranial base approach to the paraclinoid and parasellar region. Neurosurgery. 2009;64(3 Suppl):ons96-105; discussion ons-6.
22. Chang HS, Joko M, Song JS, Ito K, Inoue T, Nakagawa H. Ultrasonic bone curettage for optic canal unroofing and anterior clinoidectomy. Technical note. J Neurosurg. 2006;104(4):621–4.
23. Yonekawa Y, Ogata N, Imhof HG, Olivecrona M, Strommer K, Kwak TE, et al. Selective extradural ante-

rior clinoidectomy for supra- and parasellar processes. Technical note. J Neurosurg. 1997;87(4):636–42.
24. Kulwin C, Tubbs RS, Cohen-Gadol AA. Anterior clinoidectomy: description of an alternative hybrid method and a review of the current techniques with an emphasis on complication avoidance. Surg Neurol Int. 2011;2:140.
25. Acioly MA, Hendricks BK, Cohen-Gadol A. Extradural clinoidectomy: an efficient technique for expanding the operative corridor toward the central skull base. World Neurosurg. 2021;145:557–66.
26. Cohen-Gadol A. Intradural clinoidectomy: a tailored osteotomy for approaching the paraclinoid carotid artery and interpeduncular cisterns. World Neurosurg. 2021;146:442–7.
27. Hauser MJ, Gass H. Optic nerve pressure by aneurysm relieved by decompression of optic nerve; report of a case. AMA Arch Ophthalmol. 1952;48(5):627–31.
28. Dolenc VV. A combined epi- and subdural direct approach to carotid-ophthalmic artery aneurysms. J Neurosurg. 1985;62(5):667–72.
29. Champagne PO, Zenonos GA, Wang EW, Snyderman CH, Gardner PA. Endoscopic endonasal anterior clinoidectomy: volumetric assessment and feasibility. World Neurosurg. 2022;168:e269–77.
30. Xiao L, Xie S, Tang B, Hu J, Hong T. Endoscopic endonasal anterior clinoidectomy: surgical anatomy, technique nuance, and case series. J Neurosurg. 2019;133(2):451–61.
31. Di Somma A, Torales J, Cavallo LM, Pineda J, Solari D, Gerardi RM, et al. Defining the lateral limits of the endoscopic endonasal transtuberculum transplanum approach: anatomical study with pertinent quantitative analysis. J Neurosurg. 2018;130(3):848–60.
32. Bly RA, Ramakrishna R, Ferreira M, Moe KS. Lateral transorbital neuroendoscopic approach to the lateral cavernous sinus. J Neurol Surg B Skull Base. 2014;75(1):11–7.
33. Chen HI, Bohman LE, Loevner LA, Lucas TH. Transorbital endoscopic amygdalohippocampectomy: a feasibility investigation. J Neurosurg. 2014;120(6):1428–36.
34. Ramakrishna R, Kim LJ, Bly RA, Moe K, Ferreira M. Transorbital neuroendoscopic surgery for the treatment of skull base lesions. J Clin Neurosci. 2016;24:99–104.
35. Di Somma A, Andaluz N, Cavallo LM, Topczewski TE, Frio F, Gerardi RM, et al. Endoscopic transorbital route to the petrous apex: a feasibility anatomic study. Acta Neurochir. 2018;160(4):707–20.
36. Di Somma A, Andaluz N, Cavallo LM, de Notaris M, Dallan I, Solari D, et al. Endoscopic transorbital superior eyelid approach: anatomical study from a neurosurgical perspective. J Neurosurg. 2018;129(5):1203–16.
37. Kim EH, Yoo J, Jung IH, Oh JW, Kim JS, Yoon JS, et al. Endoscopic transorbital approach to the insular region: cadaveric feasibility study and clinical application (SevEN-005). J Neurosurg. 2021;135(4):1164–72.
38. Guizzardi G, Mosteiro A, Hoyos J, Ferres A, Topczewski T, Reyes L, et al. Endoscopic transorbital approach to the middle fossa: qualitative and quantitative anatomic study. Oper Neurosurg. 2022;23(4):e267–5.
39. De Rosa A, Di Somma A, Mosteiro A, Ferrés A, Reyes LA, Roldan P, et al. Superior eyelid endoscopic transorbital approach to the tentorial area: a qualitative and quantitative anatomic study. Front Surg. 2022;9:1007447.
40. Di Somma A, Cavallo LM, de Notaris M, Solari D, Topczewski TE, Bernal-Sprekelsen M, et al. Endoscopic endonasal medial-to-lateral and transorbital lateral-to-medial optic nerve decompression: an anatomical study with surgical implications. J Neurosurg. 2017;127(1):199–208.
41. Lim J, Sung KS, Yoo J, Oh J, Moon JH. Endoscopic transorbital extradural anterior clinoidectomy: a stepwise surgical technique and case series study [SevEN-013]. Front Oncol. 2022;12:991065.

The Sagittal Crest and Mid-subtemporal Ridge

29

Matteo de Notaris, Francesco Corrivetti, Toma Spiriev, and Lili Laleva

Introduction

The considerable interest gained in recent years by the TONES [1] led to the widespread application of the superior eyelid endoscopic transorbital approach (SETOA) for a large variety of neurosurgical pathology [2–5]. This approach has shown to be particularly suitable for accessing the lateral portion of the middle cranial fossa in a minimally invasive fashion [6, 7]. Moreover, thanks to the refinements of endoscopic technique and anatomical knowledge, SETOA can be further performed as a complementary pathway to the endoscopic endonasal approach (EEA), in the contest of combined multiportal approaches, to "overcome" the paramedian limitations of EEA [8, 9].

After careful anatomical investigations and several clinical applications of SETOA [2, 4, 10], the authors documented two key anatomical landmarks visible during the drilling of the greater sphenoid wing (GSW). These landmarks are two bony ridges. The first, named the "sagittal crest," it's a bony ridge with sagittal orientation that constantly remains unnoticed after lateral-to-medial drilling of the GSW, located between the medial temporal dura and the posterior periorbita, superior to the foramen rotundum [11]. Is worth noting that this surgical landmark is created "artificially" during the approach after drilling the lateral portion of the of the GSW, and it is not present in "native anatomy." The second, named "mid-subtemporal ridge," is a bony prominence located on the floor of the middle cranial fossa, lateral to the foramen rotundum (Figs. 29.1 and 29.2).

M. de Notaris (✉)
Laboratory of Neuroanatomy, EBRIS Foundation, European Biomedical Research Institute of Salerno, Salerno, Italy

Unit of Neurosurgery, San Giovanni di Dio and Ruggi D'Aragona Hospital, University of Salerno, Salerno, Italy

F. Corrivetti
Laboratory of Neuroanatomy, EBRIS Foundation, European Biomedical Research Institute of Salerno, Salerno, Italy

Department of Neurosurgery, San Luca Hospital, Vallo della Lucania, Salerno, Italy

T. Spiriev · L. Laleva
Department of Neurosurgery, Acibadem City Clinic University Hospital Tokuda, Sofia, Bulgaria

T. H. Schwartz et al. (eds.), *Endoscopic Transorbital Surgery of the Orbit, Skull Base and Brain*,
https://doi.org/10.1007/978-3-031-59504-2_29

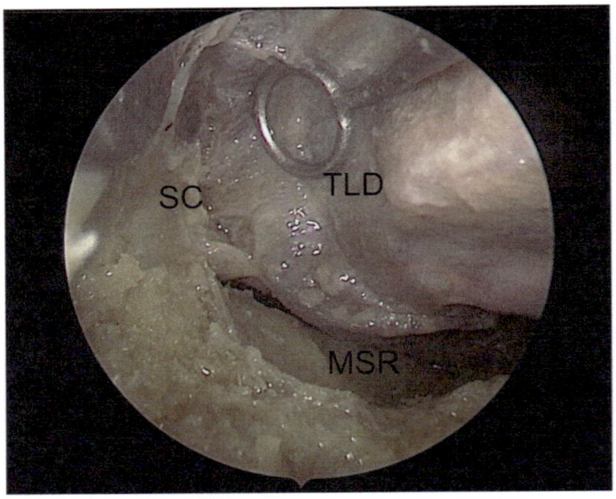

Fig. 29.1 Endoscopic phase of the trans-orbital approach presenting the sagittal crest and mid-subtemporal ridge; left side. *MSR* mid-subtemporal; *SC* sagittal crest, *TLD* temporal lobe dura

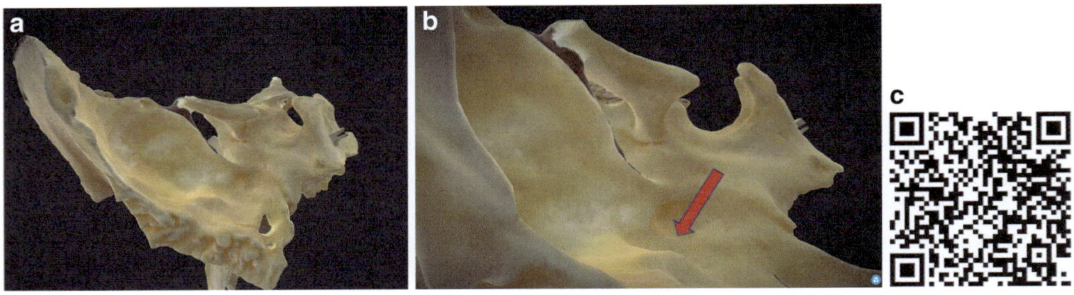

Fig. 29.2 (**a**, **b**) The mid-subtemporal ridge (MSR). The red arrow indicates the position of the MSR 3D photorealistic models from the 3D Atlas of Neurological Surgery project and Panum Institute, Department of Cellular and Molecular Medicine University of Copenhagen (published with permission https://3datlasofneurologicalsurgery.org/). The 3D models of this database represent surface scanning of anatomical specimens using a photogrammetry technique, which allows the extraction of 3D data from 2D photographs. The 3D data were processed using Blender software, and the 3D photorealistic models were uploaded to a dedicated website for 3D visualization. This allows users to see the 3D models from every desktop or mobile device, as well as some of the 3D models that can be displayed in AR mode by scanning the QR next to the Figures. (**c**) QR codes to 3D photorealistic models of the sphenoid bone

Stepwise SETOA to the Middle Cranial Fossa

The stepwise anatomy of the SETOA has been extensively described previously (Chap. 2). Briefly, the skin incision is placed in the lateral (temporal) half of the superior lid to expose the lateral orbital rim and the frontozygomatic suture. A skin flap is elevated supero-laterally, dissecting inside the sub-orbicularis plane and exposing the periosteum. Then, dissection is lead in the sub-periosteal plane toward the orbit, exposing the ventral surface of the greater and lesser sphenoid wing. The orbital content is displaced medially with a malleable retractor, providing space for the endoscopic tip and the surgical instruments. Under endoscopic visualization, the lateral orbital wall is exposed until the inferior and then the superior orbital fissures are encountered. The lateral orbital wall is widely drilled until the fascia of the temporalis muscle is exposed laterally in the temporal fossa to gain an adequate working space to proceed with the dissection deeply. The ventral aspect of the greater sphenoid wing (GSW) is drilled in a lateral-to-medial direction up to the lateral margin of the SOF, exposing the dura mater of the temporal pole.

Sagittal Crest

The sagittal crest is identified during this step of the anatomical dissection. At the end of the GSW drilling, a residual bone crest is frequently left unrecognized. This bony structure can be constantly identified. It is formed by the most medial portion of the GSW where it turns from a coronal to a sagittal plane (Fig. 29.1). Its boundaries are: (1) the base, located at the exit of the foramen rotundum, the anterior edge, that is an imaginary line passing where the GSW turns from a coronal to a sagittal plane; (2) the posterior edge that is free, pointing towards the cavernous sinus. The SC separates the medial temporal dura from the postero-lateral periorbital. It must be completely removed, biting off the apical portion and then drilling the base until the anterior aspect of foramen rotundum, to unlock the "gate" to access the cavernous sinus through an interdural approach.

It is essential to identify the SC to subsequentially separate the meningeal and periostal layers of the cavernous sinus and expose its lateral wall.

Mid-subtemporal Ridge

Drilling the ventral aspect of GSW exposes the temporal dura and allows the MCF to accede. During this step, the middle cranial fossa floor and the midtemporal ridge must be drilled and flattened to obtain a straight working space from the transorbital access, allowing the elevation of the temporal lobe and exposing the floor of the MCF. The mid-subtemporal ridge is a bone prominence located just lateral from the foramen rotundum, in the place in which the GSW turns downward to form the floor of the MCF (Figs. 29.2 and 29.3). It is essential to flatten the mid-subtemporal ridge to gain adequate working space and work inside the MC, considering the supero-inferior orientation of the SETOA, acceding the orbit from the superior eyelid, and pointing toward the MCF floor (Fig. 29.4).

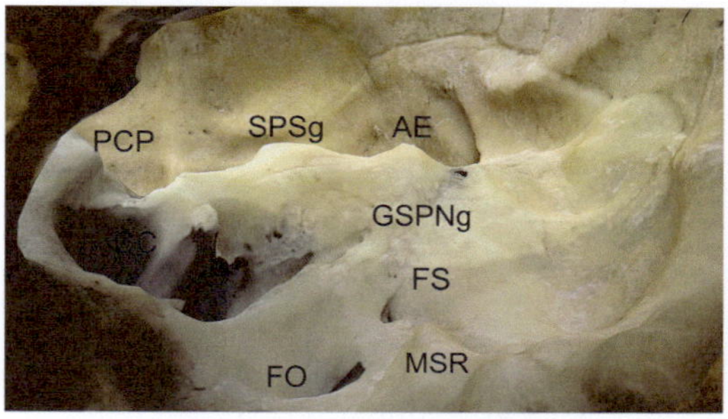

Fig. 29.3 Transorbital perspective of the bone anatomy of the middle fossa; left side. *AE* arcuate eminence, *CC* carotid canal, *FS* foramen spinosum, *GSPNg* greater superficial petrosal nerve groove, *MSR* mid-subtemporal ridge, *PCP* posterior clinoid process, *SPSg* superior petrosal sinus groove

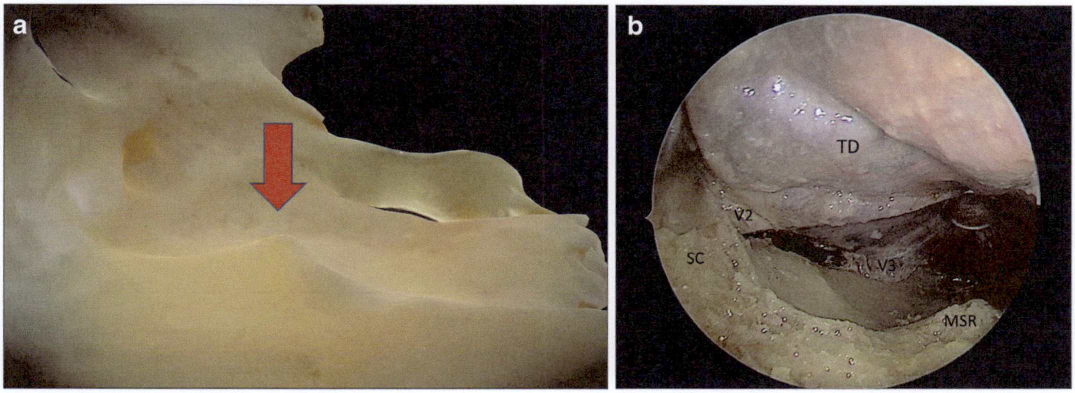

Fig. 29.4 (**a**) Mid-subtemporal ridge left side—bone anatomy middle fossa; red arrow indicating the position of the MRS. (**b**) Endoscopic transorbital perspective—left side. *MRS* mid-subtemporal ridge, *SC* sagittal crest, *TD* temporal dura, *V2* maxillary nerve, *V3* mandibulary nerve

Understanding and recognizing these "key anatomical landmarks" is fundamental for performing the SETOA.

References

1. Moe KS, Bergeron CM, Ellenbogen RG. Transorbital neuroendoscopic surgery. Neurosurgery. 2010;67:16–28.
2. Jeon C, Hong C-K, Woo KI, Hong SD, Nam D-H, Lee J-I, Choi JW, Seol HJ, Kong D-S. Endoscopic transorbital surgery for Meckel's cave and middle cranial fossa tumors: surgical technique and early results. J Neurosurg. 2018;131(4):1126–35.
3. Kong D-S, Kim YH, Hong C-K. Optimal indications and limitations of endoscopic transorbital superior eyelid surgery for spheno-orbital meningiomas. J Neurosurg. 2020;134(5):1472–9.
4. Almeida JP, Omay SB, Shetty SR, Chen Y-N, Ruiz-Treviño AS, Liang B, Anand VK, Levine B, Schwartz TH. Transorbital endoscopic eyelid approach for resection of sphenoorbital meningiomas with predominant hyperostosis: report of 2 cases. J Neurosurg. 2018;128:1885–95.
5. Dallan I, Castelnuovo P, Turri-Zanoni M, Fiacchini G, Locatelli D, Battaglia P, Sellari-Franceschini S. Transorbital endoscopic assisted management of intraorbital lesions: lessons learned from our first 9 cases. Rhinology. 2016;54:247–53.
6. Dallan I, Di Somma A, Prats-Galino A, Solari D, Alobid I, Turri-Zanoni M, Fiacchini G, Castelnuovo P, Catapano G, de Notaris M. Endoscopic transorbital route to the cavernous sinus through the meningo-orbital band: a descriptive anatomical study. J Neurosurg. 2017;127:622–9.
7. Di Somma A, Andaluz N, Cavallo LM, et al. Endoscopic transorbital superior eyelid approach: anatomical study from a neurosurgical perspective. J Neurosurg. 2018;129:1203–16.
8. Dallan I, Castelnuovo P, Locatelli D, Turri-Zanoni M, AlQahtani A, Battaglia P, Hirt B, Sellari-Franceschini S. Multiportal combined transorbital transnasal endoscopic approach for the management of selected skull base lesions: preliminary experience. World Neurosurg. 2015;84:97–107.
9. Di Somma A, Langdon C, de Notaris M, Reyes L, Ortiz-Perez S, Alobid I, Enseñat J. Combined and simultaneous endoscopic endonasal and transorbital surgery for a Meckel's cave schwannoma: technical nuances of a mini-invasive, multiportal approach. J Neurosurg. 2020;134(6):1836–45.
10. Park HH, Hong SD, Kim YH, Hong C-K, Woo KI, Yun I-S, Kong D-S. Endoscopic transorbital and endonasal approach for trigeminal schwannomas: a retrospective multicenter analysis (KOSEN-005). J Neurosurg. 2019;133(2):467–76.
11. Corrivetti F, de Notaris M, Di Somma A, Dallan I, Enseñat J, Topczewski T, Solari D, Cavallo LM, Cappabianca P, Prats-Galino A. "Sagittal crest": definition, stepwise dissection, and clinical implications from a transorbital perspective. Oper Neurosurg. 2022;22(5):e206–12. https://doi.org/10.1227/ONS.0000000000000131.

Lateral Orbital Rim Osteotomy

30

Ju Hyung Moon, Kyoung Su Sung, and Jaejoon Lim

The endoscopic transorbital approach (ETOA) through the lateral orbital corridor has become increasingly popular for anterior and middle cranial fossa lesions. Initially, ETOA was primarily used to remove lesions in the orbit and middle cranial fossa [1–3]. However, following successful clinical outcomes from early studies, its indications have expanded to include lesions in the cavernous sinus, anterior clinoid process, petrous apex, posterior fossa, infratemporal fossa, insula, and central skull base [4–11].

Despite its advantages, ETOA has several limitations that need to be overcome for safe and effective application in regions beyond the orbit and middle cranial fossa. The surgical entry site is small, and the working corridor is narrow constrained by the surrounding orbital rim and orbital contents. Retraction of the orbital contents can widen the surgical space, but this retraction should be limited to <15 mm to avoid increasing intraocular pressure [12]. Such a narrow working space can also impede the angle of attack and surgical freedom when approaching deeper surgical targets. Additionally, retraction and manipulation in the narrow working space can increase the risk of injury to the orbital contents. The crowding of surgical instruments further limits maneuverability, making it challenging to perform fine surgical dissection and bleeding control, which can hinder its use in complex skull base lesions.

To overcome this limitation, the lateral orbital rim (LOR) osteotomy can be performed as a modification of the ETOA procedure. Widening the entry site (by temporarily removing the LOR) can have significant advantages in endoscopic surgery, which by its nature involves a long working distance from the entry to the surgical target. The larger entry site can increase the angle of attack to the target site and can maximize the exposure of deep surgical targets afforded by ETOA. More space allows for enhanced surgical freedom by improving instrument maneuverability [13]. Removal of the LOR also significantly reduces the need for retraction of orbital contents and prevents injury to the globe. The addition of a LOR osteotomy creates a larger working corridor, which can improve the flow and ease of the surgical procedure and the outcome of ETOA.

J. H. Moon (✉)
Department of Neurosurgery, Endoscopic Skull Base Center, Severance Hospital, Yonsei University College of Medicine, Seoul, Republic of Korea
e-mail: MJJR80@yuhs.ac

K. S. Sung
Department of Neurosurgery, Dong-A University Hospital, Dong-A University College of Medicine, Busan, Republic of Korea

J. Lim
Department of Neurosurgery, Bundang CHA Medical Center, CHA University College of Medicine, Seongnam, Republic of Korea
e-mail: coolppeng@chamc.co.kr

T. H. Schwartz et al. (eds.), *Endoscopic Transorbital Surgery of the Orbit, Skull Base and Brain*,
https://doi.org/10.1007/978-3-031-59504-2_30

However, the necessity and effects of a LOR osteotomy remain controversial. Several reports have demonstrated that adequate surgical target exposure and acceptable manipulation of the target lesion can be achieved during ETOA without an LOR osteotomy [4, 13, 14]. The excessive tissue dissection and additional bone work involved in a LOR osteotomy have drawbacks, namely prolonged operative time and the need for orbital rim reconstruction, which may result in poor cosmetic outcomes. Therefore, LOR osteotomy should be reserved for selected cases, such as large tumors or lesions that extend beyond the orbit and middle cranial fossa and require more extensive manipulation. With anatomical knowledge and meticulous surgical technique, a LOR osteotomy can augment an ETOA without any functional or cosmetic compromise.

Operative Technique

A skin incision is made in the superior eyelid crease that extends toward the lateral canthus. To expose the LOR, the incision is extended laterally 1.5 cm from the lateral canthus to the outermost edge of the LOR. If more vertical retraction is required, the incision can be extended up to 2.4 cm from the lateral canthus without risking damage to the frontalis nerve [15]. Alternatively, an incision from the lateral canthus extending laterally along a natural fold can similarly expose the LOR. The skin incision can also originate at the eyebrow and curve down inferolaterally along the LOR to facilitate access to the superior orbital rim (Fig. 30.1a). The skin incision should be undermined laterally to expose the periosteum of the LOR. A vertical incision of the periosteum is

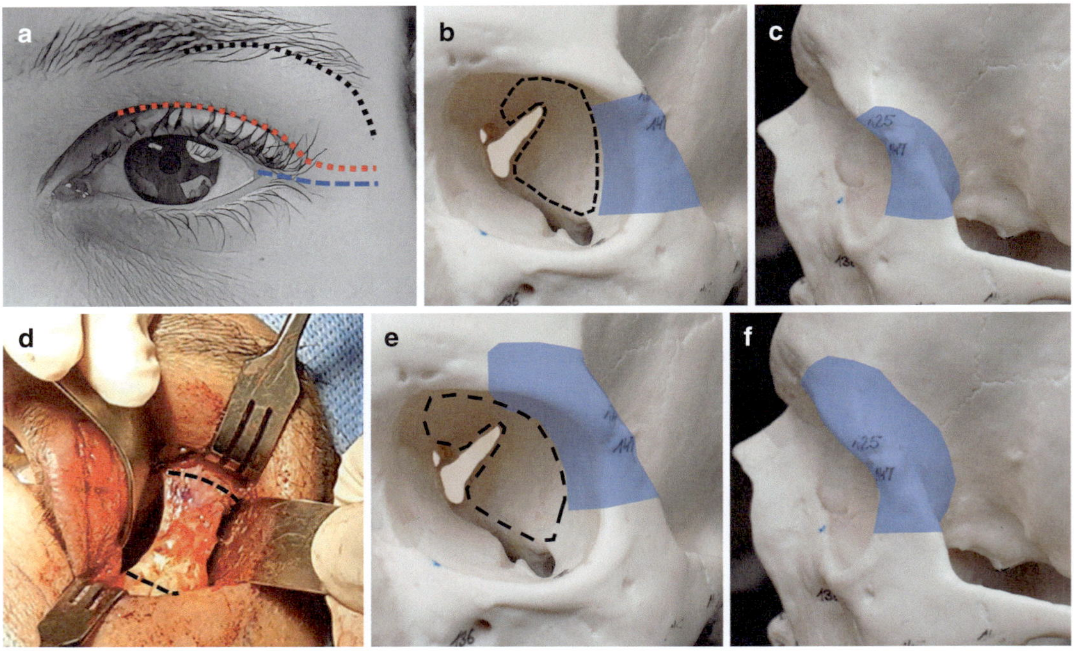

Fig. 30.1 (**a**) Illustration of skin incisions. Superior eyelid crease incision (red dotted line); Lateral canthotomy incision (blue dotted line); Eyebrow incision (black dotted line). (**b**, **c**) Illustration of LOR osteotomy of a left-sided ETOA. Intraorbital portion of the lesser and greater wing of the sphenoid that would be removed after LOR osteotomy (dashed line). (**d**) Intraoperative photograph of left-sided LOR osteotomy. Location of superior and inferior cuts of LOR (dashed line). (**e**, **f**) Illustration of SLOR osteotomy of a left-sided ETOA. Intraorbital portion of the lesser and greater wing of the sphenoid that would be removed after SLOR osteotomy (dashed line)

made at the apex of the LOR, exposing the bony orbital rim and the frontozygomatic suture. The temporalis muscle is then dissected subperiosteally and detached from the lateral orbit through to the inferior orbital fissure. The superior aspect of the zygomatic arch is approximately level with the orbital floor and the anterolateral aspect of the inferior orbital fissure. The periorbita of the lateral orbital wall is dissected from the bone with a blunt elevation of the periosteum up to the superior and inferior orbital fissures. Then, two axial cuts are then made in the LOR using a drill saw. The inferior cut is made at the level of the junction of the frontal process and the body of the zygomatic bone, which connects to the inferior orbital fissure. The inferior orbital fissure is identified in the temporal fossa with a blunt hook, and its anterolateral limit marks the site of the bone cut in the lateral orbit. The superior cut is made just above the level of the frontozygomatic suture. A posterior cut of the lateral orbital wall is made by drilling medially or laterally to combine the superior and inferior cuts. The posterior extent of this cut should approximate the zygomaticosphenoid suture (Fig. 30.1b–d). During drilling, the orbital contents should be retracted medially and protected, and generous irrigation is required to avoid heat transfer to the orbital contents. The orbital bone, including the LOR, can then be outfractured and removed. After the rim is removed, the periorbita is retracted medially, and the temporalis muscle is retracted laterally, exposing the greater and lesser wings of the sphenoid bone along with the orbital roof. To access intracranial lesions, additional bone may be removed posteriorly from the sphenoid wings using a high-speed drill and Kerrison punch (Fig. 30.1b, c).

The extent of orbital rim resection depends on the location of the lesion and can be tailored to the surgical goal. When a higher level of access is required, the superior orbital rim (SOR) can be removed along with the LOR. This procedure is called an "ETOA with superior-lateral orbital rim (SLOR) osteotomy" [11]. In this approach, the eyebrow incision provides more suitable access to the SOR. The superior cut of the orbital rim is made in the SOR medial to the supraorbital foramen to avoid injury to the supraorbital nerve. A McCarty keyhole is performed using a cutting burr to gain access to both the anterior cranial fossa and the orbit, and the dura is freed from the overlying bone through the burr hole. The burr hole is connected to the superior and inferior cuts of the orbital rim using a craniotome. After elevating the periorbita from the orbital roof and lateral orbital wall, a posterior osteotomy is performed by drilling the orbital roof and lateral orbital wall from the orbital side, combining the superior and inferior cuts. The orbital bone, including the SLOR, can then be removed, exposing the greater and lesser sphenoid wings and the frontal dura (Fig. 30.1e, f). The extent of the SLOR osteotomy can be designed to avoid injury to the frontal sinus by using a preoperative computed tomography (CT) scan to visualize the size and degree of pneumatization of the frontal sinus.

The orbital rim bone flap should be meticulously aligned and repositioned and then firmly fixed with low-profile titanium plates to improve the postoperative cosmetic outcome (Fig. 30.2). The skin incision should be closed with fine sutures in a single layer to minimize the postoperative scar.

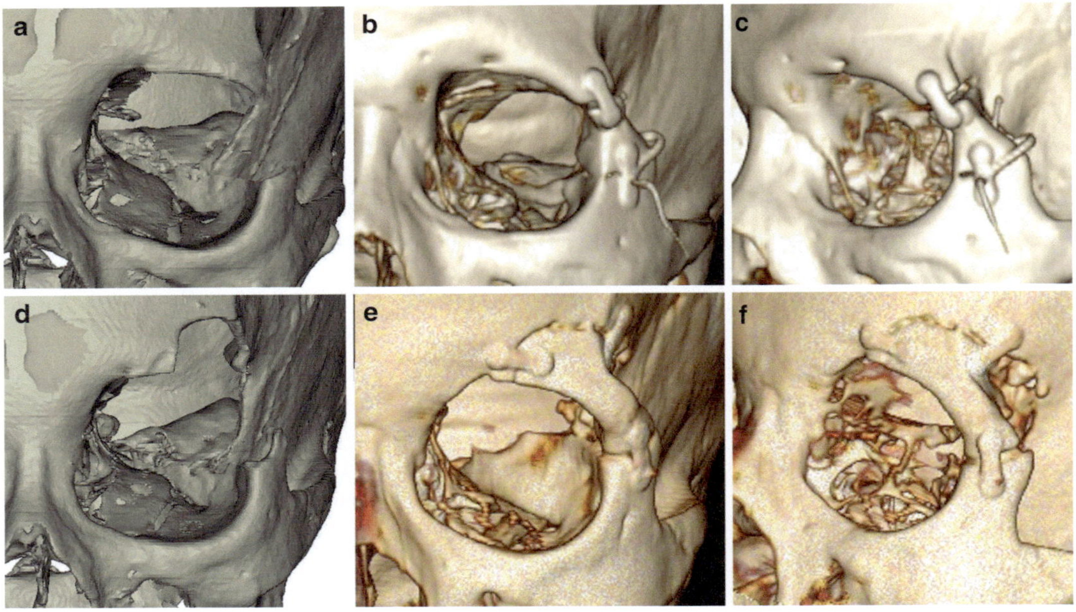

Fig. 30.2 3D computed tomography (CT) rendering showing bone removal and reconstruction. (**a**) Left-sided ETOA with LOR osteotomy. (**b**, **c**) Reconstruction using miniplates after ETOA with LOR osteotomy. (**d**) Left-sided ETOA with SLOR osteotomy. (**e**, **f**) Reconstruction using miniplates after ETOA with SLOR osteotomy

Comparison of the ETOA with and without Orbital Rim Osteotomy

ETOA combined with LOR osteotomy or SLOR osteotomy can increase the area of exposure and angle of attack to the surgical target, which provides more surgical freedom than ETOA with LOR preservation [6, 11, 13]. It can not only expand the indications for the ETOA but also improve the maneuverability of surgical instruments and reduce orbital retraction. However, an orbital rim osteotomy procedure may be more invasive and destructive, and potential difficulties in reconstruction may increase the likelihood of postoperative cosmetic problems (Table 30.1). Therefore, ETOA with orbital rim osteotomy is recommended for select cases that would significantly benefit from it.

Table 30.1 Comparison of the ETOA with and without orbital rim osteotomy

	ETOA	ETOA with LOR osteotomy	ETOA with SLOR osteotomy
Invasiveness	+	++	+++
Surgical freedom and angle of attack (horizontal)	+	+++	+++
Surgical freedom and angle of attack (vertical)	+	+	+++
Instrument maneuverability	+	++	+++
Orbital retraction	+++	+	+
Simplicity of reconstruction	+++	++	+
Probability of cosmetic problem	+	++	+++

ETOA endoscopic transorbital approach, *LOR* lateral orbital rim, *SLOR* superior-lateral orbital rim

References

1. Moe KS, Bergeron CM, Ellenbogen RG. Transorbital neuroendoscopic surgery. Neurosurgery. 2010;67(3):16–28. https://doi.org/10.1227/01.NEU.0000373431.08464.43.
2. Dallan I, Sellari-Franceschini S, Turri-Zanoni M, de Notaris M, Fiacchini G, Fiorini FR, et al. Endoscopic transorbital superior eyelid approach for the management of selected spheno-orbital meningiomas: preliminary experience. Oper Neurosurg. 2018;14(3):243–51. https://doi.org/10.1093/ons/opx100.
3. Kong DS, Young SM, Hong CK, Kim YD, Hong SD, Choi JW, et al. Clinical and ophthalmological outcome of endoscopic transorbital surgery for cranioorbital tumors. J Neurosurg. 2018;131(3):667–75. https://doi.org/10.3171/2018.3.JNS173233.
4. Jeon C, Hong CK, Woo KI, Hong SD, Nam DH, Lee JI, et al. Endoscopic transorbital surgery for Meckel's cave and middle cranial fossa tumors: surgical technique and early results. J Neurosurg. 2019;131:1126–35. https://doi.org/10.3171/2018.6.JNS181099.
5. Lopez CB, Di Somma A, Cepeda S, Arrese I, Sarabia R, Agustin JH, et al. Extradural anterior clinoidectomy through endoscopic transorbital approach: laboratory investigation for surgical perspective. Acta Neurochir. 2021;163(8):2177–88. https://doi.org/10.1007/s00701-021-04896-y.
6. Lim J, Sung KS, Yoo J, Oh J, Moon JH. Endoscopic transorbital extradural anterior clinoidectomy: a stepwise surgical technique and case series study [SevEN-013]. Front Oncol. 2022;12:991065. https://doi.org/10.3389/fonc.2022.991065.
7. Di Somma A, Andaluz N, Cavallo LM, Topczewski TE, Frio F, Gerardi RM, et al. Endoscopic transorbital route to the petrous apex: a feasibility anatomic study. Acta Neurochir. 2018;160(4):707–20. https://doi.org/10.1007/s00701-017-3448-x.
8. Noiphithak R, Yanez-Siller JC, Revuelta Barbero JM, Otto BA, Carrau RL, Prevedello DM. Quantitative analysis of the surgical exposure and surgical freedom between transcranial and transorbital endoscopic anterior petrosectomies to the posterior fossa. J Neurosurg. 2018;131(2):569–77. https://doi.org/10.3171/2018.2.JNS172334.
9. Gerges MM, Godil SS, Younus I, Rezk M, Schwartz TH. Endoscopic transorbital approach to the infratemporal fossa and parapharyngeal space: a cadaveric study. J Neurosurg. 2019;133:1948–59. https://doi.org/10.3171/2019.7.JNS191743.
10. Kim EH, Yoo J, Jung IH, Oh JW, Kim JS, Yoon JS, et al. Endoscopic transorbital approach to the insular region: cadaveric feasibility study and clinical application (SevEN-005). J Neurosurg. 2021;135:1164–72. https://doi.org/10.3171/2020.8.JNS202255.
11. Lim J, Sung KS, Kim W, Yoo J, Jung IH, Choi S, et al. Extended endoscopic transorbital approach with superior-lateral orbital rim osteotomy: cadaveric feasibility study and clinical implications (SevEN-007). J Neurosurg. 2021;137:18–31. https://doi.org/10.3171/2021.7.JNS21996.
12. Kim W, Moon JH, Kim EH, Hong CK, Han J, Hong JB. Optimization of orbital retraction during endoscopic transorbital approach via quantitative measurement of the intraocular pressure - [SevEN 006]. BMC Ophthalmol. 2021;21(1):76. https://doi.org/10.1186/s12886-021-01834-5.
13. Noiphithak R, Yanez-Siller JC, Revuelta Barbero JM, Otto BA, Carrau RL, Prevedello DM. Comparative analysis between lateral orbital rim preservation and osteotomy for transorbital endoscopic approaches to the cavernous sinus: an anatomic study. Oper Neurosurg. 2019;16(1):86–93. https://doi.org/10.1093/ons/opy054.
14. Dallan I, Di Somma A, Prats-Galino A, Solari D, Alobid I, Turri-Zanoni M, et al. Endoscopic transorbital route to the cavernous sinus through the meningo-orbital band: a descriptive anatomical study. J Neurosurg. 2017;127(3):622–9. https://doi.org/10.3171/2016.8.JNS16465.
15. Chabot JD, Gardner PA, Stefko ST, Zwagerman NT, Fernandez-Miranda JC. Lateral orbitotomy approach for lesions involving the middle fossa: a retrospective review of thirteen patients. Neurosurgery. 2017;80(2):309–22. https://doi.org/10.1093/neuros/nyw045.

Harvesting a Pericranial Flap

31

Edoardo Porto, J. Manuel Revuelta Barbero, Justin Maldonado, Alejandra Rodas, C. Arturo Solares, and Gustavo Pradilla

Abbreviations

ASB Anterior skull base
NSF Nasoseptal flap
PCF Pericranial flap

Introduction

A variety of extranasal pedicled flaps have been devised and explored for skull base reconstruction. Among these, the pericranial flap (PCF) for anterior skull base (ASB) defects and the temporoparietal fascia flap for posterior and lateral defects are the techniques most widely adopted [1, 2]. The PCF is a versatile and robust pedicled graft for skull base reconstruction that can be used in open and endoscopic procedures when a nasoseptal flap (NSF) is unavailable due to prior endonasal surgery, sinonasal malignancy, or as a second-line repair strategy ascending the *reconstructive ladder* [3].

The PCF's vascular pedicle depends on deep branches of the supraorbital and supratrochlear vessels. As such, it is a good option for the repair of the anterior ethmoid and cribiform defects [4, 5]. This flap includes the calvarial periosteum and the overlying associated areolar tissue (also called *subgaleal fascia*) and can be raised via a traditional bicoronal approach or in an endoscopic-assisted, minimally invasive manner using three small incisions. [6]. In addition, the endoscopic transorbital approach has been recently reported [7]. The pericranial flap has the relative advantages of being technically easy to dissect and raise, reliable, and having minimal cosmetic consequence and morbidity [8, 9].

The adequate length for PCFs to reconstruct defects along the sagittal plane, with a low risk of CSF leak, has been determined to be 11–12.5 cm for anterior skull base defects, 14–15.5 cm for sellar defects, and 18.50–20.5 cm for clival defects [10]. Although the PCF has been considered a technique to repair exclusively ASB defects, evidence supports its use for reconstruction of caudal defects extending to the clivus [8]. Gode et al. recently examined seven patients with large clival defects who had failed previous primary CSF leak reconstruction attempts [8]. Neither nasoseptal nor inferior turbinate flaps

E. Porto · J. M. Revuelta Barbero · J. Maldonado
G. Pradilla (✉)
Department of Neurosurgery, School of Medicine, Emory University, Atlanta, GA, USA
e-mail: eporto@emory.edu; jmrevuelta@emory.edu; jmald23@emory.edu; gpradil@emory.edu

A. Rodas · C. A. Solares
Department of Otolaryngology, School of Medicine, Emory University, Atlanta, GA, USA
e-mail: mayrarodas@ufm.edu; clementino.arturo.solares@emory.edu

T. H. Schwartz et al. (eds.), *Endoscopic Transorbital Surgery of the Orbit, Skull Base and Brain*,
https://doi.org/10.1007/978-3-031-59504-2_31

were available options for repair. The success of secondary repair with a PCF reported was 58%, suggesting that it may be a viable option in patients with clival defects who have had local flap failure.

Transcranial "Open" Technique

A bicoronal or a lateral fronto-temporal incision is performed, and elevation proceeds along the subgaleal plane (Fig. 31.1a, b). The periosteum is

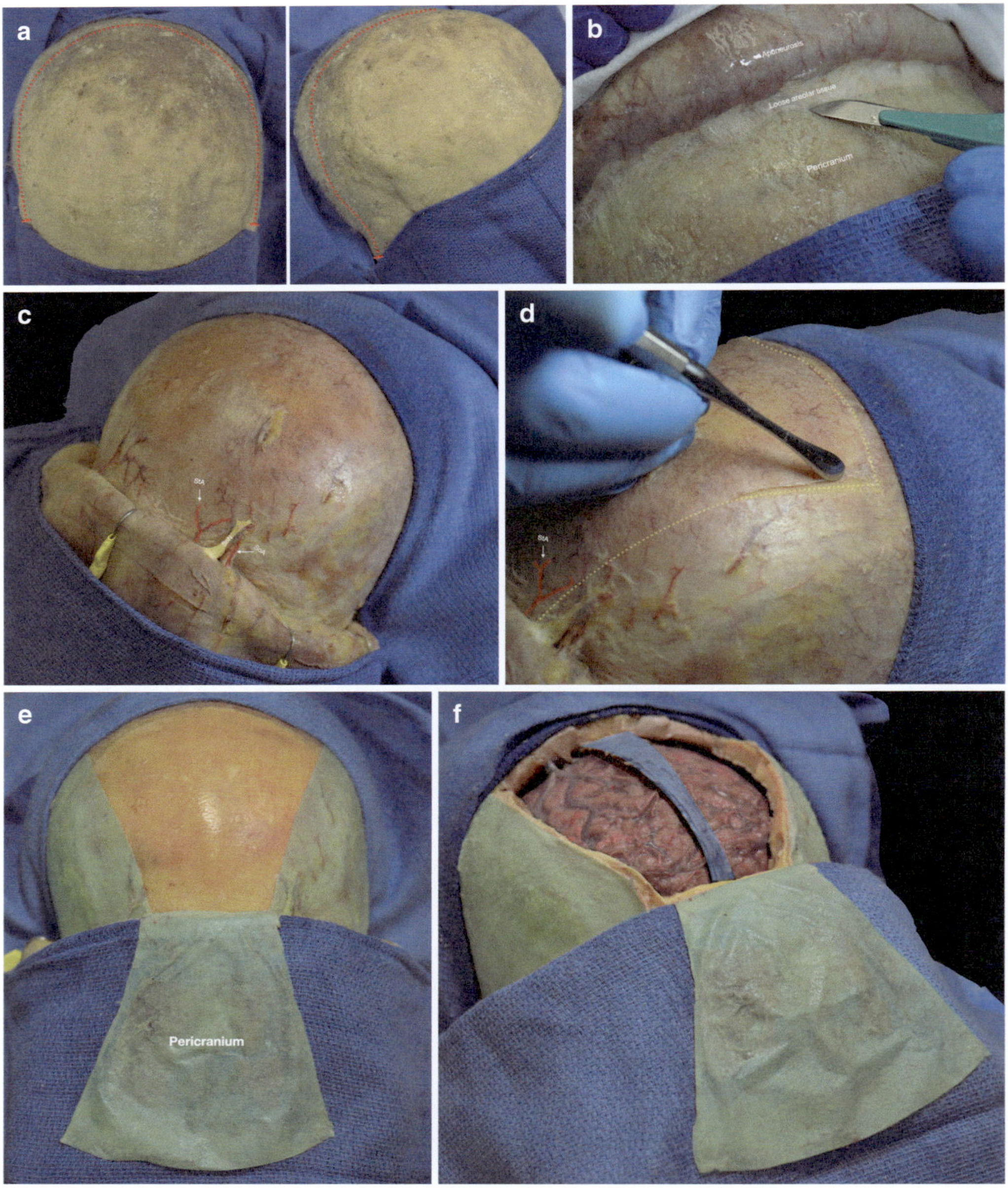

Fig. 31.1 Cadaveric dissection showing (**a**). The landmarks for a bicoronal incision, (**b**). The dissection plane to isolate the pericranium during a bicoronal approach, (**c**) the bilateral exposition of the supratrochlear (StA) and supraorbital arteries (SoA) and nerve (SoN), (**d**) the elevation of the PCF using an open technique, (**e**) the caudal rotation of the harvested PCF, (**f**) a bifrontal craniotomy and durotomy with preservation of the superior sagittal sinus, (**g**) the retraction of the frontal lobes to expose the olfactory bulbs, cribriform plates, crista galli (CG), frontal sinuses (FS) and (**h**) the apposition of the PCF on the ASB

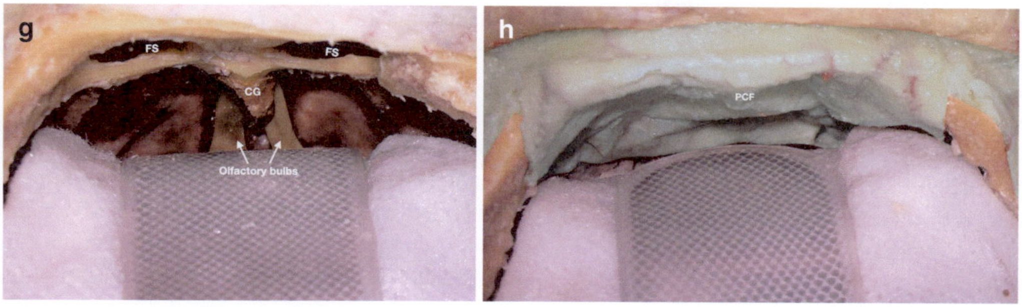

Fig. 31.1 (continued)

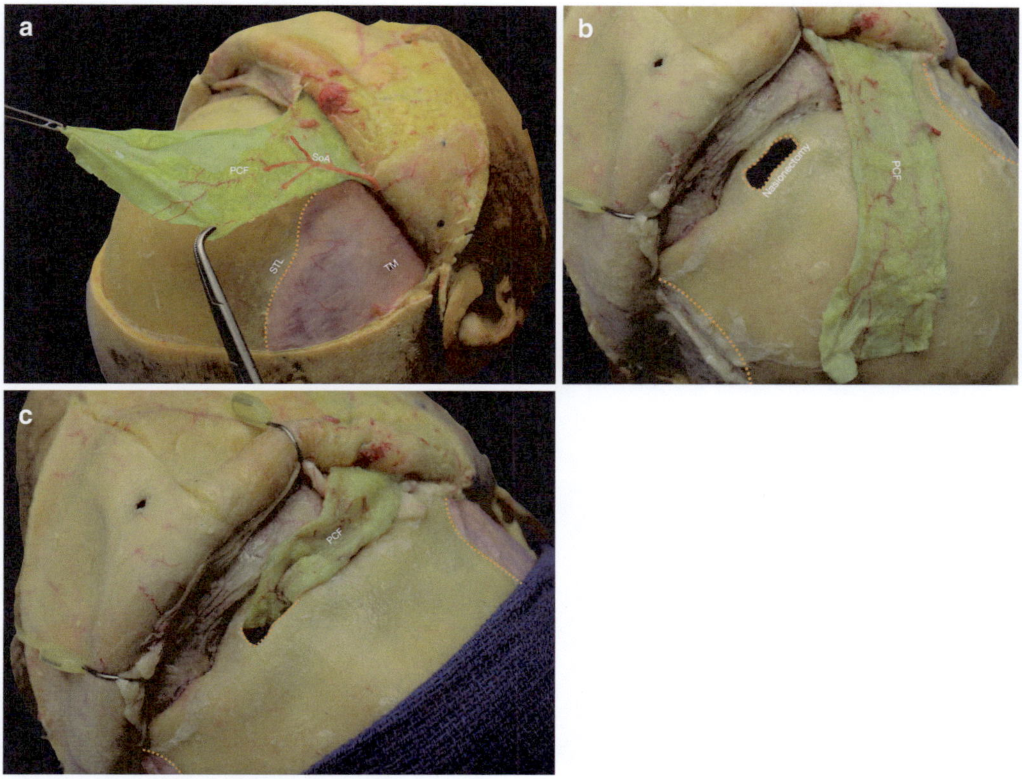

Fig. 31.2 Cadaveric dissection showing (**a**) a right-sided pedicled pericranial flap, (**b**) the drilling of the nasion to access the ASB through the frontal sinus and (**c**) the inset of the pericranial flap. *PCF* pericranial flap, *SoA* supraorbital artery, *STL* superior temporal line, *TM* temporal muscle

transected on its lateral edges at the superior attachment of the temporalis muscle bilaterally. The posterior incision can be made at the same point as the coronal incision or extended posteriorly if greater length is needed. To improve rotation, two flaps can be created. To reduce the overall size, the flap can be pedicled and supplied by the vessels of a single side [5] (Fig. 31.1c–e).

If a bilateral subfrontal craniotomy is performed and an intracranial defect of the ASB must be repaired, the flap can be directly introduced by elevating the periosteal layer of the dura mater of the ASB (Fig. 31.1f–h). Otherwise, a nasionectomy is performed to introduce this pedicled flap into the nasal cavity through the frontal sinus [4] (Fig. 31.2a–c).

Endoscopic Endonasal Technique

During the preoperative setup, the scalp should be prepped in alignment with a coronal incision for the possibility of a rescue open PCF harvesting procedure. A 2-cm midline incision is planned along with a 1-cm lateral port incision. If necessary, the supraorbital and supratrochlear arteries can be identified by Doppler ultrasound. A 1-cm horizontal glabellar incision is marked in a natural skin crease to obtain access to the nasion at a later stage (Fig. 31.3a). With the surgeon seated at the vertex of the patient and with an assistant holding retractors, an endoscopic dissection of the subgaleal plane is performed through both incisions towards the orbital rims. Subgaleal dissection posterior to the coronal plane of the incisions may also be performed to extend the length of the pericranial flap if necessary. A needle tip cautery with the tip bent at 90 degrees is recommended to incise the pericranium under direct endoscopic visualization. The PCF is then gently elevated from the cranium to preserve its integrity. The dissection is carried from posterior to anterior, narrowing down to 3 cm at the pedicle (Fig. 31.3b). Next, a 1-cm transverse glabellar incision is made in a natural skin crease and a needle-tip cautery is used to dissect down to the

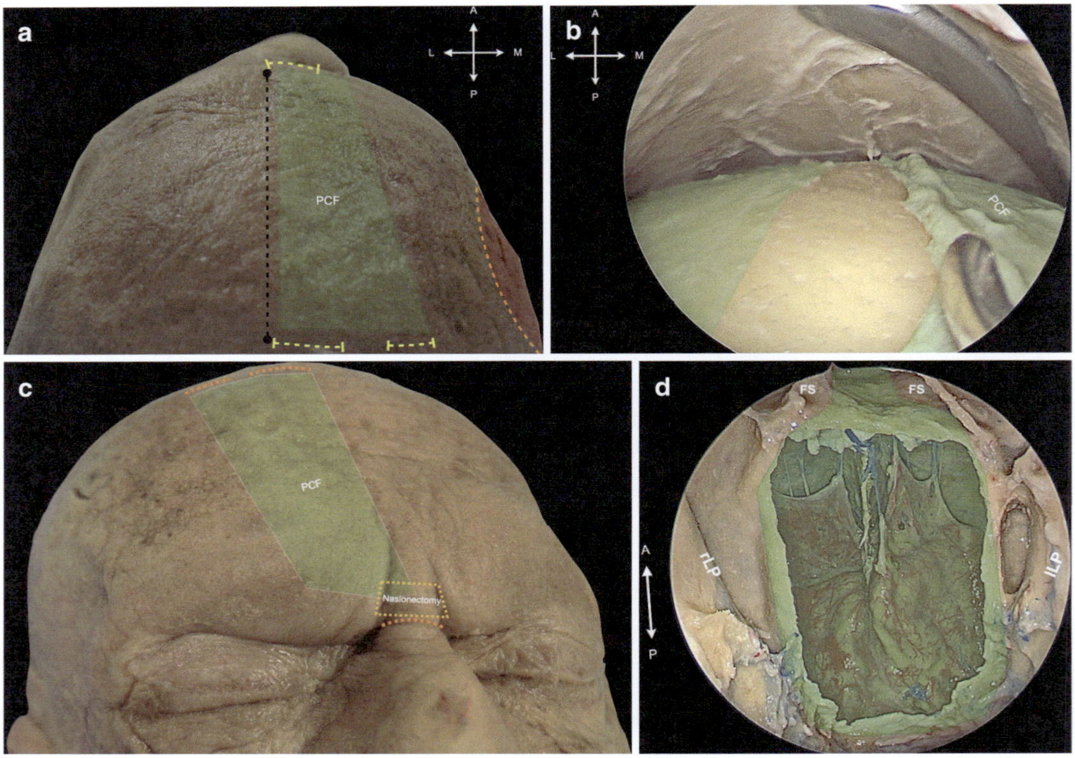

Fig. 31.3 (**a**) Schematic illustration of the PCF endoscopic harvesting technique. (**b**) Cadaveric dissection showing endoscopic elevation of the PCF from the calvaria. (**c**) Schematic illustration of the location of the nasionectomy, in yellow, and the incision, in orange, that can be performed in a natural skin crease to expose the nasion. (**d**) Cadaveric dissection showing a transcribriform approach and an ASB defect. The green shadow illustrates the position of the PCF and its pedicle coming from the frontal sinus (FS). *rLP* right lamina papyracea, *lLp* left lamina papyracea

periosteum of the nasion. This subperiosteal plane is dissected superiorly until it communicates with the subperiosteal plane of the flap dissection over the frontal bone. A 3-mm coarse diamond bur is used to drill the bone at the level of the nasion to create a defect measuring 1.5 cm. The resultant bone defect is analogous to the nasal osteotomy on a standard subfrontal approach (supraorbital osteotomy) (Fig. 31.3c). The PCF is then transposed through the glabellar incision under endoscopic visualization to prevent torsion of the vascular pedicle. The PCF is passed through the nasion bone defect and into the endonasal surgical field under endoscopic endonasal visualization. The PCF is gently flattened to cover dural edges and surrounding bone edges as an extradural extracranial onlay (Fig. 31.3d) [6].

Endoscopic Transorbital Technique

This approach is divided into an orbitonasal stage and a cranial stage [7].

Orbitonasal Stage The location of the supratrochlear and supraorbital notch or foramen can be identified with neuronavigation assistance. A transorbital superior eyelid approach is performed (Fig. 31.4a). An incision superficial to the levator aponeurosis is performed, and dissection along the avascular plane is carried out until the orbital rim is exposed (Fig. 31.4b). Subsequently, the supratrochlear and supraorbital notch or foramen and their respective arteries are identified (Fig. 31.4c). At this point in the dissection, there are two possible options in relation to the main vascular pedicle and the desired flap size: (1) Standard approach: the vascular pedicle is supplied by the supratrochlear artery only which is exposed after subgaleal dissection under the loose areolar tissue plane and extending 1.5 cm cranially from the orbital rim and 0.5 cm medial to the supraorbital artery. (2) Extended approach: the supratrochlear and supraorbital arteries comprise the vascular pedicle. In this scenario, the flap is extended 0.5 cm lateral to the supraorbital artery (Fig. 31.4d).

Cranial stage Two 2.5 cm incisions are performed along the coronal suture or further posterior, depending on the defect size. The first incision is performed medially with 2.5 cm of lateral extension. The second incision is made more laterally, with 2.5 cm of medial extension from the superior temporal line. At this stage, both incisions can be used interchangeably as the endoscopic and working channel access points. Using the first incision, subgaleal dissection under the loose areolar tissue plane is carried out in a dorso-ventral direction (toward the flap pedicle) connecting with the transorbital dissection. Second, subperiosteal dissection following the same trajectory is performed to free the flap. The periosteum is then incised along the midline under endoscopic view, starting from the posterior extent of the flap to the most anterior point. Subsequently, a lateral incision is made from the orbital segment (to allow for better visualization and control of the flap pedicle) with a posterior trajectory. Posteriorly, an incision made parallel to the coronal suture connecting both sagittal incisions must be performed to release, maintaining tethering solely by its vascular pedicle. At this point, the PCF can be extracted anteriorly through the superior eyelid incision (Fig. 31.4e). After resecting the posteromedial orbital wall fascial sheath, a 0.5-cm medial orbitotomy is created immediately below and anterior to the frontoethmoidal and sphenoethmoidal sutures, respectively (Fig. 31.4f). Finally, the pericranial flap is transposed through the medial orbitotomy into the nasal cavity and inset with the superficial surface of the flap in contact with the brain over the previously created anterior skull base defect (Fig. 31.4g).

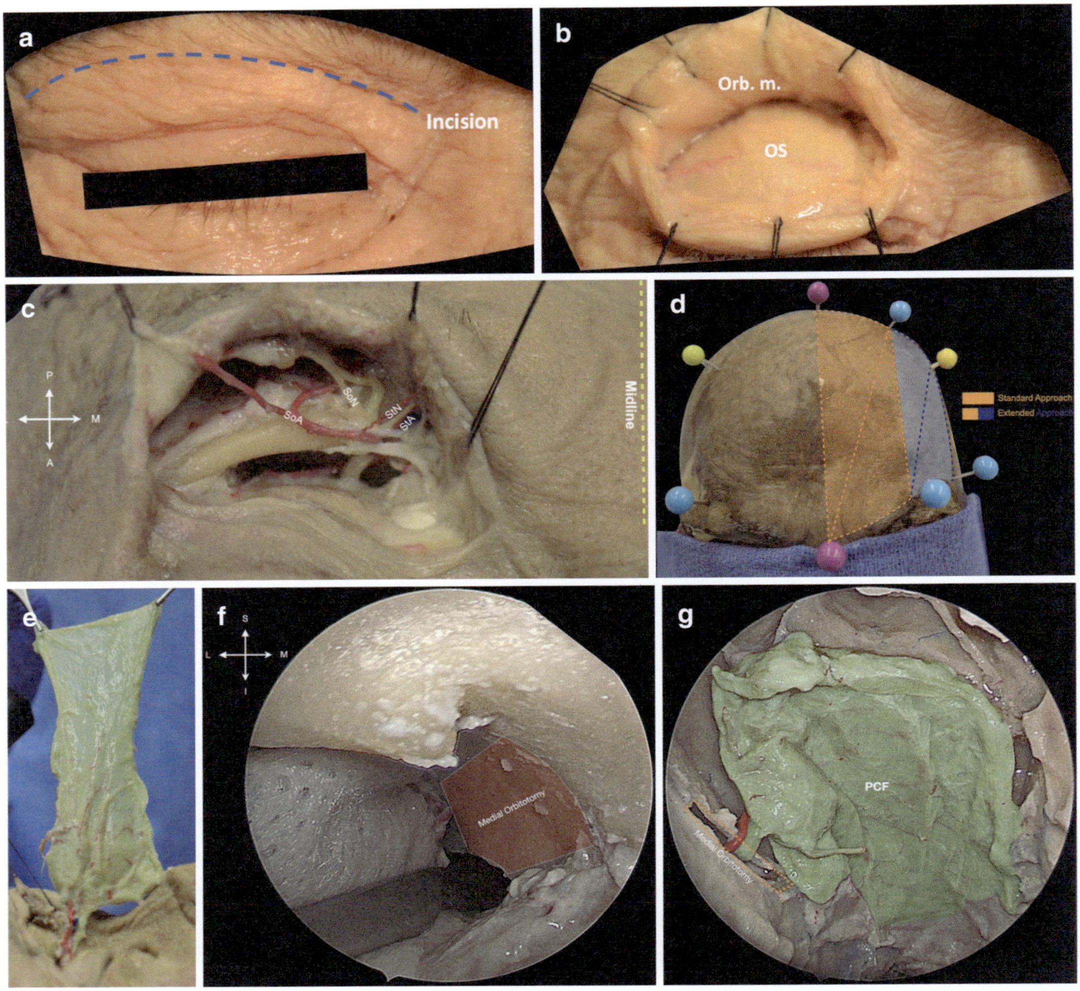

Fig. 31.4 Cadaveric dissection showing (**a**). The location of the skin incision for a transorbital superior eyelid approach (blue). (**b**) The orbitalis muscle (Orb. m.) and the orbital septum (OS) guide the dissection towards the orbital rim. (**c**) The orbital rim, along with the supraorbital artery (SoA), the supraorbital nerve (SoN), the supratrochlear artery (StA), and nerve (StN) are exposed. (**d**) Schematic illustration showing the alternatives for transorbital PCF harvesting and routing: standard approach, in orange, and extended approach (orange + blue). (**e**) Cadaveric illustration showing the extraction of the PCF through the superior eyelid incision. (**f**) Location of the medial orbitotomy to access the nasal cavity for routing of the PCF. (**g**) The PCF is routed through the medial orbitotomy and placed on the transcribriform defect

References

1. Price JC, Loury M, Carson B, Johns ME. The pericranial flap for reconstruction of anterior skull base defects. Laryngoscope. 1988;98(11):1159–64. https://doi.org/10.1288/00005537-198811000-00002.
2. Stow NW, Gordon DH, Eisenberg R. Technique of temporoparietal fascia flap in ear and lateral skull base surgery. Otol Neurotol. 2010;31(6):964–7. https://doi.org/10.1097/MAO.0b013e3181e3d33c.
3. Patel MR, Stadler ME, Snyderman CH, Carrau RL, Kassam AB, Germanwala AV, et al. How to choose? Endoscopic skull base reconstructive options and limitations. Skull Base. 2010;20(6):397–404. https://doi.org/10.1055/s-0030-1253573.
4. Gutierrez WR, Bennion DM, Walsh JE, Owen SR. Vascular pedicled flaps for skull base defect

reconstruction. Laryngosc Investig Otolaryngol. 2020;5(6):1029–38. https://doi.org/10.1002/lio2.471.
5. Yoshioka N, Rhoton AL Jr. Vascular anatomy of the anteriorly based pericranial flap. Neurosurgery. 2005;57(1):11–6.; discussion 6. https://doi.org/10.1227/01.neu.0000163477.85087.b1.
6. Zanation AM, Snyderman CH, Carrau RL, Kassam AB, Gardner PA, Prevedello DM. Minimally invasive endoscopic pericranial flap: a new method for endonasal skull base reconstruction. Laryngoscope. 2009;119(1):13–8. https://doi.org/10.1002/lary.20022.
7. Revuelta Barbero JM, Soriano RM, Bray DP, Rindler RS, Henriquez O, Solares CA, et al. The transorbital pericranial flap. World Neurosurg. 2021;152:e241–e9. https://doi.org/10.1016/j.wneu.2021.05.078.
8. Gode S, Lieber S, Nakassa ACI, Wang EW, Fernandez-Miranda JC, Gardner PA, et al. Clinical experience with secondary endoscopic reconstruction of clival defects with extracranial pericranial flaps. J Neurol Surg B Skull Base. 2019;80(3):276–82. https://doi.org/10.1055/s-0038-1668517.
9. Ahmed OH, Zhang K. Reconstruction following endoscopic endonasal skull base surgery: options and technical considerations. Curr Otorhinolaryngol Rep. 2020;8(2):147–53. https://doi.org/10.1007/s40136-020-00276-9.
10. Patel MR, Shah RN, Snyderman CH, Carrau RL, Germanwala AV, Kassam AB, et al. Pericranial flap for endoscopic anterior skull-base reconstruction: clinical outcomes and radioanatomic analysis of preoperative planning. Neurosurgery. 2010;66(3):506–12; discussion 12. https://doi.org/10.1227/01.Neu.0000365620.59677.Ff.

32 Supraorbital Versus Transorbital Keyhole Approaches: Selecting the Right Approach

Evan D. Bander, Kate U. Rosen, Joseph A. Carnevale, and Theodore H. Schwartz

Introduction

A wide range of open transcranial approaches exist to reach pathologies of the anterior and middle cranial fossa. Traditionally, pterional, subfrontal, bifrontal, orbitozygomatic and/or orbitofrontal approaches have been employed with modifications depending on the lesion location and goals of the surgery [1–4]. Open approaches rely on long incisions and extensive craniotomies that facilitate ease of resection and degrees of freedom for instruments [5] but can come at the cost of increased patient pain from temporalis muscle violation, poor cosmetic outcomes, and decreased quality of life relative to more minimally invasive approaches [6]. Furthermore, the wide exposure in these open approaches put larger territories of the exposed brain at risk from retraction, resulting in higher rates of seizure and stroke, with rates of frontal lobe contusions as high as 25% [7–10]. Advances in neurosurgical tools and technologies such as neuro-navigation and endoscopy have increased the efficacy and utilization of keyhole approaches.

Keyhole approaches leverage small incisions and craniotomies that provide the most direct trajectory to the surgical target, minimizing uninvolved brain exposure, decreasing retraction, and avoiding vital neurovascular anatomy. The addition of the endoscope has facilitated keyhole approaches by providing improved illumination with the light source at the depth of the opening, thus widening the visualization available through these small corridors. Keyhole approaches are meant to ease risk and improve comfort for the patient, but they come at the expense of decreased intraoperative flexibility and comfort for the surgeon. As such, keyhole approaches require extensive experience, have steep learning curves, and demand thoughtful case selection. The supraorbital (SOA) and lateral transorbital (LTOA) approaches have gained increasing acceptance as viable minimal access corridors to reach anterior and middle fossa skull base lesions [11–172]. While the technical steps and specifics are described elsewhere, within this chapter, we will describe the vital elements of case selection and relevant complications based on literature review.

E. D. Bander · K. U. Rosen · J. A. Carnevale
Department of Neurosurgery, Weill Cornell Medical College, New York Presbyterian Hospital, New York, NY, USA

T. H. Schwartz (✉)
Department of Neurosurgery, Weill Cornell Medicine, New York–Presbyterian Hospital, New York, NY, USA
e-mail: schwarh@med.cornell.edu

T. H. Schwartz et al. (eds.), *Endoscopic Transorbital Surgery of the Orbit, Skull Base and Brain*,
https://doi.org/10.1007/978-3-031-59504-2_32

Learning Curve and Pathologies

While the SOA and LTOA keyhole approaches are both minimally invasive and require work within or around the orbit (Fig. 32.1a), the SOA approach is primarily a neurosurgical approach with less need for a specialist co-surgeon. The medial anatomic boundary of the supraorbital nerve and frontal sinus as well as craniotomy, including removal of the orbital roof, are all techniques commonly used in open transcranial approaches. The exposure provided by the SOA comprises mostly the anterior cranial fossa. If only a microscope is used, the cribriform plate and crista galli cannot be exposed, but with endoscope assistance, these areas are easily seen (Fig. 32.1b). The additional use of the rigid endoscope and endoscopic instrumentation to improve visualization within the SOA are also well within the neurosurgical repertoire of a surgeon trained in endoscopic endonasal approaches (EEA). As such, the SOA is readily assimilated by neurosurgeons trained in transcranial and endonasal surgery. LTOA, on the other hand, provides a less familiar perspective to neurosurgeons and thus involves a steeper learning curve [173]. The LTOA exposes a different area of the skull base, namely the lesser wing of the sphenoid, the middle fossa, the cavernous sinus, and Meckel's Cave (Fig. 32.1b). The LTOA can also expose regions of the ipsilateral anterior fossa, just above the orbit, which overlaps with the SOA. LTOA generally, although not necessarily, requires a multidisciplinary approach involving a collaboration between neurosurgery and oculoplastic surgery to achieve appropriate cosmetic and orbital outcomes.

A review of the literature on SOA and LTOA was completed with 162 articles fulfilling criteria for review (Fig. 32.2) [11–172]. Given the longer history of the SOA, a wider range of pathologies have been treated compared to the LTOA. Our review identified 4733 SOA cases published in the literature. The most common pathology approached by the SOA was aneurysm cases (n = 2984; 63%) of all reported cases (Fig. 32.3). Anterior cerebral artery (ACA) aneurysms accounted for ~50% of the aneurysm cases, with middle cerebral (MCA) and internal carotid artery (ICA) aneurysms following behind.

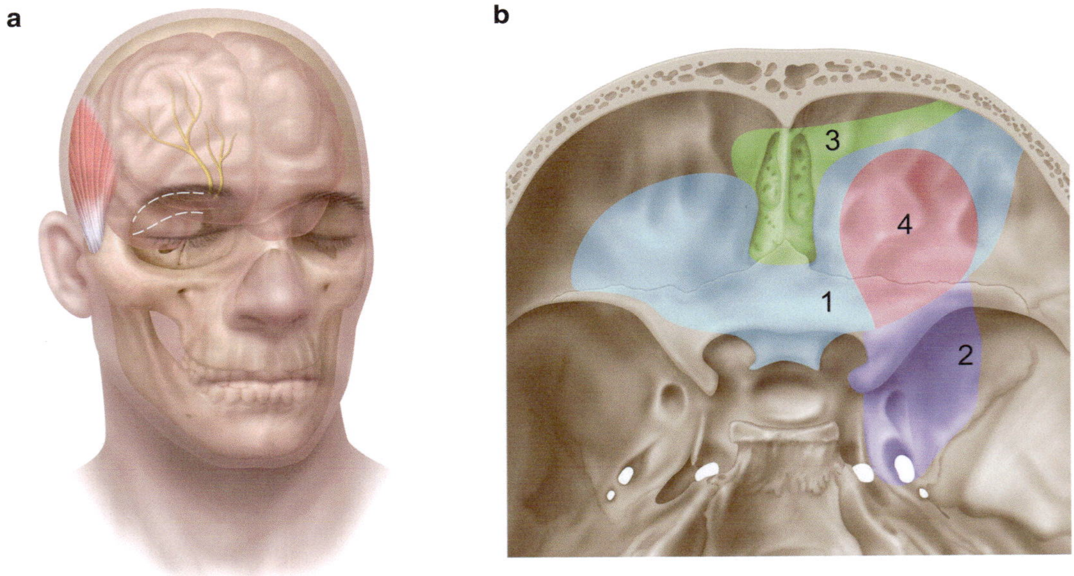

Fig. 32.1 (**a**) Supraorbital incision within the eyebrow (upper dotted line) and the lateral transorbital incision in the superior eyelid crease (lower dotted line). (**b**) Regions of the skull base exposed by (1) SOA; (2) LTOA; or (3) SOA with endoscopic assistance (4) SOA and LTOA

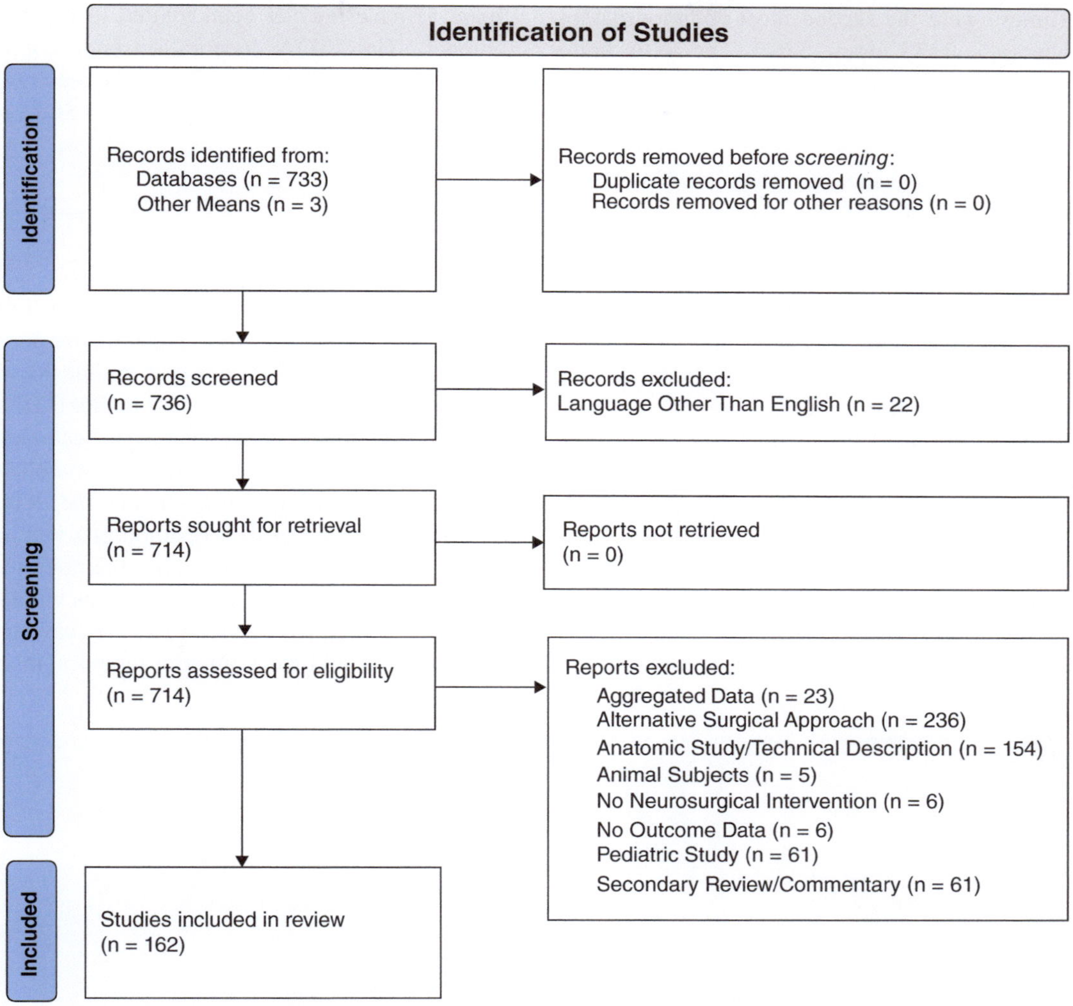

Fig. 32.2 Flow diagram of supraorbital and transorbital journal articles reviewed for inclusion in this study

Fig. 32.3 The number of cases for SOA and LTOA reported in reviewed articles separated by target pathology

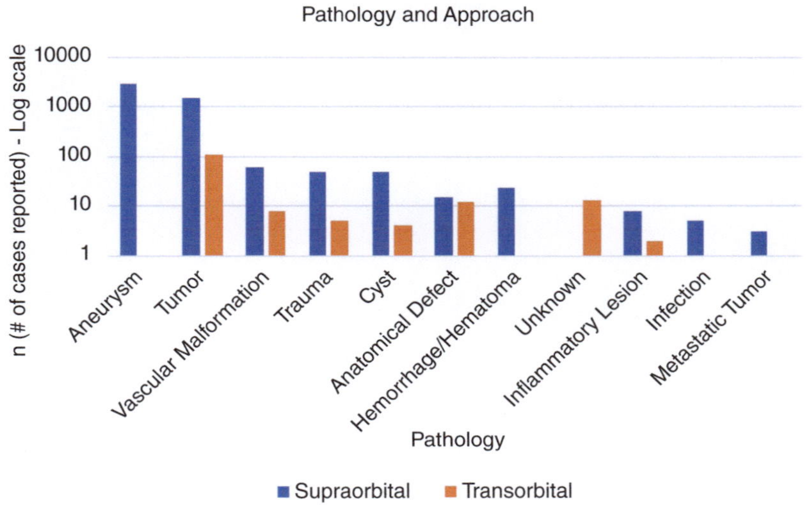

Tumors were the second most common pathology (n = 1533 cases; 32%). The SOA tumor pathologies included primarily meningiomas, craniopharyngiomas, and pituitary adenomas. As discussed above, the addition of the endoscope to the SOA can enhance visualization. However, it was used in only 35.7% of the reviewed cases in the literature, the remainder being done with the microscope alone.

The LTOA has a more limited literature, with only 156 cases for review. Tumors comprised most of the pathologies approached with this technique (71%, Fig. 32.3). Meningiomas were the most common tumor treated by the LTOA, followed by schwannomas. Anatomic defects, including cerebrospinal fluid (CSF) leak, traumatic fractures, and vascular malformations/cavernomas, have also been reported in the literature, but at lower rates. Consistent with the stages of difficulty in the LTOA reported by Di Somma, aneurysms and other vascular lesions (Stage 5) have not yet been treated using this approach. The LTOA depends on endoscopic assistance to a much larger degree than the SOA (76.3% of LTOA cases versus 35.7% for SOA, $p < 0.00001$).

Case Selection

Comparing the SOA and LTOA, case selection predominantly comes down to location. We analyzed 42 consecutive anterior and middle fossa meningioma surgeries by the senior author (THS) and generated the following volumetric heatmaps for tumor location separated by surgical approach (Fig. 32.4). As seen in the heatmaps, the SOA was primarily an approach for pathologies within the anterior cranial fossa and along the midline. The LTOA was used primarily for lesions within the middle cranial fossa, Meckel's cave, cavernous sinus, sphenoid wing, anterior temporal lobe

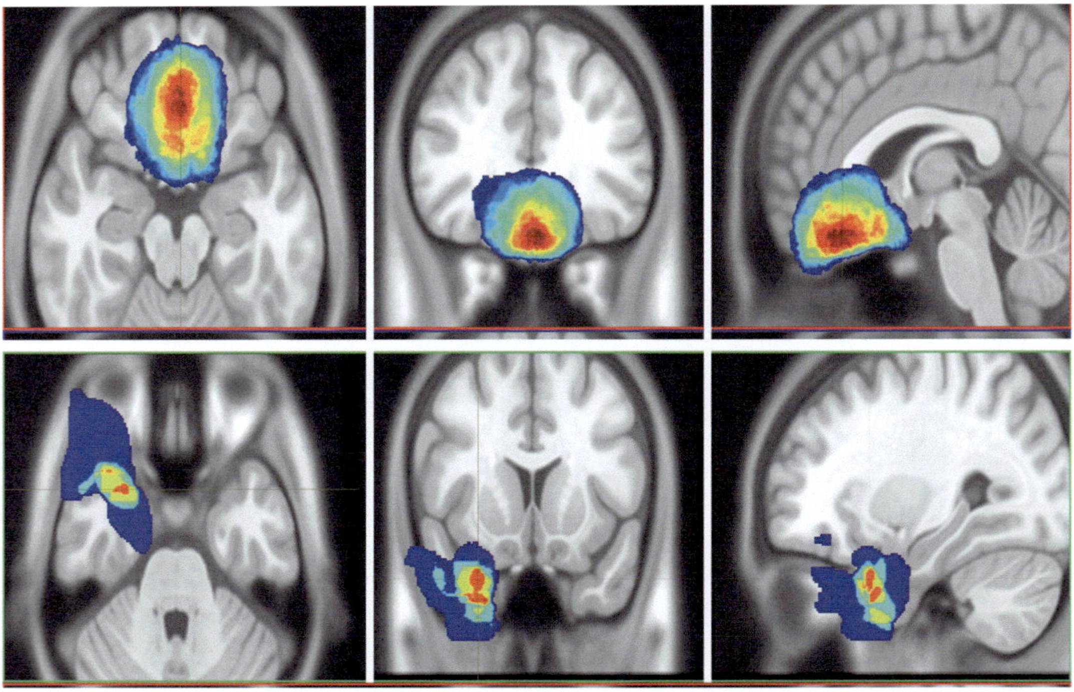

Fig. 32.4 Probabilistic heat map of tumor location by surgical approach (top row—SOA and bottom row—LTOA). The concentric rings correspond to 20%, 50%, and 80% of tumors located in this region

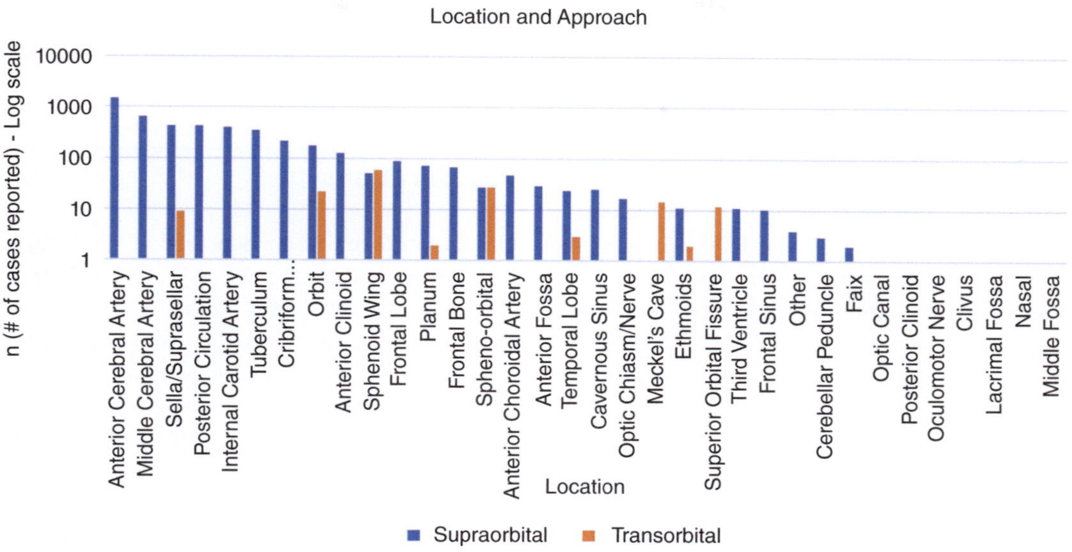

Fig. 32.5 The number of cases for SOA and LTOA reported in reviewed articles separated by the anatomic location of target

and orbit. The literature review validated these findings with the frequency of anatomic location reported in the literature displayed in Fig. 32.5.

Prior literature reviews of the SOA have demonstrated high rates (~98%) of technical success in clipping anterior circulation aneurysms [174]. The midline and interhemispheric location of ACA aneurysms makes these particularly ideal for the SOA. Similarly, regarding tumors, lesions that grow along the midline and anterior fossa were the most common targets such as the sellar/suprasellar region (9%), including craniopharyngiomas or adenomas, tuberculum/planum (8.9%) and olfactory groove (4.5%) meningiomas emanating from the cribriform plate. While many of these midline tumors can also be approached by an EEA, the SOA provides better access to lesions that extend lateral to the carotid artery or lamina papyracea [175]. The SOA can be used for olfactory groove meningiomas using angled endoscopes to gain greater visualization of the cribriform plate medially. Compared to the EEA, an SOA can offer better olfaction outcomes for olfactory groove meningiomas in patients with intact pre-operative olfaction [36]. Lesions more laterally located, such as anterior clinoid (2.6%) or those along the sphenoid wing (1%), can also be reached via an SOA. However, suppose these tumors extend below the sphenoid wing into the middle fossa. In that case, visualization under the sphenoid wing is limited and may be better approached via an open transcranial approach or LTOA. As such, they account for only a small percentage of cases reported in the literature.

The LTOA remains in its infancy relative to the supraorbital approach. While a number of anatomic and cadaveric studies have demonstrated the wide potential trajectories and targets of the LTOA, even extending as far posterior as the petrous apex [176], only 156 patient cases have been reported with pathology, location data, and outcomes. The primary lesion location treated with the LTOA has been the sphenoid wing, accounting for 38% of cases. This is followed by spheno-orbital lesions (17%), targets within the orbit (14%), Meckel's cave (9%), superior orbital fissure (SOF) (7.6%), and the sella/suprasellar (5.8%) region. The LTOA provides a direct trajectory to the middle/temporal fossa by drilling the triangular wedge of the greater wing of the sphenoid bone between the superior and inferior orbital fissures. This approach is ideal for spheno-orbital meningiomas that invade this area as it can allow for direct, minimally invasive access to this region. Middle fossa meningiomas, which lie posterior to the sphenoid wing and lateral to the cavernous sinus, are also ideal. The LTOA can expose the lateral wall of the cavernous sinus; however, only a few reports have demonstrated the use of the LTOA within the cavernous sinus [177]. The lateral to the medial trajectory of the LTOA is medially bounded by the optic nerve, anterior clinoid, internal carotid artery and cavernous sinus. This trajectory is nicely complementary to the medial/midline keyhole endoscopic endonasal approach (EEA), which is facile for midline lesions of the anterior skull base, sella, and clivus. Still, it is primarily limited in its lateral extent by neurovascular structures, including the carotid artery, cavernous sinus, and cranial nerves. The LTOA achieved similar rates of gross total resection (GTR) to the SOA for tumor cases, with rates of 73% versus 75%, respectively. Using a lateral orbital rim osteotomy with the LTOA can also increase degrees of freedom for surgical instrumentation at the target site [178]. Cases that did not use an endoscope for the LTOA were limited to the orbit, superior orbital fissure, and sphenoid wing.

Complications

Our literature review found a total of 633 complications reported for the SOA (13.4%) and 29 for the LTOA (18.6%), with no statistically significant difference between the two (p = 0.073, Fig. 32.6). The complication rates are, however, not necessarily comparable given the differences in lesion pathology and locations treated. The most common complication with the SOA was supraorbital hypoesthesia at a rate of 2% within all cases. This was followed by vasospasm and anosmia, which are likely byproducts of the lesions being treated. Ptosis occurred in 8.9% of LTOA cases, followed by periorbital edema, enophthalmos and wound complications, each occurring at a rate of 1–2%. CSF leaks occurred at a rate of 0.9% in the SOA group and 1.9% in

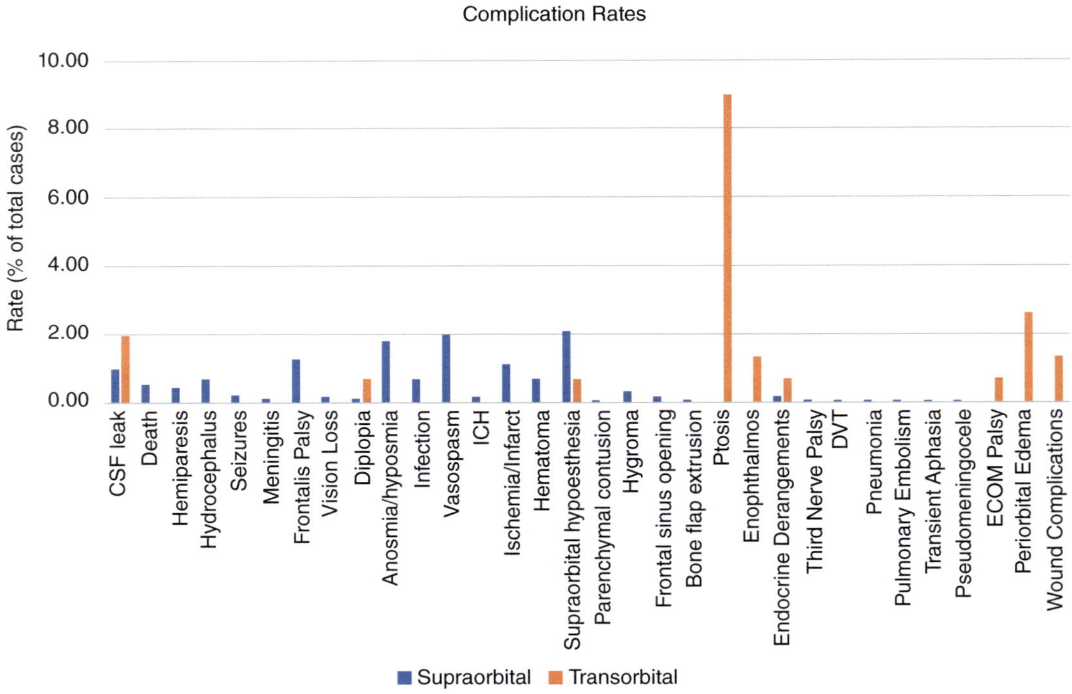

Fig. 32.6 Complication rates reported in the literature for the SOA or LTOA

the LTOA group ($p = 0.18$). These rates of complications are consistent with other prior literature reviews on the supraorbital and transorbital approaches [174, 179].

Conclusions

The SOA and LTOA are both keyhole approaches that can minimize incision length, cranial opening and brain retraction by utilizing the endoscope to increase the field of view while working through small corridors. The SOA has been utilized and studied in a variety of pathologies and has a more straightforward learning curve for neurosurgeons. However, the LTOA can provide complementary keyhole access to regions that can be difficult to reach via the SOA. The SOA offers excellent access to the anterior fossa, while the LTOA provides keyhole access to the anterior compartment of the middle fossa and its surroundings. These two approaches are both important tools in a minimally invasive skull base neurosurgeon's repertoire.

References

1. Bitter AD, Stavrinou LC, Ntoulias G, Petridis AK, Dukagjin M, Scholz M, Hassler W. The role of the pterional approach in the surgical treatment of olfactory groove meningiomas: a 20-year experience. J Neurol Surg Part B Skull Base. 2013;74:97–102.
2. Bir SC, Maiti T, Konar S, Nanda A. Comparison of the surgical outcome of pterional and frontotemporal-orbitozygomatic approaches and determination of predictors of recurrence for sphenoid wing meningiomas. World Neurosurg. 2017;99:308–19.
3. Nanda A, Maiti TK, Bir SC, Konar SK, Guthikonda B. Olfactory groove meningiomas: comparison of extent of frontal lobe changes after lateral and bifrontal approaches. World Neurosurg. 2016;94:211–21.
4. Nakamura M, Struck M, Roser F, Vorkapic P, Samii M. Olfactory groove meningiomas: clinical outcome and recurrence rates after tumor removal through the frontolateral and bifrontal approach. Neurosurgery. 2008;62:1224–32.
5. Noiphithak R, Yanez-Siller JC, Revuelta Barbero JM, Otto BA, Carrau RL, Prevedello DM. Quantitative analysis of the surgical exposure and surgical freedom between transcranial and transorbital endoscopic anterior petrosectomies to the posterior fossa. J Neurosurg. 2018;131:569–77.
6. Abergel A, Cavel O, Margalit N, Fliss DM, Gil Z. Comparison of quality of life after transnasal endoscopic vs open skull base tumor resection. Arch Otolaryngol Neck Surg. 2012;138:142–7.
7. Nair BR, Ganesh S, Moorthy RK, Rajshekhar V. Risk factors for postoperative brain contusion and early outcomes in patients with anterior skull base meningiomas undergoing unifrontal surgery: single center experience with 110 patients. Neurol India. 2022;70:2053.
8. Bander ED, Singh H, Ogilvie CB, Cusic RC, Pisapia DJ, Tsiouris AJ, Anand VK, Schwartz TH. Endoscopic endonasal versus transcranial approach to tuberculum sellae and planum sphenoidale meningiomas in a similar cohort of patients. J Neurosurg. 2018;128:40–8.
9. Komotar RJ, Starke RM, Raper DMS, Anand VK, Schwartz TH. Endoscopic endonasal versus open transcranial resection of anterior midline skull base meningiomas. World Neurosurg. 2012;77:713–24.
10. Moussazadeh N, Prabhu V, Bander ED, Cusic RC, Tsiouris AJ, Anand VK, Schwartz TH. Endoscopic endonasal versus open transcranial resection of craniopharyngiomas: a case-matched single-institution analysis. Neurosurg Focus. 2016;41:E7.
11. Johns CE, Johns CS. A case of central diabetes insipidus secondary to neurosarcoidosis. Cureus. 2020;12:e11119.
12. Cai M, He H, Zhang B, Luo L, Gong J, Li W, Huang T, Guo Y. An ectopic recurrent craniopharyngioma of the temporal lobe: case report and review of the literature. World Neurosurg. 2019;126:216–22.
13. Briggs RG, Conner AK, Chakraborty AR, Allan PG, Young IM, Teo C, Sughrue ME. An eyebrow, supracarotid triangle approach for lesions at the ventral thalamopeduncular junction: a technical report. World Neurosurg. 2020;140:e41–5.
14. Lin YJ, Chen KT, Lee CC, et al. Anterior skull base tumor resection by transciliary supraorbital keyhole craniotomy: a single institutional experience. World Neurosurg. 2018;111:e863–70.
15. Thanabalasundaram G, Soon WC, Ponnampalam A, Brydon HL. Case series of 100 supraorbital mini-craniotomies in patients with good grade aneurysmal subarachnoid haemorrhage at a single neurosurgical centre. Br J Neurosurg. 2022;36:368–71.
16. Chong CT, Chin KJ, Yip LW, Singh K. Case series: monocular visual loss associated with subarachnoid hemorrhage secondary to ruptured intracranial aneurysms. Can J Anaesth. 2006;53:684–9.
17. Bakhsheshian J, Zada G, Pham MH. Cavernous sinus hemangioma: rare vascular tumor of cavernous sinus. World Neurosurg. 2018;110:432–3.
18. Kong DS, Young SM, Hong CK, et al. Clinical and ophthalmological outcome of endoscopic transorbital surgery for cranioorbital tumors. J Neurosurg. 2018;131:667–75.
19. Zhang S, Qian C, Sun G, Li X. Clinical application of the supraorbital keyhole approach to the treatment

of unilateral-dominant bilateral frontal contusions. Oncotarget. 2017;8:48343–9.

20. Millesi M, Pichler L, Denk C, Lukas J, Matula C, Wadiura L. Clinical outcome and technical nuances after resection of orbital cavernous venous malformations-a single-center experience. World Neurosurg. 2021;153:e244–9.
21. Travers S, Bradshaw D, Siddiq F. Clip ligation of midsegment M1 artery aneurysm through a lateral supraorbital approach: 2-dimensional operative video. World Neurosurg. 2021;147:79.
22. Hage ZA, Charbel FT. Clipping of bilateral MCA aneurysms and a coiled ACOM aneurysm through a modified lateral supraorbital craniotomy. Neurosurg Focus. 2015;38:19.
23. Fischer-Szatmári T, Fülöp B, Szakács L, Gyura E, Bella Z, Barzó P. Combined simultaneous multiportal approach via minimally invasive transciliary and endoscopic endonasal approaches for tumors invading both the skull base and the sinonasal area. World Neurosurg. 2021;148:70–9.
24. Knopman J, Sigounas D, Huang C, Kacker A, Schwartz TH, Boockvar JA. Combined supraciliary and endoscopic endonasal approach for resection of frontal sinus mucoceles: technical note. Minim Invasive Neurosurg. 2009;52:149–51.
25. Park HH, Yoo J, Yun IS, Hong CK. Comparative analysis of endoscopic transorbital approach and extended mini-pterional approach for sphenoid wing meningiomas with osseous involvement: preliminary surgical results. World Neurosurg. 2020;139:e1–e12.
26. Fonseca RB, Correia AO, Vieira RS, Dos Santos JEF, Alves-Neto HR, da Silva Vieira AF, Belém DRF, Tobias-Machado M, Vidal CHF, Waisberg J. Comparative study between minimally invasive supraorbital craniotomy and pterional craniotomy for treating anterior circulation cerebral aneurysms in a low-resource setting. Sci Rep. 2021;11:5555.
27. Cha KC, Hong SC, Kim JS. Comparison between lateral supraorbital approach and pterional approach in the surgical treatment of unruptured intracranial aneurysms. J Korean Neurosurg Soc. 2012;51:334–7.
28. Wu X, Zhang S, Cheng Z, Aung TT, Fang Y, Li C. Comparison of supraorbital and pterional keyhole approach for clipping middle cerebral artery aneurysm: a Chinese population-based study. World Neurosurg. 2019;121:e596–604.
29. Chagla AS, Bhaganagare A, Kansal R, Tyagi D. Complete recovery of visual loss following surgical treatment of mucopyocele of the anterior clinoid process. J Clin Neurosci. 2010;17:670–2.
30. He H, Chen C, Li W, Luo L, Ling C, Wang H, Chen Z, Guo Y. Contralateral approach based on a preoperative 3-dimensional virtual osteotomy technique for anterior circulation aneurysms. J Stroke Cerebrovasc Dis. 2019;28:1099–106.
31. Eroglu U, Sayaci EY, Buyuktepe M, Caglar YS. Contralateral subfrontal supraorbital approach for microsurgical resection of optic canal meningioma. J Craniofac Surg. 2021;32:1830–1.
32. Pease M, Marquez Y, Tuchman A, Markarian A, Zada G. Diagnosis and surgical management of traumatic cerebrospinal fluid oculorrhea: case report and systematic review of the literature. J Neurol Surg Rep. 2013;74:57–66.
33. Jenks JD, Benson CA. Early cerebritis resulting in a first-time seizure in an otherwise healthy young man. Infect Clin Pract. 2016;24:e66–8.
34. Jakobs M, Orakcioglu B. Ectopic recurrent craniopharyngioma of the frontal bone. J Neurosurg. 2012;117:490–7.
35. Fatemi N, Dusick JR, de Paiva Neto MA, Malkasian D, Kelly DF. Endonasal versus supraorbital keyhole removal of craniopharyngiomas and tuberculum sellae meningiomas. Neurosurgery. 2009;64:269–84; discussion 284–6.
36. Banu MA, Mehta A, Ottenhausen M, Fraser JF, Patel KS, Szentirmai O, Anand VK, Tsiouris AJ, Schwartz TH. Endoscope-assisted endonasal versus supraorbital keyhole resection of olfactory groove meningiomas: comparison and combination of 2 minimally invasive approaches. J Neurosurg. 2016;124:605–20.
37. Igressa A, Pechlivanis I, Weber F, Mahvash M, Ayyad A, Boutarbouch M, Charalampaki P. Endoscope-assisted keyhole surgery via an eyebrow incision for removal of large meningiomas of the anterior and middle cranial fossa. Clin Neurol Neurosurg. 2015;129:27–33.
38. Menovsky T, Grotenhuis JA, de Vries J, Bartels RH. Endoscope-assisted supraorbital craniotomy for lesions of the interpeduncular fossa. Neurosurgery. 1999;44:106–10; discussion 110–2
39. Linsler S, Fischer G, Skliarenko V, Stadie A, Oertel J. Endoscopic assisted supraorbital keyhole approach or endoscopic endonasal approach in cases of tuberculum sellae meningioma: which surgical route should be favored? World Neurosurg. 2017;104:601–11.
40. Mallari RJ, Thakur JD, Rhee JH, Eisenberg A, Krauss H, Griffiths C, Sivakumar W, Barkhoudarian G, Kelly DF. Endoscopic endonasal and supraorbital removal of tuberculum sellae meningiomas: anatomic guides and operative nuances for keyhole approach selection. Oper Neurosurg. 2021;21:E71–e81.
41. Gazzeri R, Nishiyama Y, Teo C. Endoscopic supraorbital eyebrow approach for the surgical treatment of extraaxial and intraaxial tumors. Neurosurg Focus. 2014;37:E20.
42. Park HH, Hong SD, Kim YH, Hong CK, Woo KI, Yun IS, Kong DS. Endoscopic transorbital and endonasal approach for trigeminal schwannomas: a retrospective multicenter analysis (KOSEN-005). J Neurosurg. 2020;133:467–76.
43. Jeon C, Hong CK, Woo KI, Hong SD, Nam DH, Lee JI, Choi JW, Seol HJ, Kong DS. Endoscopic transorbital surgery for Meckel's cave and middle cranial

fossa tumors: surgical technique and early results. J Neurosurg. 2018;131(4):1126–35.
44. Zoia C, Bongetta D, Gaetani P. Endoscopic transorbital surgery for spheno-orbital lesions: how I do it. Acta Neurochir (Wien). 2018;160:1231–3.
45. Ko Y, Yi HJ, Kim YS, Oh SH, Kim KM, Oh SJ. Eyebrow incision using tattoo for anterior fossa lesions: technical case reports. Minim Invasive Neurosurg. 2001;44:17–20.
46. Paladino J, Pirker N, Stimac D, Stern-Padovan R. Eyebrow keyhole approach in vascular neurosurgery. Minim Invasive Neurosurg. 1998;41:200–3.
47. Youngerman BE, Shtayer L, Gerges MM, Larsen AG, Tomasiewicz HC, Schwartz TH. Eyebrow supraorbital keyhole craniotomy for olfactory groove meningiomas with endoscope assistance: case series and systematic review of extent of resection, quantification of postoperative frontal lobe injury, anosmia, and recurrence. Acta Neurochir (Wien). 2021;163:101–12.
48. Bhattarai R, Liang CF, Chen C, Wang H, Huang TC, Guo Y. Factors determining the side of approach for clipping ruptured anterior communicating artery aneurysm via supraorbital eyebrow keyhole approach. Chin J Traumatol. 2020;23:20–4.
49. Chandra PS, Tej M, Sawarkar D, Agarwal M, Doddamani RS. Fronto-orbital variant of supraorbital keyhole approach for clipping ruptured anterior circulation aneurysms (f-Sokha). Neurology. 2020;68:1019–27.
50. Wai YZ, Chong YY, Dusa NM, Lai YP, Lim LT. Godtfredsen syndrome - recurrent clival chondrosarcoma with 6 years follow up: a case report and literature review. BMC Neurol. 2022;22:134.
51. Toyooka T, Otani N, Wada K, Tomiyama A, Takeuchi S, Fujii K, Kumagai K, Fujii T, Mori K. Head-up display may facilitate safe keyhole surgery for cerebral aneurysm clipping. J Neurosurg. 2018;129:883–9.
52. Alessi G, Aiyer S, Nathoo N. Home-made gun injury: spontaneous version and anterior migration of bullet. Br J Neurosurg. 2002;16:381–4.
53. Shanno G, Maus M, Bilyk J, Schwartz S, Savino P, Simeone F, Goldman HW. Image-guided transorbital roof craniotomy via a suprabrow approach: a surgical series of 72 patients. Neurosurgery. 2001;48:559–67; discussion 567–8
54. Fan J, Peng Y, Qi S, Zhang XA, Qiu B, Pan J. Individualized surgical strategies for Rathke cleft cyst based on cyst location. J Neurosurg. 2013;119:1437–46.
55. Cuellar-Hernandez JJ, Valadez-Rodriguez A, Olivas-Campos R, Tabera-Tarello P, Juan-Orta DS, Segura-López R, Fleury A. Intrasellar cysticercosis cyst treated with a transciliary supraorbital keyhole approach - a case report. Surg Neurol Int. 2020;11:436.
56. Shao D, Li Y, Sun Z, Cai X, Zheng X, Jiang Z. Keyhole approach for clipping anterior circulation aneurysms: clinical outcomes and technical note. Front Surg. 2021;8:783557.
57. Lan Q, Zhang H, Zhu Q, Chen A, Chen Y, Xu L, Wang Z, Yuan L, Liu S. Keyhole approach for clipping intracranial aneurysm: comparison of supraorbital and pterional keyhole approach. World Neurosurg. 2017;102:350–9.
58. Wong AK, Wong RH. Keyhole clipping of a low-lying basilar apex aneurysm without posterior clinoidectomy utilizing endoscopic indocyanine green video angiography. Surg Neurol Int. 2020;11:31.
59. Kalani MYS, Spetzler RF, Wanebo JE. Keyhole supraorbital craniotomy for aneurysm clipping in the setting of bypass for moyamoya disease. World Neurosurg. 2016;94:442–6.
60. Revuelta Barbero JM, Rindler RS, Martin C, Orellana M, Porto E, Solares CA, Pradilla G. Keyhole supraorbital eyebrow approach for the resection of a tuberculum sellae meningioma with intraoperative endoscopic assistance. Surg Neurol Int. 2022;13:93.
61. Lin EY, Hsieh CT, Lin CS, Tsai TH, Chiang YH. Keyhole surgery for isolated pituitary stalk metastatic tumors: a case report and review of the literature. Minim Invasive Neurosurg. 2008;51:222–4.
62. Goehre F, Jahromi BR, Elsharkawy A, Lehto H, Shekhtman O, Andrade-Barazarte H, Munoz F, Hijazy F, Makhkamov M, Hernesniemi J. Lateral supraorbital approach to ipsilateral PCA-P1 and ICA-PCoA aneurysms. Surg Neurol Int. 2015;6:91.
63. Klironomos G, Mehan N, Dehdashti AR. Lateral supraorbital craniotomy for Tuberculum sella meningioma resection. J Neurol Surg B Skull Base. 2018;79:S263–s264.
64. Mori K, Yamamoto T, Nakao Y, Oyama K, Esaki T, Watanabe M, Nonaka S, Hara T, Honma K. Lateral supraorbital keyhole approach to clip unruptured anterior communicating artery aneurysms. Minim Invasive Neurosurg. 2008;51:292–7.
65. La Rocca G, Della Pepa GM, Sturiale CL, Sabatino G, Auricchio AM, Puca A, Olivi A, Marchese E, Albanese A. Lateral supraorbital versus pterional approach: analysis of surgical, functional, and patient-oriented outcomes. World Neurosurg. 2018;119:e192–9.
66. Chen HI, Bohman LE, Emery L, Martinez-Lage M, Richardson AG, Davis KA, Pollard JR, Litt B, Gausas RE, Lucas TH. Lateral transorbital endoscopic access to the hippocampus, amygdala, and entorhinal cortex: initial clinical experience. ORL J Otorhinolaryngol Relat Spec. 2015;77:321–32.
67. O'Connor KP, Bohnstedt BN. Left anterior cranial fossa dural arteriovenous fistula ligation using a supra-orbital (eyebrow) craniotomy. Neurosurg Focus. 2019;46:V3.
68. Yip CM, Lee HP, Hsu SS, Chen YT. Left orbital roof giant cell tumor of bone: a case report. Surg Neurol Int. 2018;9:127.
69. Borghei-Razavi H, Das P, Kshettry V. Left supraorbital eyebrow approach for microscopic fenestration of a neuroglial cyst. World Neurosurg. 2018;118:161.
70. Mori K, Wada K, Otani N, Tomiyama A, Toyooka T, Tomura S, Takeuchi S, Yamamoto T, Nakao Y,

Arai H. Long-term neurological and radiological results of consecutive 63 unruptured anterior communicating artery aneurysms clipped via lateral supraorbital keyhole minicraniotomy. Oper Neurosurg. 2018;14:95–103.

71. Burks JD, Conner AK, Bonney PA, Archer JB, Christensen B, Smith J, Safavi-Abbasi S, Sughrue M. Management of intracranial meningiomas using keyhole techniques. Cureus. 2016;8:e588.
72. Mariniello G, Bonavolontà G, Tranfa F, Maiuri F. Management of the optic canal invasion and visual outcome in spheno-orbital meningiomas. Clin Neurol Neurosurg. 2013;115:1615–20.
73. Dhandapani S, Sahoo SK. Median supraorbital keyhole approach for clipping ruptured distal anterior cerebral artery aneurysm: technical report with review of literature. World Neurosurg. 2018;112:73–6.
74. Marzi S, De Paulis D, Ricci A, Taddei G, Dehcordi SR, Coletti G, Maselli G, Galzio RJ. Meningioangiomatosis without neurofibromatosis type 2. World J Oncol. 2012;3:127–33.
75. Beems T, Grotenhuis JA, Wesseling P. Meningioma of the pituitary stalk without dural attachment: case report and review of the literature. Neurosurgery. 1999;45:1474–7.
76. You W, Meng J, Yang X, et al. Microsurgical management of posterior circulation aneurysms: a retrospective study on epidemiology, outcomes, and surgical approaches. Brain Sci. 2022;12(8):1066. https://doi.org/10.3390/brainsci12081066.
77. Chen HC, Tzaan WC. Microsurgical supraorbital keyhole approach to the anterior cranial base. J Clin Neurosci. 2010;17:1510–4.
78. Ivan ME, Lawton MT. Mini supraorbital approach to inferior frontal lobe cavernous malformations: case series. J Neurol Surg Cent Eur Neurosurg. 2013;74:187–91.
79. Niknejad HR, Stockx L, Wuyts J. Minimally invasive aneurysm clipping: the extent of the supraorbital approach. World Neurosurg. 2019;127:e1132–6.
80. Seaman SC, Ali MS, Marincovich A, Li L, Walsh JE, Greenlee JDW. Minimally invasive approaches to anterior skull base meningiomas. J Neurol Surg B Skull Base. 2022;83:254–64.
81. Cohen-Gadol AA. Minimally invasive clip ligation of anterior communicating artery aneurysms through the eyebrow keyhole supraorbital craniotomy: 3-dimensional operative video. Neurosurgery. 2015;11(2):360; discussion 360.
82. Santa Maria P, Bertani R, Pilon B, Ribeiro LF, Perret C, Koester S, Schiavini H, Monteiro R. Minimally invasive keyhole supraorbital craniotomy as treatment option for penetrating foreign body through orbital roof. Br J Neurosurg. 2021;26:1–4.
83. Wong RH. Minimally invasive lateral orbital wall approach for sphenocavernous meningioma resection with endoscope assistance. World Neurosurg. 2020;138:261.
84. Abdel Aziz KM, Bhatia S, Tantawy MH, Sekula R, Keller JT, Froelich S, Happ E. Minimally invasive transpalpebral "eyelid" approach to the anterior cranial base. Neurosurgery. 2011;69:195–206; discussion 206–7.
85. Tra H, Huynh T, Nguyen B. Minipterional and supraorbital keyhole craniotomies for ruptured anterior circulation aneurysms: experience at single center. World Neurosurg. 2018;109:36–9.
86. Aldea S, Gaillard S. Multiple aneurysms clipping through the eyebrow approach: 2-dimensional operative video. Oper Neurosurg. 2019;16:E78.
87. Tucker AM, Beckett JS, Martin NA. Next generation case report: supraorbital craniotomy for anterior communicating artery aneurysm clipping in annotated virtual reality environment. Oper Neurosurg. 2018;15:E73–e76.
88. Hendrix P, Fischer G, Krug J, Linnebach AC, Simgen A, Griessenauer CJ, Burkhardt BW, Oertel J. Olfactory dysfunction in patients undergoing supraorbital keyhole craniotomy for clipping of unruptured aneurysms. Clin Anat. 2020;33:316–23.
89. Bassiouni H, Asgari S, Stolke D. Olfactory groove meningiomas: functional outcome in a series treated microsurgically. Acta Neurochir (Wien). 2007;149:109–21.
90. Ved R, Mo M, Hayhurst C. Olfactory outcomes after resection of Tuberculum sella and Planum sphenoidale meningiomas via a transcranial approach. J Neurol Surg B Skull Base. 2022;83:296–304.
91. Mahmoud M, Nader R, Al-Mefty O. Optic canal involvement in tuberculum sellae meningiomas: influence on approach, recurrence, and visual recovery. Neurosurgery. 2010;67:108–18; discussion ons118-9.
92. Kong DS, Kim YH, Hong CK. Optimal indications and limitations of endoscopic transorbital superior eyelid surgery for spheno-orbital meningiomas. J Neurosurg. 2020;134:1472–9.
93. Essayed W, Al-Mefty O. Orbital cavernous venous malformation resection through supraorbital craniotomy: 2-dimensional operative video. Oper Neurosurg. 2022;22:e128.
94. Lall RR, Shafizadeh SF, Lee KH, Mao Q, Mehta M, Raizer J, Bendok BR, Chandler JP. Orbital metastasis of pituitary growth hormone secreting carcinoma causing lateral gaze palsy. Surg Neurol Int. 2013;4:59.
95. Montano N, Lauretti L, D'Alessandris QG, Rigante M, Pignotti F, Olivi A, Paludetti G, Pallini R, Fernandez E. Orbital tumors: report of 70 surgically treated cases. World Neurosurg. 2018;119:e449–58.
96. Reisch R, Marcus HJ, Hugelshofer M, Koechlin NO, Stadie A, Kockro RA. Patients' cosmetic satisfaction, pain, and functional outcomes after supraorbital craniotomy through an eyebrow incision. J Neurosurg. 2014;121:730–4.
97. Yang P, Li Y, Liu HC, Qiu E, Zhang JL, Ren J, Jiang LB, Liu HG, Kang J. Prognosis analysis and clini-

cal features of orbital cavernous venous malformations with refractory insidious onset. Front Oncol. 2021;11:745479.
98. Park J, Son W, Kwak Y, Ohk B. Pterional versus superciliary keyhole approach: direct comparison of approach-related complaints and satisfaction in the same patient. J Neurosurg. 2018;130:220–6.
99. Wu Y, Zhao Y, Yu S, Li F, Cai S, Peng C, Wang Z, Yang Y, Wang B, Yang X. Reconstruction clipping of ruptured anterior circulation aneurysms via supraorbital lateral keyhole approach. Chin Neurosurg J. 2022;8:3.
100. Berrington T, Chang B, Thomson S. Removal of a penetrating orbital and anterior fossa foreign body using an eyebrow incision. Br J Neurosurg. 2015;29:306–7.
101. Desai R, Srienc AI, Maamari RN, Custer PL, Warren DK, Chicoine MR. Removal of a penetrating tree branch in the orbitofrontal region-a unique application of an orbitofrontal craniotomy through a supraciliary brow approach. Oper Neurosurg. 2021;21:E386–e391.
102. Maus M, Goldman HW. Removal of orbital apex hemangioma using new transorbital craniotomy through suprabrow approach. Ophthalmic Plast Reconstr Surg. 1999;15:166–70.
103. Park JS, Kim H, Baik MW, Park IS. Risk factor analysis for poor outcomes in supraorbital keyhole aneurysm clipping for ruptured anterior circulation aneurysms. World Neurosurg. 2018;111:e386–94.
104. Nair BR, Ganesh S, Moorthy RK, Rajshekhar V. Risk factors for postoperative brain contusion and early outcomes in patients with anterior skull base meningiomas undergoing unifrontal surgery: single center experience with 110 patients. Neurology. 2022;70:2053–8.
105. Revuelta R, Arriada-Mendicoa N, Ramirez-Alba J, Soto-Hernandez JL. Simultaneous treatment of a pituitary adenoma and an internal carotid artery aneurysm through a supraorbital keyhole approach. Minim Invasive Neurosurg. 2002;45:109–11.
106. Seaman SC, Ali MS, Marincovich A, Osorno-Cruz C, Greenlee JDW. Single surgeon experience with minimally invasive supraorbital craniotomy versus bifrontal craniotomy for anterior skull base meningiomas. Surg Neurol Int. 2020;11:458.
107. Alam S, Ferini G, Muhammad N, et al. Skull base approaches for tuberculum sellae meningiomas: institutional experience in a series of 34 patients. Life. 2022;12(4):492. https://doi.org/10.3390/life12040492.
108. Romani R, Silvasti-Lundell M, Laakso A, Tuominen H, Hernesniemi J, Niemi T. Slack brain in meningioma surgery through lateral supraorbital approach. Surg Neurol Int. 2011;2:167.
109. Peron S, Cividini A, Santi L, Galante N, Castelnuovo P, Locatelli D. Spheno-orbital meningiomas: when the endoscopic approach is better. Acta Neurochir Suppl. 2017;124:123–8.
110. Zurita M, Candanedo C, Moscovici S, Kaye AH, Spektor S. Spontaneous symptomatic orbital meningoencephalocele in an adult patient. Case report and review of the literature. J Clin Neurosci. 2020;77:224–6.
111. Araujo JL, Ferraz VR, Vilela D, Sette M. Stab wound in the skull treated with a medial supraorbital craniotomy through an incision in the eyebrow-a minimally invasive approach. Indian J Surg. 2015;77:535–7.
112. Koppe M, Gleizal A, Orset E, Bachelet JT, Jouanneau E, Rougeot A. Superior eyelid crease approach for transobital neuroendoscopic surgery of the anterior cranial fossa. J Craniofac Surg. 2013;24:1616–21.
113. Paiva-Neto MA, Tella OI. Supra-orbital keyhole removal of anterior fossa and parasellar meningiomas. Arq Neuropsiquiatr. 2010;68:418–23.
114. Joseph V, Chacko AG. Suprabrow minicraniotomy for suprasellar tumours. Br J Neurosurg. 2005;19:33–7.
115. Avery MB, Mallari RJ, Barkhoudarian G, Kelly DF. Supraorbital and mini-pterional keyhole craniotomies for brain tumors: a clinical and anatomical comparison of indications and outcomes in 204 cases. J Neurosurg. 2021;136(5):1314–24.
116. Dossani RH, Kalakoti P, Guthikonda B. Supraorbital approach for resection of clinoidal meningioma. World Neurosurg. 2018;109:295.
117. Khanapure K, Joshi KC, Jagannatha AT, Perikal PJ, Quryshi SA, Srikantha U, Verma RG, Hegde AS. Supraorbital craniotomy for large anterior skull base meningiomas: a technical note. Asian J Neurosurg. 2019;14:767–72.
118. Delitala A, Brunori A, Russo N. Supraorbital endoscopic approach to colloid cysts. Neurosurgery. 2011;69:176–82; discussion ons182-3.
119. Oh HJ, Hwang SC. Supraorbital endoscopic evacuation for traumatic intracerebral hematomas in the frontal lobe. J Korean Neurosurg Soc. 2022;65:846–52.
120. Fernandes YB, Maitrot D, Kehrli P, Tella OI, Ramina R, Borges G. Supraorbital eyebrow approach to skull base lesions. Arq Neuropsiquiatr. 2002;60:246–50.
121. Ditzel Filho LF, McLaughlin N, Bresson D, Solari D, Kassam AB, Kelly DF. Supraorbital eyebrow craniotomy for removal of intraaxial frontal brain tumors: a technical note. World Neurosurg. 2014;81:348–56.
122. Bhattarai R, Liang C, Chen C, Wang H, Huang T, Ning X, Guo Y. Supraorbital eyebrow keyhole approach for microsurgical management of ruptured anterior communicating artery aneurysm. Exp Ther Med. 2020;20:2079–89.
123. Mitchell P, Vindlacheruvu RR, Mahmood K, Ashpole RD, Grivas A, Mendelow AD. Supraorbital eyebrow minicraniotomy for anterior circulation aneurysms. Surg Neurol. 2005;63:47–51; discussion 51.
124. Tang C, Sun J, Xue H, Yu Y, Xu F. Supraorbital keyhole approach for anterior circulation aneurysms. Turk Neurosurg. 2013;23:434–8.

125. Eroglu U, Shah K, Bozkurt M, et al. Supraorbital keyhole approach: lessons learned from 106 operative cases. World Neurosurg. 2019;124:e667–74. https://doi.org/10.1016/j.wneu.2018.12.188.
126. Chen YH, Lin SZ, Chiang YH, Ju DT, Liu MY, Chen GJ. Supraorbital keyhole surgery for optic nerve decompression and dura repair. J Neurotrauma. 2004;21:976–81.
127. Yu LB, Huang Z, Ren ZG, Shao JS, Zhang Y, Wang R, Zhang D. Supraorbital keyhole versus pterional craniotomies for ruptured anterior communicating artery aneurysms: a propensity score-matched analysis. Neurosurg Rev. 2020;43:547–54.
128. Brydon HL, Akil H, Ushewokunze S, Dhir JS, Taha A, Ahmed A. Supraorbital microcraniotomy for acute aneurysmal subarachnoid haemorrhage: results of first 50 cases. Br J Neurosurg. 2008;22:40–5.
129. Prat-Acín R, Galeano-Senabre I, Pancucci G, Evangelista R, Ayuso-Sacido A, Botella C. Supraorbital trans-eyebrow craniotomy and fluorescence-guided resection of fronto-basal high grade gliomas. Clin Neurol Neurosurg. 2013;115:1586–90.
130. Cuellar-Hernandez JJ, Olivas-Campos JR, Tabera-Tarello PM, Anokwute M, Valadez-Rodriguez A. Supraorbital transciliary keyhole approach for removal of tuberculum sellae meningioma: 3D surgical video. Surg Neurol Int. 2021;12:5.
131. Czirják S, Szeifert GT. Surgical experience with frontolateral keyhole craniotomy through a superciliary skin incision. Neurosurgery. 2001;48:145–9; discussion 149–50.
132. Hopf NJ, Stadie A, Reisch R. Surgical management of bilateral middle cerebral artery aneurysms via a unilateral supraorbital keyhole craniotomy. Minim Invasive Neurosurg. 2009;52:126–31.
133. Das AK, Mani SK, Singh SK. Surgical management of post-COVID invasive rhino-orbito-cerebral mucormycosis and its outcomes: Role of neurosurgeons in a tertiary care center. Surg Neurol Int. 2022;13:335.
134. Jee TK, Lee YW, Yeon JY, Kim KH, Jeon P, Kim JS, Hong SC. Surgical strategy for ethmoidal dural arteriovenous fistula. World Neurosurg. 2022;164:e91–8.
135. Tang R, Mao S, Lin H, Ye HB, Li DW, Chen ZN, Su KM, Zhang WT. Surgical treatment and outcomes for sinonasal and skull base phosphaturic mesenchymal tumors. Otolaryngol Head Neck Surg. 2020;162:674–82.
136. Rassi MS, Al-Mefty O. Surgical treatment of bilateral optic nerve sheath meningioma: 2-dimensional operative video. Oper Neurosurg. 2021;20:e418–9.
137. Reisch R, Perneczky A. Ten-year experience with the supraorbital subfrontal approach through an eyebrow skin incision. Neurosurgery. 2005;57:242–55; discussion 242–55.
138. Kabil MS, Shahinian HK. The endoscopic supraorbital approach to tumors of the middle cranial base. Surg Neurol. 2006;66:396–401; discussion 401.
139. Paladino J, Mrak G, Miklić P, Jednacak H, Mihaljević D. The keyhole concept in aneurysm surgery–a comparative study: keyhole versus standard craniotomy. Minim Invasive Neurosurg. 2005;48:251–8.
140. Raygor KP, Garcia J, Rutledge C, Tonetti DA, Raper DMS, Abla AA. The lateral supraorbital craniotomy approach for anterior circulation aneurysms: a modern surgical case series in the endovascular era. World Neurosurg. 2022;166:e799–807.
141. Reisch R, Stadie A, Kockro R, Gawish I, Schwandt E, Hopf N. The minimally invasive supraorbital subfrontal keyhole approach for surgical treatment of temporomesial lesions of the dominant hemisphere. Minim Invasive Neurosurg. 2009;52:163–9.
142. Kocaman U, Dalbasti T, Ozer MH, Yilmaz H, Yilmaz MB, Atci IB, Celik S. The modified lateral supraorbital approach. Br J Neurosurg. 2018;32:418–23.
143. Czirják S, Szeifert GT. The role of the superciliary approach in the surgical management of intracranial neoplasms. Neurol Res. 2006;28:131–7.
144. McLaughlin N, Ditzel Filho LF, Shahlaie K, Solari D, Kassam AB, Kelly DF. The supraorbital approach for recurrent or residual suprasellar tumors. Minim Invasive Neurosurg. 2011;54:155–61.
145. Ziai K, Shah S, Daggubati LC, Zacharia BE, Lighthall JG. The supraorbital approach via an eyebrow incision: analysis of cosmetic outcomes using the scar cosmesis assessment rating scale. J Craniofac Surg. 2022;33:307–11.
146. Hassler W, Schick U. The supraorbital approach–a minimally invasive approach to the superior orbit. Acta Neurochir (Wien). 2009;151:605–11; discussion 611–2
147. Melamed I, Merkin V, Korn A, Nash M. The supraorbital approach: an alternative to traditional exposure for the surgical management of anterior fossa and parasellar pathology. Minim Invasive Neurosurg. 2005;48:259–63.
148. van Lindert E, Perneczky A, Fries G, Pierangeli E. The supraorbital keyhole approach to supratentorial aneurysms: concept and technique. Surg Neurol. 1998;49:481–9; discussion 489-90.
149. Peng Y, Fan J, Li Y, Qiu M, Qi S. The supraorbital keyhole approach to the suprasellar and supra-intrasellar rathke cleft cysts under pure endoscopic visualization. World Neurosurg. 2016;92:120–5.
150. Wiedemayer H, Sandalcioglu IE, Wiedemayer H, Stolke D. The supraorbital keyhole approach via an eyebrow incision for resection of tumors around the sella and the anterior skull base. Minim Invasive Neurosurg. 2004;47:221–5.
151. Raza SM, Quinones-Hinojosa A, Lim M, Boahene KD. The transconjunctival transorbital approach: a keyhole approach to the midline anterior skull base. World Neurosurg. 2013;80:864–71.
152. Beseoglu K, Lodes S, Stummer W, Steiger HJ, Hänggi D. The transorbital keyhole approach: early and long-term outcome analysis of approach-related morbidity and cosmetic results. Technical note. J Neurosurg. 2011;114:852–6.

153. Marx S, Clemens S, Schroeder HWS. The value of endoscope assistance during transcranial surgery for tuberculum sellae meningiomas. J Neurosurg. 2018;128:32–9.
154. Kumar VR, Madhugiri VS, Ramesh AS, Yadav AK. Trans-ciliary minimally invasive keyhole craniotomy for skull base and vascular lesions. J Neurosci. 2015;6:636–8.
155. Ramos-Zúñiga R, Velázquez H, Barajas MA, López R, Sánchez E, Trejo S. Trans-supraorbital approach to supratentorial aneurysms. Neurosurgery. 2002;51:125–30; discussion 130–1
156. Warren WL, Grant GA. Transciliary orbitofrontozygomatic approach to lesions of the anterior cranial fossa. Neurosurgery. 2009;64:324–9; discussion 329–30
157. Bhatoe HS. Transciliary supraorbital keyhole approach in the management of aneurysms of anterior circulation: operative nuances. Neurology. 2009;57:599–606.
158. Schaberg M, Murchison AP, Rosen MR, Evans JJ, Bilyk JR. Transorbital and transnasal endoscopic repair of a meningoencephalocele. Orbit. 2011;30:221–5.
159. Lew H, Rootman DB, Nassiri N, Goh A, Goldberg RA. Transorbital approach without craniotomy to orbital tumors with extradural intracranial extension. Orbit. 2014;33:343–51.
160. Cutney C, Bernardino CR, Buono LM, Goldman WH, Maus M. Transorbital craniotomy through a suprabrow approach: a case series. Orbit. 2001;20:107–17.
161. Smith CS, Karlin JN, Cohen LM, Rootman DB. Transorbital debulking of sphenoid wing meningioma. J Craniofac Surg. 2022;33:859–62.
162. Almeida JP, Omay SB, Shetty SR, Chen YN, Ruiz-Treviño AS, Liang B, Anand VK, Levine B, Schwartz TH. Transorbital endoscopic eyelid approach for resection of sphenoorbital meningiomas with predominant hyperostosis: report of 2 cases. J Neurosurg. 2018;128:1885–95.
163. Moe KS, Bergeron CM, Ellenbogen RG. Transorbital neuroendoscopic surgery. Neurosurgery. 2010;67:16–28.
164. Ramakrishna R, Kim LJ, Bly RA, Moe K, Ferreira M. Transorbital neuroendoscopic surgery for the treatment of skull base lesions. J Clin Neurosci. 2016;24:99–104.
165. Delavari N, Staffenberg D, Riina H. Transpalpebral incision for resection of an ethmoidal dural arteriovenous fistula: 2-dimensional operative video. Oper Neurosurg. 2020;19:E606.
166. Peto I, Molcanyi M, Noureldine MHA, Bajric J, Agazzi S. Transpalpebral transorbital neuroendoscopic (TONES) repair of orbital meningoencephalocele: a technical note. Br J Neurosurg. 2021;37(6):1904–8.
167. Deshmukh VR, Hott JS, Dumont T, Nakaji P, Spetzler RF. Treatment of recurrent previously coiled anterior circulation aneurysm with minimally invasive keyhole craniotomy: report of two cases. Minim Invasive Neurosurg. 2006;49:70–3.
168. Mallari RJ, Thakur JD, Griffiths C, Krauss H, Eisenberg A, Barkhoudarian G, Kelly DF. Tuberculum sellae meningiomas in pregnancy: 3 cases treated in the second trimester and literature review. World Neurosurg. 2020;143:268–75.
169. Landeiro JA, Gonçalves MB, Guimarães RD, Klescoski J, Correa JL, Lapenta MA, Maia O. Tuberculum sellae meningiomas: surgical considerations. Arq Neuropsiquiatr. 2010;68:424–9.
170. Marenco-Hillembrand L, Bamimore MA, Webb R, Chaichana KL. Unilateral supraorbital keyhole craniotomy avoiding the frontal sinus for large and giant olfactory-groove meningiomas: a case series. World Neurosurg. 2022;170:e324–30. https://doi.org/10.1016/j.wneu.2022.11.015.
171. Feroze RA, Agarwal N, Sekula RF. Utility of calcium phosphate cement cranioplasty following supraorbital approach for tumor resection. Int J Neurosci. 2018;128:1199–203.
172. Adawi MM, Abdelbaky AM. Validity of the lateral supraorbital approach as a minimally invasive corridor for orbital lesions. World Neurosurg. 2015;84:766–71.
173. Somma AD, Kong D-S, Notaris M, Moe KS, España JCS, Schwartz TH, Enseñat J. Endoscopic transorbital surgery levels of difficulty. J Neurosurg. 2022;137:1187–90.
174. Robinow ZM, Peterson C, Waldau B, Shahlaie K. Supraorbital keyhole craniotomy via eyebrow incision: a systematic review and meta-analysis. World Neurosurg. 2022;158:e509–42.
175. Ottenhausen M, Rumalla K, Alalade AF, et al. Decision-making algorithm for minimally invasive approaches to anterior skull base meningiomas. Neurosurg Focus. 2018;44:E7.
176. Di Somma A, Andaluz N, Cavallo LM, et al. Endoscopic transorbital route to the petrous apex: a feasibility anatomic study. Acta Neurochir. 2018;160:707–20.
177. Carnevale JA, Ramirez-Loera C, Goldberg JL, Godfrey KJ, Schwartz TH. Transorbital endoscopic approach for middle fossa floor/lateral cavernous sinus meningioma: 2-dimensional operative video. Oper Neurosurg. 2022;24(3):e201–2. https://doi.org/10.1227/ons.0000000000000496.
178. Noiphithak R, Yanez-Siller JC, Revuelta Barbero JM, Otto BA, Carrau RL, Prevedello DM. Comparative analysis between lateral orbital rim preservation and osteotomy for transorbital endoscopic approaches to the cavernous sinus: an anatomic study. Oper Neurosurg. 2019;16:86–93.
179. Vural A, Carobbio ALC, Ferrari M, et al. Transorbital endoscopic approaches to the skull base: a systematic literature review and anatomical description. Neurosurg Rev. 2021;44:2857–78.

Technical Nuances: Indications for Transorbital Compared to Endoscopic Endonasal Approach

33

Hanna N. Algattas, S. Tonya Stefko, Georgios A. Zenonos, Eric W. Wang, Carl H. Snyderman, and Paul A. Gardner

Introduction

Like the endoscopic endonasal approach (EEA), transorbital approaches (TOA) have been developed as minimally invasive corridors to the skull base. While both routes have become workhorses in their regard, multiple factors, including anatomic relationships and clinical judgment, are necessary in selecting the appropriate approach. TOAs include TOES (TransOrbital EndoscopicvSurgery), supraorbital craniotomy, orbitozygomatic (OZ) modifications, lateral orbitotomy, transconjunctival, and transcaruncular approaches. The EEA can be reduced to a series of modules that build upon one another in the sagittal and coronal planes; of particular importance in gaining access to the orbit are the transcribriform and transpterygoid modules [1–3].

With any minimally invasive approach, recognition of safe corridors and regions of access is of utmost importance in avoiding severe complications. While there are anatomical regions that overlap between EEA and TOA, access trajectories and the identification of critical structures may better suit one approach over the other. The orbit has been likened to a clock face, and the location of pathologies in relation to the orbit is used to select the type of TOA [4, 5]. Lesions along the entire medial orbit can usually be managed endonasally or via a multi-portal approach after taking into consideration their relation to critical neurovascular structures.

Extending from anatomical constraints are those related to pathology. EEA and TOA are used for several neoplasms of varied origins, including dural, neural, endothelial, inflammatory, and infectious. Factors to consider when determining surgical approach include access to the tumor epicenter, tumor extension, desired extent/radicality of resection, need for early

H. N. Algattas
Department of Neurological Surgery, University at Buffalo Neurosurgery, Buffalo, USA
e-mail: halgattas@ubns.com

S. T. Stefko
Department of Ophthalmology, School of Medicine, University of Pittsburgh, Pittsburgh, PA, USA
e-mail: stefst@upmc.edu

G. A. Zenonos · P. A. Gardner (✉)
Department of Neurological Surgery, School of Medicine, University of Pittsburgh, Pittsburgh, PA, USA
e-mail: zenonosg2@upmc.edu; gardpa@upmc.edu

E. W. Wang · C. H. Snyderman
Department of Otolaryngology, School of Medicine, University of Pittsburgh, Pittsburgh, PA, USA
e-mail: wangew@upmc.edu; snydermanch@upmc.edu

T. H. Schwartz et al. (eds.), *Endoscopic Transorbital Surgery of the Orbit, Skull Base and Brain*, https://doi.org/10.1007/978-3-031-59504-2_33

devascularization, access to vascularized/reconstructive tissue, and complication reduction. Distinct from anatomy and pathology are other essential factors not to be underestimated, including functional status, morbidity assessment, familiarity with approach, availability of co-surgeons and ancillary staff, cosmetic considerations and, of course, patient preference. After accounting for these factors, possessing endonasal and transorbital options within the surgical armamentarium is extraordinarily valuable. Importantly, clinical judgment is necessary in selecting and evaluating the anatomic, pathologic, and practical considerations for either technique to increase the likelihood of optimum outcomes.

Anatomic Considerations

While endonasal approaches provide inferomedial access, most transorbital approaches, like open craniotomies, inherently provide an anterolateral to the medial corridor. Anatomy does not change, though vantage points, surgical mobility, and safe operating windows will differ (Fig. 33.1).

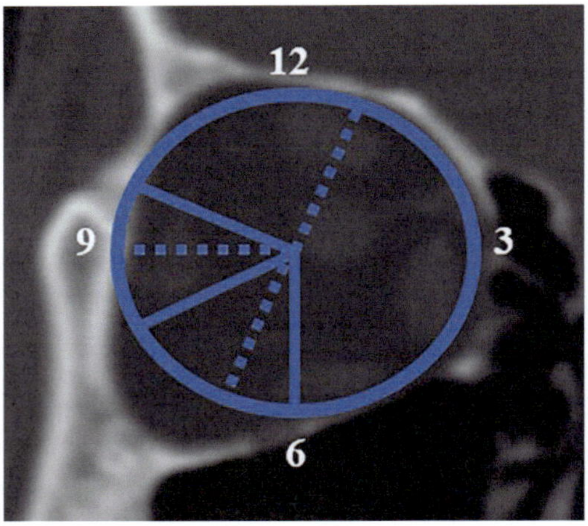

Fig. 33.1 Clock-face representation of approaches to pathologies encompassing orbit. 1 o'clock to 6 o'clock position: medial micro-orbitotomy. 1 o'clock to 7 o'clock position: endoscopic endonasal approach, 6 o'clock to 8 o'clock position: additional zygomatic osteotomy. 8 o'clock to 10 o'clock position: lateral orbitotomy. 9 o'clock to 1 o'clock position: frontotemporal craniotomy/orbitotomy

In the endonasal coronal plane, the medial half of the orbit posterior to the globe, from roof to floor, is accessible, even to the midorbit. TOAs are better suited for pathologies lateral to a line vertically bisecting the orbit via lateral orbitotomy or modified OZ approaches via an eyelid crease. In addition, the location of the lesion within the sagittal plane needs to be factored in with the coronal plane locale to determine accessibility. Lesions posterior to the globe within the orbit, especially towards the orbital apex, are well suited for endonasal management. Cardenas et al. identified the interethmoidal zone, relative to the orbit, as the region granting the largest degree of superomedial orbitectomy endonasally [6]. Further anteriorly toward the anterior ethmoids, the same coronal plane reach is limited by the cartilaginous nares, lateral nasal wall and nasolacrimal duct. Lesions anterior to the posterior table of the frontal sinus, such as nasofrontal encephaloceles and cerebrospinal fluid (CSF) leaks, may be difficult to manage purely endonasally. Multiportal approaches incorporating the medial transorbital approaches, such as transcaruncular or transconjunctival, with endoscopic assistance can be helpful for excessively anteromedial lesions [7, 8].

The endonasal limitation posteriorly is the optic nerve, which blocks access to the lateral optic canal and anterior clinoid process (ACP) [9]. The ACP is bound by three roots: the roof of the optic canal, the lesser wing of the sphenoid, and the optic strut. When the sphenoid sinus is well pneumatized, the optic strut is synonymous with the lateral optico-carotid recess from an endonasal vantage point. Complete and safe detachment of the ACP is not recommended endonasally due to the risk of injury to the optic nerve and carotid artery [10]. Cases where anterior clinoidectomy is necessary are better suited for TOAs such as lateral orbitotomy, supraorbital craniotomy, or eyelid crease-modified OZ craniotomies.

Lesions of the cavernous sinus are accessible via both approaches, but their precise location within the cavernous sinus and point of origin and the resultant displacement of cranial nerves are essential in selecting the approach [11]. The superior, posterior, and inferior compartments are well accessed endonasally, with the major risk, aside from carotid artery injury, being abducens palsy. TOAs attempting to reach these compartments require traversing cranial nerves of the superior orbital fissure (SOF). The lateral compartment of the cavernous sinus is better approached laterally (i.e., TOA) if the lesion originates laterally and due to the risk of crossing the carotid artery from the endonasal route. Importantly, the lateral wall of the cavernous sinus is composed of a dual dural layer comprising a dura propria and separate layer contiguous with the epineurium of the SOF and Meckel's cave cranial nerves. Sectioning of the meningo-orbital band (MOB) and interdural dissection between these layers is necessary to expose the lateral cavernous sinus, which can be achieved via lateral orbitotomy or eyelid OZ approaches.

Like the lateral cavernous sinus, the middle fossa is well-suited for TOAs, particularly lateral orbitotomy. Meckel's cave can be accessed via both approaches, but well-pneumatized lateral recesses certainly facilitate endonasal access. However, with inferior extension of lesions into the inferotemporal fossa (IFT) the TOAs reach limitation and limited vascular control. The IFT can be accessed via endonasal approaches with a maxillary antrostomy and transpterygoid extension. Caldwell-Luc incision and transalisphenoid approach through the ipsilateral maxillary sinus can also facilitate IFT access [12, 13]. The endonasal corridor provides superior proximal control to the internal maxillary artery within the IFT compared to TOAs, though both are options. In addition, the trajectory of the approach to Meckel's cave or the middle fossa is critical. For example, a trigeminal schwannoma that is more vertical (along V3 into the infratemporal fossa) may be more in line with an antero-medial trans-sinus approach, while a schwannoma that extends along V1 or V2 into Meckel's cave is exactly in line with a lateral orbitotomy trajectory (Fig. 33.2).

The petrous apex is a challenging location to reach due to its central location within the skull base and proximity to several critical neurovascular structures. Open craniotomy with anterior petrosectomy through Kawase's rhomboid provides one such vantage point [14]. The endonasal corridor via a transclival and transpterygoid accesses the most anterior aspect of the petrous apex and the petrous base but is limited in reaching the more posterolateral aspects of the petrous bone, which are better accessed via open craniotomy or TOA [3, 15]. However, coupling with a contralateral transmaxillary approach extends access capabilities. Accessing the petrous apex via a purely transorbital approach is technically challenging and may provide limited exposure to more extensive pathologies [16]. The TOA may carry greater risk to the greater superficial petrosal nerve (GSPN) due to the limited ability to elevate the middle fossa dura from a posterior to the anterior direction [17]. Ultimately, the evaluation of medial-lateral location along the petrous apex will help guide the decision between EEA and TOA.

Where TOAs gain superiority is with most purely orbital lesions. Both extraconal and intraconal lesions of the orbit are well accessed via the various orbital approaches. Still, there is a need for endonasal approaches for lesions located in the posterior orbit, medially between the medial and inferior recti, either extraconal or intraconal. However, with intraconal lesions that require sectioning of either the medial or inferior rectus, there is limited ability for reconstruction of the musculature from an endonasal approach and adding a transconjunctival approach to manage the muscle, either via retraction or detachment and re-attachment, is key for full access. In this manner, the endonasal approach is well suited for orbital lesions where displacement of the medial or inferior recti is the only manipulation necessary for their resection.

The last anatomic consideration that should be mentioned is, broadly, lesions within intraparenchymal brain locations. The primary consideration for intraparenchymal lesions is their relationship to functional neural tissue and the necessity of vascular control. Midline lesions are inherently better suited for the endonasal approach. Examples are those along the anterior

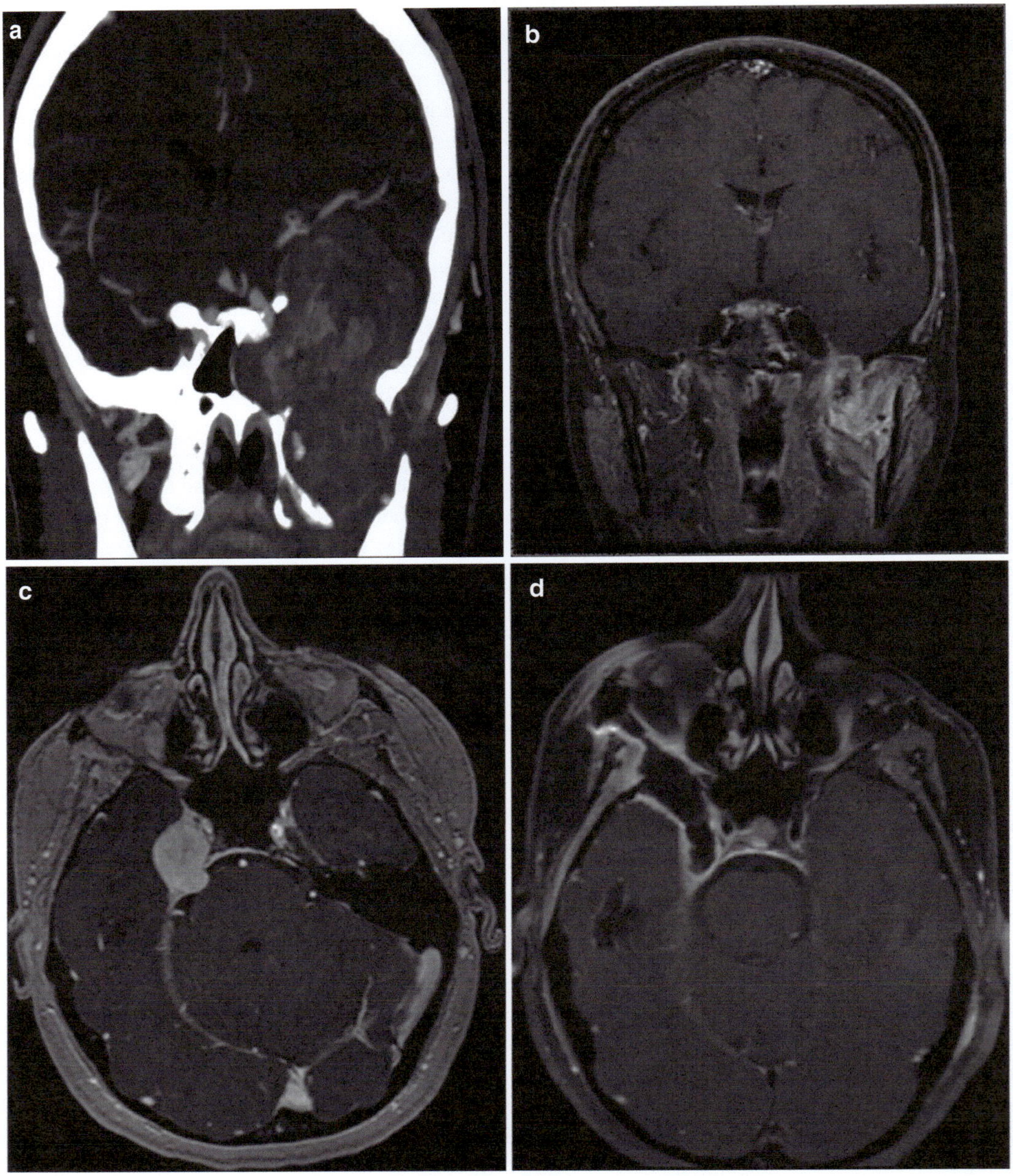

Fig. 33.2 (**a**) Coronal CTA showing a V3 schwannoma involving Meckel's cave. The vertical dimension of the tumor is well suited for an anteromedial approach such as EEA and anterior transmaxillary (Caldwell Luc, transalisphenoid) approach. (**b**) Immediate postoperative post-contrast T1-weighted coronal MRI showing complete resection via this approach. (**c**) Axial post-contrast T1 weighted MRI image shows a growing schwannoma involving Meckel's cave and V2, perfectly in line with the trajectory of a lateral orbitotomy approach (LOA). (**d**) Postoperative, post-contrast, T1-weighted MRI showing complete removal via LOA

cranial fossa, suprasellar space, or extending through the retrochiasmatic corridor into the third ventricle. Lesions of the temporal pole or anterior or lateral frontal lobe are better approached via lateral orbitotomy, supraorbital craniotomy or eyelid crease, respectively.

Pathologic Considerations

While anatomy guides the selection of approach, pathology guides the technique employed and the extent of resection. Furthermore, when selecting between two minimally invasive options, such as the EEA and TOA, preservation of olfactory and ocular function must be considered. While there are myriad pathologies to consider, this discussion will be limited to the major culprits: meningioma, schwannoma, hemangioma, CSF leak and encephalocele, sinonasal tumors, and lesions requiring optic nerve decompression.

While classified based on their dural pedicle, meningiomas can arise from any dural surface within the central nervous system, making each unique. It is well-accepted that, typically, meningiomas of the skull base are more indolent (most often WHO grade I) than those of the cerebral convexity, falx, and parasagittal space (WHO grade II) [18]. One theory for this variation is the immune micro-environment, with skull base meningiomas demonstrating elevated oncolytic gamma-delta T cells. In contrast, convexity meningiomas have elevated oncogenic mast cells and neutrophils [19]. Thus, given that lesions requiring EEA or TOA are more likely to be WHO grade I, the first preoperative consideration should be the planned extent of resection. This decision is not straightforward and needs to be weighed along with the patient's age, life expectancy, preoperative functional status, nutritional status, comorbidities, anesthetic risk, social factors, and much more. Furthermore, radiographic factors weigh into this equation and include tumor vascularity, predicted tumor consistency, extent of dural involvement, bone involvement, and reconstruction options. In addition, with the increasing advances in radiation, including stereotactic radiosurgery, treatment of residual radiation is a well-accepted option.

A common location for skull base meningiomas is the anterior cranial fossa (ACF), either along the olfactory groove, planum sphenoidale, or tuberculum sella. The primary benefit of the endonasal approach along the ACF is early devascularization of the dural pedicle and wide bony removal [20]. Preoperative olfactory function must be considered, particularly with olfactory groove and planum meningiomas. When olfaction is present, a supraorbital craniotomy may be more appropriate, depending on the patient's preference; however, open approaches require frontal lobe manipulation or retraction and have an increased incidence of postoperative seizure and FLAIR changes on MRI [21, 22]. A special consideration for any endonasal approach is the presence of comorbid obstructive sleep apnea (OSA) requiring continuous positive airway pressure (CPAP) ventilation. In large skull base reconstructions, as is the case for olfactory groove meningiomas approached endonasally, CPAP should be avoided for several weeks postop given the risk of CSF leak, reconstruction failure, and tension pneumocephalus. Though not an absolute contraindication, in patients with severe OSA in whom Simpson Grade I resection with extensive bony and dural resection is not indicated, TOA may be a better option [20]. For extensive tumors, some argue for a combined approach with endonasal and supraorbital craniotomy for resection [23].

Lateral extension or origin of meningiomas begin favoring TOA, particularly those of the anterior clinoid or sphenoid wing. Anteriorly, the EEA is limited to the mid-orbit in the coronal plane; posteriorly, the ACP is not well-accessed via endonasally and places undue risk on the optic nerve. Furthermore, complete resection typically requires anterior clinoidectomy, which is not safe endonasally and better suited for eyelid crease-modified OZ approaches. Sphenoid wing meningiomas are prime for TOA and inappropriate targets for the EEA. Special consideration needs to be given toward sphenocavernous and spheno-orbito-cavernous meningiomas, which extend into multiple compartments that may include the sellar and suprasellar spaces, orbit, posterior fossa, and cavernous sinus. Gross total resection (GTR) is not possible for these lesions, and staged approaches, which may include radiosurgery, are often necessary. The order of approach depends on the patient presenting symptoms. Those who present with vision loss and oculomotor deficits may require TOA first for debulking and lateral cavernous sinus cranial nerve decompression; in severe vision loss cases, the endonasal approach can then be used to achieve 360-degree decompression of the optic nerve. Commonly, patients may present with hyperprolactinemia due to compression of the pituitary gland or early optic neuropathy due to optic nerve compression. These patients may benefit from endonasal debulking first. Staging is generally preferred over multiple weeks to avoid disrupting cranial nerve microvasculature and causing circumferential dissection or inflammation around the nerves.

Separate discussion is necessary to further discuss those lesions located near the canalicular portion of the optic nerve or within the optic nerve sheath (i.e., meningiomas). Pure nerve sheath meningiomas do not have any intracranial or intradural extension but rather have a classic circumferential appearance around the optic nerve in the orbit. Radiotherapy has historically been used to control meningiomas and lesions in close proximity, or intertwined, with the optic nerve in this location [24]. While surgical resection portends high visual morbidity, the role of optic nerve decompression in conjunction with radiotherapy has not been well addressed [25]. Selecting between the EEA and TOA for optic nerve decompression again relies on the extent of disease and location [26]. The TOA approach is useful for significant disease burdens lateral to the optic nerve, where the primary vector of compression is directed from lateral to medial. In such cases, anterior clinoidectomy and unroofing of the optic canal may improve visual acuity. Compression from a medial vector and extending into the intracanalicular segment of the optic is better approached endonasally given the ability to decompress a long nerve segment and safely biopsy any exophytic portion when necessary. These lesions may also occur bilaterally, in which the endonasal approach can allow bilateral decompressions in the same surgical setting rather than requiring two separate lateral approaches.

Schwannomas may be mistaken for skull base meningiomas, but their dumb-bell-shaped appearance paired with intradural and extradural extension should raise suspicion. One of the most important factors in selecting between EEA and TOA is the location of the schwannoma. Those exiting the foramen rotundum originate from V2, whereas those from foramen ovale originate from V3 origin. Location along the course of the nerve is also essential. Purely extradural V3 schwannomas commonly enter the infratemporal fossa and are better suited for endonasal resection with maxillary antrostomy and a possible transalisphenoid approach. Similarly, extradural V2 schwannomas may be appropriate for endonasal resection with transpterygoid approach. More proximal location of trigeminal schwannomas, towards Meckel's cave, is better suited for TOA since the trajectory from an endonasal corridor is fraught with risk due to the adjacent carotid artery and the lateral orbitotomy trajectory is directly in line with the tumor.

Orbital cavernous hemangiomas (OCH) are the most common benign orbital lesions in adults, typically intraconal. They are comprised of endothelial-lined vascular channels surrounded by a fibrous cap and require surgical resection when causing symptoms such as diplopia, vision loss, or significant proptosis. The predominant factor determining the approach is location. While OCHs may occur anywhere along the orbit, they have a predilection for the intraconal, middle third, often lateral to the optic nerve [27, 28]. Given that arterial supply within the middle third of the orbit is lateral to the optic nerve, this relationship makes sense [27]. While the middle and posterior third of the orbit are feasibly approached endonasally, lesions lateral to the optic nerve and/or ophthalmic artery branches are best approached via TOA. Lateral orbitotomy is often appropriate; however, large series have made judicious use of the transcutaneous/transconjunctival anterior orbitotomy [29]. When pos-

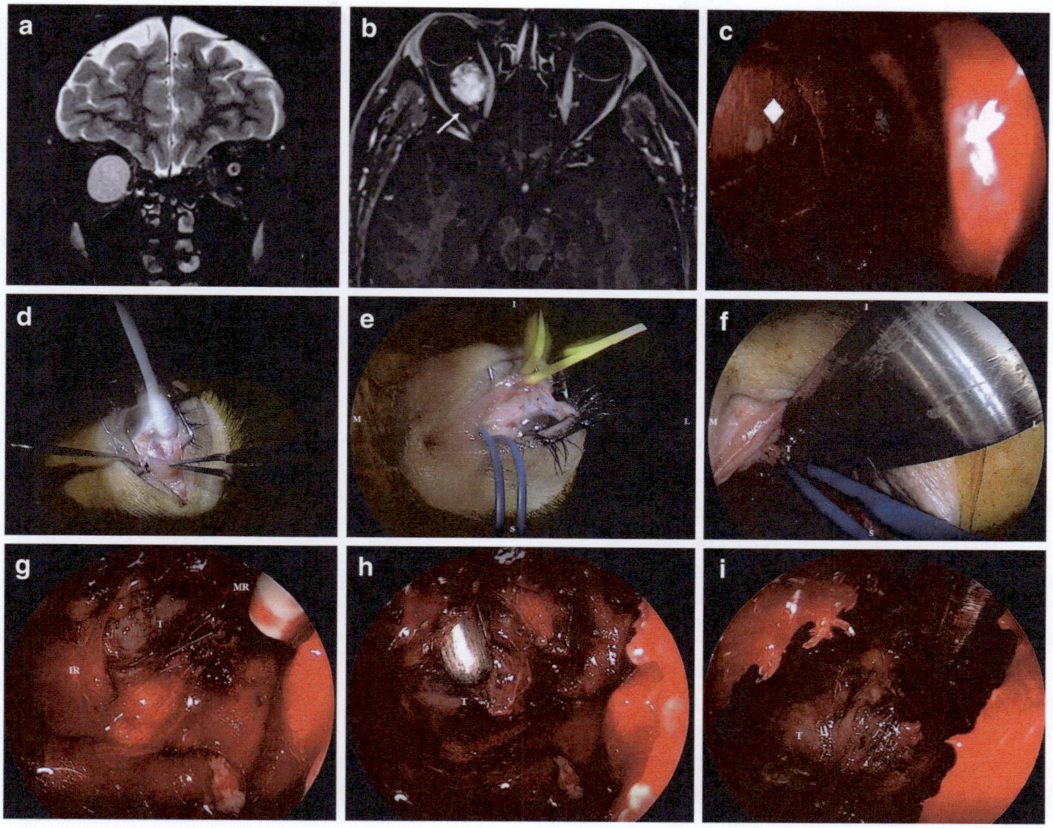

Fig. 33.3 A 40-year-old man presented with right-sided proptosis, vision loss, and diplopia with right lateral gaze. (**a**) Coronal T2-weighted MRI demonstrating hyperintense intraconal hemangioma within the quadrant between medial and inferior recti with resultant mass effect on the optic nerve (white arrow). (**b**) Axial T1-weighted and contrasted MRI with the heterogeneous but intense enhancement of hemangioma located lateral to medial rectus, causing the right optic nerve displacement. (**c**) Endonasal view after sphenoidotomy, ethmoidectomy, and removal of lamina papryacea for medial orbital decompression with periorbita revealed (white diamond). (**d**) Transcaruncular approach with identification of medial rectus (black arrow). (**e**) Identification of inferior lateral rectus (yellow vessel loop) and medial rectus (blue vessel loop) to allow mobilization of the eye within orbit. (**f**) Dissection of hemangioma via transcaruncular approach prior to resection from endonasal cavity. (**g**) Endonasal view after the opening of periorbita, identification of medial and inferior recti, and then identification and dissection of hemangioma. (**h**) Transorbital assistance for delivery of tumor via transcaruncular approach as viewed from endonasal view. (**i**) Final dissection and ultimately delivery of tumor via endonasal route. *I* inferior, *IR* inferior rectus, *L* lateral, *M* medial, *MR* medial rectus, *S* superior, *T* tumor

teriorly located, toward within the orbit, they can take a 'pear-shaped' appearance due to the bony confinement of the orbital apex, and they should remain in the differential [30]. Depending on the relation to the neurovascular structures at the orbital apex, an endonasal approach may be more appropriate, particularly because the ophthalmic originates inferomedially relative to the optic nerve at the orbital apex and may suggest the OCH arises closer to that location (Fig. 33.3) [31]. This consideration of the location of the tumor relative to the optic nerve perfectly illustrates the clock analogy, with the approach selected to avoid any manipulation or crossing of the optic nerve.

Sinonasal malignancies often involve the orbit via direct invasion, perineural spread or adjacent extension. Naturally, a tumor that originates in the nasal corridor and compresses the orbit can usually be managed completely or mostly endonasally. However, tumors whose margin extends laterally to the midorbit or anterior to the globe are best managed with a combined EEA and TOA. Pure V1 involvement with perineural invasion of a sinus or cutaneous malignancy can usually be managed with a TOA alone.

Lastly, a non-neoplastic entity requiring discussion is a spontaneous CSF leak and encephalocele. Common locations for spontaneous leaks include the cribriform (bordering the olfactory sulcus of nasofrontal recesses), the lateral recess of the sphenoid, and Meckel's cave. The EEA is commonly preferred for the repair of these defects due to the presence of several reconstruction options, including the nasoseptal flap and free mucosal grafts (i.e., middle turbinate or nasal floor grafts). The lateral TOA (LTOA) has shown success in repairing lateral recess defects with a shorter working distance and without the need to sacrifice the sphenopalatine artery; however, as the authors accurately report, reconstruction focuses on muscle patches and sewn grafts rather than vascularized reconstruction methods [32]. Laterally located leaks of Meckel's cave can be considered for TOA in select situations. Special attention should be given to cribriform leaks, particularly those located exceptionally anteriorly. These can be challenging to approach endonasally due to access limitations and require angled endoscopy. Very anterior defects in the frontal sinus or near the nasofrontal duct may be most easily managed via a medial TOA, though an EEA can still be used for many of these. True multi-portal surgery is often helpful in these cases, with endoscope-assisted medial TOAs to provide dual access to these locations [33, 34].

Conclusion

EEA, TOA, and their variations have significant merit as minimally invasive options limiting morbidity for a variety of diseases of the skull base and orbit. A thorough understanding of anatomy and pathology is necessary for EEA and TOA selection. Importantly, the disease should be viewed in the unique context of each patient to help assess the goals of the surgery. It is worth noting, however, that surgical experience with each approach should represent a substantial consideration when selecting an approach. Both approaches have a learning curve and require a certain degree of facility not only for the primary surgeon(s) but also for appropriate co-surgeon involvement, dedication, and ancillary staff experience. When necessary, both approaches can be combined for unique multi-portal surgical solutions.

References

1. Kassam A, Snyderman CH, Mintz A, Gardner P, Carrau RL. Expanded endonasal approach: the rostrocaudal axis. Part I. Crista galli to the sella turcica. Neurosurg Focus. 2005;19(1):E3.
2. Kassam A, Snyderman CH, Mintz A, Gardner P, Carrau RL. Expanded endonasal approach: the rostrocaudal axis. Part II. Posterior clinoids to the foramen magnum. Neurosurg Focus. 2005;19(1):E4.
3. Kassam AB, Gardner P, Snyderman C, Mintz A, Carrau R. Expanded endonasal approach: fully endoscopic, completely transnasal approach to the middle third of the clivus, petrous bone, middle cranial fossa, and infratemporal fossa. Neurosurg Focus. 2005;19(1):E6.
4. Paluzzi A, Gardner PA, Fernandez-Miranda JC, Tormenti MJ, Stefko ST, Snyderman CH, et al. "Round-the-clock" surgical access to the orbit. J Neurol Surg Part B Skull Base. 2015;76(1):12–24.
5. Cockerham KP, Bejjani GK, Kennerdell JS, Maroon JC. Surgery for orbital tumors. Part II: transorbital approaches. Neurosurg Focus. 2001;10(5):E3.
6. Cárdenas Ruiz-Valdepeñas E, Kaen A, González-Martínez E, Gardner PA, Wang EW, Snyderman CH, et al. Endoscopic endonasal superomedial orbitectomy: how far is safe and possible? Laryngoscope. 2020;130(5):1151–7.
7. Koutourousiou M, Gardner PA, Stefko ST, Paluzzi A, Fernandez-Miranda JC, Snyderman CH, et al. Combined endoscopic endonasal transorbital approach with transconjunctival-medial orbitotomy for excisional biopsy of the optic nerve: technical note. J Neurol Surg Rep. 2012;73(1):52–6.
8. Ogawa T, Nishimura K, Takahashi Y, Iwami K, Yasumura T, Yo K, et al. Incisionless facial resection for Kadish stage C olfactory neuroblastoma: transcaruncular approach with combined endonasal and skull base surgery. Clin Case Reports. 2020;8(8):1494–501.
9. Setty P, Fernandez-Miranda JC, Wang EW, Snyderman CH, Gardner PA. Residual and recurrent disease fol-

lowing endoscopic endonasal approach as a reflection of anatomic limitation for the resection of midline anterior skull base meningiomas. Oper Neurosurg. 2021;21(4):207–16.

10. Champagne PO, Zenonos GA, Wang EW, Snyderman CH, Gardner PA. Endoscopic endonasal anterior clinoidectomy: volumetric assessment and feasibility. World Neurosurg. 2022;168:e269–e77.
11. Fernandez-Miranda JC, Zwagerman NT, Abhinav K, Lieber S, Wang EW, Snyderman CH, et al. Cavernous sinus compartments from the endoscopic endonasal approach: anatomical considerations and surgical relevance to adenoma surgery. J Neurosurg. 2018;129(2):430–41.
12. Truong HQ, Sun X, Celtikci E, Borghei-Razavi H, Wang EW, Snyderman CH, et al. Endoscopic anterior transmaxillary "transalisphenoid" approach to Meckel's cave and the middle cranial fossa: an anatomical study and clinical application. J Neurosurg. 2018;130(1):227–37.
13. Lin BJ, Ju DT, Hsu TH, Chen YA, Chung TT, Liu WH, et al. Quantitative comparison of endoscopically assisted endonasal, sublabial and transorbital transmaxillary approaches to the anterolateral skull base. Clin Otolaryngol. 2021;46(1):123–30.
14. Tummala RP, Coscarella E, Morcos JJ. Transpetrosal approaches to the posterior fossa. Neurosurg Focus. 2005;19(2):E6.
15. Van Gompel JJ, Alikhani P, Tabor MH, van Loveren HR, Agazzi S, Froelich S, et al. Anterior inferior petrosectomy: defining the role of endonasal endoscopic techniques for petrous apex approaches. J Neurosurg. 2014;120(6):1321–5.
16. Di Somma A, Andaluz N, Cavallo LM, Topczewski TE, Frio F, Gerardi RM, et al. Endoscopic transorbital route to the petrous apex: a feasibility anatomic study. Acta Neurochir. 2018;160(4):707–20.
17. Topczewski TE, Di Somma A, Pineda J, Ferres A, Torales J, Reyes L, et al. Endoscopic endonasal and transorbital routes to the petrous apex: anatomic comparative study of two pathways. Acta Neurochir. 2020;162(9):2097–109.
18. Magill ST, Young JS, Chae R, Aghi MK, Theodosopoulos PV, McDermott MW. Relationship between tumor location, size, and WHO grade in meningioma. Neurosurg Focus. 2018;44(4):E4.
19. Zador Z, Landry AP, Balas M, Cusimano MD. Landscape of immune cell gene expression is unique in predominantly WHO grade 1 skull base meningiomas when compared to convexity. Sci Rep. 2020;10(1):9065.
20. Algattas HN, Wang EW, Zenonos GA, Snyderman CH, Gardner PA. Endoscopic endonasal surgery for anterior cranial fossa meningiomas. J Neurosurg Sci. 2021;65(2):118–32.
21. Goldschmidt E, Chabot JD, Algattas H, Lieber S, Khattar N, Nakassa ACI, et al. Seizure risk following open and expanded endoscopic endonasal approaches for intradural skull base tumors. J Neurol Surg Part B Skull Base. 2020;81(6):673–9.
22. de Almeida JR, Carvalho F, Vaz Guimaraes Filho F, Kiehl TR, Koutourousiou M, Su S, et al. Comparison of endoscopic endonasal and bifrontal craniotomy approaches for olfactory groove meningiomas: a matched pair analysis of outcomes and frontal lobe changes on MRI. J Clin Neurosci. 2015;22(11):1733–41.
23. Banu MA, Mehta A, Ottenhausen M, Fraser JF, Patel KS, Szentirmai O, et al. Endoscope-assisted endonasal versus supraorbital keyhole resection of olfactory groove meningiomas: comparison and combination of 2 minimally invasive approaches. J Neurosurg. 2016;124(3):605–20.
24. de Melo LP, Arruda Viani G, de Paula JS. Radiotherapy for the treatment of optic nerve sheath meningioma: a systematic review and meta-analysis. Radiother Oncol. 2021;165:135–41.
25. Maza G, Subramaniam S, Yanez-Siller JC, Otto BA, Prevedello DM, Carrau RL. The role of endonasal endoscopic optic nerve decompression as the initial management of primary optic nerve sheath meningiomas. J Neurol Surg Part B Skull Base. 2019;80(6):568–76.
26. Di Somma A, Cavallo LM, de Notaris M, Solari D, Topczewski TE, Bernal-Sprekelsen M, et al. Endoscopic endonasal medial-to-lateral and transorbital lateral-to-medial optic nerve decompression: an anatomical study with surgical implications. J Neurosurg. 2017;127(1):199–208.
27. McNab AA, Selva D, Hardy TG, O'Donnell B. The anatomical location and laterality of orbital cavernous haemangiomas. Orbit. 2014;33(5):359–62.
28. McNab AA, Wright JE. Cavernous haemangiomas of the orbit. Aust N Z J Ophthalmol. 1989;17(4):337–45.
29. Yan J, Wu Z. Cavernous hemangioma of the orbit: analysis of 214 cases. Orbit. 2004;23(1):33–40.
30. Kloos R, Mourits D, Saeed P, Mourits M. Orbital apex cavernous hemangioma–beware of the pear! Acta Ophthalmol. 2013;91(4):e328–9.
31. Chen L, White WL, Xu B, Tian X. Transnasal transsphenoid approach: a minimally invasive approach for removal of cavernous haemangiomas located at inferomedial part of orbital apex. Clin Experiment Ophthalmol. 2010;38(5):439–43.
32. Alves-Belo JT, Mangussi-Gomes J, Truong HQ, Cohen S, Gardner PA, Snyderman CH, et al. Lateral transorbital versus endonasal transpterygoid approach to the lateral recess of the sphenoid sinus-a comparative anatomic study. Oper Neurosurg. 2019;16(5):600–6.
33. Noiphithak R, Yanez-Siller JC, Nimmannitya P, Rukskul P. Transorbital endoscopic approach for repair of frontal sinus cerebrospinal fluid leaks: case-series. Laryngoscope. 2021;131(8):1753–7.
34. Lee WJ, Hong SD, Woo KI, Seol HJ, Choi JW, Lee JI, et al. Combined endoscopic endonasal and transorbital multiportal approach for complex skull base lesions involving multiple compartments. Acta Neurochir. 2022;164(7):1911–22.

Transorbital Approaches to the Skull Base Triangles

34

Doo-Sik Kong

It is critical for surgeons to have thorough knowledge of the anatomical complexity of the skull base and associated neurovascular structures. This has been made possible with the advent of a better understanding of skull base anatomy from the transorbital perspective, as well as the development of better instrumentation [1]. Essential neurovascular structures are occasionally distorted or displaced by surgical pathologies or congenital variations. In these situations, anatomical triangles surrounded by important landmarks guide surgeons during complex skull base procedures. Knowledge of skull base triangles combined with neurosurgical navigation is essential to achieve successful surgical dissection, minimize surgical risks, and ensure surgical safety.

The chosen surgical corridor guides the surgeon to the surgical field and provides confidence in the localization of the skull base during dissection [1]. However, anatomical triangles in the skull base provide safe pathways to enter the cavernous sinus. These have been described under the microscope from a transcranial surgical view. This is also a top-down approach. Because endoscopic transorbital surgery only allows a very small surgical window to access the skull base and also provides an anteromedial or anterolateral surgical corridor, it remains unclear whether these important anatomical triangles can still serve as landmarks to guide surgeons under the endoscopic view. Here, we show the representative anatomical triangles as they appear from the endoscopic transorbital perspective to guide surgeons and inform endoscopic dissection in the middle cranial fossa (Fig. 34.1).

D.-S. Kong (✉)
Department of Neurosurgery, Samsung Medical Center, Sungkyunkwan University, Seoul, South Korea

T. H. Schwartz et al. (eds.), *Endoscopic Transorbital Surgery of the Orbit, Skull Base and Brain*,
https://doi.org/10.1007/978-3-031-59504-2_34

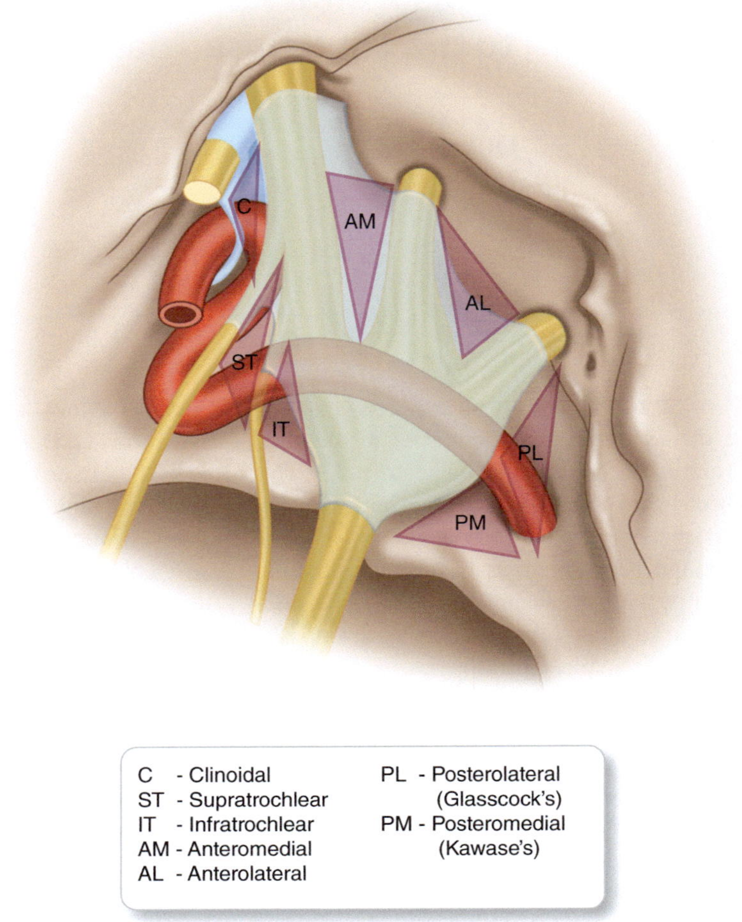

Fig. 34.1 Illustration describing the cavernous sinus triangle

Clinoidal Triangle

The clinoidal triangle is bordered by the optic strut anteriorly, the roof of the cavernous sinus posteriorly, and the optic nerve within the optic canal medially [2]. From the transorbital perspective, this clinoidal triangle can be exposed after the removal of the anterior clinoid process. To remove the anterior clinoidal process via the transorbital route requires significant experience with transorbital surgical technique. After drilling the greater and lesser sphenoid bones, the orbital roof connected to the optic canal located on the medial side of the superior orbital fissure is opened, and the base of the anterior clinoid process with a triangular shape is exposed. Careful drilling of the anterior clinoid process exposes the extradural segment of the internal carotid artery (Fig. 34.2).

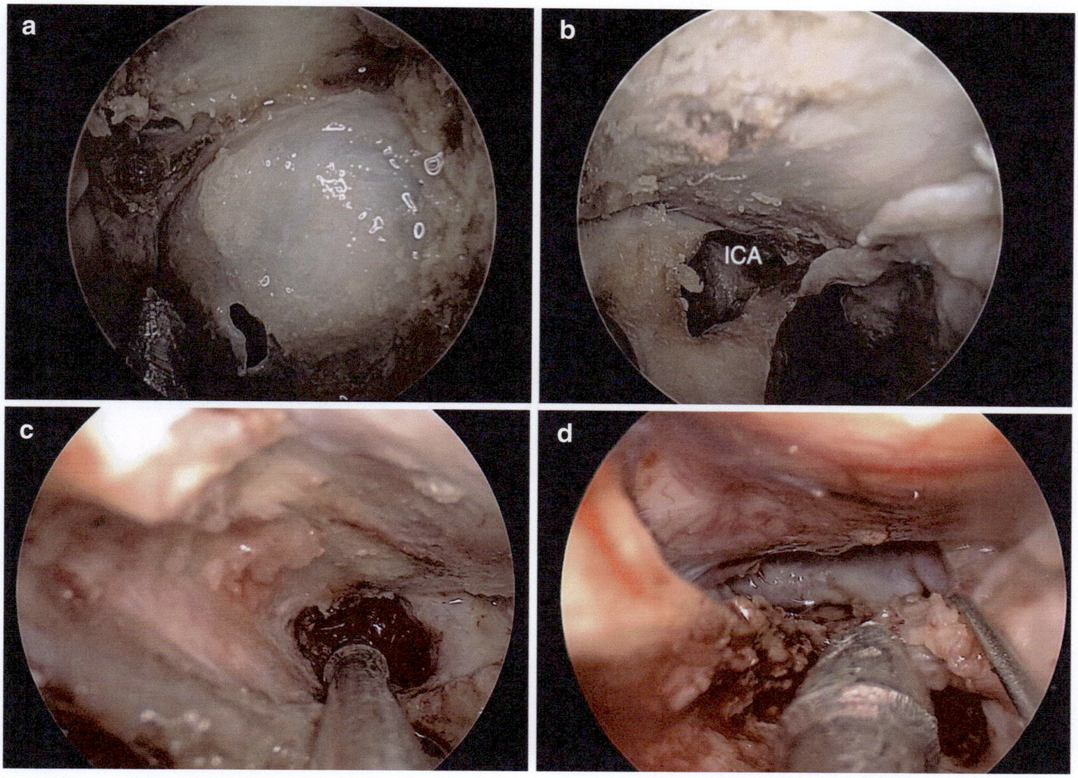

Fig. 34.2 Clinoidal triangle in the transorbital view. (**a**) The base of the anterior clinoidal process is seen after the removal of the greater and lesser sphenoid bone (cadaver specimen). (**b**) After removal of the anterior clinoidal process and opening of the dura, the clinoidal segment of the internal carotid artery is exposed. (**c**) In a patient with a clinoidal meningioma, the extradural optic canal is exposed after removal of the anterior clinoidal process. (**d**) After incision of the dura and removal of the tumor, ascending internal carotid artery with an ophthalmic branch is exposed

Mullan's Anteromedial Triangle

Mullan's anteromedial triangle is defined by the ophthalmic nerve (V1), maxillary nerve (V2), and a line between the foramen rotundum and the superior orbital fissure [3]. This triangle is the most commonly used route for accessing Meckel's cave lesions using the endoscopic transorbital approach. As the long axis of this triangle runs from anterior to posterior, the surgical corridor of the endoscopic transorbital approach is aligned with this triangle. Anatomically, the anteromedial triangle provides a wider surgical window than the anterolateral triangle (Fig. 34.3).

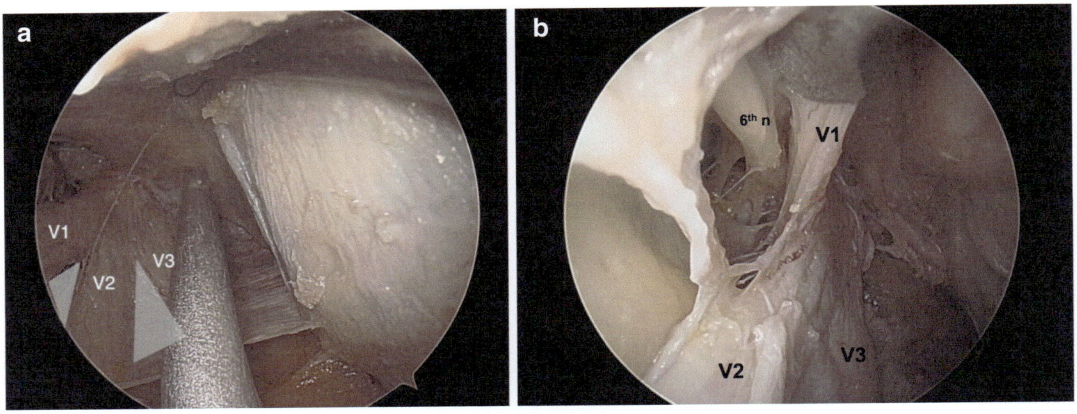

Fig. 34.3 Anteromedial and anterolateral triangle. (**a**) Anteromedial triangle between the V1 and V2 nerve. (**b**) Approaching Meckel's cave or the cavernous sinus via the anteromedial triangle exposes the 6th nerve

Anterolateral Triangle

The anterolateral triangle is bordered by the maxillary nerve (V2), the mandibular nerve (V3), and a line connecting foramen rotundum and ovale. When lesions involve the foramen ovale or the infratemporal fossa or widen the foramen ovale, the surgical corridor can be selected by the endoscopic transorbital view. Representative lesions requiring this corridor include meningoencephaloceles near the foramen rotundum or ovale and V2 or V3-origin trigeminal schwannomas extending into the infratemporal fossa or sphenoid sinus. Compared with the anteromedial triangle, this area is located on the floor of the middle cranial fossa and the transorbital approach should be directed downward. To do so, an inferior transconjunctival incision combined with the release of the lateral canthal ligament may be helpful. In addition, more downward drilling of the temporal fossa is required, and the temporal fossa should be flattened, just as the base of the sphenoid sinus is flattened during endoscopic endonasal surgery for sellar or clival lesions. More angled and longer instruments may be needed to reach the bottom of the lesion.

Kawase's Triangle

Kawase's triangle, also known as the posteromedial triangle, is formed by the mandibular nerve (V3), the greater superior petrosal nerve, the arcuate eminence, and the petrous ridge [4]. This surgical corridor is designed to access Meckel's cave and petroclival lesions, especially petrous apex bony lesions, using an anterior petrosal approach. To perform a successful anterior petrosal approach, a superolateral orbital rim osteotomy is essential to obtain sufficient working space. Unlike other surgical corridors, access via this route requires upward elevation of the temporal dura. The feasibility of the anterior petrosal approach for endoscopic transorbital surgery is still being clarified (Fig. 34.4).

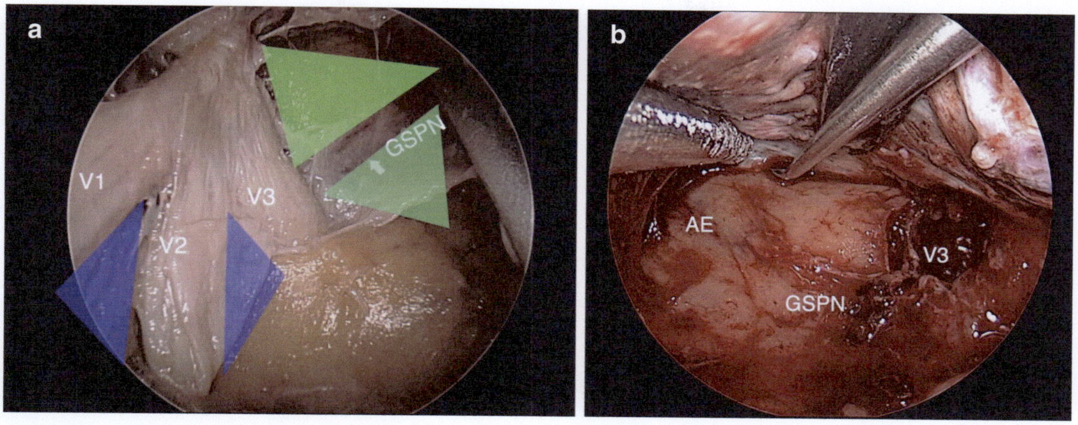

Fig. 34.4 Cadaver specimen describing the anteromedial, anterolateral, posteromedial (Kawase's) and posterolateral triangles. (**a**) Kawase's triangle is bordered by the lateral margin of the V3 nerve, the greater superficial petrosal nerve, arcuate eminence, and the petrous ridge. (**b**) Transorbital view of the petrous apex. *V1* the ophthalmic branch of the trigeminal nerve, *V2* the maxillary nerve, *V3* the mandibular nerve, *GSPN* the greater superficial petrosal nerve, *AE* the arcuate eminence

Parkinson's Triangle

The Parkinson's triangle, or the infratrochlear triangle, is bordered by the trochlear nerve, the ophthalmic nerve (V1), and the dural fold between the entries of the two nerves in the dura. Because this triangle is located in the upper lateral wall of the cavernous sinus, it is not easy to view the deep structures with a 0-degree endoscopic view. The angled endoscopic view through this triangle introduces access to the posterior compartment of the cavernous sinus and the posterior portion of the cavernous internal carotid artery, such as the meningohypophyseal trunk. In cases where the cavernous sinus is invaded by ACTH or GH-producing adenomas, surgical resection through this route provides a potential alternate strategy (Fig. 34.5).

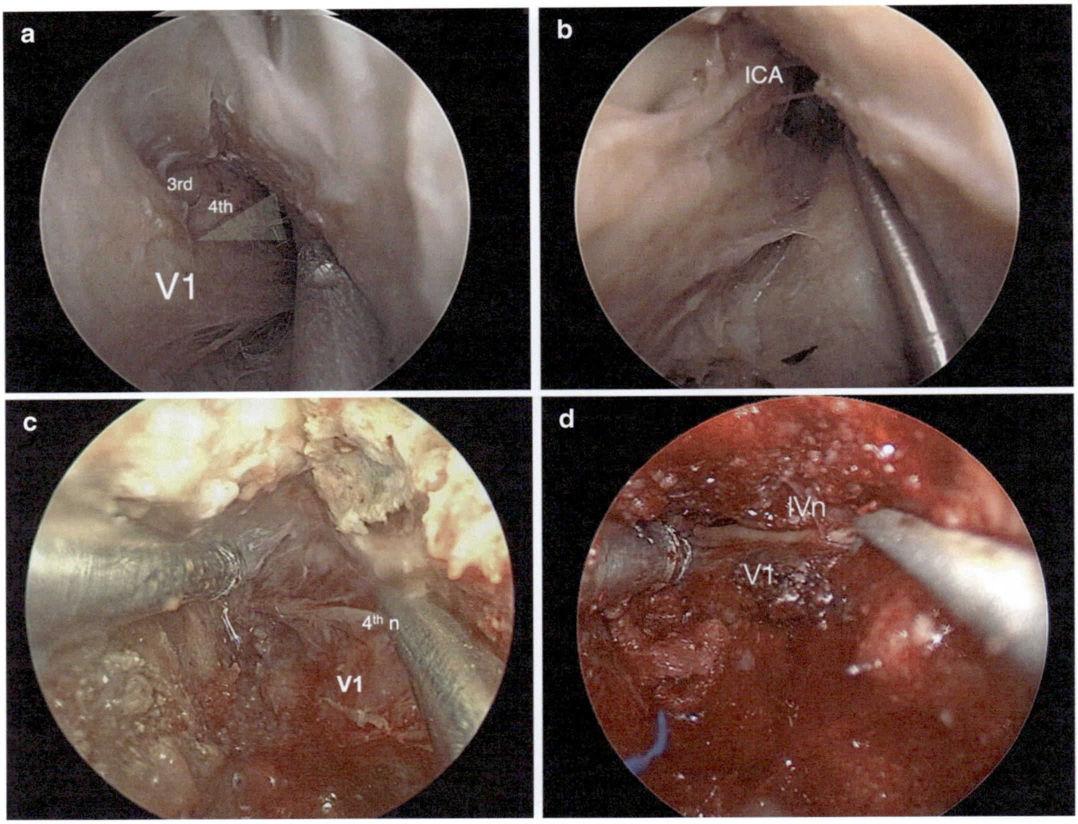

Fig. 34.5 Parkinson triangle. (**a**) Parkinson triangle is defined as the 4th nerve, V1 nerve, and dural fold. (**b**) Along this route, the internal carotid artery and its posterior compartmental structures are encountered. C&D, Endoscopic transorbital view of the Parkinson's triangle. Parkinson's triangle between the 4th nerve and the V1 nerve

Conclusions

Although skull base lesions can distort normal anatomy, comprehensive knowledge of normal anatomy is indispensable to recognize this distortion. For approaches to the cavernous sinus, understanding the triangles for safe entry is critical, equally for transcranial and transorbital surgery.

References

1. Hendricks BK, Benet A, Lawrence PM, Benner D, Preul MC, Lawton MT. Anatomical triangles for use in skull base surgery: a comprehensive review. World Neurosurg. 2022;164:79–92.
2. Isolan GR, Krayenbuhl N, de Oliveira E, Al-Mefty O. Microsurgical anatomy of the cavernous sinus: measurements of the triangles in and around it. Skull Base. 2007;17(6):357–67.
3. Alalade AF, Mensah E, Morosanu CO, Kumar A, Gurusinghe NT, Roberts GA. Skull base neurosurgery eponyms: a review of notable anatomical landmarks. World Neurosurg. 2022;168:26–42.
4. Fukaya R, Yoshida K, Ohira T, Kawase T. Trigeminal schwannomas: experience with 57 cases and a review of the literature. Neurosurg Rev. 2010;34(2):159–71.

Multi-Portal Approaches to the Skull Base: Expanding Indications

35

Brandon Lucke-Wold, Christopher Bergeron, Kris S. Moe, and Jeremy N. Ciporen

Introduction

Skull base tumors are frequently located in different compartments, thereby portending the need for combined skull base surgical approaches. Neuroendoscopy plays a major role in addressing the complexities of these tumors [1]. Multi-portal approaches to the skull base have grown over the past several years since the seminal papers introducing transorbital and multi-portal approaches to the skull base were first published [2]. The original TONES manuscript introduced the clinical application of transorbital approaches to the skull base [3]. This concept and clinical application were expanded with the Multi-Portal Approaches to the Central Skull Base paper in 2010 [4]. The concept of endoscopic multi-portal approaches to the central skull base highlighted the importance of versatility in addressing these complex tumors [5].

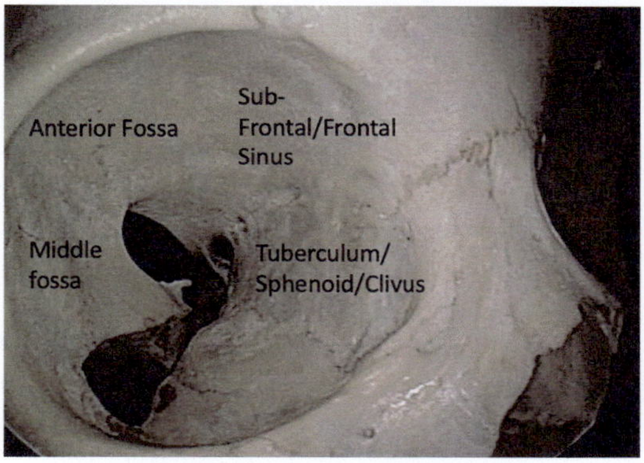

Fig. 35.1 Transorbital skull base access points

The "clock face" transorbital corridors described by Moe defined these minimally invasive passages to the anterior and middle fossa and the frontal and sphenoid sinuses (Fig. 35.1).

Endoscopic multi-portal techniques were developed to optimize microsurgical bi-manual dissection with the advantages of an enhanced field of visualization added by neuro-endoscopy [6]. The optimization of the four-handed microsurgical dissection techniques and visualization thereby lead to safer surgery and closes the gap between open and endoscopic microsurgical skull base techniques [7].

B. Lucke-Wold
Department of Neurosurgery, University of Florida, Gainesville, FL, USA

C. Bergeron
Division of Otolaryngology/Division of Neurosurgery, Scripps Clinic and Scripps Green Hospital, La Jolla, CA, USA
e-mail: Bergeron.chris@scrippshealth.org

K. S. Moe
Division of Facial Plastic Surgery, Departments of Otolaryngology and Neurological Surgery, University of Washington School of Medicine, Seattle, WA, USA
e-mail: krismoe@uw.edu

J. N. Ciporen (✉)
Department of Neurosurgery, Scripps Clinic Medical Group-Scripps Green Hospital, La Jolla, CA, USA
e-mail: ciporen.jeremy@scrippshealth.org

T. H. Schwartz et al. (eds.), *Endoscopic Transorbital Surgery of the Orbit, Skull Base and Brain*,
https://doi.org/10.1007/978-3-031-59504-2_35

Endoscopic Endonasal approaches began within the central skull base from the clivus, sella, parasellar, tuberculum, planum and cribriform. These approaches have expanded laterally to access the middle fossa, pterygopalatine and posterior fossa [8]. Despite the improved access, there were continued anatomic limitations to visualization and microsurgical access to pathology extending superiorly and lateral to critical structures such as the optic nerves, optic chiasm, and carotid arteries. Multi-portal skull base approaches involving the orbit provide improved and safer access to these challenging regions [9]. These combined minimally invasive approaches minimize the morbidity as presented in the recent case series. Endoscopic endonasal and multi-portal endoscopic approaches compliment open skull base techniques and add the skull base surgeon's skill set to optimize outcomes [10].

Recent manuscripts have stated the importance of multi-portal skull base techniques [11]. These manuscripts demonstrate the value of laboratory concept to practical application and adoption of multi-portal approaches to the skull base by the international community since the original manuscript published in 2010 [12].

Multi-portal and transorbital techniques have been widely adopted and recognized internationally with improved appreciation of anatomy [13]. In this chapter, we highlight these approaches to inspire the reader to study these approaches. Even if the approaches are not utilized, the study of them provides an improved 3D understanding of complex skull base anatomy (Figs. 35.6 and 35.7). In planning skull base surgery, advanced imaging and visualization are necessary to perform the operation safely. To achieve adequate visualization, one must have an advanced knowledge of the neuroanatomy and its relationship to the pathology being addressed [14]. This enables the surgeon to address the surgery's oncologic and reconstructive dimensions. The scope of this chapter is to highlight the use of the TOA precaruncular, supraorbital and sublabial Caldwell Luc ports in combination with the well-established EEEA.

The limitations of the EEA when dealing with lateral extension of anterior skull base meningiomas, and the limitations of the supraorbital eyebrow approach for medial skull base drilling and reconstruction, can be overcome by a judicious, anatomically based combination of both approaches [15].

Combined Expanded Endoscopic Endonasal and Transorbital Precaruncular Approach

The expanded endoscopic endonasal approach (EEEA) is the work horse approach for endoscopic anterior skull base surgery (Fig. 35.2) [8].

These approaches have been expanded laterally to the trans-ptyergoid approach and inferiorly to address C2 pathology. Skull base pathology frequently transcends regions anatomically limited by bone, arteries and/or cranial nerves. Multi-portal approaches have evolved over the last decade whereby the portal approaches complement the EEEA. There are many challenges to the EEEA approach. As the dissection extends posteriorly toward the posterior fossa, there is a natural coning-down effect. This principal challenge makes bi-manual surgical techniques more difficult. Visualization is critical, and the need for suction and the use of multiple instruments to safely manage tumors, especially those that are vascular, is limited through the EEEA approach alone [16]. Chordomas and clival meningiomas typically encase brainstem perforating vessels and cranial nerves. While the EEEA approach is very effective, a transorbital port may be considered to provide an offset view (Fig. 35.3) [17]. This offers an improved dimensional view of the tip of instruments as it relates to critical anatomy.

The medial transorbital approach (TOA) via a precaruncular approach was applied to multiple skull base pathologies by Moe et al. In 2010, our report defined the anatomy and utilization of this approach to complement the EEEA (Fig. 35.3) [4]. Further studies have demonstrated the ergonomic advantages and improved degrees of free-

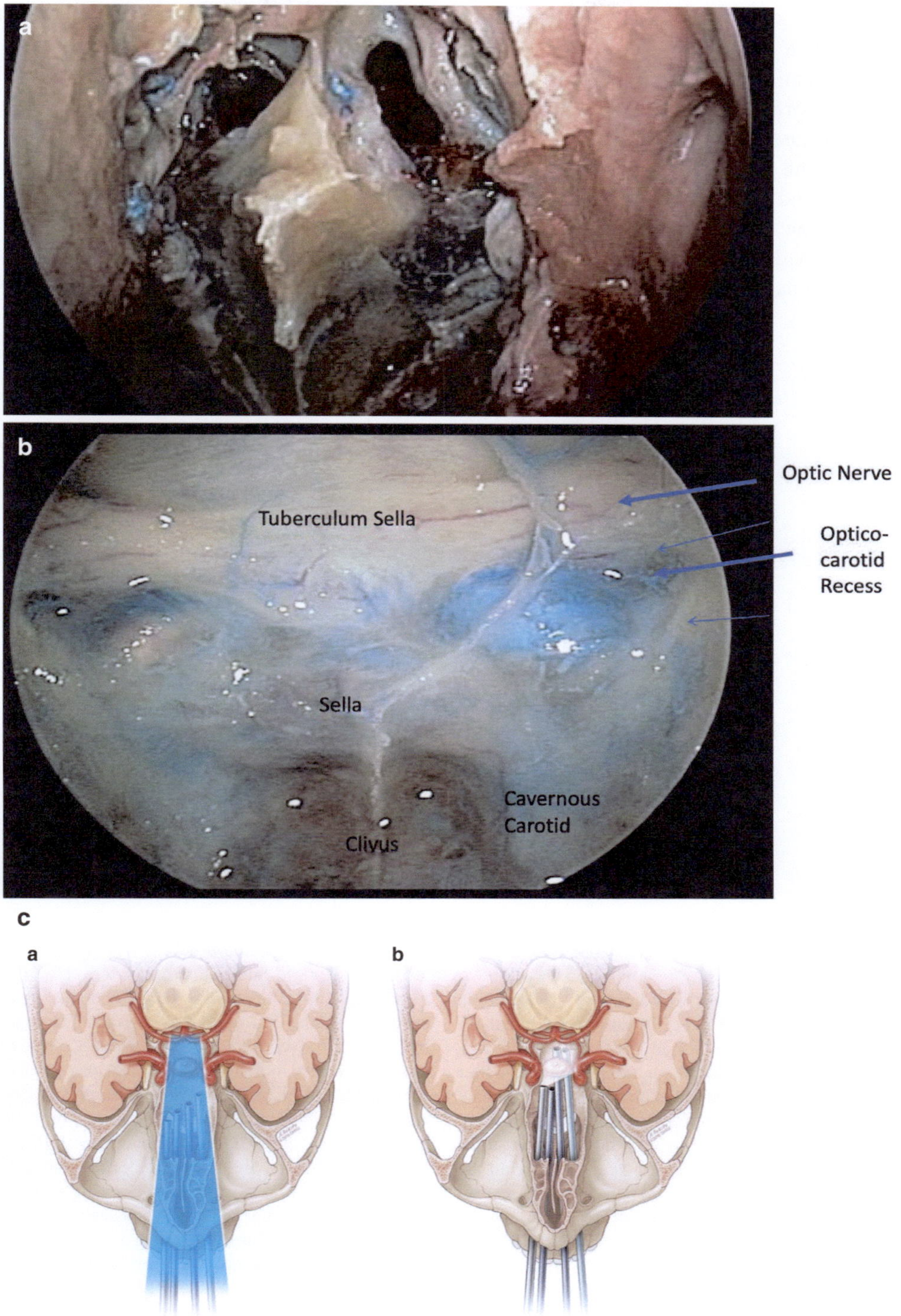

Fig. 35.2 (**a**) Expanded endoscopic endonasal approach with view of sphenoid sinus showing bilateral ostia. The bilateral nares approach provides sufficient opportunity to develop nasoseptal flap as well as to further operate beyond the sphenoid. (**b**) Expanded endoscopic endonasal approach showing posterior sphenoid sinus and relevant anatomy. (**c**) Expanded endoscopic endonasal approach to the sphenoid, clivus, sella, tuberculum. Bi-Nares and bi-manual four-handed technique

dom gained when these approaches are combined. The description of this multiport approach is detailed in the figures below. In planning, it is important to recognize that the fronto-ethmoidal suture defines the region of access [18]. Above the frontal ethmoidal suture to the frontal sinus and sub-frontal region are accessed, whereas below the frontal ethmoidal suture, access is gained to the sphenoid sinus, clivus, sella, cavernous sinus, parasellar region, and tuberculum.

Recent manuscripts have stated the importance of multi-portal skull base techniques [11]. These manuscripts demonstrate the value of laboratory concept to practical application and adoption of multi-portal approaches to the skull base by the international community since the original manuscript published in 2010 [12].

> *The judicious combination of transcranial and endoscopic-transnasal approaches warrants highest chances of achieving satisfactory tumors resection with a reduced risk of complications* [19].

Fig. 35.3 (**a**) Precaruncular approach showing caruncular lateralization for increased visualization. (**b**) Appreciated anatomy of anterior ethmoidal artery (AEA), fronto-ethmoidal suture (FES), instrument (IN), lamina papyricea (LP), and periorbita (PO) with the precaruncular approach. (**c**) Upon further dissection periorbita, fronto-ethmoidal suture, and lamina papyricea are better visualized as exposure is extended down to the optic canal (OC). (**d**) Bone schematic showing increased working angles with combined approach and appreciation of opened lamina papyracea, optic canal, superior orbital fissure, sphenoid, sphenoid ostia, and middle turbinate. (**e**) Right transorbital view through the defect in the medial orbital wall. An ethmoidectomy, middle turbinectomy has been performed, in addition to the removal of the face of the sphenoid and the bone over the sella and tuberculum. *C* clivus, *EAC* ethmoidal air cells, *LICA* left internal carotid artery, *P* pituitary. (**f**) Right transorbital view (0° endoscope) of the sella, suprasellar and parasellar regions. The tuberculum has been removed and the dura opened. Multi-portal access TOA and EEEA. *ACoA* anterior communicating artery, *LACA* left anterior cerebral artery, *LICA* left internal carotid artery, *LON* left optic nerve, *OC* optic chiasm, *P* pituitary, *RACA* right anterior cerebral artery, *RICA* right internal carotid artery, *ON* right optic nerve. (**g**) Right transorbital view (0° endoscope) of the sella, suprasellar and parasellar regions. The tuberculum has been removed and the dura opened. An endonasal trans-sphenoidal port is used for the instrument. Multi-portal TOA and EEEA access. *ACoA* anterior communicating artery, *LACA* left anterior cerebral artery, *LICA* left internal carotid artery, *LON* left optic nerve, *OC* optic chiasm, *P* pituitary, *RACA* right anterior cerebral artery, *RICA* right internal carotid artery, *ON* right optic nerve. (**h**) Right transorbital view (0° endoscope) of brainstem and posterior circulation. The clival dura has been opened. An endonasal trans-sphenoidal port is used for the instrument. Multi-portal TOA and EEEA access. *BA* basilar artery, *BS* brainstem, *Ill* third cranial nerve, *LAICA* left anterior inferior cerebellar artery, *LICA* left internal carotid artery, *LPCA* left posterior cerebral artery, *LSCA* left superior cerebellar artery, *P* pituitary, *RICA* right anterior inferior cerebellar artery, *RPCA* right posterior cerebral artery, *RSCA* right superior cerebellar artery

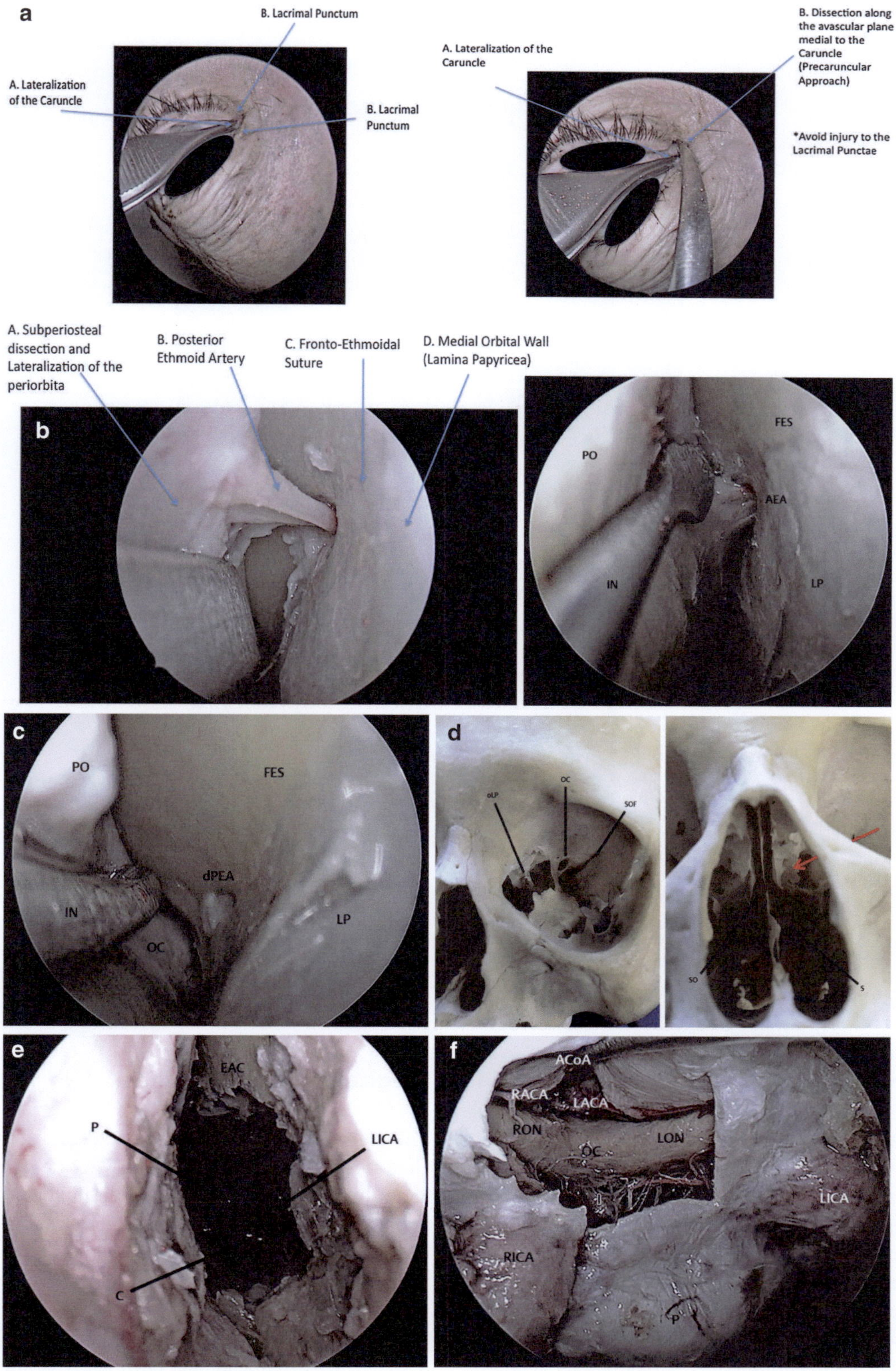
a
B. Lacrimal Punctum
A. Lateralization of the Caruncle
B. Lacrimal Punctum
A. Lateralization of the Caruncle
B. Dissection along the avascular plane medial to the Caruncle (Precaruncular Approach)
*Avoid injury to the Lacrimal Punctae
A. Subperiosteal dissection and Lateralization of the periorbita
B. Posterior Ethmoid Artery
C. Fronto-Ethmoidal Suture
D. Medial Orbital Wall (Lamina Papyricea)
b
PO
FES
AEA
IN
LP
c
PO
FES
dPEA
IN
OC
LP
d
oLP
OC
SOF
SO
S
e
EAC
P
LICA
C
f
ACoA
RACA
LACA
RON
LON
OC
LICA
RICA
P

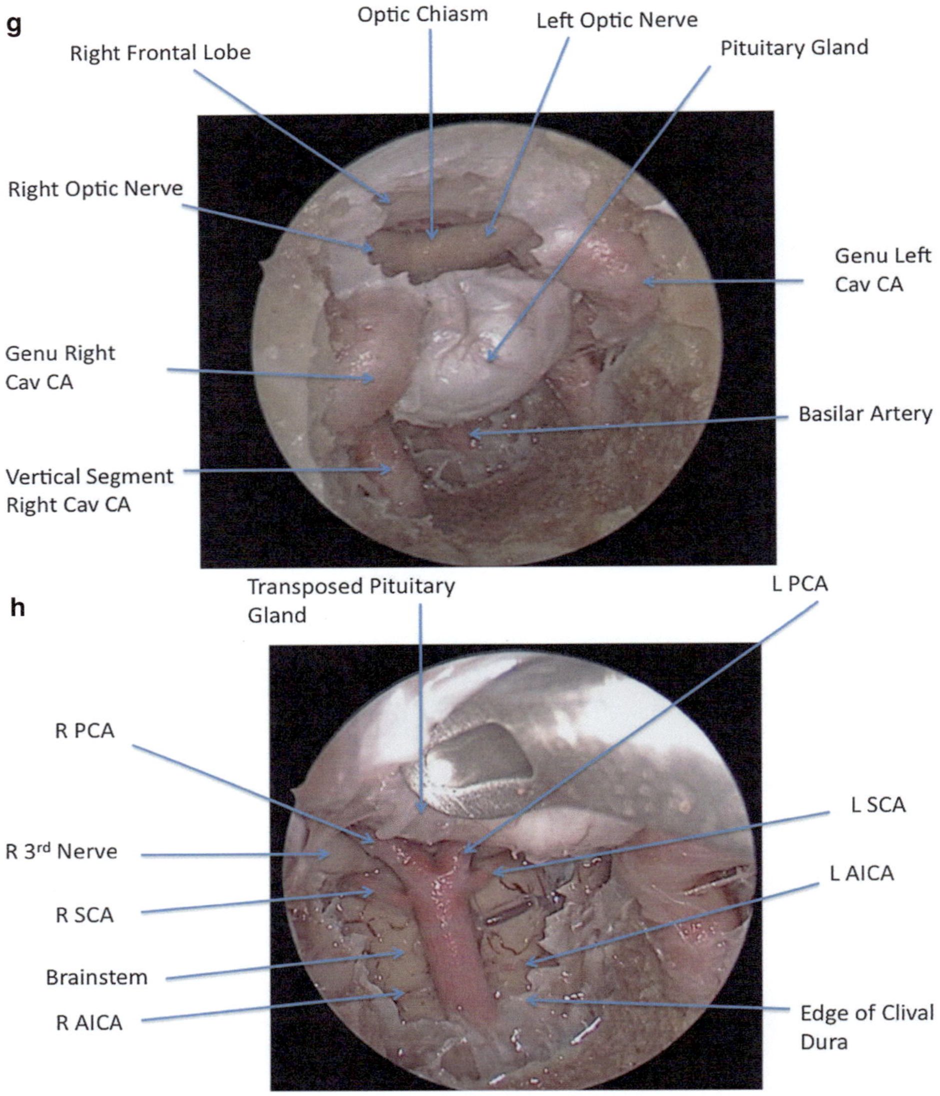

Fig. 35.3 (continued)

Transorbital Precaruncular Port

Patient Positioning

The patient should be positioned supine with the head secured by either Mayfield or gel donut. The head should be neutral with a slight turn toward the surgeon at 15°. The body should be resting neutral with no need for a bump. The endotracheal tube should be maintained midline and reflected toward the feet with a flexible adaptor.

Surgical Technique

The corneal shield is at the surgeon's discretion. Care must be taken to avoid injury to the cornea and orbit. Caruncles should be identified and lateralized with pick-up to reveal superior and inferior lacrimal ducts (Fig. 35.4). Incision should be made with Colorado tip bovie along avascular plane medial to caruncle.

At this point scissors should be used to further dissect the avascular plane. Of note, it is impor-

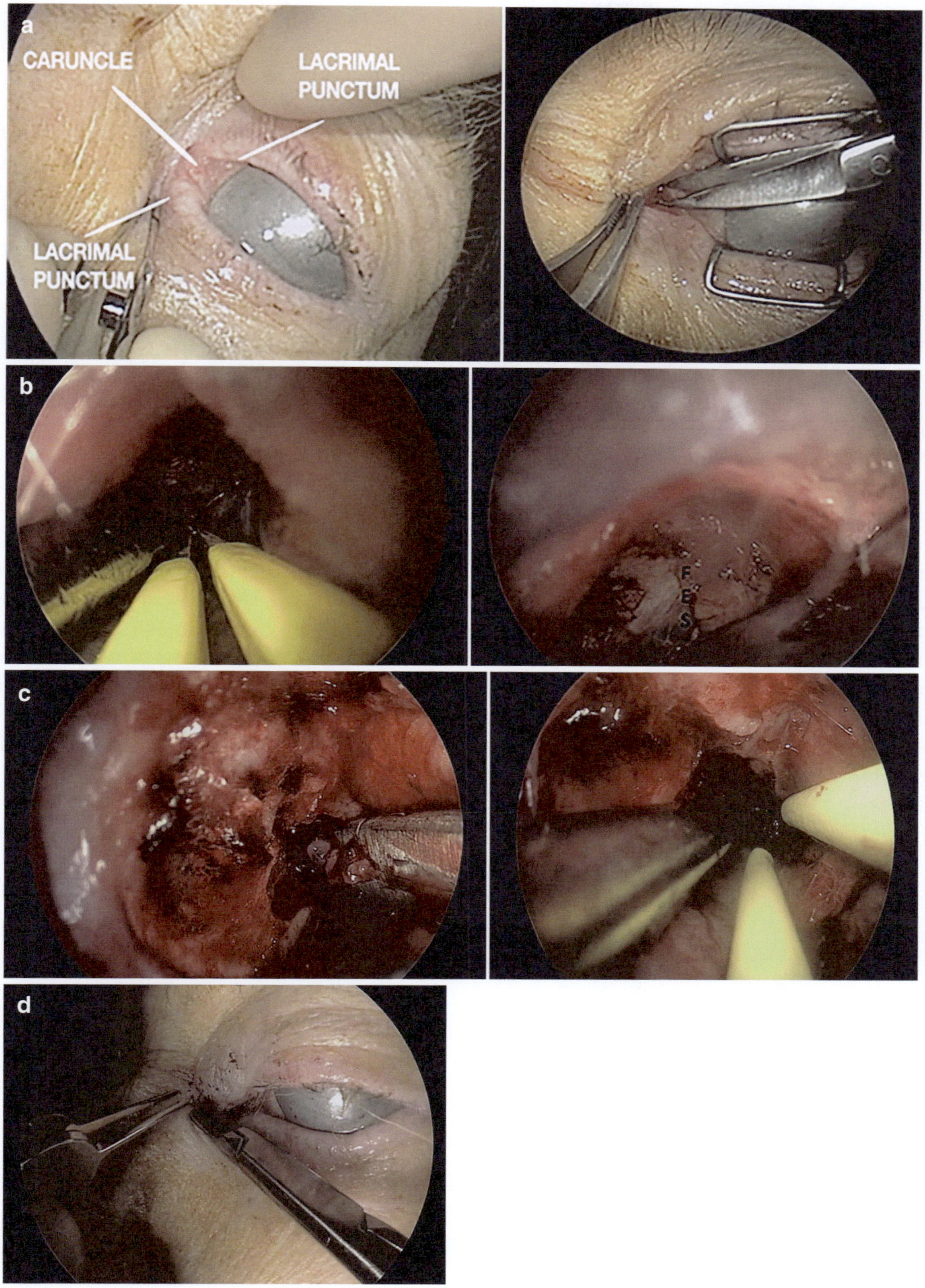

Fig. 35.4 (**a**) Identification of the precaruncular approach and access to the medial lamina papyracea. (**b**) Once access to the lamina papyracea is gained, the anterior and posterior ethmoid arteries are coagulated. The FES (fronto-ethmoidal suture) identified. (**c**) Access and removal of the meningioma. Suction and bipolar utilized for tumor resection and hemostasis. Bimanual microdissection through the Transorbital port along the vertical, lateral to medial axis. (**d**) Closure of the caruncle with 4-0 monocryl suture

tant to avoid lacrimal sac by remaining posterior to lacrimal impression. The trajectory will be towards the medial orbital wall and a periosteum can be used to establish the plane. The periorbita must be always maintained. The fronto-ethmoidal suture should be identified, and dissection continued along the suture. Once the anterior and posterior ethmoidal arteries are identified, they should be coagulated and divided to increase exposure.

The intraoperative perspective in Fig. 35.4 highlights the minimally invasive nature of the precaruncular approach. These figures also demonstrate how the surgeon can function as a two-handed microsurgeon. When utilizing minimal access approaches for tumor resection, both suction and coagulation must be utilized. In these figures, one can see how the bipolar can be easily utilized along the vertical access parallel to the periorbita. With gentle lateral to medial angulation, this meningioma was able to be safely removed. The pressure on the orbit should always be monitored. The minimal closure techniques of closing caruncle are also demonstrated.

Figures 35.5 and 35.6 demonstrate how the multi-portal TOA and EEEA approach can be utilized to improve the degrees of freedom in addressing vascular or neoplastic processes involving the posterior fossa, clivus sella cavernous sinous and parasellar regions. The precaruncular port allows one to remove the endoscope from the nose. The transorbital port create more room for instruments via the EEEA. This port also offers an offset view of the tip of instruments and aneurysm clips if needed, as opposed to the less angled view from the EEEA alone. These points are highlighted in Fig. 35.5.

The transorbital approach is a versatile approach. Key findings utilizing the approach are highlighted in Table 35.1. Briefly, Kempton and colleagues have shown the feasibility of the approach for the repair of medial orbital wall fractures in cadavers [20]. Yoon's group trialed in trauma patients and had great success in repair in 36 medial orbit fractures [21]. Zhou was able to show adequate mesh placement with an expanded incision [22]. The approach has also been used for transfers to aid in oculomotor palsy [23], and for anterior ethmoidal artery ligation in settings of trauma [24]. Hakim showed use in the treatment of medial orbital tumors [25]. Lubbe and colleagues describe the use of the combined endoscopic and precaruncular with success for sphenoid pathology and CSF leak [26]. Others have expanded the approach to show use for the anterior central skull base lesions [1, 4]. Our group has also shown the feasibility of posterior circulation and cavernous carotid arteries for

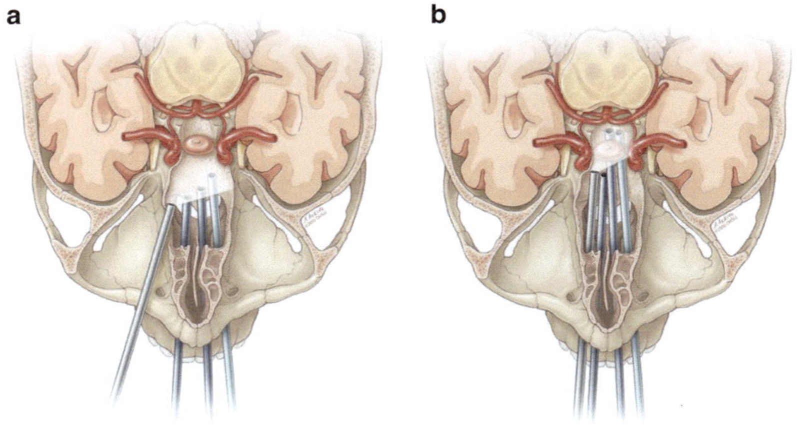

Fig. 35.5 (**a**, **b**) A Multi-portal technique illustrated utilizing the medial precaruncular port complimenting the EEEA and improving endoscope and instrument degrees of freedom. (**b**) Depicts the EEEA approach and the coning-down effect as the dissection proceeds posteriorly. Degrees of instrument and endoscope freedom are limited compared to adding the precaruncular approach

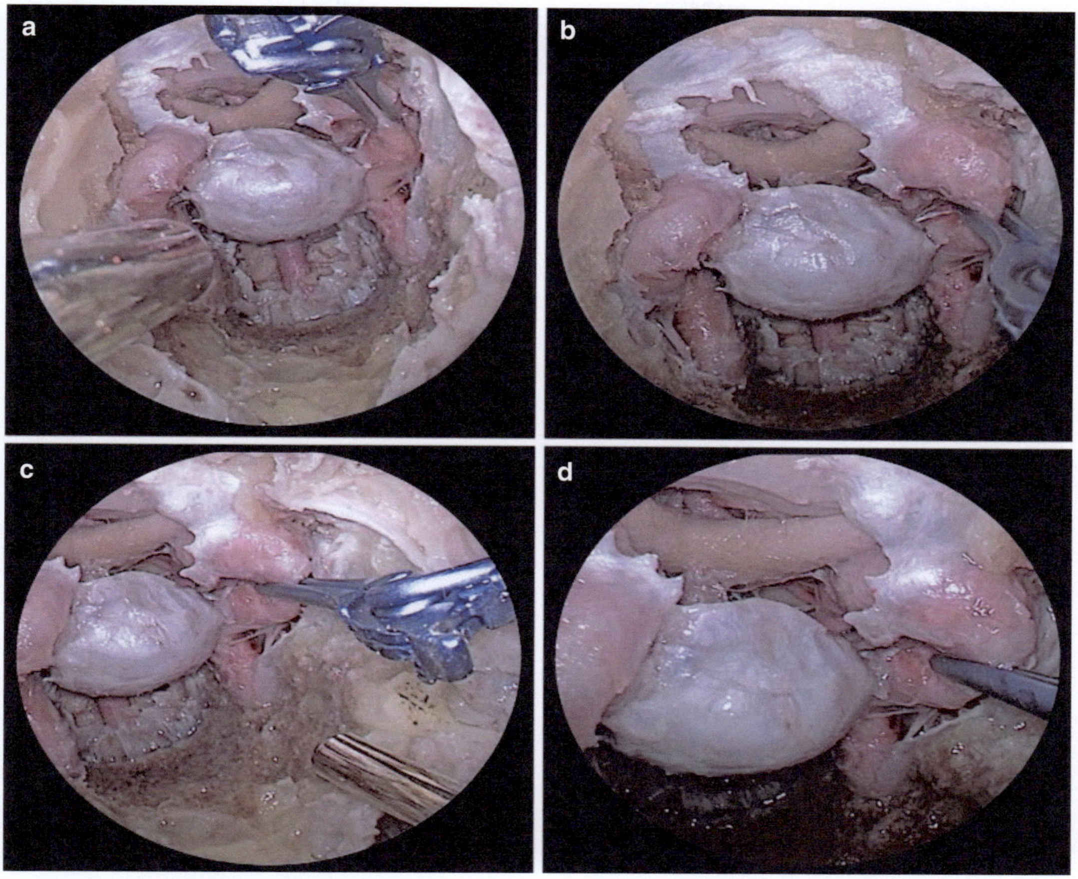

Fig. 35.6 (**a–d**) Endoscopic Endonasal view inline view. (**c** and **d**) Endoscopic right transorbital port provides an offset view demonstrating improved visualization and spatial relationship of the tip of the aneurysm clip and carotid artery. Multi-portal Transorbital approach has also demonstrated improved degrees of freedom of instruments

Table 35.1 Supporting literature

Study	Type	Approach	Outcomes
Cornelis and Lubbe [24]	Cadaveric	Precaruncular	Showed feasibility for treating epistaxis
Moe [3]	Cadaveric and case series	Precaruncular	Better cosmetic results and healing for medial cantopexy and orbital lesions
Saxena et al. [27]	Case series	Precaruncular and lateral	Oculomotor palsy treatment via anchoring globe to medial orbital wall (93% success rate)
You et al. [21]	Case series	Precaruncular	Successful orbital blowout fracture repair in 36 patients with good cosmesis
Lubbe et al. [26]	Case report	Contralateral Precaruncular	CSF leak repair of sphenoid sinus defect

(continued)

Table 35.1 (continued)

Study	Type	Approach	Outcomes
Kempton et al. [20]	Cadaveric	Retrocaruncular	Showed potential approach for medial orbital wall fractures
Ciporen et al. [29]	Cadaveric	Transphenoidal and precaruncular	Successful access for cavernous carotid aneurysms
Ciporen et al. [28]	Cadaveric	Dual precaruncular with endoscopic endonasal vs. endoscopic endonasal	Dual approach increases the visualization of posterior circulation pathology
Ciporen et al. [4]	Cadaveric	Precaruncular vs. endoscopic endonasal vs. supraorbital	Precaruncular provided more direct visualization and access to the pituitary gland, optic chiasm, and ipsilateral cavernous carotid compared to the other two approaches
Zhou et al. [22]	Case series	Endoscopic Transconjunctival inferior fornix and precaruncular	In 84 patients, repair of combined medial and orbital floor fractures was obtained. Of those with diplopia, 32/33 improved
Gillham et al. [30]	Simulation study	Combined endoscopic endonasal and precuruncular	Perfusion simulation model for training otolaryngology and neurosurgery residents/fellows' key endoscopic skill sets
Moe et al. [31]	Cadaveric and case series	Transorbital endoscopic	Successful anterior fossa CSF leak repair in 10 individuals
Nannavecchia et al. [1]	Cadaveric	Precaruncular vs. lateral retrocanthal	Precaruncular is a better approach to visualize optic nerve and frontal sinus pathology whereas lateral retrocanthal is safer for reaching anterior and middle cranial fossa
Hakim and Sieg [25]	Case series	Lateral orbitotomy, transconjunctival, and precaruncular approaches	Orbital tumors can be successfully reached and visualized with precaruncular approach

potential use with aneurysms, vessel injury control, or vessel reconstruction [28–30]. The approach has also been used for cerebrospinal fluid leak repair [31] and more recently the resection of a medial sphenoid wing meningioma [32]. The approach is versatile, with quick recoveries and the ability to be combined with multiport techniques to enhance exposure. Early clinical work has been promising for a multitude of pathologies as highlighted.

> *The multiportal combined transorbital transnasal endoscopic approach is a safe and effective procedure for management of selected complex skull base lesions that is able to capitalize on the advantages and overcome the limitations of each single approach* [33].

The Supraorbital Port (Eyebrow Incision)

Patient Positioning

The patient is positioned supine with the head raised above the plane of the heart. The head is extended to facilitate frontal lobe relaxation with gravity and CSF egress. The head is turned based on the pathology. Head rotation away from the surgeon is greater for midline pathology while the opposite is true for the more lateral approaches.

The supraorbital craniotomy was popularized in 2005. The indications for utilization, safety,

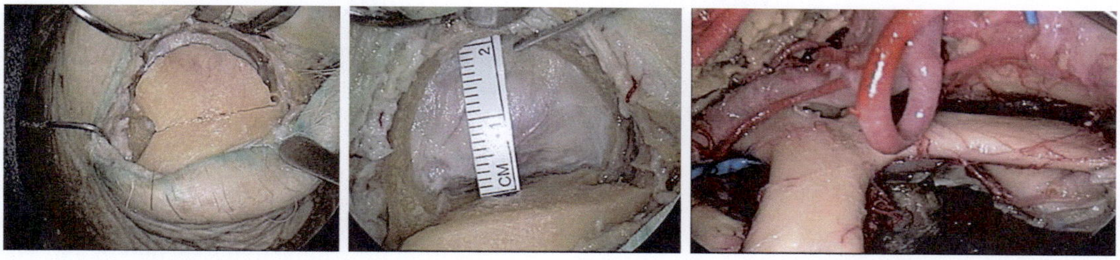

Fig. 35.7 Supraorbital craniotomy through an eyebrow incision. Care was taken to remain lateral to the supraorbital nerve and foramen. The orbicularis muscles are reflected inferiorly as the pericranium is incised superiorly and based inferiorly. A 2 × 3 cm craniotomy is made with a pterional bur hole. The endoscopic view demonstrates the access to the anterior skull base and parasellar region. Craniotomy can be adjusted for use as an endoscopic visualization versus a working port for instruments

and efficacy have been well described [34]. Surgical technique of the supraorbital keyhole craniotomy. The supraorbital approach can be achieved through an eyebrow incision or a trans-palpebral incision [35]. Pathology involving the anterior skull base, parasellar area, and cerebral artery aneurysms have been approached [36].

Incision is made in the unshaven eyebrow through the skin with a 15-blade scalpel. The Colorado needle bovie carries the incision through subcutaneous tissue. The orbicularis oculi and temporalis muscles and pericranium are preserved. Incision and dissection should remain lateral to the supraorbital nerve to avoid the supraorbital nerve. Care is also taken laterally to avoid the frontal branch of the facial nerve. The orbicularis muscle is maintained intact as the subgalea plane is dissected, preserving the pericranium. The skin is retracted with blunt fishhooks or sutures and secured to a retractor system attached to the headframe. The pericranium is opened medially, superiorly, and laterally based frontally on its blood supply. The craniotomy dimensions are based on the pathology, however, given the soft tissue restrictions, it is usually limited to a 2 × 3 cm craniotomy (Fig. 35.7). The burr hole is made laterally for cosmetic/reconstructive purposes. The floor of the craniotomy is drilled flush with the anterior fossa. An orbitotomy may be incorporated as needed. Care is taken regarding the frontal sinus, which may play a role in patient selection, for one must consider reconstruction requirements when selecting a surgical approach. The craniotomy size may be smaller if utilized more as an endoscopic viewing port complimenting the expanded endonasal trans-tuberculum approach for tumors with significant parasellar extension. If it is going to be utilized as a working port, then the dimensions above should be considered. A guide to keyhole approaches is that the opening in the dura and location at which the dissection is being performed be able to accommodate an open bipolar to obtain hemostasis [37]. This endoscopic multiportal approach skull base pathology extends suprasellar and lateral to the optic nerve and/or carotid artery [38]. Examples would be tuberculum sella meningiomas with lateral extension, giant pituitary adenomas and craniopharyngiomas [39]. This combined minimally invasive approach is complimentary. The validation of this approach has been in the reported experience of leaders in the field of skull base surgery.

> *The limitations of the EEA when dealing with lateral extension of anterior skull base meningiomas, and the limitations of the supraorbital eyebrow approach for medial skull base drilling and reconstruction, can be overcome by a judicious, anatomically based combination of both approaches [15].*

Caldwell-Luc Port (Sublabial Incision)

The Caldwell-Luc operation was initially described in the nineteenth century [40]. The technique gains access to the maxillary sinus via

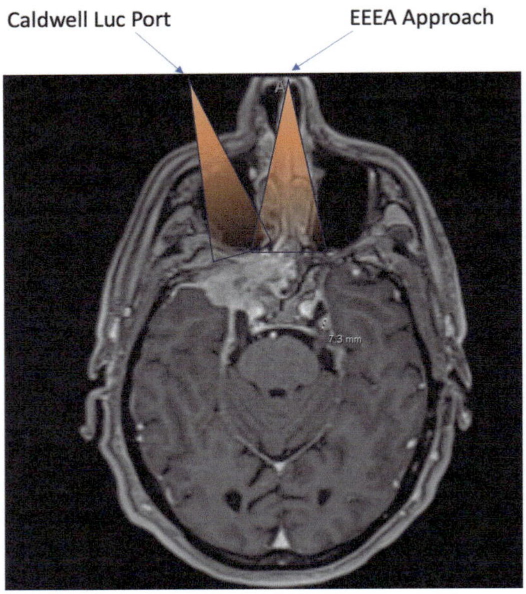

Fig. 35.8 Multiportal Caldwell-Luc & EEEA highlighted. The improved degrees of freedom and endoscopic visualization for more lateral skull base pathology. Improved access to the ptyergopalatine fossa, infratemporal fossa and posterior fossa

the canine fossa. It has been utilized to treat odontogenic and sinus pathology. Much like the precuruncular TOA or the supraorbital approach, it is a well-established and safe as a stand-alone operation [41]. This has made it a good addition to the endoscopic skull base multi-portal armamentarium (Fig. 35.8). This technique can be utilized as an instrument and/or enhanced endoscopic visualization port. This is like the TOA or supraorbital craniotomy approach for complex skull base tumors. The advantage of utilizing this endoscopic port in combination with the EEEA is in addressing pathology involving the maxillary sinus, ptyergopalatine or infratemporal fossa. The approach allows for more degrees of surgical freedom, enhances visualization, and minimizes intra-nasal tissue trauma of surgery. As this port compliments the bilateral traditional EEEA it can also be utilized with a unilateral EEEA on the ipsilateral side of the pathology. The port allows for more effective bimanual dissection, vascular control and addressing the pathology for resection. The Caldwell-Luc has been reported to be performed in short surgical time, reduced post-op healing time and post-op morbidity [42]. Little et al. demonstrated that the endoscopic Caldwell-Luc provided benefits when compared to the endoscopic endonasal-transmaxillary [43].

The surgery is performed via a sublabial incision overlying the canine fossa. The incision extends from the canine to the second molar. The mucoperiostium is elevated. Care is taken to avoid the infraorbital nerve and the dental roots. The antrostomy is performed with a drill thereby accessing the antrum of the maxillary sinus. The antrum is widened by a Kerrison as needed. The antrostomy is smaller for use as an endoscopic port alone and widened instrument access.

> *Multiportal Approaches have been incorporated by skull base centers in training their residents and fellows. "The future skull base surgeon must be well trained and knowledgeable in all surgical portals to the skull base to select the safest, least invasive, most direct approach that offers the optimum exposure to handle a complex skull base pathology. The multi-portal/corridor philosophy is often adopted to achieve superior surgical and clinical outcomes"* [44].

Conclusion

The introduction of TONES and Multi-portal endoscopic approaches to the skull base (2010) has led to a growing body of knowledge and experience that has validated these approaches in practice. Endoscopic multi-portal techniques to the skull base are considered, by teaching institutions, as critical to the training of future generations of skull base surgeons. They allow the skull base surgeon to work through minimal access ports for tumors of the skull base that transcend compartments. Multi-portal approaches allow skull base surgeons to tailor the approach to the patient and their pathology with less normal tissue disruption and minimize complications. These techniques have been demonstrated to improve degrees of freedom for bimanual dissection and visualization and overcome some limitations of a single approach. Multi-portal approaches are versatile. The foundation has been established for further innovations.

References

1. Nannavecchia BA, Ganau M, Cebula H, et al. Endoscopic transorbital approaches to anterior and middle cranial fossa: a laboratory investigation on surgical anatomy and potential routes. J Neurol Surg B Skull Base. 2021;82(4):443–9.
2. Elhadi AM, Zaidi HA, Yagmurlu K, et al. Infraorbital nerve: a surgically relevant landmark for the pterygopalatine fossa, cavernous sinus, and anterolateral skull base in endoscopic transmaxillary approaches. J Neurosurg. 2016;125(6):1460–8.
3. Moe KS, Bergeron CM, Ellenbogen RG. Transorbital neuroendoscopic surgery. Neurosurgery. 2010;67(3 Suppl Operative):ons16-28.
4. Ciporen JN, Moe KS, Ramanathan D, et al. Multiportal endoscopic approaches to the central skull base: a cadaveric study. World Neurosurg. 2010;73(6):705–12.
5. Aref MH, Youssef AS. Training the skull base surgeon of the future: a comprehensive approach. J Neurosurg Sci. 2018;62(6):627–35.
6. Borghei-Razavi H, Truong HQ, Fernandes-Cabral DT, et al. Minimally invasive approaches for anterior skull base meningiomas: supraorbital eyebrow, endoscopic endonasal, or a combination of both? Anatomic study, limitations, and surgical application. World Neurosurg. 2018;112:e666–74.
7. Martinez-Perez R, Requena LC, Carrau RL, Prevedello DM. Modern endoscopic skull base neurosurgery. J Neurooncol. 2021;151(3):461–75.
8. Di Somma A, Langdon C, de Notaris M, et al. Combined and simultaneous endoscopic endonasal and transorbital surgery for a Meckel's cave schwannoma: technical nuances of a mini-invasive, multiportal approach. J Neurosurg. 2020;134(6):1836–45.
9. Dallan I, Castelnuovo P, Locatelli D, et al. Multiportal combined transorbital transnasal endoscopic approach for the management of selected skull base lesions: preliminary experience. World Neurosurg. 2015;84(1):97–107.
10. Lee WJ, Hong SD, Woo KI, et al. Combined endoscopic endonasal and transorbital multiportal approach for complex skull base lesions involving multiple compartments. Acta Neurochir. 2022;164(7):1911–22.
11. Han X, Yang H, Wang Z, et al. Endoscopic transorbital approach for skull base lesions: a report of 16 clinical cases. Neurosurg Rev. 2023;46(1):74.
12. de Lara D, Ditzel Filho LF, Prevedello DM, et al. Endonasal endoscopic approaches to the paramedian skull base. World Neurosurg. 2014;82(6 Suppl):S121–9.
13. Cavallo LM, Solari D, Cappabianca P. Multiportal approach to the skull base: one key, multiple gates. World Neurosurg. 2015;84(3):630–1.
14. Lee MH, Hong SD, Woo KI, et al. Endoscopic endonasal versus transorbital surgery for middle cranial fossa tumors: comparison of clinical outcomes based on surgical corridors. World Neurosurg. 2019;122:e1491–504.
15. Fernandez-Miranda JC, Zwagerman NT, Abhinav K, et al. Cavernous sinus compartments from the endoscopic endonasal approach: anatomical considerations and surgical relevance to adenoma surgery. J Neurosurg. 2018;129(2):430–41.
16. Matano F, Passeri T, Abbritti R, et al. Eyebrow incision with a crescent-shaped orbital rim craniotomy for microscopic and endoscopic transorbital approach to the anterior and middle cranial fossa: a cadaveric study and case presentation. Brain Spine. 2022;2:100891.
17. Zoia C, Mantovani G, Muther M, et al. Through the orbit and beyond: current state and future perspectives in endoscopic orbital surgery on behalf of the EANS frontiers committee in orbital tumors and the EANS skull base section. Brain Spine. 2023;3:102669.
18. Guizzardi G, Prats-Galino A, Mosteiro A, et al. Multiportal combined endoscopic endonasal and transorbital pathways: qualitative and quantitative anatomic studies of the "connection" skull base areas. Oper Neurosurg (Hagerstown). 2023;24(5):e342–50.
19. Silveira-Bertazzo G, Li R, Rejane-Heim TC, et al. Endoscopic approaches to skull base malignancies affecting the anterior fossa. J Neurosurg Sci. 2021;65(2):169–80.
20. Kempton SJ, Cho DC, Thimmappa B, Martin MC. Benefits of the retrocaruncular approach to the medial orbit: a clinical and anatomic study. Ann Plast Surg. 2016;76(3):295–300.
21. You HJ, Kim DW, Dhong ES, Yoon ES. Precaruncular approach for the reconstruction of medial orbital wall fractures. Ann Plast Surg. 2014;72(6):652–6.
22. Zhou G, Tu Y, Yu B, Wu W. Endoscopic repair of combined orbital floor and medial wall fractures involving the inferomedial strut. Eye (Lond). 2021;35(10):2763–70.
23. Sadagopan KA, Wasserman BN. Managing the patient with oculomotor nerve palsy. Curr Opin Ophthalmol. 2013;24(5):438–47.
24. Cornelis MM, Lubbe DE. Pre-caruncular approach to the medial orbit and landmarks for anterior ethmoidal artery ligation: a cadaveric study. Clin Otolaryngol. 2016;41(6):777–81.
25. Hakim SG, Sieg P. Resection of medial orbital tumours via lateral orbitotomy and minimally invasive microscopic, transconjunctival and precaruncular approaches. Br J Oral Maxillofac Surg. 2022;60(4):519–21.
26. Lubbe DE, Douglas-Jones P, Wasl H, Mustak H, Semple PL. Contralateral precaruncular approach to the lateral sphenoid sinus—a case report detailing a new, multiportal approach to lesions, and defects in the lateral aspect of well-pneumatized sphenoid sinuses. Ear Nose Throat J. 2020;99(1):62–7.
27. Saxena R, Sinha A, Sharma P, et al. Precaruncular approach for medial orbital wall periosteal anchoring of the globe in oculomotor nerve palsy. J AAPOS.

2009;13(6):578–82. https://doi.org/10.1016/j.jaapos.2009.11.003. PMID: 20006821.
28. Ciporen JN, Lucke-Wold B, Dogan A, Cetas J, Cameron W. Endoscopic endonasal transclival approach versus dual transorbital port technique for clip application to the posterior circulation: a cadaveric anatomical and cerebral circulation simulation study. J Neurol Surg B Skull Base. 2017;78(3):235–44.
29. Ciporen J, Lucke-Wold B, Dogan A, Cetas JS, Cameron WE. Dual endoscopic endonasal transsphenoidal and precaruncular transorbital approaches for clipping of the cavernous carotid artery: a cadaveric simulation. J Neurol Surg B Skull Base. 2016;77(6):485–90.
30. Gillham HE, Lucke-Wold B, Dogan A, Cetas J, Cameron WE, Ciporen JN. Development of a cadaveric multiport model of posterior circulation aneurysm clipping for neurosurgery and otolaryngology residents. J Vis Exp. 2021;(175).
31. Moe KS, Kim LJ, Bergeron CM. Transorbital endoscopic repair of cerebrospinal fluid leaks. Laryngoscope. 2011;121(1):13–30.
32. Goncalves N, Lubbe DE. Transorbital endoscopic surgery for sphenoid wing meningioma: long-term outcomes and surgical technique. J Neurol Surg B Skull Base. 2020;81(4):357–68.
33. Dallan I, Locatelli D, Turri-Zanoni M, et al. Transorbital endoscopic assisted resection of a superior orbital fissure cavernous haemangioma: a technical case report. Eur Arch Otorrinolaringol. 2015;272(12):3851–6.
34. Reisch R, Perneczky A. Ten-year experience with the supraorbital subfrontal approach through an eyebrow skin incision. Neurosurgery. 2005;57(4 Suppl):242–55; discussion 242–255.
35. Abdel Aziz KM, Bhatia S, Tantawy MH, et al. Minimally invasive transpalpebral "eyelid" approach to the anterior cranial base. Neurosurgery. 2011;69(2 Suppl Operative):ons195-206; discussion 206-7.
36. Lin BJ, Ju DT, Hsu TH, et al. Endoscopic transorbital approach to anterolateral skull base through inferior orbital fissure: a cadaveric study. Acta Neurochir. 2019;161(9):1919–29.
37. Nanda A, Sonig A. The expansive realm of skull base neuroendoscopy. World Neurosurg. 2014;82(3–4):e423–5.
38. Bove I, Cheok S, Ruzevick JJ, Zada G. Endoscopic endonasal and keyhole surgery for skull base meningiomas. Neurosurg Clin N Am. 2023;34(3):393–402.
39. Cappabianca P, Cavallo LM, Esposito F, De Divitiis O, Messina A, De Divitiis E. Extended endoscopic endonasal approach to the midline skull base: the evolving role of transsphenoidal surgery. Adv Tech Stand Neurosurg. 2008;33:151–99.
40. Masterson L, Al Gargaz W, Bath AP. Endoscopic Caldwell-Luc technique. J Laryngol Otol. 2010;124(6):663–5.
41. Schroeder HW. Indications and limitations of the endoscopic endonasal approach for anterior cranial base meningiomas. World Neurosurg. 2014;82(6 Suppl):S81–5.
42. Elhadi AM, Almefty KK, Mendes GA, et al. Comparison of surgical freedom and area of exposure in three endoscopic transmaxillary approaches to the anterolateral cranial base. J Neurol Surg B Skull Base. 2014;75(5):346–53.
43. Little AS, Nakaji P, Milligan J. Endoscopic endonasal transmaxillary approach and endoscopic sublabial transmaxillary approach: surgical decision-making and implications of the nasolacrimal duct. World Neurosurg. 2013;80(5):583–90.
44. Youssef AS, Yang A, Getz AE, Mizuho I, Labib M. Clival chordoma: endoscopic bilateral transmaxillary approach. J Neurol Surg B Skull Base. 2019;80(Suppl 4):S371.

36 Reconstruction and Postoperative Care After Transorbital Skull Base and Brain Surgery

Kris S. Moe

Part I: Reconstruction

The transorbital neuroendoscopic approaches were created with the goal of minimal tissue disruption. As such, little reconstruction is typically required at the end of the procedure. An additional benefit of these techniques is that the orbital contents function as a vascularized tissue layer that, depending on the approach used, may buttress any exposed dura and may obviate the need for further reconstruction.

In general, the need for orbital reconstruction is based on the potential for alterations in appearance or function. The primary factor to take into consideration is the presence and magnitude of a CSF leak. Small CSF leaks are typically sealed by the adjacent periorbita or orbital fat. For larger leaks, a layered repair is typically undertaken using allograft or synthetic materials. If the leak extends beyond the orbit to a site that may drain into the middle ear or nasal cavity (sphenoid, ethmoid, or frontal sinuses), those defects are repaired in a standard fashion. For the sinonasal cavities, this may include a pedicled septal mucosa flap or similar repair.

K. S. Moe (✉)
Division of Facial Plastic Surgery, Departments of Otolaryngology and Neurological Surgery, University of Washington School of Medicine, Seattle, WA, USA
e-mail: krismoe@uw.edu

The other major factor to consider pertains to the volume and location of bone removal. Each wall of the orbit has unique topographical, structural, and functional characteristics and should thus be assessed independently. Resection of orbital bone may result in loss of structural support, particularly in the medial wall or floor of the orbit or in loss of globe projection as provided by the greater wing of the sphenoid. Secondary effects of bone removal may be herniation of orbital contents to obstruct sinus drainage pathways or possibly extraocular muscle dysfunction. Though the literature suggests these are not common occurrences, they should be considered to prevent complications.

A measure that can help judge changes in orbital volume is the pre and postoperative use of exophthalmometry (Chap. 1, Fig. 1.10). This technique is straightforward to learn using a handheld device. Used preoperatively, it can document preexisting asymmetries in the globe position, which can then be pointed out to the patient. This can also be performed with the patient supine under general anesthesia at the beginning of a procedure and again at the end of an operation to demonstrate changes in globe position. We have found that a typical transorbital endoscopic procedure lasting several hours will result in 2–3 mm of proptosis due to edema at the end of the procedure, which resolves within 1–2 weeks after surgery. If reconstruction of the orbital bone is performed, the goal should be to

T. H. Schwartz et al. (eds.), *Endoscopic Transorbital Surgery of the Orbit, Skull Base and Brain*,
https://doi.org/10.1007/978-3-031-59504-2_36

bring the globe to this position rather than achieve symmetry with the contralateral side. Failure to achieve mild proptosis may result in enophthalmos when the edema resolves.

The use of *endoscopy* for visualization during reconstruction can greatly improve outcomes. As we have discussed elsewhere [1–3], endoscopy provides superior field illumination, image magnification (important when surveilling for entrapment of orbital contents), and multiple monitor viewing so the entire surgical team can observe the procedure and participate effectively.

Navigation guidance with mirror-image overlay (MIO) has also been demonstrated to improve outcomes in orbital reconstruction [2], particularly for larger defects of the medial wall and floor (Fig. 36.1). The principle of this technology is the use of the orbital component of the CT scan to provide a template for orbital wall reconstruction. As navigation is used for earlier parts of the procedure, this does not require additional technology. The implant is positioned as desired, and the surface of the implant is then swept with the navigation probe to confirm that its shape conforms to the original CT contours. If the original contours were altered by pathology, the contralateral orbit can be used as the template. This is done by reversing the contralateral image and superimposing it over the affected side. If the contours of the implant do not conform to the CT plan, it is adjusted to the appropriate shape and then navigated again. This technology is a feature available in several commercial systems' software.

When small surface area bone defects are present, these can be reconstructed with a thin (0.25 mm) polydiaxanone (*PDS*) sheet. This material provides an excellent glide surface that will not adhere to the orbital contents, which dissolves, leaving behind a thin, non-adherent tissue surface. For somewhat larger defects, the thicker (0.5 mm) sheet may be used to span the defect (Fig. 36.2). For defects that may be topographically more complex, such as the medial wall or floor, larger defects may be reconstructed with thin titanium mesh (sheeting) over which a layer of thin PDS is then placed. Bare titanium should not be used alone, as orbital fat can herniate through the mesh and interfere with muscle function. Titanium mesh is available as pre-bent implants or custom-made implants. Our preference is to use pre-bent implants that are then adjusted with in-situ contouring according to a navigation-based plan.

When possible, the technique of orbital "*preconstruction*" should be used [3]. If the region of bone reconstruction can be anticipated at the beginning of the procedure, the implant is placed into the region and shaped as necessary. It is then replaced to span the defect when needed at the end of the procedure.

The following provides greater details on reconstruction for specific regions of the orbit.

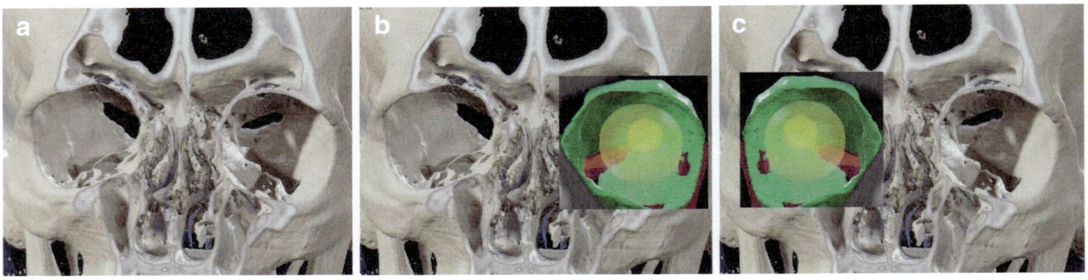

Fig. 36.1 Mirror-image overlay navigation. Reconstruction of right orbit when normal anatomy is altered by pathology. (**a**), Preoperative CT. (**b**), normal (left) orbit highlighted, (**c**), normal orbit reversed as mirror-image and superimposed over the abnormal orbit. The construct can now serve as a reconstruction template for navigation. If preoperative orbit anatomy was normal, navigation is performed without the need for mirror-imaging

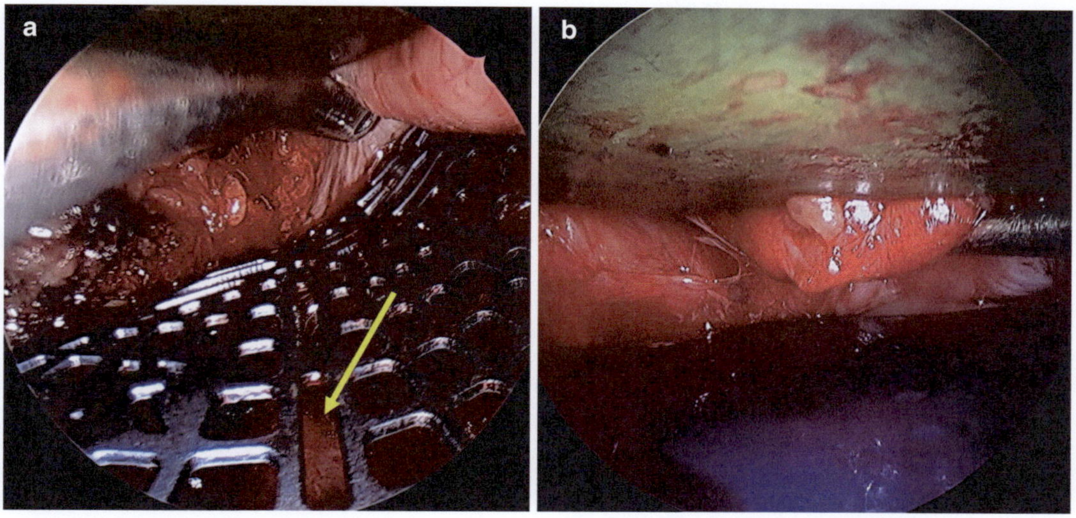

Fig. 36.2 Placement of titanium mesh and resorbable PDS sheet across right orbital floor defect. (**a**) Implant is placed in position, and the periorbita is then lifted circumferentially to eliminate the possibility of entrapment. The yellow arrow points to the infraorbital nerve seen through the implant. (**b**) Implant lined with PDS sheet. Orbital contents retracted with a malleable retractor and periosteal elevator

Roof

As with all regions of the orbit, the bone defect should be inspected for abrupt or raised edges that could possibly impede the motion of the levator or superior rectus muscles across its surface. Any such areas should be either removed or smoothed with a diamond burr.

There are two regions in the roof with distinct considerations: the region comprising the floor of the frontal sinus, and posterior to that, the area under the frontal lobe of the brain. It is not generally necessary to reconstruct the region underlying the brain, even when most of the bone has been removed. While pulsatile exophthalmos may occur, this is temporary and typically resolves within 1–2 weeks after surgery. We have not had a case of permanent pulsatile exophthalmos or proptosis due to the lack of reconstruction of this region.

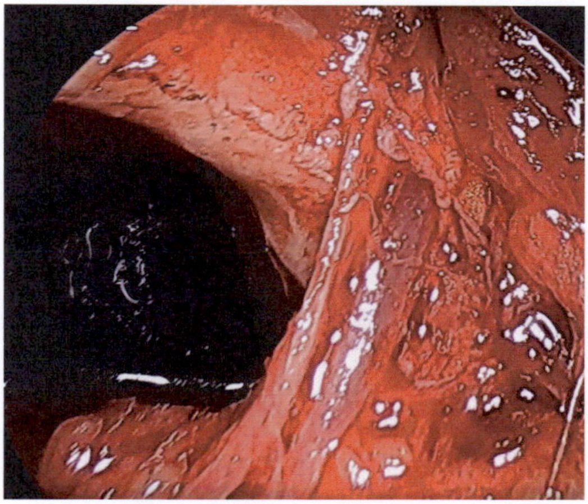

Fig. 36.3 Orbit roof reconstruction. A sheet of 0.25 mm PDS (blue) has been placed in a right orbital roof defect to prevent herniation of the orbital contents into the frontal outflow tract. The supratrochlear neurovascular pedicle is visible anterior and medial to the implant

If the bone constituting the floor of the frontal sinus has been removed, the region of the frontal outflow tract at the anterior medial sinus floor should be inspected. If there is concern for potential obstruction of this region by orbital contents, either due to a narrow segment or disruption of the periorbital with herniation of fat, a layer of 0.25 mm PDS sheet is placed within the orbit across the defect to restore compartmentalization (Fig. 36.3).

Medial Wall

Reconstruction of the medial wall should ensure that, as above, there are no sharp bone edges that could restrict muscle movement over the area. The next consideration is the degree of herniation of orbital contents into the ethmoid sinuses. Significant herniation of the medial rectus muscle is a potential cause of postoperative diplopia, while the displacement of orbital fat could obstruct the ethmoid sinuses or maxillary antrum (outflow tract). Small defects in the lamina papyracea do not typically require repair if the periorbita is intact. If there is content herniation, a layer of thin PDS sheet will suffice. For mid-sized defects, a layer of thick PDS sheet may be adequate. For large or near-total lamina defects or defects extending to the orbit floor, it is desirable to place a construct that can be contoured to match the original topography. For these applications, we prefer titanium mesh lined with thin PDS, as described above. It may be necessary to place the implant up to the frontoethmoid suture, in which case the ethmoid neurovascular pedicles will be exposed (Fig. 36.4). These can be cauterized with bipolar forceps and transected if needed for adequate exposure. Navigation guidance of the reconstruction can be performed for shape confirmation. Once the implant is placed, it is important to view it circumferentially to be certain that no orbital contents are trapped between the implant and the adjacent bone. Any entrapment can lead to restricted function of the extraocular muscles and result in postoperative diplopia.

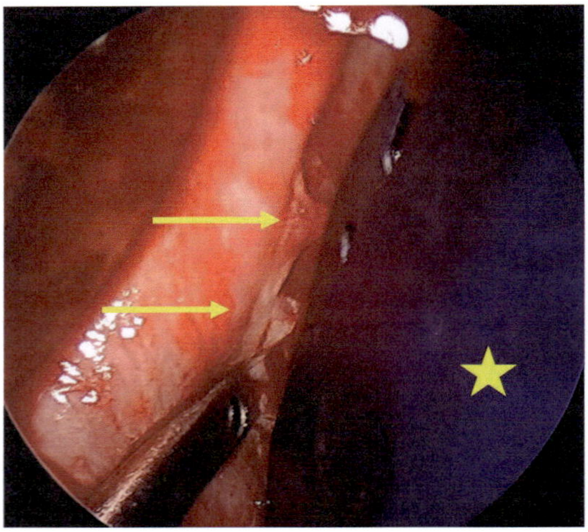

Fig. 36.4 Extended right medial orbit reconstruction. A 0.25 mm thick sheet of PDS (yellow star) is placed to cover a titanium mesh implant spanning defect in the right lamina papyracea. It is important that the implant spans the entire defect without entrapment of orbital contents. The anterior and central neurovascular pedicles (yellow arrows) are visible and superior to the titanium implant. A suction Freer elevator is used to check implant circumferentially for content entrapment

Floor

The orbit floor may be topographically complex, with a spoon shape when viewed from the sagittal perspective. It also bears much of the load of the orbital contents. Restoration of contour and structure is important in this region.

Similar to the medial wall, small defects can be repaired with a PDS sheet. This material is challenging to contour; however, we limit its use to mostly flat regions. For larger defects, titanium mesh lined with PDS is used as it can be effectively shaped to match the preoperative topography. Pre-shaped implants are effective for this, with tailoring performed to match the individual's anatomy as needed. Again, navigation guidance is very helpful, particularly when the medial wall is also involved. Care should be taken to span the entire bone defect, particularly at the orbital apex (Fig. 36.2), and place the implant superior to the infraorbital nerve without compression at any point along its course. It is also important to be certain that the edges of the implant do not rise off the bone at the orbital apex, as this could impede muscular motion over the construct.

Lateral Wall

The lateral wall plays a significant role in maintaining the projection of the orbital contents, given the substantial volume of the greater wing of the sphenoid bone. If a large component of this bone is removed, replacement of the volume should be undertaken to prevent postoperative enophthalmos. As discussed above, when an

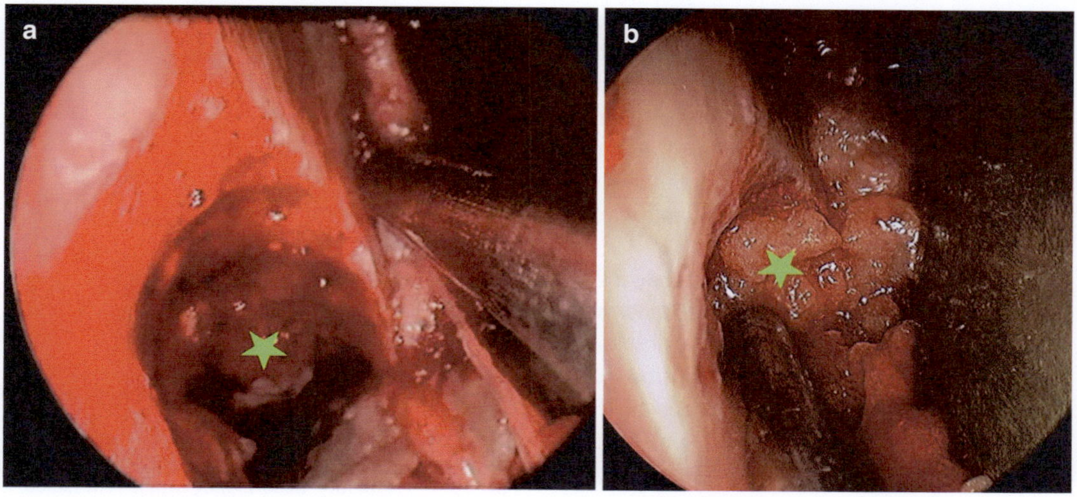

Fig. 36.5 Lateral wall reconstruction, right orbit. (**a**) Defect in the greater wing of the sphenoid bone for repair of lateral sphenoid sinus encephalocele. Star indicates encephalocele. (**b**) Fat graft placed in right lateral orbital wall defect. Orbital contents displaced medial with the malleable retractor. The star indicates a fat graft within the bone defect

approach to the middle or posterior cranial fossae is anticipated, exophthalmometry can be performed at the beginning of the procedure and again at the time of reconstruction to guide the type of reconstruction to be performed. As noted, the goal should be approximately 2 mm of proptosis of the surgical site at the conclusion to compensate for intraoperative edema.

For small defects in the bone, the concern is not orbital volume; rather it is providing a platform of appropriate topography over which the lateral rectus muscle will glide. Defects less than 1 cm can typically be spanned with a fat graft (Fig. 36.5) or a thin PDS sheet. If a dural defect and CSF leak are present, a fat graft and fibrin glue are typically sufficient, given the vascularized buttress provided by the orbital contents. For larger bone defects that cause a significant increase in orbital volume and allow lateral herniation of the lateral rectus muscle, a more substantial reconstruction is performed. When a dural defect and CSF leak are present, these are repaired with a multi-layer construct as described above. This should include a fat graft to obliterate dead space, which can then be covered with a thick PDS sheet. We rarely use permanent (titanium or other) constructs in the lateral orbit as the wall is not weight-bearing. As noted earlier, it is essential to be certain that there are no rough bone edges exposed that will interfere with functional range of motion of the musculature.

Before concluding the procedure, it is important to perform forced ductions regardless of which quadrant of the orbit was accessed. This test of extraocular muscle passive function ensures that the orbital contents are not entrapped by the reconstruction or by abrupt bone contours. It is done by gently grasping the conjunctiva adjacent to the limbus and rotating the globe vertically and horizontally. After a prolonged procedure, resistance is often felt at the extremes of motion, but this is generally symmetric. If focal resistance in a single direction is encountered, the reconstruction should be inspected endoscopically again to rule out entrapment or malposition of the repair.

Soft Tissue Support: The Lateral Canthus

Soft horizonal tissue support of the eyelids is provided primarily by the lateral and medial canthal tendons, and the superior support by the levator aponeurosis. The levator muscle and aponeurosis are not intentionally disrupted as part of these procedures; they should be reconstructed appropriately if this occurs. Likewise, the medial transorbital portal is posterior to the medial canthal tendon, and neither this nor the components of the lacrimal system are disrupted intentionally as part of the medial approach.

For extended lateral approaches that involve the removal of the lateral orbital rim and/or lateral orbital wall deep to that, it is possible to disrupt the attachment or integrity of the lateral canthus as a component of the approach. If this occurs, repair must be considered. This is especially true for elderly patients who may have preexisting diminished support of the lateral canthus and lower eyelid due to laxity of the lateral retinaculum, weakness of the orbicularis oculi muscle, or actual preexisting ectropion. Failure to restore this support can lead to postoperative ectropion, which can be highly symptomatic and lead to functional and esthetic complaints.

To determine lateral canthal integrity, the lateral junction of the upper and lower eyelids can be gently grasped with forceps and displaced medially. If there is no firm attachment to the orbital wall, re-attachment is undertaken. The type of reconstruction depends on the region of the disrupted lateral canthus. If only the superior or inferior limb of the lateral canthus is disrupted, the canthus can be reconstituted with a 5-0 permanent or dissolving suture. If the canthus is completely detached, transorbital lateral canthopexy [4] is undertaken. This is done by placing a suture through the deep side of the canthus at the junction of the eyelids. A second suture is placed through the lateral aspect of the inferior tarsus. Two holes are drilled through the lateral orbital rim inferior to the frontozygomatic suture to enter the orbit slightly superior and deep to the original canthal attachment. The two sutures in the lateral canthus are then externalized through the orbital rim holes and tied together with sufficient tension to provide adequate lid support.

The final consideration at the end of the operation is to determine the need for a temporary tarsorrhaphy stitch (Fig. 36.6). Occasionally, with prolonged procedures, particularly when the conjunctiva is exposed during the approach, moderate-to-significant conjunctival edema (chemosis) may occur. Mild chemosis is not uncommon and is treated with ophthalmic ointment postoperatively. However, if the edema is more pronounced, it may prevent the eyelids from closing fully. This may, in turn, lead to conjunctival exposure postoperatively, which can be a source of worsening chemosis. To prevent this problem, a temporary tarsorrhaphy stitch may be placed. This is positioned at the point of maximal edema either at the lateral or medial limbus. Placement over the pupil should be avoided as this would prevent monitoring vision and pupil shape/size during the perioperative period. The tarsorrhaphy stitch is removed 2–4 days after surgery or at the first postoperative visit when the edema has diminished.

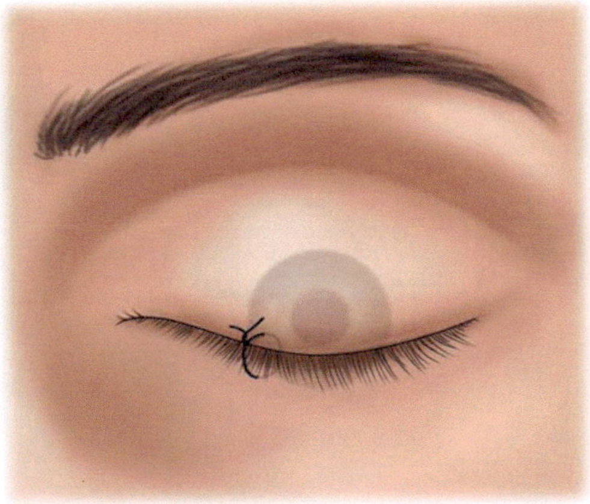

Fig. 36.6 Temporary tarsorrhaphy stitch. The stitch is placed at the medial or lateral limbus so the eye can still be opened to check pupil size, shape and symmetry

Part II: Postoperative Care

Postoperative care involves assuring the recovery from two components of the procedure: access to the target for instrumentation and visualization (collateral damage) and instrumentation of the pathology. Trauma from the latter depends on the location, type, and severity of the underlying condition. It is cared for postoperatively in the same manner as it would if an open approach had been undertaken. This will be discussed elsewhere in the book as relevant to the treatment of specific pathology.

Care of the periorbital issues encountered after transorbital neuroendoscopic surgery is unique to this group of procedures [3] and may be less familiar to some surgical specialties. The goals of postoperative care are to rule out intraoperative complications, monitor the patient for postoperative issues, and assure a comfortable, rapid, full recovery.

During the initial perioperative period, studies and examinations are obtained as indicated by the underlying pathology. The patient's gross visual acuity, pupil symmetry and extraocular muscle function are checked once the patient has regained an adequate level of consciousness to cooperate. This is rechecked every 1–2 h for the first 12 h and as indicated thereafter. We do not routinely obtain a postoperative CT scan unless indicated by the underlying pathology. A wrapped cold pack is placed over the eye for roughly 20 min per hour for the first 48 h. The ophthalmic ointment is placed at least twice daily for 5–7 days, and lubricating eye drops are used every 2–4 h as needed. If a temporary tarsorrhaphy stitch was placed as described above, it is removed when the chemosis has subsided, typically 2–5 days after surgery. For lengthy procedures, a course of steroids may be considered if not contraindicated. If the patient remains in the hospital, this can be given intravenously for 48 h. Alternatively, a 5-day oral course may be given. Antibiotics are not indicated for the approach itself, as it is sterile, unless the sinonasal cavities are entered.

The first postoperative clinic follow-up typically occurs 1 week after surgery. At this time, the patient's symptoms are monitored, and a visual exam is performed. The patient will often complain of reduced visual acuity due to edema and the use of ophthalmic ointment. Extraocular muscle function may be reduced, but the excursion should not be interrupted abruptly. Any non-absorbable periorbital sutures are typically removed at this time. The patient is seen again approximately 2 weeks after surgery for similar purposes. At that time the patient is examined for diplopia, globe dystopia, and evidence of eyelid malposition. If diplopia is present, the patient is taught physical therapy consisting of a range of motion exercises. The patient is then seen at 1- and 3-month time points after surgery and thereafter as indicated. At the 3-month visit, exophthalmometry may be considered to check the globe position within 2 mm of the contralateral side (Chap. 1, Fig. 1.10).

The most concerning complication of transorbital surgery, which is extremely rare, is blindness. Should this be noted on emergence from anesthesia, an emergent ophthalmology consult and CT scan should be obtained. Further care should be provided based on the underlying etiology. Another rare complication that can occur within the first 2 weeks of surgery is retrobulbar hematoma. This may present with diminished visual function upon emergence or later with decreased vision, increasing orbital pain and proptosis. This is an emergency, again requiring an ophthalmology consultation and tonometry if available. If unavailable, canthotomy and cantholysis should be performed, and an emergent CT scan may be obtained.

New onset of diplopia that did not exist before surgery may be either expected due to manipulation of the pathology or an unexpected complication. In the latter case, it is important to determine whether this is due to injury of a cranial nerve, or muscle dysfunction due to retraction or impingement/entrapment by the reconstruction material. A CT scan may be helpful if the examination does not determine the etiology. Other than muscle entrapment, which is also rare but should be relieved surgically, other sources of diplopia can be observed postoperatively, as most will respond spontaneously. Failure of diplopia to resolve spontaneously, unless the diagnosis is clear, warrants an ophthalmology consultation.

Postoperative globe dystopia is extremely rare and would most likely be due to malposition of the orbital reconstruction material. Postoperative eyelid malposition is also uncommon. The patient must be examined to determine the etiology of the malady. The most common source would be disruption with failure to reconstruct one of the eyelid support mechanisms, typically the lateral canthus, as described above. In addition, preexisting eyelid laxity may be exacerbated by postoperative edema and necessitate eventual correction. Alternatively, unfavorable scarring may cause retraction on an eyelid, such as the lateral canthus pulling away from the globe from failure to provide adequate support. These issues can generally be corrected with minor procedures.

References

1. Bevans S, Moe KS. Advances in orbital reconstruction. In: Moe KS, editor. Trauma in facial plastic surgery. Facial plastic surgery clinics of North America, vol. 25. Amsterdam: Elsevier; 2017. p. 479–644.
2. Bly R, Liu J, Cjudekova M, Chang SH, Moe KS. Computer-guided orbital reconstruction improves surgical outcomes. JAMA Facial Plast Surg. 2013;15(2):113–20.
3. Miller C, Rly RA, Moe KS. Endoscopic orbital and periorbital approaches in minimally disruptive skull base surgery. J Neurol Surg Pt B Skull Base. 2020;81(4):459–71. PMID: 33072486.
4. Moe KS, Linder T. The lateral transorbital canthopexy for correction and prevention of ectropion: report of a procedure, grading system, and prospective study. JAMA Facial Plast Surg. 2000;2:9–15.

Part X

Complications of Transorbital Surgery

Surgical Complications After Endoscopic Transorbital Surgery

37

Doo-Sik Kong

Introduction

Assessment of surgical complications is critical because it can improve the safety and quality of patient treatment. Unexpectedly, recent advances in various surgical techniques and the introduction of newly developed instruments may have contributed to an increase in new morbidity and mortality, as never previously reported. For instance, significant advances in endonasal endoscopic surgery have introduced applications for extensive indications such as anterior cranial fossa meningioma, clivus, and posterior fossa tumors, resulting in an increased incidence of postoperative cerebrospinal fluid (CSF) leak, which was uncommon in the pre- endoscopic surgery era.

Pathway-Related Morbidities

Dr. Moe et al. described two types of surgical complications: those caused by the creation and use of the pathway to the target and those incurred during the manipulation of the pathology. Manipulation-associated complications may be difficult to minimize other than using adequate exposure, appropriate instrument selection, and gentle manipulation of the tumor. However, a pathway-associated complication, the so-called damage to the surrounding tissue caused by creating and transiting the approach, is collateral damage, and every effort should be made to bring this damage to nothing. In endoscopic transorbital surgery, pathway-related complications include perioperative swelling, partial and transient ptosis, mechanical sores or electrical burns on the eyelid, ocular dysfunction, CSF leak, corneal keratitis, and enophthalmos. Before overcoming the learning curve, many surgeons struggle with unfamiliar anatomical knowledge about the orbit and the limited use of instruments under a narrow endoscopic field. As a result, lengthy operation time is closely associated with long-time retraction of the orbit, resulting in ocular dysfunction, periorbital swelling, transient ptosis, or mechanical sores on the eyelid. Therefore, the duration of retraction should be shortened or intermittent release (once every 10 min) of retracting the orbit must be emphasized to reduce associated morbidities. In our consecutive series of 100 cases of endoscopic transorbital surgery (unpublished), we encountered 3 cerebrospinal fluid leaks, 5 wound problems, 62 periorbital swelling, 13 transient ptosis, 7 ocular dysfunctions, and one case of enophthalmos.

D.-S. Kong (✉)
Department of Neurosurgery, Samsung Medical Center, Sungkyunkwan University, Seoul, South Korea

T. H. Schwartz et al. (eds.), *Endoscopic Transorbital Surgery of the Orbit, Skull Base and Brain*,
https://doi.org/10.1007/978-3-031-59504-2_37

Cerebrospinal Fluid Leaks

We experienced postoperative CSF leaks in only three patients after meningioma removal. It is believed that the removal of the meningioma leaves a large dural defect. The three cases of postoperative CSF leak (less than 3%) were treated with a slight compressive eye patch in one patient and postoperative lumbar drainage in two patients. No additional re-do surgery for reconstruction was required for any patient. Compared to endonasal endoscopic surgery, a relatively low incidence of CSF leak in endoscopic transorbital surgery is because the eye globe naturally blocks the high pressure of CSF leaks. The transorbital approach does not use a natural corridor such as the nasal cavity but creates a new working space by removing the greater sphenoid bone. Consequently, it is possible that the newly created space between the orbit and temporal dura is completely closed. After our experience of CSF leaks after meningioma removal, we routinely obtain fat tissue grafts from the abdomen and place the fat tissue into an inlay and onlay dura mater to fill out the dead space. There have been no reports of CSF leaks after the removal of any lesions other than meningiomas.

Wound Problems

Most wound problems are mechanical sore from long-standing operations, electrical burns from the electro-cauterization or endoscopic light, bacterial infection, and allergic reactions (Fig. 37.1). The skin of the eyelid is very thin, and long-standing retraction of the eyelid should be avoided. In addition, a lengthy operation is closely associated with long-time compression of the eyelid by the endoscope itself, the shaft of a drill, or the heating injury of an ultrasonic cavitation aspirator. Cosmetically, scarring of the eyelid is one of the most lethal complications. Care must be taken regarding the frequent release of retraction of the eyelid and inspection of possible causes of compression. In addition, a longer skin incision over the lateral canthus (less than 2 cm) can relieve pressure on the skin.

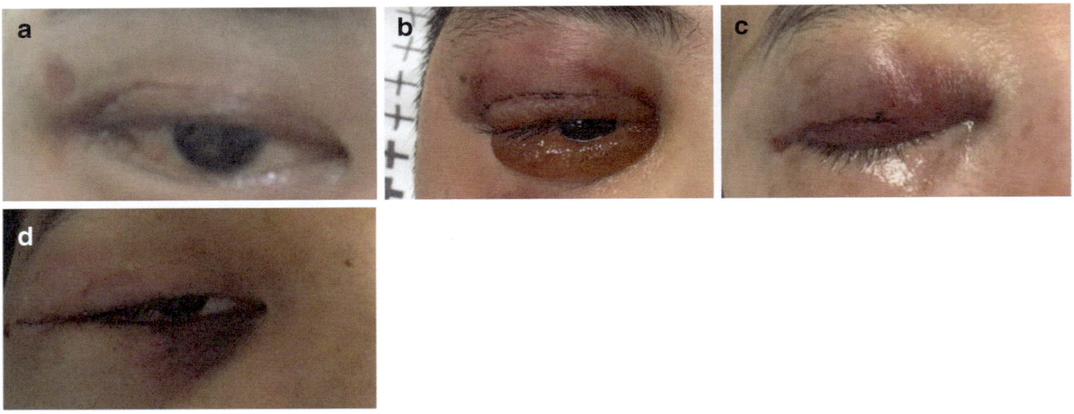

Fig. 37.1 Possible wound problems as complications of endoscopic transorbital surgery. (**a**) (First), electrical burns; (**b**) (Second), skin infection; (**c**) (Third), periorbital swelling with inflammation; (**d**) (Fourth), purpura with partial ptosis resulted from excessive orbital retraction

Periorbital Swelling, Transient Ptosis, and Ocular Dysfunction

Periorbital swelling is a common complication. This complication is also associated with long operative time. As surgeons will become familiar with this approach, the incidence and degree of periorbital swelling will decrease. With variations in transorbital surgery, osteotomy of the lateral or superolateral orbital rim may be added to obtain an adequate working space. In these situations, excessive retraction of the eyelid and temporalis muscle can lead to more frequent periorbital swelling. Ptosis is the most fearful situation that a surgeon and patient can experience. Postoperative transient ptosis occurs commonly but is usually spontaneously relieved (Fig. 37.2). In a majority of cases, it shows temporary and partial ptosis, which is related to periorbital swelling. It should be differentiated from complete ptosis, caused by injury of the oculomotor nerve or levator muscle. Usually, complete ptosis should be ruled out in cases of eyelid wrinkling disappearance or forced attempts to open the eye using the eyebrows. In addition, complete ptosis due to oculomotor nerve palsy shows a decreased levator function test result and significant limitation of adduction, elevation, and depression of the eye. Postoperative ocular dysfunction can result from excessive retraction of the orbit without any neurological deficits. Ocular dysfunction due to retraction of the extraocular muscle should be differentiated from that due to cranial nerve palsies.

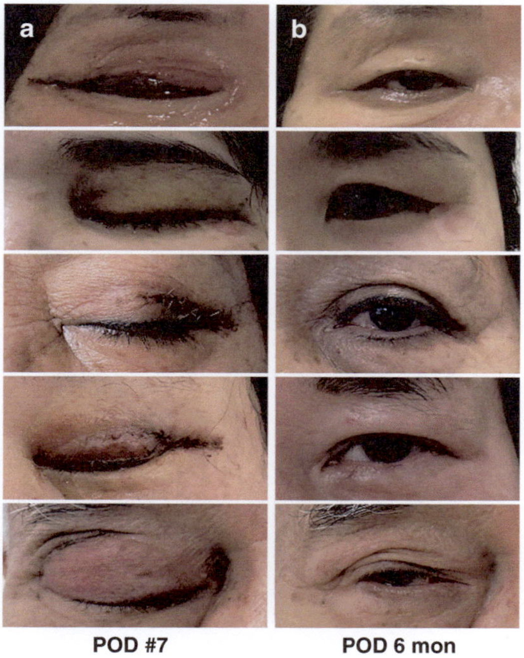

Fig. 37.2 Postoperative ptosis immediately after transorbital surgery. (**a**) (Left), complete ptosis immediately after surgery; (**b**) (Right), At the 6-month follow-up, ptosis was fully recovered

Newly Developed Enophthalmos

Postoperative enophthalmos, depression of the eye, is a very rare complication of transorbital surgery. In my personal series of approximately 130 cases of endoscopic transorbital surgery, only one patient experienced symptomatic enophthalmos. However, in patients with multiple orbital wall fractures due to trauma or accident, postoperative enophthalmos is a possible complication, because fracture of the bone supporting the eyeball or simultaneous fractures of the medial and lateral orbital walls are closely associated with postoperative enophthalmos. Therefore, orbital floor reconstruction with an alloplastic resorbable polydioxanone sheet or titanium mesh should be considered in trauma patients or combined endonasal and transorbital surgery cases.

Manipulation-Associated Complications

In neurosurgery, manipulation-associated complications refer to cranial nerves or brain parenchymal injuries. Cranial nerve palsies (oculomotor, trochlear, trigeminal, and abducens nerves) are representative complications after trigeminal schwannomas removal. Therefore, diplopia, facial sensory changes, and mastication difficulties should be carefully examined. In addition, newly developed corneal keratopathy may not be a rare complication from an ophthalmological perspective. In our series, 7 of the 50 patients with trigeminal schwannoma experienced postoperative corneal keratopathy (unpublished). One of the pathway-related complications, such as scratching or scarring of the cornea during surgery, might cause this complication. To prevent this pathway-related morbidity, a corneal protector or temporary suture, so-called tarsorrhaphy, is recommended during surgery. However, despite these attempts, corneal keratopathy can occur due to damage to the ophthalmic branch of the trigeminal nerve. This complication is more likely to occur in trigeminal schwannomas that involve the orbit. As described above, permanent ptosis due to oculomotor nerve palsy is accompanied by ocular dysfunction or enophthalmos. In rare cases, more serious complications, such as stroke or brain injury, may occur. It is important to discuss the potential risks and benefits of endoscopic transorbital surgery with a qualified surgeon before deciding whether to perform the procedure.

Conclusions

Endoscopic transorbital surgery is a minimally invasive procedure that involves reaching the brain through the orbit using an endoscope. It is used to treat various conditions, such as meningioma, schwannoma, and trauma. Overall, the potential risks and complications of endoscopic transorbital surgery are generally low; however, it is important to discuss them with colleagues before the procedure.

Part XI

Future Applications of Transorbital Surgery

38 Robotic Transorbital Surgery: Concepts and Future Directions

Tae Hoon Roh

Introduction

Brief History of Surgical Robots

In 1921, Josef Čapek invented the word "robot" for the first time in his brother's play *Rossum's Universal Robots*. The Czech word "robota," which means "labor," is where the name robot originates [1, 2]. Since then, its definition has changed, and it may today be described as a technical system that can carry out particular duties automatically in accordance with a set or customizable program. The robotic systems currently employed in surgery are not, strictly speaking, robots, but rather instrument-handling devices. Telemanipulators are systems that can complete certain operations remotely. These are master-slave systems that obey the surgeon's voice or hand commands rather than carrying out tasks automatically [3].

The first recorded robotic surgery performed on humans took place in the field of neurosurgery. This dates back to 1985 when the first robotic surgical system, the Unimation Puma 200 (an acronym for Programmable Universal Machine for Assembly), was used to conduct computed tomography (CT) guided stereotactic brain surgery [4]. This system, which utilizes a robot to accurately identify surgical sites, continues to be implemented in current devices such as ROSA (Robotic Stereotactic Assistance) and Kymero for precise tissue biopsy or electrode insertion [5] (Fig. 38.1). These surgical robots fall under the category of supervisory-controlled robots, which, while possessing the advantage of high precision, have the drawback of being highly limited in their functionality. The robots commonly used recently, on the other hand, are of the telesurgical or master-slave type, and their advantage lies in dexterity enhancement. However,

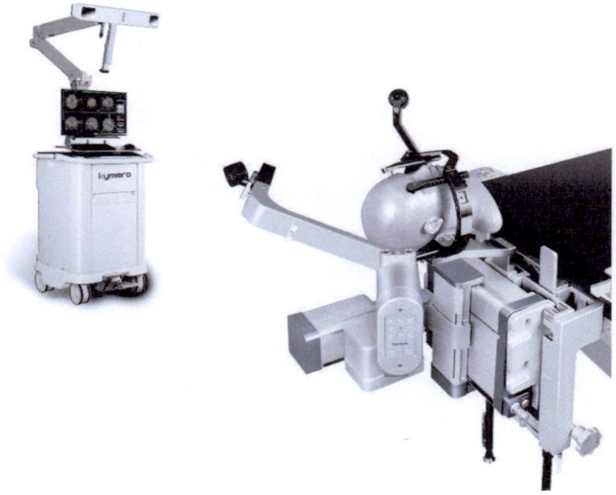

Fig. 38.1 Kymero (Kohyoung, Suwon, South Korea) is stereotactic robotic guidance fully integrated with proprietary neurosurgical navigation technology, delivering pinpoint accuracy on a larger scale. [With permissions from Kohyoung Technologies, Suwon, South Korea]

T. H. Roh (✉)
Department of Neurosurgery, Ajou University Hospital, Ajou University School of Medicine, Suwon, Gyeonggi-Do, Republic of Korea
e-mail: throh@ajou.ac.kr

T. H. Schwartz et al. (eds.), *Endoscopic Transorbital Surgery of the Orbit, Skull Base and Brain*,
https://doi.org/10.1007/978-3-031-59504-2_38

they have the disadvantage of not being able to perform surgery while feeling subtle sensations at the fingertips [6]. With the development of advanced robotic systems, surgeons are now able to perform complex procedures with greater precision and control [7].

Evolution of Master-Slave System Robots

In 1993, a voice-controlled robotic arm equipped with an endoscope named AESOP® was developed. This system was composed of two parts: a robotic arm that holds an endoscope attached to the instrument rail of the operating table and a computer system with a surgeon-specific voice control system [3]. The purpose of this system is to improve image stability, avoid needless accidental movements of the endoscope, and reduce the medical personnel required in the operating room. The system has been used for hundreds of thousands of minimally invasive surgical procedures in gastrointestinal, urologic, thoracic, cardiac, and pituitary surgery [8].

Computer Motion developed the ZEUS® system to improve surgeon dexterity during minimally invasive procedures [3]. It comprises two physically separate subsystems: a control console connected to three robotic arms attached to the operating table. The computer system acts as an electromechanical interface and can filter tremors and scale down movements. Clinical experience began in cardiovascular surgery, gynecology, and prostatectomies. Marescaux's team in Strasbourg published 25 telerobotic cholecystectomies in 2001, which led to the first transcontinental robot-assisted laparoscopic cholecystectomy [9, 10]. Fiberoptic technology made it possible to perform the first transatlantic cholecystectomy on September 7, 2001 [11]. Telesurgery has passed the test, and it is now possible to envision its practical application to surgery in hostile or difficult to reach environments. In 2003, Intuitive Surgical acquired Computer Motion.

The da Vinci® robotic system (Intuitive Surgical, Sunnyvale, CA) is composed of three components: a surgeon console, a patient trolley, and an imaging system [12]. The patient trolley is composed of three arms and four arms, while the surgeon console is composed of a binocular stereoscopic vision system that transmits the image from the endoscope 12 mm in diameter. Two handles or joysticks transmit the surgeon's hand movements to control the instruments and the lens. The Intuitive Surgical da Vinci® surgical was originally designed for cardiovascular surgery but was later extended to colorectal, bariatric, urology, gynecology, otolaryngology, and other disciplines [3].

Examples of Master-Slave Robotic Usage in Brain and Skull Base Surgery

Transoral Robot Surgery (TORS)

TORS is a surgical procedure that has been developed rapidly since its introduction in 2005 and is now widely used to access areas such as the oropharynx, hypopharynx, supraglottis, and glottis [13–15]. TORS has been shown to be safe and effective and has reduced morbidity and quality of life in head and neck surgery. It has also reduced the need for adjuvant therapy and has a lower rate of positive margins than traditional approaches. In high-volume centers, TORS is used to preserve laryngopharyngeal function without compromising oncologic outcomes.

TORS is often attempted in skull base surgeries as well. Clinical studies performing TORS in neurosurgery using devices like Da Vinci have been reported. Petrov and colleagues reported a case where a C2 Chordoma was removed en bloc using Da Vinci [16]. However, in this case, bone curettage was performed using an ultrasonic aspirator, and spine instrumentation after tumor removal was conducted manually without a robot. Therefore, it is questionable whether it can be truly called robotic surgery in the strictest sense. Lee and colleagues used the da Vinci Surgical System in two cadaver heads with neck and clavicles intact. It provided superb illumination and 3D depth perception, allowing for better cephalad visualization and the ability to suture the dura mater in a deep, dark corridor. The authors concluded that transoral robotic surgery holds great potential for decompression of the CCJ as well as resection of both extra- and intradural tumors of this region [17].

Chauvet et al. [18] aimed to confirm the feasibility of an innovative TORS using the da Vinci Surgical System for patients with sellar tumors. The main outcome measure was sellar accessibility using the robot, and results showed that four patients underwent TORS for resection without the need for a second surgery. In all four cases, the operation was performed via TORS, with a mean operative time of 2 h 43 min, and no rhinological side effects or complications occurred. Side effects specific to TORS included minor sore throat, transient hypernasal speech, and 1 case of delayed otitis media. The mean length of hospital stay and mean follow-up were 8.25 days and 82 days, respectively. This technique is feasible and constitutes an innovative neurosurgical technique that may avoid the adverse side effects and technical disadvantages of the classic transsphenoidal route.

Robotic Brain Surgery

Akbaş et al. conducted a study presenting the advantages and disadvantages of the most common robotic surgical system, the da Vinci Xi system, in the supracerebellar transtentorial approach to the mesial temporal region [19]. Four formalin-fixed human cadaveric head specimens with colored silicone dye injected into their vessels were used. Results showed that the robotic system can be used in difficult approaches and narrow regions with a wider exposure and superior image quality than with the microscopic approach, improving the surgeon's ergonomics. However, the shortcomings of robotic systems are examined, and innovative solutions are offered. Future research and development of these systems and related instruments are necessary to ensure their wider implementation in neurosurgery.

Robotic Intraventricular Surgery

NeuRobot is a micromanipulator system with a rigid neuroendoscope and three micromanipulators developed for less invasive and telecontrolled neurosurgery [20, 21]. It was used to simulate four intraventricular neurosurgical procedures in three fixed cadaver heads and successfully performed a third ventriculostomy in a patient with obstructive hydrocephalus [22].

The Introduction of Endoscopy and the Development of the Transorbital Approach in Neurosurgery

The use of endoscopy in the field of neurosurgery was highly limited. This was largely due to the intricate manipulation required during brain surgery, necessitating the use of a surgical microscope, which made it challenging to operate in confined spaces with an endoscope. Additionally, the cranial cavity is a considerably restricted space; even if a hole is drilled for access, the static nature of the hole implies that movement is limited with a rigid, non-flexible endoscope. The instruments required for manipulation also had limitations when performing surgery through straight instruments. Furthermore, since the cranial cavity is filled with brain tissue, endoscopy in brain surgery was confined to certain intraventricular procedures [23].

However, as endoscopy began to be utilized in minimally invasive approaches, neurosurgeons also became accustomed to endoscopic surgeries [24]. Thanks to the efforts of several pioneers, the transorbital approach has gained traction. The endoscopic transorbital approach has grown in popularity as the standard surgical approach for the middle cranial fossa, posterior cranial fossa, cavernous sinus regions, and some intra-axial lesions [25–28].

Potential Use of Robotics in the Transorbital Approach

Transorbital surgery, a relatively recent innovation compared to other surgical methods, holds significant potential for application in robotic surgery. Utilizing the space occupied by orbital fat, a relatively ample area can be secured, enabling access to most of the skull base, from the anterior, middle, to the posterior cranial fossa. However, there have been no reported cases where the transorbital approach has been implemented in actual surgery.

In the context of orbital lesions, the Da Vinci Xi robotic system has recently been used to perform decompression of orbital fat in patients with Grave's disease [29].

Preclinical studies have used the orbit in conjunction with other regions as a surgical corridor. For instance, both orbits and the transnasal corridor have been used to access the nasopharynx, sellar, and anterior skull base [30]. Bly et al. [31]. examined the feasibility of robotic transorbital and transnasal approaches to reach sella and parasellar target locations. Using computer analysis on 10 computed tomography scans, they determined approach trajectories, angles between robotic tools, and distances to specified skull base target locations. Multiportal analyses revealed that the angles between two robotic tools were 14.7, 28.3, and 52.0°. The addition of medial and superior transorbital portals improved the skull base trajectory angles by 21 and 27°.

Distinct Requirements for Transorbital Surgery Robots Compared to Other Fields

Comparing Intraperitoneal Robotic Systems and Transorbital Surgical Methods

Surgical operations utilizing the Da Vinci system often involve the manipulation and elevation of soft tissues, followed by dissection via electrocautery through a monopolar coagulator. However, in brain surgery, there is little to no soft tissue to grasp and lift. A majority of brain tumor surgeries employ an ultrasonic aspirator, a device that requires an electrical system for operation.

Entry Point Constrained to Bone

In Da Vinci surgeries, a trocar is used to create an entry point through which instruments are passed. This serves as a pivot or fulcrum point [32]. While the entry point in the abdomen is fixed, some movement is possible. In the case of abdominal surgery, this fulcrum point allows the inserted endoscope or instrument to move like a lever. However, such a fulcrum point does not exist in transorbital surgery. If a hole perfectly fitting the instrument is drilled into the bone, a rigid instrument cannot change its direction from that position. The thicker the bone through which the instrument passes, the more limited the movement of the rigid instrument becomes. As a result, it is necessary for instruments in transorbital surgery to be capable of internal articulation.

Narrow Entry Point for Instruments

The diameters of the Da Vinci robot's endoscope are 8.5 and 12 mm. The robotic arms are 5 and 8 mm [33]. Therefore, once the endoscope is inserted, there is no room left for the robotic arm. Moreover, the minimum angle between the robotic arms can be problematic in tight spaces. In the supraorbital keyhole approach, the size of the craniotomy is only 25 × 15 mm [34]. According to one study, visualization is limited when craniotomy is less than 40 mm, and an endoscope and instruments can only be inserted when it is over 50 mm [35]. Even if all instruments are inserted, they are too close together, making manipulation difficult. In experimental results, even a 60 mm craniotomy size was difficult to manipulate, and a craniotomy size of over 70 mm was necessary for smooth movement. This is significantly larger than the bone size in a transorbital approach [33].

In the transorbital approach, an entry larger than 20 mm can be secured by removing the lateral orbital rim through osteotomy or using a modified supraorbital approach [36, 37]. Increasing orbital retraction without removing the orbital rim can raise intraocular pressure, leading to potential vision loss [38].

To overcome these problems, it appears that single-port robotic instruments or a multiportal approach should be used. In the case of Da Vinci Single Port (SP), a single port with a diameter of 25 mm can accommodate one stereoscopic endoscope and three instruments.

Lack of Internal Space for Robotic Arm Movement

In the case of the abdominal or thoracic cavity, space is secured by insufflating carbon dioxide gas. For the thyroid, gas is insufflated under the skin to expand it and create space [39].

On the other hand, the intracranial space consists of brain tissue, cerebrospinal fluid (CSF), and tumor mass. The only way to secure space for visualization and movement inside is to drain the CSF. When operating on lesions in the temporal pole, middle cranial fossa, or posterior cranial fossa, additional intracranial space can be secured by draining the CSF. Theoretically, there is 50 ml of CSF in the ventricles and 50 ml in the subarachnoid space, so if all of this is drained, about 100 cc of space can be secured. However, this is still insufficient for the current robotic arms like Da Vinci to enter. When brain edema is present, it's often difficult to secure space even if a lot of CSF is drained. Especially when the tumor is not removed, the intracranial pressure (ICP) is often higher than normal, making it difficult to secure enough space.

In skull base surgery, it has traditionally been a principle to remove as much of the skull base bone as possible to secure space. The same principle applies in transorbital surgery, which involves removing the orbital rim and grinding the sphenoid ridge bone. Retracting the orbital contents, especially fat and the temporalis muscle, can secure a pathway for the instruments to enter. However, in cases where the surgical site is right behind the orbit, such as with a sphenoid ridge meningioma, the space is limited, and there may not be enough room for the instruments to move.

A Significant Amount of Bone Work

The lateral orbital wall, sphenoid ridge, and the posterior frontal bone must be drilled out to perform a transorbital approach. The extensive bone work implies two difficulties. A robot capable of drilling is needed to perform bone resection using a drill. However, bone drilling is a task that requires a high degree of tactile feedback, which is currently technically difficult to incorporate into a robot. It is thought to be risky to perform drilling with only visual feedback. Otherwise, the robot arm must incorporate tools like a bone-cutter or rongeur, which can apply strong force. Developing a drill with a motor attached to the end of the instrument is required. Still, there are currently technical limitations to mounting a small drill capable of delivering sufficient force at the end of the robot [32].

The other issue is the difficulty of securing a clear field of view. Even if a robot that drills under endoscope visualization is made, bone dust continuously flies off during drilling, necessitating continuous irrigation. Therefore, unlike endoscopic surgery, robotic surgery makes it extremely cumbersome, if not virtually impossible, to remove and clean the endoscope in the middle of the procedure. Therefore, a continuous irrigation and clearing system must be established. Using a round bur, if the flute is large, the suction can frequently get blocked due to large bone dust.

High Risk of Bleeding

The brain is a hypervascular organ that receives 20% of the cardiac output. The dura mater, which wraps the brain, is also highly vascular, and many brain tumors are hypervascular. During brain tumor surgery, there tends to be relatively high bleeding, which often obscures the surgical field. Continuous blood suction and coagulation of the bleeding site are necessary to maintain visibility. The currently used robots do not have suction equipment, and it's challenging to use materials like surgical patties, which gently press the brain for hemostasis and simultaneously suck in blood to maintain visibility.

For brain surgery, it would be necessary to be able to identify and coagulate the bleeding focus using bipolar forceps equipped with suction and irrigation channels. Especially, since the endoscope cannot be removed and wiped when blood is on the tip, it should be washed away through irrigation.

Overcoming the Challenges in Transorbital Robotic Surgery

Robot-Assisted Surgery with Master-Slave System

Endoscope-Holding Robot

Holding an endoscope throughout surgery is a highly fatiguing task for the operator and restricts the movement of one hand, making intricate procedures difficult. Particularly in transorbital approaches, which require more drilling compared to endonasal ones, the usage of endoscopic holders is common, often resorting to passive endoscopic holding robots. When an assistant holds the endoscope, collisions with the surgeon frequently occur, and it is difficult to adjust the direction as desired by the surgeon. Therefore, a robotic endoscopic system that the surgeon can directly control is necessary (Fig. 38.2). Proposed methods include controlling the endoscope through the movement of the head [40], using a joypad [41, 42], facial movements [43], or through a head-mounted display [44].

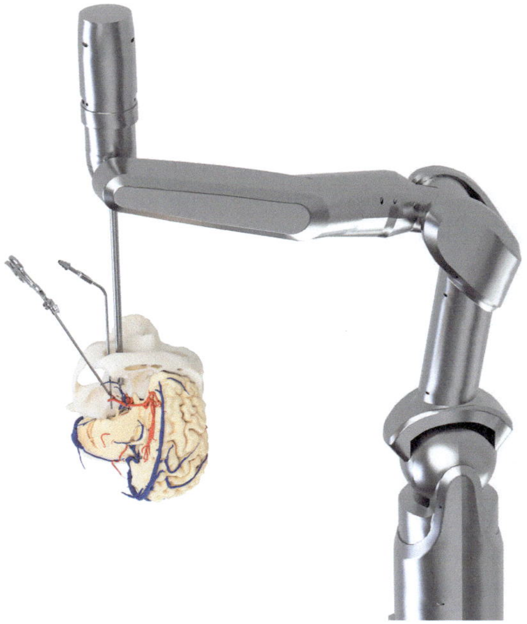

Fig. 38.2 A robotic endoscope holder

Micro-Single Port Robotic System

Currently, the surgical robot that uses the narrowest passage is the Da Vinci Single Port system (Fig. 38.3). In the future, the development of a micro-single port robotic system capable of sophisticated operations through an active cannula will enable microsurgeries like pituitary surgeries.

Robotic Arms with Actuator

The development of advanced robotic arms equipped with specialized tools is essential for the future of robotic surgery. Key examples include the drill-attached robotic arm and the ultrasonic-aspirator-attached robotic arm, both designed for precise bone and tumor resection. The drill-attached robotic arm features motors at the end, enabling accurate control over the drilling process. This precision reduces the risk of human error and improves patient outcomes in bone surgeries like craniotomies. The ultrasonic-aspirator-attached robotic arm uses highfrequency vibrations to emulsify and remove tumors. This method is particularly useful in neurosurgery, where precision and minimal invasive-

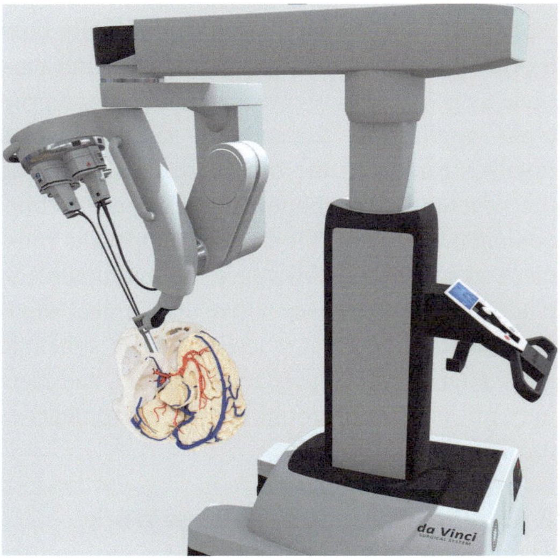

Fig. 38.3 Da Vinci single port robotic surgical system

ness are critical. The actuators ensure steady and controlled movements, enhancing the safety and effectiveness of these procedures. These robotic arms not only improve surgical precision and safety but also reduce the physical strain on surgeons by automating complex tasks. Continued advancements in these technologies promise to make complex surgeries more accessible and efficient. In summary, the development of drill-attached and ultrasonic-aspirator-attached robotic arms with advanced actuators is a vital step toward the future of robotic surgery, transforming surgical practices for better safety and efficiency.

Tactile Feedback

The absence of tactile feedback complicates the use of robotic surgical devices. Visual feedback on movements can partially overcome this issue. The robotic arms of the da Vinci system have incorporated pressure sensors to enhance the safety of dissection. In the future, a robotic grasper that provides tactile feedback will be introduced to the master-slave system, enabling more precise surgeries [45]. If a robotic hand capable of precise movements and modeled after a human hand is developed, it will allow surgeons at a distance to perform any surgery [46].

Autonomous Robots

Autonomous Bone Drilling Robot

The next step in surgeon-controlled endoscopes is to have artificial intelligence automatically create the optimal viewpoint [47]. Allowing users to switch instantly between autonomous and master-slave modes will eliminate the need for an assistant during surgery.

Autonomous Bone Drilling Robot

If a robot capable of performing craniotomy as planned while receiving navigation feedback, similar to a milling machine processing metal, is developed, the entire surgical process could be replaced by robotic surgery. A robot capable of performing a mastoidectomy has already been developed [48]. Until this is possible, drilling must be done manually before starting robotic surgery.

Autonomous Humanoid Robot

The ultimate stage of robotic development is the fully autonomous humanoid robot. Achieving this milestone suggests that all other preceding challenges have been successfully addressed. Considering the rapid advancements in artificial intelligence, it seems only a matter of time before this becomes a reality.

Future Perspectives in Robotic Surgery Simulation

3D Printing Simulation

3D printing has changed surgical simulation. Using diagnostic cross-sectional imaging and specialized software, several groups have built high-fidelity 3D-printed brain tumor and skull base models [49, 50]. These models are mostly used in surgical simulation as high-fidelity drylab training platforms. In the simulation environment, trainees can learn hard activities like transsphenoidal and transorbital approaches using a 3D-printed model. Cost, availability, and resemblance to normal brain parenchyma are current drawbacks, but they may be solved in the future. These bench-top models could also be used by skilled neurosurgeons for surgical rehearsal [51]. In difficult tumors, the best way to remove the tumor must be found. 3D-printed models help patients and doctors visualize tumor locations [52]. These models can also be used to simulate whether robotic surgery is possible.

Virtual Reality (VR) Simulation

In the Da Vinci Surgical System, if the robotic arms are replaced with virtual arms that can be operated, and medical images are reconstructed into three dimensions for manipulation, it would transform into a virtual surgery platform. VR simulation has been shown to improve basic skill acquisition and familiarize novices with the robotic console. However, higher-fidelity models like human cadavers, live animals, or ex vivo animal organs are used for more advanced procedural modeling. These are closer to patient operations, but ethical concerns and increased prices limit access. Thus, higher-fidelity procedure-specific VR simulation has resurged [53]. These models have demonstrated promise in teaching operational anatomy and procedural processes, but larger research is needed. Procedure-specific VR simulation cannot replace wet lab instruction without further development. Nevertheless, whole-procedure VR simulation is intriguing, and new innovations like patient-specific features are possible.

Conclusions

As of now, there are no clinical studies on the transorbital approach, and only some preclinical studies using cadavers exist. The robots currently in use are thought to be unsuitable for performing transorbital surgery. Nevertheless, the areas with the highest potential for introducing robots in brain surgery are the endonasal and transorbital approaches, which currently use endoscopes.

The future of robotic neurosurgery is promising, with ongoing research and development aimed at improving the safety, efficacy, and accessibility of robotic technology. Areas of focus include the development of more advanced robotic systems, the integration of artificial intelligence and machine learning, and the expansion of robotic technology to more surgical fields and procedures.

References

1. Borumandi F, Heliotis M, Kerawala C, Bisase B, Cascarini L. Role of robotic surgery in oral and maxillofacial, and head and neck surgery. Br J Oral Maxillofac Surg. 2012;50:389–93.
2. Kalan S, Chauhan S, Coelho RF, Orvieto MA, Camacho IR, Palmer KJ, Patel VR. History of robotic surgery. J Robot Surg. 2010;4:141–7.
3. Pugin F, Bucher P, Morel P. History of robotic surgery: from AESOP® and ZEUS® to da Vinci®. J Visc Surg. 2011;148:e3–8.
4. Gajjar AA, Huy Dinh Le A, Swaroop Lavadi R, Boddeti U, Barpujari A, Agarwal N. Evolution of robotics in neurosurgery: a historical perspective. Interdiscip Neurosurg. 2023;33:101721.
5. Cho K, Chang WS, Kim HD, Chang JW, Kim SH, Lee JS, Kang H-C. Robot-assisted stereoelectroencephalography for pediatric epilepsy surgery: the first case in Korea. Ann Child Neurol. 2021;29:205–8.
6. Karas CS, Chiocca EA. Neurosurgical robotics: a review of brain and spine applications. J Robot Surg. 2007;1:39–43.
7. Fomenko A, El Idrissi FE, Aji N, Outani O, Benkirane K, Moujtahid H, Al-Salihi MM, Serletis D. Introduction and history of robotics in neurosurgery. Cham: Springer; 2022. p. 1–10.
8. Nathan C-AO, Chakradeo V, Malhotra K, D'Agostino H, Patwardhan R. The voice-controlled robotic assist scope holder AESOP for the endoscopic approach to the Sella. Skull Base. 2006;16:123–31.
9. Marescaux J, Rubino F. The ZEUS robotic system: experimental and clinical applications. Surg Clin N Am. 2003;83:1305–15.
10. Marescaux J, Leroy J, Gagner M, Rubino F, Mutter D, Vix M, Butner SE, Smith MK. Transatlantic robot-assisted telesurgery. Nature. 2001;413:379–80.
11. Marescaux J, Leroy J, Rubino F, Smith M, Vix M, Simone M, Mutter D. Transcontinental robot-assisted remote telesurgery: feasibility and potential applications. Ann Surg. 2002;235:487.
12. Gharagozloo F, Patel VR, Giulianotti PC, Poston R, Gruessner R, Meyer M. Robotic surgery. Cham: Springer; 2021. https://doi.org/10.1007/978-3-030-53594-0.
13. Weinstein GS, O'Malley BW Jr, Hockstein NG. Transoral robotic surgery: supraglottic laryngectomy in a canine model. Laryngoscope. 2005;115:1315–9.
14. Mercante G, Ruscito P, Pellini R, Cristalli G, Spriano G. Transoral robotic surgery (TORS) for tongue base tumours. Acta Otorhinolaryngol Ital. 2013;33:230–5.
15. Faulkner J, Arora A, Swords C, Cook E, Rajangam A, Jeannon J-P. Preclinical evaluation of a novel robotic system for transoral robotic surgery. Clin Otolaryngol. 2021;46:869–74.
16. Petrov D, Spadola M, Berger C, Glauser G, Mahmoud AF, O'Malley B, Malhotra NR. Novel approach using ultrasonic bone curettage and transoral robotic surgery for en bloc resection of cervical spine chordoma: case report. J Neurosurg Spine. 2019;30(6):788–93.
17. Lee JYK, O'Malley BW, Newman JG, Weinstein GS, Lega B, Diaz J, Grady MS. Transoral robotic surgery of craniocervical junction and atlantoaxial spine: a cadaveric study: laboratory investigation. J Neurosurg Spine. 2010;12:13–8.

18. Chauvet D, Hans S, Missistrano A, Rebours C, Bakkouri WE, Lot G. Transoral robotic surgery for sellar tumors: first clinical study. J Neurosurg. 2017;127:941–8.
19. Akbaş A, Tuğcu B, Ekşi MŞ, Erkan B, Canbolat Ç, Pamir MN, Gungor A. Robotic surgical approach to the mesial temporal region: a preliminary three-dimensional cadaveric study of technical feasibility. World Neurosurg. 2020;144:e40–52.
20. Davies B, Starkie S, Harris SJ, Agterhuis E, Paul V, Auer LM (2000) Neurobot: a special-purpose robot for neurosurgery. In: Proceedings 2000 ICRA. Millennium Conference. IEEE International Conference on Robotics and Automation. Symposia Proceedings (Cat. No.00CH37065), p. 4103–8.
21. Hongo K, Goto T, Miyahara T, Kakizawa Y, Koyama J, Tanaka Y. Telecontrolled micromanipulator system (NeuRobot) for minimally invasive neurosurgery. In: Nimsky C, Fahlbusch R, editors. Medical technologies in neurosurgery. Vienna: Springer; 2006. p. 63–6.
22. Takasuna H, Goto T, Kakizawa Y, Miyahara T, Koyama J, Tanaka Y, Kawai T, Hongo K. Use of a micromanipulator system (NeuRobot) in endoscopic neurosurgery. J Clin Neurosci. 2012;19:1553–7.
23. Schwartz TH, Ss Y, Fw C, Goodman RR, Goodman RR. Third ventriculostomy: post-operative ventricular size and outcome. Minim Invasive Neurosurg. 1996;39:122–9.
24. Younus I, Gerges MM, Gerges MM, Uribe-Cardenas R, Morgenstern PF, Kacker A, Tabaee A, Anand VK, Schwartz TH. The slope of the learning curve in 600 consecutive endoscopic transsphenoidal pituitary surgeries. Acta Neurochir. 2020;162:2361–70.
25. Jung I-H, Yoo J, Choi S, Lim SH, Ko J, Roh TH, Hong JB, Kim EH. Endoscopic transorbital approach to the cavernous sinus: cadaveric anatomy study and clinical application (SevEN-009). Front Oncol. 2022;12:962598.
26. Kim EH, Yoo J, Jung I-H, Oh JW, Kim J-S, Yoon JS, Moon JH, Kang S-G, Chang JH, Roh TH. Endoscopic transorbital approach to the insular region: cadaveric feasibility study and clinical application (SevEN-005). J Neurosurg. 2021;135:1164–72.
27. Lim J, Sung KS, Yoo J, Oh J, Moon JH. Endoscopic transorbital extradural anterior clinoidectomy: a stepwise surgical technique and case series study [SevEN-013]. Front Oncol. 2022;12:991065.
28. Moe KS, Bergeron CM, Ellenbogen RG. Transorbital neuroendoscopic surgery. Neurosurgery. 2010;67:16–28.
29. Wang Y, Sun J, Liu X, Li Y, Fan X, Zhou H. Robot-assisted orbital fat decompression surgery: first in human. Transl Vis Sci Technol. 2022;11:8.
30. Faulkner J, Naidoo R, Arora A, Jeannon JP, Hopkins C, Surda P. Combined robotic transorbital and transnasal approach to the nasopharynx and anterior skull base: feasibility study. Clin Otolaryngol. 2020;45:630–3.
31. Bly RA, Su D, Lendvay TS, Friedman D, Hannaford B, Ferreira M, Moe KS. Multiportal robotic access to the anterior cranial fossa: a surgical and engineering feasibility study. Otolaryngol Head Neck Surg. 2013;149:940–6.
32. Hamza H, Baez VM, Al-Ansari A, Becker AT, Navkar NV. User interfaces for actuated scope maneuvering in surgical systems: a scoping review. Surg Endosc. 2023;37(6):4193–223. https://doi.org/10.1007/s00464-023-09981-0.
33. Marcus HJ, Hughes-Hallett A, Cundy TP, Yang G-Z, Darzi A, Nandi D. da Vinci robot-assisted keyhole neurosurgery: a cadaver study on feasibility and safety. Neurosurg Rev. 2015;38:367–71.
34. Bhatoe HS. The supraorbital keyhole approach: how I do it. Acta Neurochir. 2015;157:2127–7.
35. Thakre AA, Bailly Y, Sun LW, Van MF, Yeung CK. Is smaller workspace a limitation for robot performance in laparoscopy? J Urol. 2008;179:1138–43.
36. Altay T, Patel BCK, Couldwell WT. Lateral orbital wall approach to the cavernous sinus: laboratory investigation. J Neurosurg. 2012;116:755–63.
37. Alzhrani GA, Gozal YM, Sherrod BA, Couldwell WT. A modified lateral orbitotomy approach to the superior orbital fissure: a video case report and review of anatomy. Oper Neurosurg. 2019;16:685–91.
38. Kim W, Moon JH, Kim EH, Hong C-K, Han J, Hong JB. Optimization of orbital retraction during endoscopic transorbital approach via quantitative measurement of the intraocular pressure – [SevEN 006]. BMC Ophthalmol. 2021;21:76.
39. Kim HY, Choi YJ, Yu H-N, Yoon SZ. Optimal carbon dioxide insufflation pressure during robot-assisted thyroidectomy in patients with various benign and malignant thyroid diseases. World J Surg Oncol. 2012;10:202.
40. Bucher JN, Bruewer K, Dietz LJ, Trebesius N, Hidding J, Wysocki M, Schoenberg MB, Werner J, Karcz K. A robotic camera holder controlled by head movements: exploring this new robot-surgeon interface. Surg Innov. 2020;27:499–506.
41. Amin MSA, Aydin A, Abbud N, et al. Evaluation of a remote-controlled laparoscopic camera holder for basic laparoscopic skills acquisition: a randomized controlled trial. Surg Endosc. 2021;35:4183–91.
42. Mittal R, Sbaih M, Motson RW, Arulampalam T. Use of a robotic camera holder (FreeHand®) for laparoscopic appendicectomy. Minim Invasive Ther Allied Technol. 2020;29:56–60.
43. Nishikawa A, Hosoi T, Koara K, et al. FAce MOUSe: a novel human-machine interface for controlling the position of a laparoscope. IEEE Trans Robot Autom. 2003;19:825–41.
44. Zinchenko K, Komarov O, Song K-T. Virtual reality control of a robotic camera holder for minimally invasive surgery. In: 2017 11th Asian Control Conference (ASCC); 2017, p. 970–5.
45. Chen T, Saadatnia Z, Kim J, Looi T, Drake J, Diller E, Naguib HE. Novel, flexible, and ultrathin pressure feedback sensor for miniaturized intraventricular neurosurgery robotic tools. IEEE Trans Ind Electron. 2021;68:4415–25.

46. Kim U, Jung D, Jeong H, Park J, Jung H-M, Cheong J, Choi HR, Do H, Park C. Integrated linkage-driven dexterous anthropomorphic robotic hand. Nat Commun. 2021;12:7177.
47. Wagner M, Bihlmaier A, Kenngott HG, et al. A learning robot for cognitive camera control in minimally invasive surgery. Surg Endosc. 2021;35:5365–74.
48. Danilchenko A, Balachandran R, Toennies JL, Baron S, Munske B, Fitzpatrick JM, Withrow TJ, Webster RJI, Labadie RF. Robotic mastoidectomy. Otol Neurotol. 2011;32:11–6.
49. Park C-K. 3D-printed disease models for neurosurgical planning, simulation, and training. J Korean Neurosurg Soc. 2022;65:489–98.
50. Graffeo CS, Perry A, Carlstrom LP, Link MJ, Morris J. A model is worth 1000 pictures: applications of 3D-modeling in skull base surgery neuroanatomy education. J Neurol Surg Part B Skull Base. 2020;81(1):1–272.
51. Kondo K, Harada N, Masuda H, et al. A neurosurgical simulation of skull base tumors using a 3D printed rapid prototyping model containing mesh structures. Acta Neurochir. 2016;158:1213–9.
52. Dho Y-S, Lee D, Ha T, et al. Clinical application of patient-specific 3D printing brain tumor model production system for neurosurgery. Sci Rep. 2021;11:7005.
53. Roh TH, Oh JW, Jang CK, Choi S, Kim EH, Hong C-K, Kim S-H. Virtual dissection of the real brain: integration of photographic 3D models into virtual reality and its effect on neurosurgical resident education. Neurosurg Focus. 2021;51:E16.

Future Applications: New 3D Training Model for Endoscopic Endonasal and Transorbital Approach

39

Won-Jae Lee and Doo-Sik Kong

Introduction

Endoscopic techniques in skull base surgery have become imperative for accessing and managing various skull base diseases [1–3]. Comprehensive understanding of the relevant anatomy and experienced surgical skills areessential, as the skull base has a complex and unique anatomy surrounded by numerous critical neurovascular structures [3]. Skull base surgeries have little margin of error. Constant surgical training is important for surgeons who perform delicate skull base surgeries. For trainees, mastering endoscopic surgical techniques has distinct challenges, such as a steep learning curve, impaired depth perception, and ergonomics [4, 5]. Recently, we developed and validated a patient-specific three-dimensional (3D)-printed simulation surgical training model for endoscopic endonasal (EEA) and transorbital (TOA) approaches [6]. The major purpose of the 3D simulation model is to help trainees familiarize themselves with the unique viewing angle of the endoscope and develop basic skills for endoscopic surgery. Advances in 3D-printing technology have made elaborate and realistic virtual simulations possible. The model clearly demonstrates the complex anatomy and associated pathologies of the skull base.

This study is an extension of our previously published work on 3D-printed simulation models. In the following sections, we describe a new 3D training model (Anatdel, Medical IP, Seoul, Republic of Korea) for the EEA and TOA procedures. The new model provides better tactile and color feedback to operators. The texture of the bones and soft tissues has beens improved to increase the fidelity of the human body. The various modules of the EEA and TOA procedures were simulated using the model to evaluate anatomical and surgical realism.

Development and Evaluation of the 3D-Printed Simulation Model

In this study, a three-dimensional (3D) model of the human skull base was created from medical imaging data, including computed tomography (CT) and magnetic resonance imaging (MRI). The imaging data were saved in Digital Imaging and Communications in Medicine format and imported into a dedicated software program (MEDIP PRO, Medical IP, Seoul, Republic of Korea) for 3D modeling. The skull, eyeballs, brain, brain stem, cranial nerves, venous sinus, and arterial anatomies were segmented from the surrounding structures according to a grayscale, and tissues with a certain level of gray were con-

W.-J. Lee · D.-S. Kong (✉)
Department of Neurosurgery, Sungkyunkwan University School of Medicine, Samsung Medical Center, Seoul, South Korea
e-mail: kds026@skku.edu

T. H. Schwartz et al. (eds.), *Endoscopic Transorbital Surgery of the Orbit, Skull Base and Brain*,
https://doi.org/10.1007/978-3-031-59504-2_39

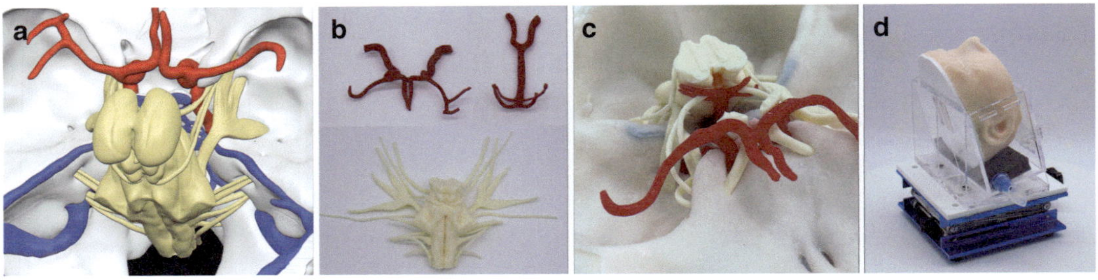

Fig. 39.1 Three-dimensional (3D) image reconstructed from patient neuroimaging data using dedicated software (**a**). Neurovascular structures were made via a molding process using silicone (**b**), and then the products were assembled into the 3D-printed skull model (**c**). The simulation model is installed on a dedicated pedestal (**d**)

verted into 3D images using a software algorithm. CT angiography was used to reconstruct the 3D cerebral vessel model, while 3D proton density-weighted images were used to create the 3D cranial nerve model. The resulting images were converted into 3D stereolithography files and processed for printing (Fig. 39.1a). The physical model was printed on a 1:1 scale using 3D printing equipment. The skull model was created using a PolyJet process for additive manufacturing on J850 Prime printers (Stratasys, Eden Prairie, MN, USA). Silicone was applied to the relevant surface of the skull model to mimic the nasal mucosa and the periosteum. Soft tissues such as the eyeballs, brain, cranial nerves, and arteries were made using silicone via molding. The molds were printed using a fused filament fabrication method with acrylonitrile butadiene styrene copolymer. Finally, the individual pieces of soft tissue were assembled into a skull model (Fig. 39.1b, c). The final simulation models were developed through an iterative process involving the prototype version of the model. Careful assessment of soft tissue sensations, bone-like drilling properties, and color feedback during endoscopic visualization was performed. Various virtual simulations of different surgical approaches, including EEA and TOA, were tested on the model to, enhancesurgical realism. To ensure ergonomic suitability for endoscopic skull base surgery (ESBS), the simulation model was installed on a dedicated pedestal (Fig. 39.1d).

Surgical Simulation Procedures

EEA Procedure

The surgical simulation was performed by experienced neurosurgeons using a rigid endoscope, 4 mm in diameter, with 0° and 30° lenses, and a 4K camera recording system (Stryker, CA, USA). A standard binostril transsphenoidal approach was used on the model (Fig. 39.2). The reconstructed anatomy of the nasal cavity, the texture of the nasal mucosa, and the optimal bone intensity of the nasal turbinate were carefully evaluated. After elevation of the nasoseptal flap, the sphenoid rostrum was removed, and a wide sphenoidotomy was performed. The bony landmarks of the sellar floor were identified, and the anterior skull base was drilled according to the extent of the surgical procedure to be simulated. The dura was incised, and the intradural structures were identified and color-coded according to their nature. To expose the central skull base, the anterior wall of the cavernous sinus (CS), clivus, and dorsum sellae, as well as the bone covering the paraclival internal carotid artery (ICA) were optimally drilled.

TOA

The same simulation model used for the EEA procedure (shown in Fig. 39.3) was used for the

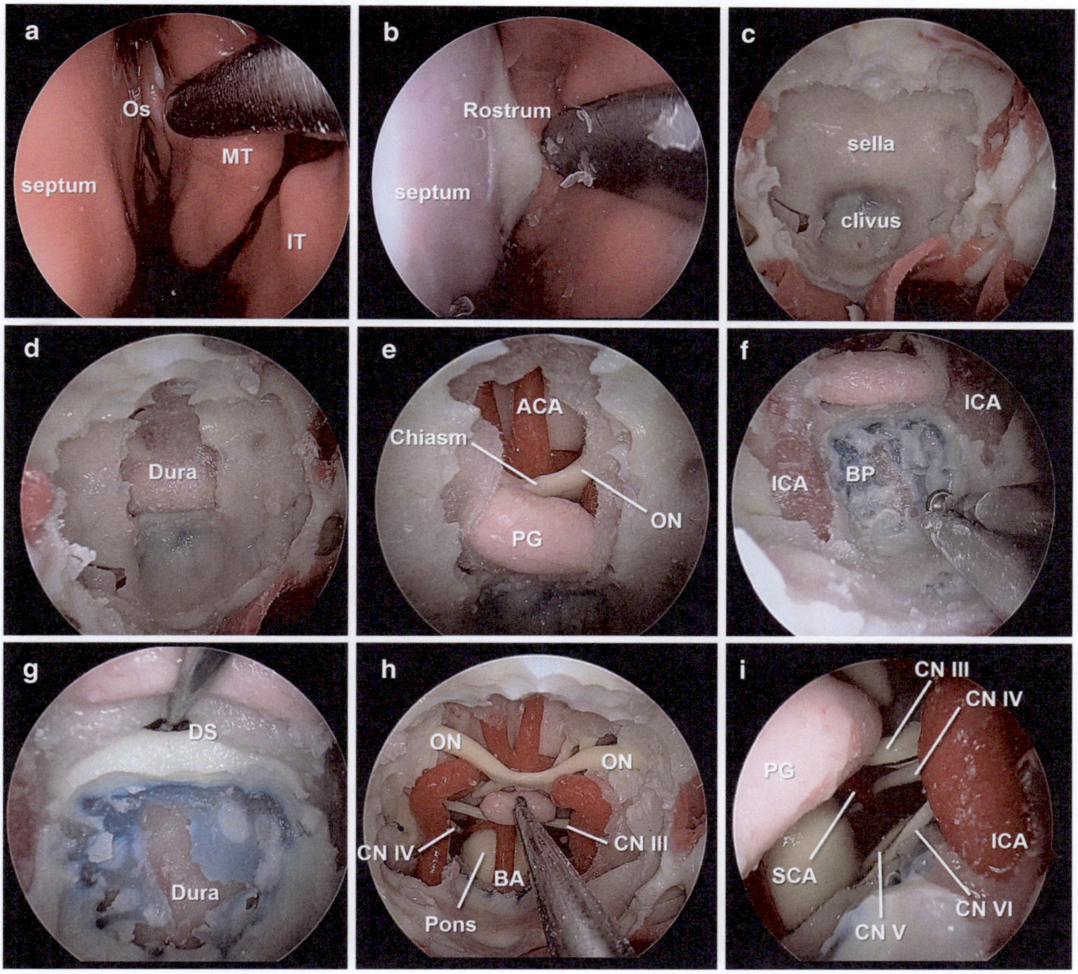

Fig. 39.2 Stepwise dissection procedure of the endoscopic endonasal approach using the simulation model. Structures of the intranasal cavity were identified under endoscopic visualization (**a**). The nasoseptal flap was elevated from the nasal septum (**b**). Wide sphenoidotomy was performed (**c**) and the anterior skull base was drilled to expose the dura of the sella and tuberculum sella (**d**). Dura was opened, and intradural structures were identified (**e**). The clivus, dorsum sellae, and posterior clinoid process were removed (**f**, **g**), and the neurovascular structures of the sella and parasellar areas were identified (**h**, **i**). *MT* middle turbinate, *IT* inferior turbinate, *Os* ostium of the sphenoid sinus, *ACA* anterior cerebral artery, *ON* optic nerve, *PG* pituitary gland, *ICA* internal carotid artery, *BP* basilar plexus, *DS* dorsum sellae, *BA* basilar artery, *CN* cranial nerve, *SCA* superior cerebellar artery

superior eyelid transorbital approach (TOA) (Fig. 39.3). On the model, a skin incision was made along the superior eyelid crease, and the periorbita was raised from the ocular surface of the greater sphenoid wing (GSW). Care was taken to preserve the temporalis muscle during the drilling of the GSW. The frontal and temporal dura were exposed, and the bone comprising the lateral border of the superior orbital fissure was completely removed. The temporal lobe dura was peeled off from the lateral wall of the CS, and the cranial nerves passing through the CS were identified. The horizontal portion of the GSW was drilled maximally to reach the

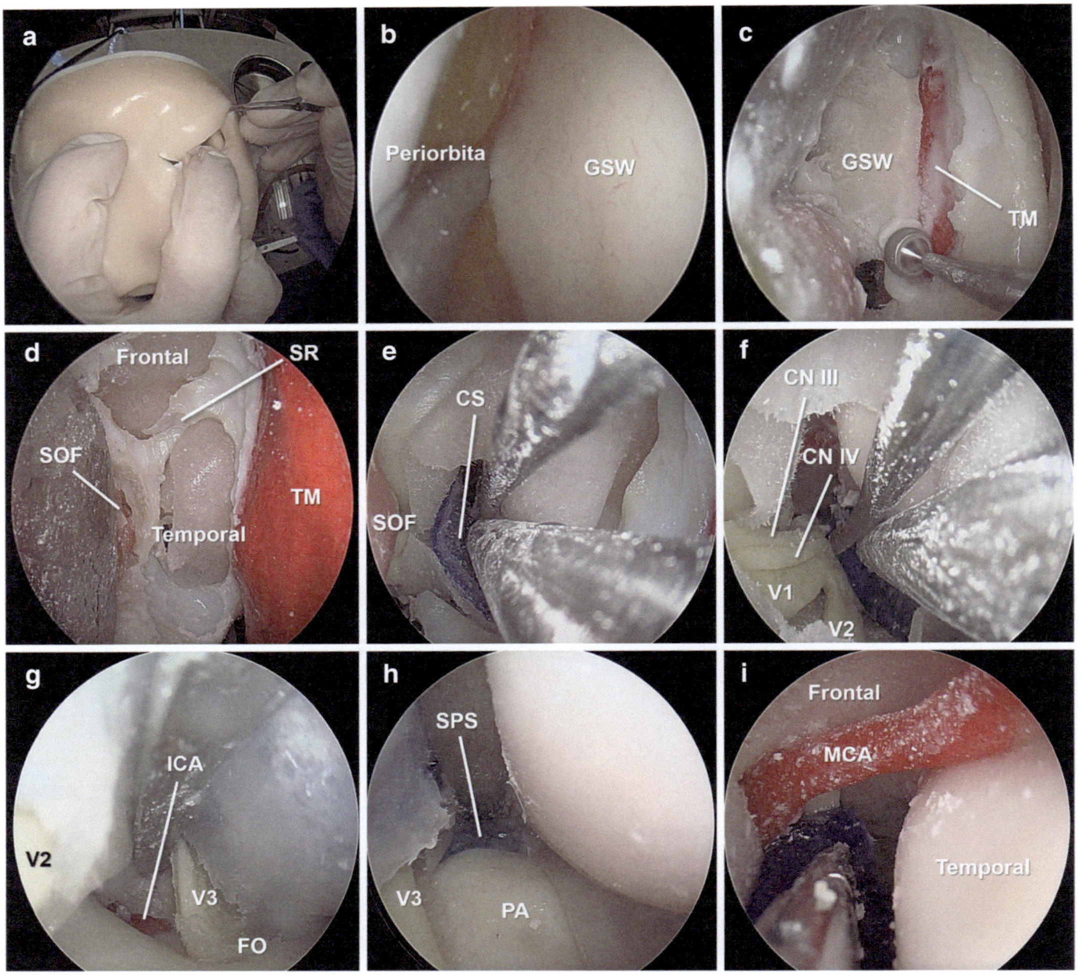

Fig. 39.3 Stepwise dissection procedure of the endoscopic transorbital approach using the simulation model. The superior eyelid incision was made on the simulation model (**a**). Subperiosteal elevation of the periorbita was performed (**b**) and the ocular surface of the greater sphenoid wing was drilled (**c**). Frontal and temporal dura was exposed, and the bone composing the lateral border of the superior orbital fissure was completely resected (**d**). The lateral wall of the cavernous sinus (CS) was colored in blue to mimic the venous sinus (**e**). Cranial nerves passing through the CS were identified (**f**). The space between the foramen rotundum and the foramen ovale (anterolateral triangle), and between the foramen ovale and the petrous ridge (posteromedial or Kawase's triangles) were identified via transorbital corridors (**g**, **h**). Intradural dissection allowed exposure of the middle cerebral artery through the Sylvian fissure (**i**). *GSW* greater sphenoid wing, *TM* temporalis muscle, *SOF* superior orbital fissure, *SR* sphenoidal ridge, *CS* cavernous sinus, *CN* cranial nerve, *V1* ophthalmic branch of the trigeminal nerve, *V2* maxillary branch of the trigeminal nerve, *ICA* internal carotid artery, *V3* mandibular branch of the trigeminal nerve, *FO* foramen ovale, *SPS* superior petrosal sinus, *PA* petrous apex, *MCA* middle cerebral artery

petrous apex. Transorbital corridors allowed identification of the anterolateral triangle between the foramen rotundum and foramen ovale and the posteromedial or Kawase triangles between the foramen ovale and petrous ridge.

Role of the 3D-Printed Surgical Training Model in ESBS

The applications of 3D-printed simulators are numerous and include preoperative planning, patient counseling, and trainee education [7, 8].

One of the critical attributes for a successful endoscopic skull base surgery (ESBS) is the ability to perceive the 3D spatial relationships of the skull base from 2D neuroimaging. This skill has traditionally been developed through surgical training, anatomical knowledge, and real-world experience. However, ESBS poses several challenges, such as unfamiliar anatomy, difficult hand-eye coordination, and a narrow operative field, which can make it difficult for some surgeons to perform successfully [9]. To address these challenges, 3D-printed skull base simulators offer a risk-free opportunity for additional education and training outside of the operating room, allowing trainees to refine their skills and gain confidence without risking patients' health. While many skull base diseases are atypical, standardized 3D-printed simulators can help surgeons become proficient in this high-stakes surgery [10]. Recently, endoscopic transorbital surgery has emerged as a new field in neurosurgery. Our 3D-printed model is the first physical model designed for the transorbital approach (TOA) procedure simulation. Beyond just anatomical modeling, our simulator provides an opportunity to develop a better understanding of the ergonomics of ESBS, experience depth perception, and master the manipulation of surgical instruments under endoscopic visualization. This can ultimately contribute to improving patient safety and clinical outcomes by enhancing the procedural performance of surgeons in actual surgery [11, 12].

Future Perspective

The use of high-resolution 3D-printed simulators for simulation-based training may provide trainees with additional opportunities to practice delicate surgical procedures outside of on-the-job training, potentially increasing their autonomy in challenging cases [13]. The customizability of 3D printing technology allows for the easy design of multiple case-specific simulators using a simple imaging process [6, 14]. Patient-specific 3D-printed simulators may supplement surgical training on a wider scale in fields where access to cases is limited [15]. In the future, efforts will be made to provide realistic and reliable haptic feedback to operators by identifying the best material for increasing the fidelity of replicating real human organs, with the aim of providing an alternative training platform for cadaveric dissection.An annual hands-on course on 3D simulators is available to provide a systematic training program using the model, and data obtained from each workshop can be used for functional improvement of the model. The low cost and high fidelity of 3D technology may facilitate its wide adoption in education and training. Collaboration between industries and academic institutions may produce synergies for the development of future models for ESBS training [16]. 3D models are valuable tools that can contribute to learning in the diverse fields of neurosurgery.

References

1. Wang EW, Zanation AM, Gardner PA, Schwartz TH, Eloy JA, Adappa ND, et al. ICAR: endoscopic skull-base surgery. Int Forum Allergy Rhinol. 2019;9(S3):S145–65. https://doi.org/10.1002/alr.22326.
2. Verillaud B, Bresson D, Sauvaget E, Mandonnet E, Georges B, Kania R, et al. Endoscopic endonasal skull base surgery. Eur Ann Otorhinolaryngol Head Neck Dis. 2012;129(4):190–6. https://doi.org/10.1016/j.anorl.2011.09.004.
3. Locatelli D, Pozzi F, Turri-Zanoni M, Battaglia P, Santi L, Dallan I, et al. Transorbital endoscopic approaches to the skull base: current concepts and future perspectives. J Neurosurg Sci. 2016;60(4):514–25.
4. Masalha MA, VanKoevering KK, Latif OS, Powell AR, Zhang A, Hod KH, et al. Simulation of cerebrospinal fluid leak repair using a 3-dimensional printed model. Am J Rhinol Allergy. 2021;35(6):802–8. https://doi.org/10.1177/19458924211003537.
5. Davids J, Manivannan S, Darzi A, Giannarou S, Ashrafian H, Marcus HJ. Simulation for skills training in neurosurgery: a systematic review, meta-analysis, and analysis of progressive scholarly acceptance. Neurosurg Rev. 2021;44(4):1853–67. https://doi.org/10.1007/s10143-020-01378-0.
6. Lee WJ, Kim YH, Hong SD, Rho TH, Kim YH, Dho YS, et al. Development of 3-dimensional printed simulation surgical training models for endoscopic endonasal and transorbital surgery. Front Oncol. 2022;12:966051. https://doi.org/10.3389/fonc.2022.966051.

7. Low CM, Morris JM, Price DL, Matsumoto JS, Stokken JK, O'Brien EK, et al. Three-dimensional printing: current use in rhinology and endoscopic skull base surgery. Am J Rhinol Allergy. 2019;33(6):770–81. https://doi.org/10.1177/1945892419866319.
8. Narayanan V, Narayanan P, Rajagopalan R, Karuppiah R, Rahman ZA, Wormald PJ, et al. Endoscopic skull base training using 3D printed models with pre-existing pathology. Eur Arch Otorrinolaringol. 2015;272(3):753–7. https://doi.org/10.1007/s00405-014-3300-3.
9. Park CK. 3D-printed disease models for neurosurgical planning, simulation, and training. J Korean Neurosurg Soc. 2022;65(4):489–98. https://doi.org/10.3340/jkns.2021.0235.
10. Wen G, Cong Z, Liu K, Tang C, Zhong C, Li L, et al. A practical 3D printed simulator for endoscopic endonasal transsphenoidal surgery to improve basic operational skills. Childs Nerv Syst. 2016;32(6):1109–16. https://doi.org/10.1007/s00381-016-3051-0.
11. Meling TR, Meling TR. The impact of surgical simulation on patient outcomes: a systematic review and meta-analysis. Neurosurg Rev. 2021;44(2):843–54. https://doi.org/10.1007/s10143-020-01314-2.
12. Xu JC, Hanna G, Fong BM, Hsu FPK, Cadena G, Kuan EC. Ergonomics of endoscopic skull base surgery: a systematic review. World Neurosurg. 2021;146:150–5. https://doi.org/10.1016/j.wneu.2020.11.026.
13. Hsieh TY, Cervenka B, Dedhia R, Strong EB, Steele T. Assessment of a patient-specific, 3-dimensionally printed endoscopic sinus and skull base surgical model. JAMA Otolaryngol Head Neck Surg. 2018;144(7):574–9. https://doi.org/10.1001/jamaoto.2018.0473.
14. Baskaran V, Strkalj G, Strkalj M, Di Ieva A. Current applications and future perspectives of the use of 3D printing in anatomical training and neurosurgery. Front Neuroanat. 2016;10:69. https://doi.org/10.3389/fnana.2016.00069.
15. Weinstock P, Rehder R, Prabhu SP, Forbes PW, Roussin CJ, Cohen AR. Creation of a novel simulator for minimally invasive neurosurgery: fusion of 3D printing and special effects. J Neurosurg Pediatr. 2017;20(1):1–9. https://doi.org/10.3171/2017.1.PEDS16568.
16. Saleh Y, Piper R, Richard M, Jeyaretna S, Cosker T. Designing a 3D printed model of the skull-base: a collaboration between clinicians and industry. J Med Educat Curri Develop. 2022;9:23821205221080703. https://doi.org/10.1177/23821205221080703.

Index

T. H. Schwartz et al. (eds.), *Endoscopic Transorbital Surgery of the Orbit, Skull Base and Brain*, https://doi.org/10.1007/978-3-031-59504-2

N

O

P